Clinical Pharmacy Pocket Companion

T0174423

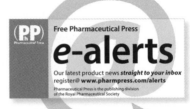

Clinical Pharmacy Pocket Companion

SECOND EDITION

Alistair Howard Gray

BSc (Hons), Dip Clin Pharm, MRPharmS
Clinical Services Lead Pharmacist
East Lancashire Hospitals NHS Trust

Jane Wright

BSc (Hons), Dip Clin Pharm, IPresc, MRPharmS
Specialist Clinical Pharmacist
Lancashire Care NHS Foundation Trust

Lynn Bruce

BSc, Dip Clin Pharm, IPresc, MRPharmS
Medical Assessment Unit Lead Pharmacist
East Lancashire Hospitals NHS Trust

Jennifer Oakley

MPharm, Dip Clin Pharm, IPresc, MRPharmS
Antimicrobial and Critical Care Pharmacist
East Lancashire Hospitals NHS Trust

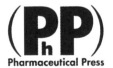

Pharmaceutical Press

Contents

Preface

Welcome to the second edition of the *Clinical Pharmacy Pocket Companion*. It is a measure of the support and demand from users of the first edition that a second edition (and hopefully future editions) of this book exists. Feedback and suggestions from people using the book have informed how this edition is laid out, what new entries have been included and what has been removed. Please continue to let us know what you think at phpeditorial@rpharms.com.

The aim of the *Clinical Pharmacy Pocket Companion* is to provide the user with a range of tools, suggestions and advice to assist in the provision of effective pharmaceutical care. The book has three main purposes.

Firstly as an *aide-mémoire*, the *Companion* helps to resolve routine queries arising from therapeutic drug monitoring, electrolyte disturbances, management of disease states and perioperative drug administration as well as more obscure problems. It complements existing literature, bridging the gap between the patient's bedside and the dispensary library. It brings together useful information not easily found in other reference sources, and previously not available in one text.

Secondly, there are prompts to seek out local information, for instance laboratory ranges and various drug policies. The action of actively seeking out this information supplements the user's continuing professional development. The references also provide further reading suggestions to explore a subject further.

Finally, space is provided at the end of each entry and section to record personal information, for example, passwords, websites and prompts from one's own experience of clinical practice.

The second edition

The way each entry has been created has changed. The first edition was written mainly by the authors with support from five contributors; for the second edition entries have been written or reviewed by many different people. Our contributors were approached because they are experts in a particular clinical field and include various professors, doctors and even a couple of presidents; and they aren't all pharmacists – a dietician and a clinical psychologist have contributed. What they all have in common was a desire to share their expertise with other healthcare professionals who have an interest in clinical pharmacy to benefit patients.

Where practical all non-essential, less clinical entries have been removed, including the hotly debated *Regimen or regime?* (For the record, a *regimen* (pronounced like 'regiment' without the 't') is a prescribed course of action, e.g. exercise, diet or pharmacological intervention, with a desired outcome. A *regime* is a method of government. The terms are commonly mixed up in the vernacular, in professional journals and in presentations!).

Refer-to-Pharmacy

The book is aimed at anyone associated with delivering pharmaceutical care (or medicines optimisation) in both a hospital setting and in community pharmacy. Some entries lend themselves more to secondary care by their very nature; however most apply to both disciplines. With the advent of various commissioned services in primary care to improve medicines adherence, e.g. New Medicine Service, Discharge Medication Review, Medicines Use Review, the clinical aspect and consultation skills of a community pharmacist's role are rightly becoming even more crucial.

With the advent of schemes such as Refer-to-Pharmacy (www.elht.nhs.uk/refer), which actively facilitates the referral of patients from the hospital pharmacy team to their community pharmacy for postdischarge pharmaceutical care, this book provides essential tips, knowledge and skills to community pharmacists consulting with patients referred to them. At the time of writing such referral schemes are in their infancy, and for more information visit www.rpharms.com/referraltoolkit to read the Royal Pharmaceutical Society's *Hospital referral to community pharmacy toolkit* to see how a referral scheme can be implemented in your health economy.

How to use the *Clinical Pharmacy Pocket Companion*

In the print edition the thumbnail cut-outs allow quick access to any letter of the alphabet. Subjects have been sited intuitively, e.g. treatment of hyperkalaemia is under 'P' for potassium. There is some cross-referencing and some information is repeated for ease of use; for example, the calculation of ideal body weight is included wherever it is needed and as an entry in its own right.

The list of contents is displayed alphabetically as laid out in the book, and there is also a full index at the back of the book.

Where doses appear, unless otherwise stated, they relate to adults.

The *Injectable Drugs Guide*

This is the sister publication of the *Clinical Pharmacy Pocket Companion* by these authors, available in print form or via www.MedicinesComplete.com. The *Injectable Drugs Guide* was published between editions of the *Clinical Pharmacy Pocket Companion* and rather went under the radar.

The *Injectable Drugs Guide* is an A–Z of approximately 300 injectable drugs in monograph format, each covering the following topics:

- pretreatment checks
- dosing regimens

- preparation and administration
- compatibility and stability information
- monitoring requirements during treatment
- side effects, interactions and pharmacokinetic information.

The *Injectable Drugs Guide* is designed to support the National Patient Safety Agency risk assessment process and each drug has a risk rating.

The book provides a holistic approach to injectable medicines to meet the needs of the many disciplines involved in the clinical use of injectables, and to those providing advice about injectable drug use.

Some sample entries can be viewed at www.pharmpress.com (search for *Injectable Drugs Guide*) and we have included the *omeprazole monograph* in this book to illustrate the benefit this one-stop shop of a book can bring to doctors, nurses and pharmacists.

About the authors

Alistair Gray is from Sunderland. He studied pharmacy at Sunderland Polytechnic, graduating in 1988 with first-class honours, and then completed his pre-registration year with Boots in Newcastle-upon-Tyne. He continued working for Boots in a variety of pharmacy and store management positions in the north-west of England. In 2002 he changed disciplines and became Community Services Pharmacist at Queens Park Hospital in Blackburn. He completed a Diploma in Clinical and Health Services Pharmacy at the University of Manchester in 2008 and subsequently became Clinical Services Lead Pharmacist for East Lancashire Hospitals NHS Trust in 2009, based at the now renamed Royal Blackburn Hospital. In 2012 he received the Royal Pharmaceutical Society's Medicines Safety Award for work in Transfer of Care. His interest in this area has continued, resulting in him conceiving what has become the Refer-to-Pharmacy scheme.

Alistair is married with two children and loves spending time with his family. He follows Formula One motor racing closely and enjoys reading, eating out, going to the movies, playing the guitar and song writing (best bits at https://soundcloud.com/Al_Chemist).

Jane Wright, after working for 18 years in the Civil Service, attended the University of Manchester to study pharmacy. Jane graduated in 1994 and did her pre-registration year at the Royal Preston Hospital. For the next 10 years Jane worked in Blackburn hospitals in a variety of clinical roles, her last being Clinical Services Manager with responsibility for education and training. In 1999 she obtained a Diploma in Clinical and Health Services Pharmacy at the University of Manchester. She moved to Lancashire Care NHS Foundation Trust in April 2005 where she was employed as Lead Pharmacist for East Lancashire until retirement in October 2014. Since then she has returned to work part-time as a non-medical prescriber in the Memory Assessment Service at Lancashire Care NHS Foundation Trust.

Jane is married and in her spare time enjoys playing with Molly and Polly (two very lively dogs).

Lynn Bruce studied pharmacy at Aston University. The first 20 years of her working life were based in secondary care variously as medicines information pharmacist, clinical pharmacy lead, clinical economist and latterly in various management positions. She migrated across the divide to primary care in 1997, becoming primary care group and then primary care trust prescribing advisor. Hospital clinical pharmacy beckoned her back to secondary care in

2002: she is now Pharmacy Team Leader on the Medical Assessment Unit at the Royal Blackburn Hospital.

Lynn is married and, when she's not writing pharmacy books, loves studying wild life and travelling and is addicted to puzzles of all types.

Jennifer Oakley is from the Wirral, Merseyside. She studied pharmacy at Liverpool John Moore's University, graduating in 2007 with a first-class honours degree, and was jointly awarded the local Royal Pharmaceutical Society of Great Britain branch prize in 2007. She then went on to complete her Postgraduate Clinical Diploma whilst undertaking a residency at Wirral University Teaching Hospitals. Meeting her future husband led her to Lancashire where she has worked in several roles, currently as an Antimicrobial and Critical Care Pharmacist at East Lancashire Hospitals.

Jenny is recently married and enjoys travelling the world and visiting exotic places.

Contributors

James Andrews
MPharm, MRPharmS
Practice Pharmacist, The Guildowns Group Practice
Lead Pharmacist for the West, Virgin Care

Sotiris Antoniou
MSc, Dip Mgt, IPresc, MRPharmS, FFRPS
Consultant Pharmacist
Cardiovascular Medicine, Barts Health NHS Trust

Nina Barnett
MSc, IPresc, FRPharmS, FFRPS, JP
Consultant Pharmacist, Care of Older People
NHS Specialist Pharmacy Service and
London North West London Hospitals NHS Trust

Victoria Bithell
BSc, MPsychol, CPsychol, AFBPsS
Registered Clinical Psychologist
Wirral Hospice St John's

Mark Borthwick
BPharm (Hons), MSc, FRPharmS, FFRPS
Consultant Pharmacist: Critical Care
Oxford University Hospitals NHS Trust

Annette Clarkson
MPharm, Dip Clin Pharm, MRPharmS
Specialist Clinical Pharmacist Antimicrobials and Infection Control
Nottingham University Hospitals NHS Trust, Nottingham, UK

Ailsing Considine
MPharm, Dip Clin Pharm, IPresc, MRPharmS
Senior Clinical Pharmacist Liver and Private Patient Services
Kings College Hospital NHS Foundation Trust

Sian Davison
MPharm, Dip Clin Pharm, IPresc, MRPharmS
Specialist Clinical Pharmacist, Medical Admissions Unit
East Lancashire Hospitals NHS Trust

Peter Foxon
MPharm, Dip Clin Pharm, MRPharmS
Senior Clinical Pharmacist Antibiotics
Nottingham University Hospitals

Patricia Ging
BPharm, MPSI, MSc, MRPharmS
Transplant/Pulmonary Hypertension Pharmacist
Pharmacy Department, Mater Misericordiae University Hospital,
Dublin, Republic of Ireland

Niamh Gormley
MPharm
Clinical Pharmacist
UHND Pharmacy Department, University Hospital of North Durham

Jill Gray
MPharm, Dip Clin Pharm, MRPharmS
Specialist Pharmacist
East Lancashire Hospitals NHS Trust

Dan Greer
BPharm, MSc, Dip Clin Pharm
Pharmacist Lecturer/Practitioner
University of Leeds/Leeds Teaching Hospitals

Susan Holgate
MPharm, Dip Clin Pharm, MRPharmS
Specialist Clinical Pharmacist
East Lancashire Hospitals NHS Trust

Nikki Holmes
MPharm, PGDipPsychPharm, IPresc, MCMHP, MRPharmS,
RegPharmNZ
Head of Pharmacy – Forensic Directorate
Nottinghamshire Healthcare NHS Foundation Trust

Sally James
BSc (Hons), MSc, MRPharmS
Divisional Pharmacist for Medicine
Royal Liverpool Hospital

Kevin Johnson
MPharm, Dip Clin Pharm, IPresc
Senior Clinical Pharmacist
Emergency Assessment Unit
Salford Royal Hospitals Foundation Trust

Shelley Jones
MSc, MPharm, IPresc, MRPharmS
Clinical Pharmacy Team Leader, Neurosciences
Kings College Hospital NHS Foundation Trust

Roger Knaggs
BSc (Hons), BMedSci, PhD, MRPharmS
Associate Professor in Clinical Pharmacy Practice
School of Pharmacy, University of Nottingham
Advanced Pharmacy Practitioner – Pain Management
Nottingham University Hospitals NHS Trust

Hannah Macfarlane
MPharm (Hons), PGDipPsychPharm, MCMHP, MRPharmS
Senior Clinical Pharmacist and Clinical Tutor
Birmingham and Solihull MHFT and Aston University

Lloyd Mayers
MPharm, Clin Dip Pharm, MRPharmS
Specialist Pharmacist Respiratory Medicine and Interstitial Lung
Disease
North Bristol NHS Trust

Catherine McKenzie
BSc, PhD, FFRPS, FRPharmS
Consultant Pharmacist in Critical Care
Guy's and St Thomas' NHS Foundation Trust

Debra Morris
BPharm, MRPharmS
Senior Clinical Pharmacist and Clinical Tutor
Salford Royal Foundation Trust/University of Manchester

Anna Murphy
MSc, DPharm, IPresc, MRPharmS
Honorary Visiting Professor, Department of Pharmacy, DeMontfort
University
Consultant Respiratory Pharmacist
University Hospitals of Leicester NHS Trust

Anne Neary
BSc (Hons), Dip Clin Pharm, IPresc, MRPharmS
Senior Pharmacist for Antimicrobials and Infectious Diseases
Royal Liverpool University Hospital

Lelly Oboh
BPharm, Dip Clin Pharm, IP, FRPharmS
Consultant Pharmacist, Care of Older People
Guy's and St Thomas' NHS Foundation Trust

Smita Ojha
BPharm (Hons), Dip Clin Pharm, IPresc, MRPharmS
Directorate Pharmacist for Stroke, Care of Elderly and Rehabilitation
East Lancashire Hospitals NHS Trust

Simon Purcell
MPharm, Dip Clin Pharm, IPresc, MRPharmS
Lead Pharmacist, Haematology and Aseptic Services
Wirral University Teaching Hospital NHS Foundation Trust

Christine Randall
BPharm, MRPharmS
Senior Medicines Information Pharmacist
North West Medicines Information Centre/Yellow Card Centre
North West

Viki Richards
MPharm, Dip Clin Pharm, MRPharmS
Advanced Primary Care Pharmacist
East Lancashire Clinical Commissioning Group

Victoria Ruszala
MPharm, Clin Dip Pharm
Specialist Pharmacist, Diabetes and Endocrinology
North Bristol NHS Trust

Christine Sluman
BSc (Hons), Dip Clin Pharm, MRPharmS
Highly Specialised Renal Pharmacist
North Bristol NHS Trust

Victoria Smith
MPharm, Dip Clin Pharm, MRPharmS
Specialist Clinical Pharmacist
East Lancashire Hospitals NHS Trust

Lynsey Stephenson
MPharm, DipClinPharm, IP, PGCCE
Senior Clinical Trials Pharmacist
UHND Pharmacy Department, University Hospital of North Durham

Katherine Stirling
BPharm (Hons), Dip Clin Pharm, IPresc, MRPharmS
Consultant Pharmacist Anticoagulation and Thrombosis
Leeds Teaching Hospitals NHS Trust

Dave Thornton
BSc (Hons), Dip Clin Pharm, IPresc, MRPharmS
Principal Pharmacist, Clinical Services
University Hospital Aintree

Alan Timmins
MSc, FFRPS, MRPharmS
Principal Pharmacist – Clinical Services
Victoria Hospital, Kirkcaldy

Mark Tomlin
BPharm, MSc (Biopharmacy), PhD, IPresc, FRPharmS, FFRPS
Consultant Pharmacist: Critical Care
Southampton General Hospital

Steve Wanklyn
MSc, IPresc, MRPharmS
Consultant Pharmacist in Palliative and End of Life Care; Joint Chair
London Opioid Safety and Improvement Group; Member PallE8
London Cancer North and East
Guy's and St Thomas' NHS Foundation Trust; Trinity Hospice;
St Joseph's Hospice; Richard House Children's Hospice

Jennifer Wilding
BSc (Hons) Applied Human Nutrition (Dietetics)
Nutrition Support Lead Dietitian
East Lancashire Hospitals NHS Trust

Rachel M Wilson
MPharm, Dip Clin Pharm, IPresc, MRPharmS
Specialist Clinical Pharmacist
East Lancashire Hospitals NHS Trust

Verity Woodhall
BSc (Hons), Dip Clin Pharm, MRPharmS
Lead Clinical Pharmacist for Musculoskeletal and Dermatology
Newcastle upon Tyne Hospitals NHS Foundation Trust

Antony Zorzi
BPharm, MSc, Dip Clin Pharm, IPresc
Lead Pharmacist, Antimicrobials and Respiratory
Pharmacy Department, Musgrove Park Hospital
Taunton and Somerset NHS Foundation Trust

ABCD² scoring system

Background

The ABCD² score is a validated risk assessment tool designed to identify individuals at high early risk of subsequent stroke after a transient ischaemic attack (TIA). Assessing people rapidly can minimise the chances of a full stroke occurring, as there is a 20% risk of a full stroke within the first 4 weeks after a TIA.[1,2]

SCORING SYSTEM

Clinical feature	Score
A − Age (≥60 years)	1
B − Blood pressure at presentation (≥140/90 mmHg)	1
C − Clinical features: unilateral weakness	2
speech disturbance without weakness	1
D − Duration of symptoms: ≥60 minutes	2
10−59 minutes	1
D − Diabetes mellitus	1
Total ABCD² score	0−7

Interpretation[3,4]

Early risk of stroke after TIA: 2-day risk of stroke:

Scores 0−3: low risk, 1%
Scores 4−5: moderate risk, 4.1%
Scores 6−7: high risk, 8.1%

- People with a score of ≥4 are regarded as being at a higher risk of early stroke. Aspirin 300 mg daily should be started immediately and specialist assessment (exclusion of stroke mimics, identification of vascular treatment, identification of likely causes) and investigation should happen (in a TIA clinic) within 24 hours of onset of symptoms.
- People with a score of ≤3 are considered at lower risk but should also start aspirin 300 mg daily and have specialist assessment and investigation within a maximum of 7 days of onset of symptoms

REFERENCES
1 Intercollegiate Stroke Working Party. Royal College of Physicians (2012). *National Clinical Guideline for Stroke*, 4th edn. https://www.rcplondon.ac.uk/sites/default/files/national-clinical-guidelines-for-stroke-fourth-edition.pdf (accessed 13 December 2014).
2 NICE (2008). Clinical guideline 68. *Stroke: Diagnosis and initial management of acute stroke and transient ischaemic attack (TIA)*. https://www.nice.org.uk/guidance/cg68 (accessed 13 December 2014).

3 Rothwell PM *et al.* (2007). Effect of urgent treatment of transient ischaemic attack and minor stroke on early recurrent stroke (EXPRESS study): a prospective population-based sequential comparison. *Lancet* 370: 1432–1442.

4 Coull A *et al.* (2004). Early risk of stroke after a TIA or minor stroke in a population-based incidence study. *BMJ* 328: 326–328.

ACE inhibitor-induced cough

Chronic cough is a well-described class effect of angiotensin-converting enzyme (ACE) inhibitors.[1] The cough is typically dry and is associated with a tickling or scratching sensation in the throat. Reports vary; 5–35% of patients who receive ACE inhibitors develop a dry cough, sometimes severe enough to require discontinuation of the drug.[1,2]

ACE inhibitor cough is considered a class effect that may occur with any ACE inhibitors and is not dose-dependent. Cough may occur within hours of the first dose of medication, or its onset can be delayed for weeks to months after the initiation of therapy. Treatment with ACE inhibitors may sensitise the cough reflex, thereby potentiating other causes of chronic cough.[3] Although cough usually resolves within 1–4 weeks of cessation of therapy with the offending drug, in a subgroup of individuals cough may linger for up to 3 months.

Women and those of black or Asian ethnicity have been reported to be at increased risk of ACE inhibitor cough.

Mechanisms of cough from ACE inhibitors

The inhibition of ACE prevents the conversion of angiotensin I to angiotensin II, with consequent salutary benefits via the renin–angiotensin system in pathological states. ACE inhibitor cough is thought to be linked to the suppression of ACE, which is proposed to result in an accumulation of substances normally metabolised by ACE: bradykinin and substance P. However, the development of cough may result from a more complex cascade of events than originally believed. Bradykinin has been shown to induce the production of arachidonic acid metabolites and nitric oxide, and there is some evidence that these products, which are subject to regulation by other pathways, may promote cough through proinflammatory mechanisms.[3,4]

Can angiotensin II receptor blockers be used in patients with a history of ACE inhibitor cough?

Theoretically, angiotensin II receptor blockers (ARBs) should not induce cough as they do not directly inhibit ACE activity or inhibit the breakdown of bradykinin. Indeed, ARBs have been associated with a low incidence of cough in patients with a history of ACE inhibitor cough, e.g. the frequency of cough with losartan was lower than with lisinopril (29 versus 72%, $P < 0.01$), and similar to hydrochlorothiazide (34%).[5]

Treatment of ACE inhibitor cough

The only uniformly effective intervention for ACE inhibitor-induced cough is the cessation of therapy with the offending agent. In cases in which the continuation of an ACE inhibitor is necessary despite cough, cromoglicate, baclofen, theophylline and local anaesthetics have been reported to be of some benefit, although none has been subjected to large-scale trials.[6,7]

Since the use of ACE inhibitors is now widespread, it is vitally important that practitioners consider identifying cases of ACE inhibitor-induced cough. Available studies indicate that, in the great majority of patients, those who develop these adverse reactions from ACE inhibitors can tolerate ARBs. The cardiovascular benefits and potential reduction in mortality from use of these drug classes are important and significant. Therefore, in a risk–benefit assessment, consideration should be given to the cautious alternative use of ARBs in the management of patients who develop cough from ACE inhibitors.

REFERENCES

1 Visser LE *et al.* (1995). Angiotensin converting enzyme inhibitor associated cough: a population-based case-control study. *J Clin Epidemiol* 48: 851–857.

2 Elliott WJ (1996). Higher incidence of discontinuation of angiotensin converting enzyme inhibitors due to cough in black subjects. *Clin Pharmacol Ther* 60: 582–588.

3 Dicpinigaitis PV (2006). Angiotensin-converting enzyme inhibitor-induced cough: ACCP evidence-based clinical practice guidelines. *Chest* 129(1 Suppl): 169S–173S.

4 Trifilieff A *et al.* (1993). Kinins and respiratory tract diseases. *Eur Respir J* 6: 576–587.

5 Lacourciere Y *et al.* (1994). Effects of modulators of the renin–angiotensin–aldosterone system on cough. Losartan Cough Study Group. *J Hypertens* 12: 1387–1393.

6 Allen TL, Gora-Harper ML (1997). Cromolyn sodium for ACE inhibitor-induced cough. *Ann Pharmacother* 31: 773–775.

7 Luque CA, Vazquez Ortiz M (1999). Treatment of ACE inhibitor-induced cough. *Pharmacotherapy* 19: 804–810.

Acetylcysteine for nebulisation

Acetylcysteine injection is sometimes used in an unlicensed capacity as a mucolytic.[1]

The adult dose is 3–5 mL of acetylcysteine 20% injection, or 6–10 mL of a 10% solution through a face mask or mouthpiece, nebulised three or four times daily with air (use of concentrated oxygen causes degradation).

Acetylcysteine reacts with some materials, e.g. rubber, iron, copper and nickel, so ensure the nebuliser does not contain these. Nebulisation equipment should be cleaned immediately after use with hot water and left to air dry.

Acetylcysteine may induce bronchospasm. As a precaution this can be avoided by either administration of a lower dose, diluting 1 mL of acetylcysteine 20% injection in 5 mL sodium chloride 0.9% and nebulising 3–4 mL, or preadministering a nebulised bronchodilator. Alternatively 1–10 mL of a 20% solution or 2–20 mL of a 10% solution may be given by nebulisation every 2–6 hours.

REFERENCE

1 *Martindale: The Complete Drug Reference* (2014). www.medicinescomplete.com (accessed 27 January 2015).

Acute kidney injury

Overview	
Definition	Clinically acute kidney injury (AKI) is characterised by a rapid reduction in kidney function over hours or days, resulting in a failure to maintain fluid, electrolyte and acid–base homeostasis. Untreated this can lead to pulmonary oedema, hyperkalaemia and metabolic acidosis. AKI is defined when one of the following criteria is met.[1] • Increase in serum creatinine of ≥26 micromol/L within 48 hours • Increase in serum creatinine of ≥50% from baseline (the lowest serum creatinine value recorded within 3 months of the event), which is known or presumed to have occurred within the past 7 days • Fall in urine output to <0.5 mL/kg/hour for >6 consecutive hours in adults and >8 hours in children
Causes	**Prenal AKI** (≈80% of cases) Blood flow to the kidney is reduced which, if left untreated, can lead to ischaemic injury to the kidney (known as acute tubular necrosis or ATN). Common causes of prerenal AKI include: • hypotension • dehydration • sepsis • significant blood loss, e.g. gastrointestinal bleeding • cardiac or liver failure • severe burns Some medications may cause prerenal AKI, such as NSAIDs, ACE inhibitors, ARBs and diuretics (see 'Further reading' for more detailed information). **Postrenal AKI** (≈10% of cases) Obstruction to urine outflow from the kidneys occurs. Common causes of postrenal AKI include: • benign prostatic hypertrophy • bladder or prostate cancer • abdominal tumours compressing the urinary tract • renal stones Some medications may cause postrenal AKI, either through deposition of crystals (e.g. aciclovir or cytotoxic agents) or through blood clots after bleeding (e.g. antiplatelet or anticoagulant therapy)

Intrinsic AKI ($\approx$10% of cases)

Damage occurs to the kidney itself, often immunological in origin.

Common causes of intrinsic AKI include:
- acute interstitial nephritis (AIN) – a hypersensitivity reaction that may often be drug-related, e.g. proton pump inhibitors (PPIs) and penicillins
- myeloma – through deposition of light chains in the kidney
- autoimmune renal disease, including lupus and vasculitis
- rhabdomyolysis – due to the renal toxicity of myoglobin from muscle breakdown

Risk factors	- Age >75 years - Chronic kidney disease - Cardiac failure - Peripheral vascular disease - Liver disease - Diabetes mellitus - Nephrotoxic medications, including iodinated radiological contrast media - Hypovolaemia - Sepsis - Surgical procedures

Diagnostic tests	- Drug history
	- Vital signs (temperature, heart rate, blood pressure)
	- Biochemistry (urea and electrolytes)
	- Full blood count
	- Urine dipstick $\pm$ microscopy
	- Microbiology:
	  - Urine culture
	  - Blood culture
	- Urine output
	- Hydration status, including jugular venous pressure
	
	More specific renal investigations are dependent upon the clinical presentation and may include:
	- renal immunology
	- urinary biochemistry (electrolytes, osmolality)
	- renal tract ultrasound within 24 hours (if renal tract obstruction is suspected)
	- kidney biopsy

Staging	The severity of AKI can be classified into three stages.[2] **Stage 1:** serum creatinine increase of $\geq$26 micromol/L within 48 hours **or** increase to $\geq$1.5–1.9 times baseline; urine output <0.5 mL/kg/hour for >6 consecutive hours **Stage 2:** serum creatinine increased to $\geq$2–2.9 times baseline; urine output <0.5 mL/kg/hour for >12 hours **Stage 3:** serum creatinine increased to $\geq$3 times baseline **or** increased to $\geq$354 micromol/L **or** commenced on renal replacement therapy, irrespective of stage; urine output <0.3 mL/kg/hour for >24 hours **or** anuria for 12 hours

Treatment goals	AKI has a poor prognosis, with the mortality ranging from 10% to 80%. depending upon the patient population studied. Even small increases in serum creatinine are associated with worse patient outcomes, including prolonged hospital stay and increased morbidity and mortality.[3]
	The goals of AKI treatment are:
	• Prevention
	• Early identification and assessment
	• Appropriate hydration
	• Avoid hypotension (systolic blood pressure <110 mmHg)
	• Prompt treatment of infection and other medical conditions
	• Stop nephrotoxic drugs
	• Adjust doses of renally excreted drugs
Treatment options	• Identify and treat potential causes, e.g. underlying sepsis
	• Assess volume status and give appropriate intravenous fluid therapy
	• Use potassium-containing solutions (e.g. Hartmann's) cautiously due to the risk of exacerbating hyperkalaemia
	• Daily observations, fluid balance, body weight and urine output should be monitored to ensure appropriate fluid therapy and avoid overload
	• Medication review:
	• Discontinue/avoid all nephrotoxic medications
	• Discontinue antihypertensive medications if patient is hypotensive
	• Adjust medication doses as necessary
	• Administer vasopressors and/or inotropes to increase blood pressure where appropriate
	• Manage biochemical complications, e.g. treatment of hyperkalaemia and/or metabolic acidosis
	• Give renal replacement therapy

Pharmaceutical care and counselling

Assess	• Ensure a detailed drug history is taken, including OTC, herbal and recently stopped medications
	• Fluid status
	• Medication review
Essential intervention	Many drugs can precipitate AKI and all nephrotoxic medications or medications that may affect renal haemodynamics should be stopped or avoided, e.g. NSAIDs, ACE inhibitors and diuretics.
	Advise on suitable alternatives where appropriate
Essential intervention	Review the side-effect profile of all medicines to identify potential causes of ATN or interstitial nephritis, e.g. amphotericin, PPIs
Essential intervention	Discontinue non-essential medications where appropriate until AKI has resolved, e.g. statins
Essential intervention	Advise on appropriate drug dosing in AKI.
	Many pharmacokinetic parameters, including volume of distribution, clearance and protein binding, are altered in AKI.
	Drug doses need to be adjusted appropriately with the correct assessment of kidney function to reduce toxicity. Examples include dose reduction of renally excreted drugs such as digoxin or gabapentin, or use of alternative agents that are less renally excreted, e.g. switching from morphine to fentanyl

Secondary intervention	Advise on the appropriate use of intravenous fluids (see *Fluid balance* entry).
	Provide recommendations around fluid restriction and minimum infusion volumes for drugs used in fluid-overloaded patients
Continued monitoring	Daily assessment of renal function and review of medication doses as renal function improves.
	Consider reintroduction of non-causative medications once AKI has resolved
Counselling	Counsel a patient regarding any medication changes prior to discharge, in particular any causative agents that have now been stopped.
	Advise patients about any medications to be avoided in future (e.g. OTC NSAIDs).
	Advise patients receiving medications that put them at risk of AKI to seek medical advice if they become acutely unwell or think they might be dehydrated.
	Provide accurate discharge information to general practitioners, including changes to medication, medicines to be restarted after discharge (and when this should occur) and any counselling provided
Further reading	Shaw S *et al.* (2012). Acute kidney injury – diagnosis, staging and prevention. *Clin Pharmacist* 4: 98–102.
	Shaw S *et al.* (2012). Acute kidney injury – management. *Clin Pharmacist* 4: 103–106.

REFERENCES

1 NICE (2013). *Acute Kidney Injury: Prevention, detection and management up to the point of renal replacement therapy. NICE guidelines CG169.* www.nice.org.uk/guidance/CG169 (accessed 7 September 2014).
2 Kidney Disease: Improving Global Outcomes (2012). *Clinical Practice Guideline for Acute Kidney Injury* www.kdigo.org/clinical_practice_guidelines/pdf/KDIGO%20AKI%20Guideline.pdf (accessed 7 September 2014).
3 UK Renal Association (2011). *Clinical Practice Guidelines: Acute Kidney Injury,* 5th edn. http://www.renal.org/docs/default-source/guidelines-resources/Acute_Kidney_Injury_-_Final_Version_08_March_2011.pdf?sfvrsn=0 (accessed 7 September 2014).

Addison's disease

Overview

Definition	Addison's disease occurs when the adrenal glands do not produce enough cortisol and, in some cases, aldosterone. There are two types of adrenal insufficiency: primary and secondary.
	Primary adrenal insufficiency (Addison's disease) is caused by adrenal gland malfunction.
	Secondary adrenal insufficiency is much more common than primary adrenal insufficiency and is due to pituitary malfunction and a lack of adrenocorticotrophic hormone (ACTH)[1]

A

Risk factors	Addison's disease has a prevalence of 93–140 per million people and annual incidence of 4.7–6.2 per million people in western populations
Differential diagnosis	The onset of Addison's disease is often insidious. Its usual symptoms (such as fatigue, lethargy, weakness and low mood) are non-specific and highly prevalent in the general population, and overlap with many other common conditions, including: • depression • chronic fatigue syndrome • anorexia nervosa • type 1 diabetes • gastrointestinal disorders
Diagnostic tests	About half of patients with Addison's disease are diagnosed only after an acute adrenal crisis. A diagnosis of Addison's disease is made by laboratory tests, firstly to determine whether levels of cortisol are insufficient and then to establish the cause. A short Synacthen test is the investigation of choice to confirm or exclude Addison's disease. 250 micrograms of tetracosactide (an analogue of corticotropin) is administered by intramuscular or intravenous injection and three blood samples for serum cortisol are taken immediately, at 30 minutes and at 60 minutes. A normal response is a rise in serum cortisol level to above 500 nmol/L at 30 minutes or 60 minutes. A level less than 100 nmol/L indicates a high likelihood of adrenal insufficiency. A plasma ACTH concentration should be measured, as a raised concentration will distinguish Addison's disease from secondary adrenal insufficiency. Once the diagnosis of Addison's disease is made, further investigations are needed to determine the underlying cause
Treatment goals	Replacing or substituting the adrenal hormones
Treatment options	• Hydrocortisone • Prednisolone • Fludrocortisone

Pharmaceutical care and counselling[1,2]

Essential intervention	Cortisol is replaced orally with hydrocortisone tablets, usually given once or twice daily. If aldosterone is also deficient, it is replaced with oral doses of fludrocortisone acetate taken once a day. Patients receiving aldosterone replacement therapy are usually advised to increase their salt intake. The doses of each of these medications are adjusted to meet the needs of individual patients
Essential intervention	The usual replacement dose of hydrocortisone is 15–25 mg/day, given in two or three divided doses. Fludrocortisone is given in a single dose of 50–200 micrograms a day. Doses do not have to be matched to meals so patients can take to suit their lifestyle
Secondary intervention	Medication may need to be increased (doubled or tripled) during times of stress, infection or injury. This should be given parenterally if a patient cannot tolerate the drug orally. A patient with an acute adrenal crisis needs urgent hospital admission for intravenous fluid, parenteral hydrocortisone and treatment of the precipitating cause

A

Continued monitoring	There are no objective measures for assessing the effectiveness of treatment. Monitor for signs of:
	• Overreplacement: hypertension, thin skin, striae, easy bruising, glucose intolerance, hyperglycaemia, electrolyte abnormalities
	• Underreplacement: symptoms of Addison's disease, including fatigue, postural hypotension, nausea, weight loss and salt craving
Further reading	NICE (2010). *Clinical Knowledge Summaries: Addison's Disease.* http://cks.nice.org.uk/addisons-disease#!topicsummary (accessed 10 October 2014).

REFERENCES

1 Vaidya B, Chakera AJ (2009). Addison's disease. *BMJ* 339: b2385.
2 Baker AJK, Wass AJH (2009). A patient's journey. Addison's disease. *BMJ* 339: b2384.

Adrenaline: nebulised

Adrenaline has a sympathomimetic action at alpha- and beta-adrenoceptors. It causes increased cardiac contraction, blood flow to skeletal muscle, hyperglycaemia, oxygen consumption and relaxation of bronchial smooth muscle.[1]

In patients with severe croup, nebulised adrenaline may be used for rapid relief alongside corticosteroid treatment. Croup is an inflammation of the respiratory tract that usually occurs in childhood.

Method of administration for children
1 month–12 years[1,2,3,4]

1 Use 400 microgram/kg (max. 5 mg) of 1:1000 (1 mg/mL) adrenaline solution.
2 Dilute with sterile sodium chloride 0.9% solution.
3 Rinse the mouth with water to prevent ingestion.
4 Monitor closely.
5 Repeat after 30 minutes if necessary.
6 The effects will last for 2–3 hours.
7 Monitor for recurrence of obstruction.

REFERENCES

1 Martindale (2014). *The Complete Drug Reference.* Medicines Complete: Martindale. www.medicinescomplete.com (accessed 30 July 2014).
2 NHS Greater Glasgow and Clyde (2008). *Croup.* NHS Greater Glasgow and Clyde: Emergency department, The Royal Hospital for Sick Children. http://www.clinicalguidelines.scot.nhs.uk/Emergency%20Medicine/YOR-AE-008%20Croup.pdf (accessed 30 August 2014).
3 National Institute for Health Research (2006). *The Safety of Nebulization with 3 to 5 ml of Adrenaline (1:1000) in Children: An evidence based review.* NHS: University of York. http://www.crd.york.ac.uk/CRDWeb/ShowRecord.asp?ID=12006003026#.U_CSUWOGe20 (accessed 30 August 2014).
4 BMJ group. *British National Formulary for Children.* London: Pharmaceutical Press; 2014.

Adverse drug reactions

Definition of ADRs

An adverse drug reaction (ADR) is a response to a drug that is noxious and unintended and which occurs at doses normally used in humans for the prophylaxis, diagnosis or therapy of disease or for the modification of a physiological function.[1]

This definition was introduced by the WHO in the 1970s and excludes events such as errors in drug administration and instances of intentional and unintentional poisoning or overdose, which other definitions may include.

In July 2012, new pharmacovigilance legislation came into effect across the EU and was transposed into UK law in the Human Medicines Regulations 2012.[2] The legislation[3] defines adverse reactions as being noxious and unintended effects resulting not only from the authorised use of a medicinal product at normal doses, but also from medication errors and uses outside the terms of the marketing authorisation, including the misuse and abuse of the medicinal product.

The terms 'adverse effect' and 'adverse reaction' tend to be used interchangeably and the term 'side effect' tends to be used for minor, predictable ADRs. In practice, use of the word 'effect' describes the problem from the drug perspective, whereas 'reaction' describes the patient perspective. 'Adverse events', however, are not necessarily related to drug therapy but, in terms of a medicine's use, they describe any adverse effect that occurred during drug therapy. For example, if a patient slipped on ice and fractured a hip, this could be perceived as an adverse event.

Classification of ADRs

Traditionally ADRs have been classified into two distinct categories. Type A reactions may be predicted from the pharmacological actions of the drug and are usually dose-dependent. They tend to be classified as mild (although important from the patient's perspective), have low mortality and may be alleviated by a reduction in dose. Examples of type A reactions include bradycardia with beta-blockers, hypoglycaemia with a sulphonylurea, dry mouth with antimuscarinics and drowsiness with benzodiazepines. In some instances, patients will become tolerant to these ADRs once their bodily systems have adjusted to the effects of the drug, e.g. drowsiness with gabapentin is usually transient. Type A reactions may be precipitated by factors leading to increased plasma concentrations of drug, for example, hepatic or renal impairment, drug–drug interactions or dosage form design. The ageing process may also contribute to the development of type A reactions because of important effects on the metabolism and excretion of drugs, increasing sensitivity to drug stimulation of receptors and altered homeostatic mechanisms.

Conversely, type B reactions tend to be more bizarre in nature as they are idiosyncratic, unpredictable and unrelated to the pharmacological action of a drug. Type B reactions appear to affect only susceptible individuals and, because they may be less common, can lead to drug withdrawals after marketing. These reactions are not dose-dependent and have a higher mortality rate than type A reactions. Anaphylactic reactions to penicillin, hepatotoxicity with sulfasalazine and malignant hyperthermia after anaesthetics are examples of type B reactions.

It is also important to consider the effect of dosage form with regard to ADRs. Almost all medicinal products contain excipients that may precipitate type B reactions.

This classification is frequently under review, primarily because the two groups are somewhat restrictive. Further subtypes for ADR classification have been suggested, including categories for ADRs caused by long-term use of a drug, drug–drug interactions, or overdose and those resulting in carcinogenicity or teratogenicity.

The timing of type B reactions cannot always be predicted either. Angioedema associated with ACE inhibitors and anaphylactic reactions with infliximab may not always occur at the start of treatment.

ADRs affect the public's confidence in medicines

The press love bad news; unfortunately, medicines provide plenty of subject matter. Over the last decade the ADRs of a number of medicines have made it into the national press. Following the withdrawal of rofecoxib in 2004, the debate over cyclooxygenase 2 (COX-2) inhibitors made repeated national headlines. Other medicines to hit the headlines include adverse effects of ketamine abuse, muscle adverse effects of statins, cardiac ADRs with NSAIDs, fatalities associated with tramadol, and the MMR vaccine debate, which continues to have real impact on public health.

Information sources on ADRs

The BNF is a useful starting point, but to explore the likelihood of an ADR, further information is readily available. A first option would be the SPC, which contains information about adverse effects, and where available, how commonly the ADR in question occurs. Commonly used and useful reference sources include:

- *Martindale*[4]
- *American Hospital Formulary Service*[5]
- *Adverse Drug Reactions*[6]
- *Meyler's Side Effects of Drugs*[7]
- *Davies's Textbook of Adverse Drug Reactions*.[8]

Periodical publications such as *Drug Safety Update* from the MHRA are also useful for bringing current issues about the adverse effects of drugs to healthcare professionals' attention. For more detailed

A

medicines information, your local UK Medicines Information centre will provide you with a high level of expert knowledge in this area.

Information sources on adverse drug–drug interactions

Vigilance for potential adverse drug–drug interactions of clinical significance is a key role for the pharmacist. As with ADRs, the BNF is limited but is a useful starting point for checking and investigating the effects of individual drug interactions. The commonly used specialist references are *Stockley's Drug Interactions*[9] and Hansten and Horn's *Drug Interactions: Analysis and Management*.[10]

Adverse drug–food interactions

There are a number of well-documented drug–food interactions, such as those with grapefruit juice (see *Grapefruit juice–drug interactions*). Patients taking warfarin should be advised to avoid cranberry products since there are several documented reports of the effects of warfarin being enhanced by cranberry. Patients taking MAOIs should be advised to avoid foods containing significant amounts of tyramine, e.g. mature cheese or yeast extracts, since MAOIs can potentiate the pressor effect of tyramine, causing a dangerous increase in blood pressure. See *Food–drug interactions* for further information.

ADRs to complementary medicines

Significant numbers of patients take herbal or homeopathic medicines. Since these medicines are not regulated in the same way as licensed medicines, there is less information regarding their quality assurance, safety or efficacy. The content of complementary medicines may vary significantly in terms of potency, content of active ingredient and the range of excipients. Furthermore, herbal medicines can be adulterated with heavy metals, corticosteroids, sildenafil and many other things. There can also be significant interactions between standard therapies and herbal medicines, e.g. St John's wort interacts with digoxin, warfarin and oral contraceptives. Other significant interactions include gingko biloba, vitamin E and ginger interacting with warfarin, and devil's claw interacting with digoxin.

It is difficult to ascertain the significance or incidence of adverse effects with complementary medicines because the majority of reactions go unreported, few clinical trials have collected data in a structured manner and patients often actively or passively choose not to disclose use of complementary medicines when consulting their doctor. There is a perception that complementary medicines are safe because of their 'natural origin', which creates a false sense of security. As few patients volunteer information about herbal medicines during medication history taking, it is important to ask about their use.

Information sources for complementary medicines-related ADRs include *Herbal Medicines*[11] and the *Natural Medicines Comprehensive Database*.[12]

Identifying ADRs

Timing

Many ADRs occur soon after a medicine is started; however, not all
reactions occur instantly, e.g. angioedema with ACE inhibitors can
occur at any time during treatment and recur at infrequent intervals;
gum hyperplasia with phenytoin occurs after a long period of
treatment; and drug-induced parkinsonism can develop after months
of treatment. Oculogyric reactions associated with metoclopramide
can occur very soon after administration, as can seizures with
ciprofloxacin.

Some ADRs develop after a patient has stopped taking the drug
responsible, so identification of the culprit should not be limited to
the medicines that the patient is currently taking. A classic example is
cholestatic jaundice and hepatitis associated with flucloxacillin, which
can occur up to several weeks after completion of treatment. Patients
can be exposed to unnecessary investigations and treatment because
of a failure to consider recent therapies. When assessing causality, the
suspect drug's half-life should be considered; for example, the
half-lives of amiodarone and leflunomide are very long, and
significant plasma concentrations persist for long periods after
cessation of therapy.

Dose

It is important to understand the pharmacology of a drug suspected of
causing an ADR in order to differentiate between type A and type B
reactions. Type A reactions are dose-related and may well respond to
a reduction in dose. Of particular concern are medicines that have a
narrow therapeutic window, where a small change in drug concentration separates lack of efficacy and toxicity, e.g. gentamicin, digoxin,
theophylline, lithium, phenytoin and ciclosporin. The risk of type A
reactions should be considered for elderly patients who, due to
reduced metabolic and excretory pathways, may accumulate high
concentrations of some drugs.

The dose of a medicine is not important for type B reactions;
withdrawal of the drug is usually required for resolution of these
reactions.

De-challenge and re-challenge

If symptoms improve when a drug is withdrawn or dose reduced, it is
suggestive that the drug was responsible. A drug re-challenge may
confirm or deny the association. Clearly, it is not safe to do this in all
circumstances and the risks to the patient associated with re-exposure
should be carefully balanced against the importance of identifying the
true cause of the reaction.

Other medical conditions

When attempting to ascertain the cause of a new symptom, consider
other non-drug possibilities, in particular the patient's concurrent
disease state. For example, syndrome of inappropriate secretion of

A

antidiuretic hormone (SIADH) in a patient taking an antidepressant could be due to a lung tumour secreting antidiuretic hormone. Similarly, jaundice in a patient taking cyproterone could be related to gallstones or hepatitis.

The placebo effect has a significant impact on ADRs. In clinical trials, where adverse events are recorded for all patients, reactions to the placebo are often similar to those for the active drug.

Documentation and communication

When a patient suffers an ADR, it is important that the drug and its specific effect are documented in the patient's case notes and communicated to the general practitioner, community pharmacist and to the patient. This is vital to prevent inadvertent re-exposure to the drug. If a patient is intolerant to a drug but has not suffered a severe ADR, this should be fully documented to avoid life-saving therapy being withheld should the need arise. For example, many patients who consider themselves to be allergic to penicillin are merely intolerant to the drug, e.g. suffer unpleasant gastrointestinal effects.

At-risk patients

Elderly patients are vulnerable to ADRs. The complex effects of the ageing process alter drug metabolism and excretion as well as altering organ sensitivity to drugs such as benzodiazepines. Elderly patients often have multiple pathologies with multiple drug therapies and are therefore at significantly increased risk of a drug–drug or drug–disease interaction.

Since the elderly have decreased functional and homeostatic reserve, they are more susceptible to the effects of many drugs, for example, antihypertensives. One method of avoiding or reducing this problem in the elderly is to use a lower starting dose and increase the dose gradually.

It is not only elderly patients who may suffer from polypharmacy: as evidence-based medicine grows, more and more patients will be taking complex medication regimens for diseases including congestive cardiac failure, post myocardial infarction and HIV infection.

Neonates and infants are at risk of ADRs because of the immaturity of their metabolic systems. In particular, neonates should not be prescribed chloramphenicol as it reaches toxic levels sooner and less predictably than in older children, causing cardiovascular collapse. This is referred to as the grey-baby syndrome.

Population genetic variation (polymorphism) is one reason for the wide variability in response to drugs between individuals. Some polymorphisms increase the risk of ADRs: cytochrome P450 isoenzymes, e.g. CYP2D6, dictate codeine metaboliser status with ultrarapid metabolisers at risk of opioid adverse effect; human leukocyte antigens, e.g. presence of the HLA-B*1502 allele, increases the risk of Stevens–Johnson syndrome with carbamazepine in individuals of Han Chinese or Thai origin; non-cytochrome P450 metabolising enzymes, e.g. thiopurine S-methyl transferases (TPMT) catalyses metabolism of azathioprine and 6-mercaptopurine; TPMT status is used as a predictor of drug toxicity, particularly myelotoxicity. Ethnicity may have a bearing on risk of ADRs, with some medications, for example rosuvastatin, requiring lower doses in patients of Asian origin. Few drugs are dosed on a gender basis, although alcohol intoxication, the neuropsychiatric effects of mefloquine and ACE inhibitor-induced cough all have increased incidence in women.

Patients with a history of ADRs/allergies also have a higher risk of experiencing a further ADR. Hepatic disorders, thyroid dysfunction and renal disorders all contribute to alterations in pharmacokinetic handling of medicines and the risks of accumulation or increases in blood concentrations should be monitored.

Preventing and managing ADRs

The basic principles are:

- Is the patient's drug therapy appropriate?
- Do the benefits of therapy outweigh the possible risks?
- Is a safer alternative available?
- Is there a potential for drug–drug or drug–disease interactions?
- Is the patient particularly vulnerable?
- Does the drug have a narrow therapeutic window?
- Is the patient on the lowest effective dose?

Fringe benefits of ADRs

In a number of instances, ADRs aren't necessarily bad news. Table A1 gives some examples of this.

TABLE A1
Fringe benefits of adverse drug reactions

Drug	ADR	Fringe benefit
Codeine	Causes constipation in many patients	Is sometimes used 'off-label' to treat diarrhoea
Erythromycin	Stimulates motilin receptors in the gut, which can cause diarrhoea in some patients	In the intensive care setting, where a patient's gut motility may be significantly impaired following prolonged intravenous feeding, intravenous erythromycin can be used 'off-label' to stimulate gut motility
Hyoscine	Can cause dry mouth	In patients with drooling hyoscine can be used to dry up secretions
Minoxidil	As an antihypertensive it can cause excess hair growth in patients	It has been marketed as an over-the-counter medicine for male-pattern baldness
Nifedipine	Causes postural hypotension due to its vasodilatory effects	Used to help relieve the symptoms of Raynaud's phenomenon
Phenytoin	Causes gum hyperplasia	Has been investigated in the healing of wounds
Sildenafil	Originally tested as a drug for cardiovascular disease; however, interesting side effects became apparent	Used to treat erectile dysfunction

A

In practice

Be proactive in looking for ADRs: make your interest known to
medical and nursing staff. Patients and their carers are a vastly
underused source of information about medicines and this aspect of
care should be actively discussed with them. Monitor the high-risk
drugs closely; these drugs are the ones that put patients' health
at risk.

'Black-triangle' drugs are those most recently marketed and their
use must be closely observed for adverse reactions and even
'expected' ADRs should be reported (see *Yellow Card scheme* entry).

Education is a key factor in monitoring adverse reactions and
it is important that both the patient and the pharmacist are aware
of the adverse effects of the medicines they are using. Finally, if we
are ever to learn and keep learning about ADRs: report, report
and report.

ADRs and drugs that cause them

Table A2 gives an indication of some ADRs and their causative agents.

TABLE A2

Examples of adverse drug reactions and drugs that cause them

ADRs	Drugs causing the ADR
Central nervous system disorders	
Agitation, excitation and irritability	Antihistamines, caffeine, omeprazole, SSRIs, theophylline, vigabatrin
Confusion	Antimuscarinics, benzodiazepines, cimetidine, levodopa, quinolone antibiotics, tramadol, tricyclic antidepressants
Drowsiness	Antiepileptic drugs, antihistamines, MAOIs, opioids, tricyclic antidepressants
Headache	Glyceryl trinitrate/nitrates, nifedipine, proton pump inhibitors, nicorandil, tramadol, leukotriene receptor antagonists, COX-2-selective inhibitors
Insomnia	Caffeine, theophylline, flupentixol, ephedrine, nicotine patches, levodopa, bupropion, statins, corticosteroids
Sleep disturbances	Beta-blockers, nicotine patches, levodopa, varenicline
Mood disturbances	Isotretinoin, bupropion, COX-2-selective inhibitors, ACE inhibitors, progestogens
Convulsions	Amphotericin, baclofen, bupivacaine, clozapine, ciclosporin, fluoxetine, foscarnet, ganciclovir, beta-lactam antibiotics, mefloquine, methylphenidate, mianserin, opioids, theophylline, tramadol
Eye disorders	
Cataracts	Corticosteroids
Retinal disorders	Hydroxychloroquine
Visual disturbances	Tricyclic antidepressants, digoxin, vigabatrin

TABLE A2
(Continued)

ADRs	Drugs causing the ADR
Nose disorders	
Disturbances of smell	Nifedipine, diltiazem
Disorders of the mouth and throat	
Dry mouth	Tricyclic antidepressants, hyoscine, antipsychotics, opioids, alpha-blockers, SSRIs, oxybutynin
Gingival hyperplasia	Phenytoin, calcium-channel blockers, ciclosporin, ethosuximide
Oral thrush	Antibiotics, inhaled steroids
Taste disturbances	Metronidazole, ACE inhibitors, penicillamine, terbinafine, quinolone antibiotics, allopurinol
Sore throat/mouth ulcers	NSAIDs, carbimazole, nicorandil, ACE inhibitors, methotrexate
Cough	ACE inhibitors, gabapentin, mycophenolate, nitrofurantoin
Disorders of the ear	
Vertigo	Bupropion, opioids, benzodiazepines, amiodarone
Deafness	Aminoglycosides, furosemide, macrolide antibiotics
Tinnitus	NSAIDs, mefloquine, COX-2-selective inhibitors, aminoglycosides
Disorders of the heart	
Hypertension	Ciclosporin, corticosteroids, erythropoietin, fludrocortisone, MAOIs, NSAIDs, sevoflurane, tramadol, etoricoxib
Hypotension	Beta-blockers, amiodarone, baclofen, benzodiazepines, calcium-channel blockers, cannabinoids, desmopressin, disopyramide, diuretics, enoximone, flecainide, iloprost, interleukins, lidocaine, MAOIs, opioids, phenytoin, procainamide, quinidine, sildenafil, teicoplanin, tricyclic antidepressants, vasodilators
Bradycardia	Amiodarone, beta-blockers, digoxin, opioids, sumatriptan
Tachycardia	Beta-2 agonists, digoxin, tricyclic antidepressants, theophylline, mirabegron
Irregular heart beat	Terfenadine, amiodarone, digoxin, quinine, SSRIs, mefloquine, opioids, calcium-channel blockers
Disorders of the muscles and joints	
Joint disease	Beta-blockers, quinolone antibiotics, SSRIs, omeprazole, cephalosporins
Cold extremities	Beta-blockers
Muscle cramps/pains	Beta-2 agonists, ACE inhibitors, cholesterol-lowering agents, terbinafine, corticosteroids, quinolone antibiotics
Tendon rupture	Quinolone antibiotics, corticosteroids
Limb oedema	NSAIDs, calcium-channel blockers, corticosteroids

(continued)

A

TABLE A2
(Continued)

ADRs	Drugs causing the ADR
Breathing disorders	
Shortness of breath/ worsening of asthma	Beta-blockers (including eye drops), NSAIDs, ACE inhibitors, tramadol, omeprazole, amiodarone, methotrexate
Disorders of skin	
Hair loss	Cytotoxics, lithium, anticoagulants, proton pump inhibitors, leflunomide, vigabatrin, mefloquine, ACE inhibitors
Facial or excessive hair growth	Danazol, phenytoin, tibolone, corticosteroids, minoxidil
Flushing	Nitrates, calcium-channel blockers, nicorandil, vancomycin, opioids, ACE inhibitors
Oedema	Corticosteroids, NSAIDs
Pigmentation/ discoloration	Oral contraceptives, antimalarials, minocycline, amiodarone, phenothiazines
Acne-like eruptions	Steroids, danazol, isoniazid, progestogens, phenytoin
Photosensitivity	Chlorpromazine, tetracyclines, amiodarone, proton pump inhibitors, NSAIDs, quinolone antibiotics
Exacerbation of psoriasis	Beta-blockers, NSAIDs, antimalarials, lithium
Urticaria	Aspirin, opioids, penicillins
Disorders of the gastrointestinal tract	
Anorexia/weight loss	Tricyclic antidepressants, digoxin, sulfasalazine, metronidazole, SSRIs, ciprofloxacin, leflunomide, donepezil
Weight increase	Gabapentin, danazol, finasteride, mirtazapine, tricyclic antidepressants, oestrogens/progestogens, corticosteroids, varenicline
Heartburn/dyspepsia	NSAIDs, ACE inhibitors, corticosteroids, alendronate, risedronate, SSRIs
Nausea and vomiting	Antibiotics, levodopa, methotrexate, opioids, SSRIs
Flatulence	Lactulose, acarbose, statins, captopril, bulk-forming laxatives
Gastrointestinal upset	NSAIDs, prednisolone, SSRIs
Abdominal pain	Clofibrate (gallstones), macrolide antibiotics, cephalosporins, mefloquine, stimulant laxatives, dabigatran
Constipation	Aluminium-containing antacids, antipsychotics, iron salts, opioids, tricyclic antidepressants, verapamil
Diarrhoea	Acarbose, antibiotics, leukotriene receptor antagonists, magnesium-containing antacids, misoprostol, mefloquine
Jaundice/abnormal liver function tests	Statins, SSRIs, antipsychotics, tricyclic antidepressants, cyproterone, methotrexate, co-amoxiclav, flucloxacillin
Disorders of hormonal regulation	
Gynaecomastia	Oestrogens, spironolactone, H_2-receptor antagonists, tricyclic antidepressants, calcium-channel blockers
Period problems	Oral contraceptives, danazol, medroxyprogesterone, spironolactone, tamoxifen, antipsychotics

TABLE A2
(Continued)

ADRs	Drugs causing the ADR
Disorders of the urinary tract	
Impotence	Beta-blockers, antiepileptic drugs, cimetidine, spironolactone, ACE inhibitors
Urinary retention	Tricyclic antidepressants, trihexyphenidyl, antihistamines, benzodiazepines
Urinary frequency	Diuretics, levodopa, alpha-blockers, lithium
Urine discoloration	Dantron, levodopa, senna, rifampicin, imipenem, sulfasalazine
Cystitis	Tiaprofenic acid, cyclophosphamide
Biochemical disorders	
Hypercalcaemia	Calcipotriol, calcium, ciclosporin, danazol, diuretics, oestrogens, lithium, tamoxifen, vitamin D
Hyperkalaemia	Ciclosporin, heparins, fluconazole, indometacin, penicillins, potassium-sparing diuretics, trimethoprim
Hypocalcaemia	Antiepileptic drugs, corticosteroids
Hypokalaemia	Amphotericin, beta-lactam antibiotics, diuretics, levodopa
Hyponatraemia	Amiloride, antiepileptic drugs, antidepressants, cisplatin, cyclophosphamide, diuretics
Blood disorders	
Agranulocytosis	Aspirin and NSAIDs, allopurinol, beta-lactam antibiotics, cephalosporins, cocaine, colchicine, co-trimoxazole, dapsone, fluconazole, metronidazole, mianserin, nitrofurantoin, penicillamine, ranitidine, rifampicin, sertraline, sulfasalazine, thiazide diuretics, tricyclic antidepressants
Anaemias	Amphotericin, auranofin, azathioprine, cisplatin, co-trimoxazole, cyclophosphamide, flucytosine, ganciclovir, corticosteroids, NSAIDs, lamivudine, levodopa, losartan, penicillamine, phenindione, sulphonamides, dabigatran
Leukopenia	Allopurinol, amphotericin, antiepileptic drugs, azathioprine, beta-lactam antibiotics, carbamazepine, cimetidine, chloramphenicol, colchicine, co-trimoxazole, flucytosine, gold salts, griseofulvin, mesalazine, methotrexate, mianserin, mycophenolate, phenelzine, quinolone antibiotics, rifampicin, tamoxifen
Thrombocytopenia	Abciximab, aspirin and NSAIDs, aminophylline, antiepileptic drugs, azathioprine, beta-lactam antibiotics, chloramphenicol, co-trimoxazole, ethambutol, ganciclovir, gold salts, heparin, mesalazine, methotrexate, mianserin, nitrofurantoin, omeprazole, quinidine, quinine, rifampicin, sulphonamides, teicoplanin, terbinafine, trimethoprim, valproic acid
Infections and infestations	
Upper respiratory tract infections	Infliximab, etanercept
Sinusitis	Infliximab
Conjunctivitis	Infliximab

REFERENCES

1 WHO (1970). International drug monitoring – the role of the hospital – a WHO report. *Drug Intell Clin Pharm* 4: 101–110.

2 Human Medicines Regulations (2012). http://www.legislation.gov.uk/uksi/2012/1916/contents/made (accessed 12 October 2014).

3 Directive 2010/84/EU of the European Parliament and of the Council of 15 December 2010 amending, as regards pharmacovigilance, Directive 2001/83/EC on the Community code relating to medicinal products for human use. http://ec.europa.eu/health/files/eudralex/vol-1/dir_2010_84/dir_2010_84_en.pdf (accessed 12 October 2014).

4 Brayfield A (ed.) (2014) *Martindale: The Complete Drug Reference*, 38th edn. London: Pharmaceutical Press.

5 McEvoy GK *et al.* (eds) (2014). *American Hospital Formulary Service*. Bethesda, MD: American Society of Health-System Pharmacist.

6 Lee A (2005). *Adverse Drug Reactions*, 2nd edn. London: Pharmaceutical Press.

7 Aronson JK (ed.) (2006). *Meyler's Side Effects of Drugs*, 15th edn. London: Elsevier.

8 Davies DM *et al.* (eds) (1999). *Davies's Textbook of Adverse Drug Reactions*, 5th edn. London: Chapman and Hall.

9 Baxter K, Preston C (eds) (2013). *Stockley's Drug Interactions*, 10th edn. London: Pharmaceutical Press.

10 Hansten PD, Horn JT (eds) (2014). *Drug Interactions: Analysis and management*. St Louis, MO: Wolters Kluwer Health.

11 Barnes J (2013). *Herbal Medicines*. 4th edn. London: Pharmaceutical Press.

12 *Natural Medicines Comprehensive Database*. http://naturaldatabase.therapeuticresearch.com/ (accessed 12 October 2014).

Anaemias

Anaemia is a reduction in the red blood cell (RBC) mass[1] and is one of the most common conditions in the world.[2] It is not a diagnosis – it is a symptom that can arise from many different pathologies. Therefore, it is important to determine the cause of the anaemia to ensure appropriate therapy is given.[1]

The WHO has defined anaemia in adults as being when haemoglobin is less than 130 g/L for males and less than 120 g/L for non-pregnant females.[3] Low haemoglobin can be a result of increased haemoglobin loss or a reduction in haemoglobin synthesis.

Anaemia can be subdivided into the following categories: microcytic anaemia, megaloblastic anaemia and haemolytic anaemia. Microcytic anaemia includes: iron-deficiency anaemia, anaemia of chronic disease and sideroblastic anaemia. Megaloblastic anaemia includes: folate deficiency and vitamin B_{12} deficiency. Haemolytic anaemia includes sickle cell disease, thalassaemia and autoimmune haemolytic anaemia.[2]

Investigations

It is important to establish the cause of the anaemia to ensure appropriate treatment is commenced. Investigations will include a full blood count, which will show the haemoglobin concentration and the RBC count. The size, shape and colour of the RBCs may be assessed as well as the mean corpuscular volume (MCV) that is used to determine the type of anaemia. The 'normal' laboratory results for various anaemias are shown in Table A3.

TABLE A3
Laboratory results for different anaemias[1]

Type of anaemia	Consistent laboratory tests
Iron-deficiency (microcytic)	Reduced serum iron
	Reduced haematocrit
	Reduced haemoglobin
	Reduced ferritin
	Reduced mean cell volume
	Reduced mean cell haemoglobin concentration
	Increased total iron-binding capacity (TIBC)
Pernicious (megaloblastic)	Reduced haematocrit
	Reduced haemoglobin
	Normal serum iron
	Increased mean cell volume
	Reduced RBC count
	Reduced serum vitamin B_{12} (N.B. antibiotics can give a 'false low')
Folate deficiency (megaloblastic)	Reduced haematocrit
	Reduced haemoglobin
	Normal serum iron
	Increased mean cell volume
	Reduced RBC count
	Reduced serum folate
Anaemia of renal failure or chronic disease	Reduced haematocrit
	Reduced haemoglobin
	Reduced reticulocyte count

Iron-deficiency anaemia

Iron deficiency is the most common cause of anaemia and may arise from:

- inadequate iron absorption, e.g. malabsorption or inadequate intake
- increased physiological demand
- blood loss (the most common cause in the western world).

Signs and symptoms

These will vary with the degree of anaemia, as well as the time over which the anaemia developed. They include tiredness, pallor, fainting, palpitations, tachycardia and worsening or precipitation of angina and/or cardiac failure.

Food containing iron

These include red meat, fish, eggs, baked beans, pulses such as kidney beans and lentils, dried apricots and fortified cereals. In healthy adults, 10% of dietary iron intake is absorbed from the duodenum and the jejunum.[2]

Treatment

Treatment involves the appropriate management of the underlying cause and iron replacement therapy to correct the anaemia and replenish body stores.[4] The oral dose of elemental iron for iron-deficiency anaemia should be 100–200 mg daily. Therefore, the cost-effective treatment of choice is oral administration of ferrous sulphate 200 mg three times a day. For prophylaxis 200 mg once or twice a day may be given. Although other iron compounds are available, haemoglobin regeneration rate is little affected by the type of ferrous salt used provided sufficient iron is given; however, there is little evidence to suggest other ferrous salts offer important advantages.

Modified-release preparations are not recommended because they tend to release the iron in the lower gut, where absorption is poor.[5]

Ascorbic acid (250–500 mg with the iron preparation) is sometimes prescribed to aid the absorption of iron.[4]

The amount of elemental iron contained in different oral preparations is shown in Table A4.

TABLE A4
Iron content of proprietary preparations[5]

Preparation	Amount	Amount of ferrous iron
Ferrous fumarate	210 mg	68 mg
Ferrous gluconate	300 mg	35 mg
Ferrous sulfate	300 mg	60 mg
Ferrous sulfate, dried	200 mg	65 mg
Ferrous sulfate, dried	325 mg	105 mg
Sodium feredetate	190 mg/5 mL	27.5 mg/5 mL
Polysaccharide–iron complex		100 mg/5 mL

For people intolerant or not responding to oral iron, there are parenteral iron therapies available (see *Iron: guidance on parenteral dosing and administration* entry).

Timing of dose

Oral iron should ideally be taken on an empty stomach to achieve maximum absorption; however, many patients experience gastrointestinal side effects, in which case the dose may be given after food.[5]

Adverse reactions

Iron preparations are associated with unpleasant side effects, including nausea, epigastric pain, constipation and diarrhoea, which can lead to poor adherence. If side effects occur the iron dose could be reduced or an alternative preparation trialled with a lower dose of elemental iron.[5]

Patients should be counselled that accidental ingestion of iron can be very dangerous or fatal, especially in children, and they should seek immediate medical advice if this occurs.

Duration of treatment

When a patient has been started on iron replacement therapy, the haemoglobin level should be expected to rise by about 20 g/L every 3 weeks, although this varies from patient to patient.[5] Oral iron should be continued for 3 months after the iron deficiency has been corrected so that stores are replenished; the patient's full blood count should be checked after this time.[4,5]

Megaloblastic anaemias

These are macrocytic anaemias and the major causes are vitamin B_{12} deficiency and/or folate deficiency.[2]

Vitamin B_{12} deficiency

This may arise from decreased supply (reduced intake or absorption) or increased demand (greater metabolic consumption, destruction or excretion).[1] Causes include veganism, poor-quality diet or a congenital or acquired lack of intrinsic factor, e.g. gastrectomy.

Treatment

Vitamin B_{12} deficiency is treated by giving intramuscular injections of hydroxocobalamin. At the start of treatment 1 mg is given three times a week for 2 weeks and then 1 mg every 3 months. If there is neurological involvement, 1 mg is given on alternate days until no further improvement, and then every 2 months.[5] In the majority of patients the duration of treatment is normally lifelong.[2]

Folate-deficiency anaemia

Folate requirements vary with age and are increased in conditions with high metabolic rates and/or an increased rate of cell division. Folate is abundant in virtually all food sources, especially fresh green vegetables, yeast and liver. For this reason most people in Britain have an adequate intake. A daily intake of 200 micrograms is recommended. The body stores about 5–10 mg of folate and deficiency can occur within 3–4 months of reduced intake.[1]

Causes

Folic acid deficiency can be caused by inadequate dietary intake or malabsorption, alcoholism and rapid cell turnover. During pregnancy deficiency can occur, partly due to inadequate diet, partly due to the transfer of folate to the fetus, and partly due to increased folate degradation.

Some drugs, such as antiepileptic drugs, sulfasalazine, trimethoprim and methotrexate, may alter folate metabolism, resulting in folate deficiency.[1]

Treatment

Before commencing treatment with folic acid as monotherapy, vitamin B_{12} deficiency must be excluded, as folic acid treatment may correct the anaemia but allow neurological disease to develop.

Folic acid 5 mg daily is given for 4 months to replenish body stores. In the case of malabsorption it may be necessary to increase the dose to 15 mg daily. Long-term folate supplementation is rarely necessary because most causes of folate deficiency are self-limiting or will yield to a short course of treatment.[5]

In pregnancy, for prevention of neural tube defects, women at low risk should take 400 micrograms daily of folic acid. This should be taken before conception and until week 12 of pregnancy. Pregnancies at high risk of neural tube defects include: couples where either partner has a neural tube defect (or has a family history of neural tube defects), or a previous pregnancy has been affected by a neural tube defect in women with malabsorption states, e.g. coeliac disease, diabetes mellitus, sickle cell anaemia or taking antiepileptic drugs. In this group women should be advised to take folic acid 5 mg daily if they wish to become pregnant (or are at risk of becoming pregnant) and continue until week 12 of pregnancy. Women with sickle cell disease should continue taking their normal dose of folic acid 5 mg daily (or increase the dose to 5 mg daily) and continue this throughout pregnancy.[5]

Anaemia of chronic disease

This includes anaemia associated with inflammatory diseases, e.g. arthritis, malignancy and inflammatory bowel disease, and anaemia associated with chronic kidney disease and heart failure. As the anaemia accompanies many different diseases, symptoms are non-specific and can vary from person to person. The patient will display symptoms of the chronic condition and general symptoms of anaemia.[2]

Treatment

Treatment is dependent upon the underlying cause of anaemia. Oral iron tends to be ineffective as patients have a functional iron deficiency rather than an actual iron deficiency.[2] Erythropoietins are used in the treatment of symptomatic anaemia associated with erythropoietin deficiency in chronic renal failure.[5]

REFERENCES

1 Alldredge BK *et al.* (eds) (2012). *Koda-Kimble & Young's Applied Therapeutics: The Clinical Use of Drugs,* 10th edn. London: Lippincott, Williams and Wilkins.

2 Walker R, Whittlesea C (eds) (2012). *Clinical Pharmacy and Therapeutics,* 5th edn. Edinburgh: Churchill Livingstone.

3 WHO (2008). *Worldwide Prevalence of Anaemia 1993–2005.* http://www.who.int/vmnis/publications/anaemia_prevalence/en/ (accessed 30 October 2014).

4 Goddard AF *et al.* (2011). Guidelines for the management of iron deficiency anaemia. *Gut* 60: 1309–1316.

5 Joint Formulary Committee (2014). *British National Formulary* (68th edn). London: BMJ Group and Pharmaceutical Press.

Angioedema: drug causes and treatment   **A**

Angioedema is swelling in the deep dermal layers of the skin and is
seen as part of both allergic and non-allergic reactions. It can affect
any part of the body but most commonly affects the eyes, lips,
genitals, hands and feet. In severe cases, when the insides of the
mouth and throat are affected, it can be life-threatening. The swelling
is non-pitting and either erythematous or skin-coloured. Angioedema
has been associated with a wide range of drugs.[1,2]

Drug-induced angioedema can be split into three main categories:

1 immediate hypersensitivity (allergic)
2 NSAID/aspirin-induced (non-allergic, intolerance, pseudoallergy)
3 ACEI-related (non-allergic).

Immediate hypersensitivity

Immediate hypersensitivity angioedema is an IgE-mediated allergic
response that is characterised by angioedema and/or urticaria (raised
itchy erythematous swellings) with systemic symptoms (e.g.
hypotension) that can result in life-threatening anaphylaxis.[3]

Treatment

The treatment is antihistamines and corticosteroids either orally or
intravenously depending on the severity of the reaction.[4,5]

NSAID/aspirin-induced

NSAID/aspirin-induced angioedema is generally non-allergic, and is
often described as an 'intolerance' or 'pseudoallergic'.

NSAID intolerance has a prevalence of 0.3–0.9% in the general
population. It occurs in 2–23% of patients with asthma and can
induce or aggravate clinical symptoms in 20–40% of patients with
chronic idiopathic urticarial angioedema.

Clinical features of NSAID-induced angioedema (rhinitis,
bronchospasm, urticaria and angioedema) are similar to those of
immediate hypersensitivity angioedema and generally occur within
minutes to a few hours of NSAID exposure.

Non-selective NSAIDs interfere with arachidonic acid metabolism
by inhibiting COX-1 and 2 pathways, resulting in overproduction of
leukotrienes and reduction of prostaglandin E_2. Consequences
include increased microvascular permeability, oedema and
degranulation of mast cells. This mechanism is pharmacological
rather than immunological, meaning that individuals with
NSAID-induced angioedema are likely to react to multiple structurally
and chemically unrelated NSAIDs, often on first exposure.

NSAIDs displaying strong COX-1 inhibition are more likely to cause
intolerance than those displaying preferential COX-2 inhibition (e.g.
meloxicam), selective COX-2 inhibition (e.g. celecoxib) or very weak
COX-1/COX-2 inhibition (e.g. paracetamol). However, the small

A

percentage of individuals cross-intolerant to NSAIDs and paracetamol are more likely to be intolerant to COX-2-selective NSAIDs.

The only reliable test for NSAID sensitivity is oral challenge.

Treatment

Treatment is antihistamines and corticosteroids. Patients should be warned to avoid NSAIDs as a class until safe alternatives can be confirmed.

ACEI-related angioedema

This is usually localised to the head and neck. Onset is often sudden and may be associated with pain or heat, but rarely with urticaria or erythema. Swelling lasts for 1–3 days, leaving no visible signs. It occurs in up to 0.7% of patients taking an ACEI and is fatal in approximately 0.1% of these cases.

Risk factors include black race (increased three- or four-fold), female gender, past history of angioedema, previous drug rash, smoking, age >65 years, seasonal allergies, recent initiation of an ACEI (first week of therapy), obesity, upper-airway surgery or trauma, sleep apnoea and immunosuppression in cardiac and renal transplant recipients.

About one in four cases occurs during the first month of taking an ACEI. The remaining cases develop many months or even years after treatment begins; this often leads to ACEIs being overlooked as a cause. Continuing administration tends to lead to more severe attacks. Episodes may recur for up to 3 months after an ACEI is stopped.

ACE inhibition decreases bradykinin degradation. Increased bradykinin levels dilate blood vessels, mediate inflammation, increase vascular permeability and activate nociceptors. High plasma levels of bradykinin are found in individuals taking ACEIs during acute episodes of angioedema. However, impaired bradykinin degradation by ACEIs is not the only factor involved, as angioedema appears inconsistently and in just a small percentage of patients. These additional factors are yet to be established.

ACEI-related angioedema is usually diagnosed after exclusion of other causes. No reliable tests can differentiate ACEI-related angioedema from angioedema due to other causes.

Treatment

Basic symptomatic emergency treatment is required. Although antihistamines and steroids are often used, evidence suggests that they are not very effective. In acute life-threatening situations, use of fresh frozen plasma has been tried. ACEIs must be stopped following an episode of angioedema and are contraindicated in patients with a history of chronic angioedema of any aetiology. Referral is only indicated if symptoms recur 3 months after stopping treatment.

Icatibant, a bradykinin inhibitor, is licensed for acute attacks of hereditary angioedema in patients with C1-esterase inhibitor deficiency but in 2014 failed to be granted a licence in the EU for ACEI-related angioedema.

REFERENCES

1 NHS Choices (2014). *Angioedema*. http://www.nhs.uk/conditions/Angioedema/Pages/Introduction.aspx (accessed 7 October 2014).

2 Clinical Knowledge Summaries (2012). *Angio-oedema and Anaphylaxis*. http://cks.nice.org.uk/angio-oedema-and-anaphylaxis (accessed 7 October 2014).

3 British Association of Dermatologists (2012). *Urticaria and Angioedema. Patient Information*. http://www.bad.org.uk/library-media/documents/Urticaria%20and%20Angioedema%20Update%20Sept%202012%20-%20lay%20reviewed%20May%202012.pdf (accessed 7 October 2014).

4 Powell RJ *et al.* (2007). BSACI guidelines for the management of chronic urticaria and angio-oedema. *Clin Exp Allergy* 37: 631–650.

5 Inomata N (2012). Recent advances in drug-induced angioedema. *Allergol Int* 61: 545–557.

Antibiotic choice

Ultimately the initial choice of antibiotic is dependent on the severity of the infection and the type of bacteria likely to be causing the infection. Antibiotic choice can be driven by laboratory culture results; however, it is often necessary to initiate antibiotic therapy before the results of cultures are known. The information here aims to aid in decision making but bacterial resistance rates vary by locality and therefore it is important to consult local guidelines.

Severity of infection

When treating a severe systemic infection it is essential antibiotics are given via the intravenous route; in sepsis this should be within the first hour of diagnosis.[1] For many mild and moderate infections the oral route is preferred. Many antibiotics do not have an oral and intravenous equivalent and therefore this can restrict choice, even when laboratory cultures are available.

Disease factors

Certain bacteria will colonise particular body areas, e.g. abdominal infections are more likely to be caused by Gram-negative aerobic or anaerobic bacteria, whereas skin infections are more likely to be caused by Gram-positive bacteria. The antibiotic choice should reflect this.

If the patient is currently, or has previously been, a carrier of MRSA, then this should affect your antibiotic choice. If a Gram-positive infection is suspected, the empirical antibiotic choice should cover MRSA, e.g. vancomycin. Certain antibiotics, such as quinolones, which will select for MRSA, should be avoided in MRSA carriers.

If the patient is currently, or has previously tested, positive for *Clostridium difficile* (polymerase chain reaction or toxin), certain antibiotics should be avoided if possible. Examples include co-amoxiclav, cephalosporins, clindamycin and quinolones, which will all select for *Clostridium difficile*.[2]

A

Previous history

It is important to know the medical history of the patient being treated. If the patient has had recent hospital admissions then the antibiotic history should be reviewed. If the person has had multiple infections within the past year with repeated courses of antibiotics, he or she is at risk of multiresistant infections. Review the patient notes and previous cultures before deciding on the antibiotic.

Site of infection

Antibiotics, like any drug, have variable rates of absorption and distribution. It is important that the antibiotic reaches therapeutic levels in the desired tissues. Many antibiotics cannot penetrate the blood–brain barrier, even when it is inflamed. Therefore, even when guided by culture results, the distribution of individual antibiotics should be taken into account. Summary of Product Characteristics will give information on antibiotic distribution.

Renal function

Many antibiotics are renally excreted and therefore dosage reductions are needed in renal impairment. Certain antibiotics, like the aminoglycosides, are nephrotoxic and for patients in acute kidney injury should be avoided where possible, or given with appropriate dose reductions and monitoring.

Reviewing

Regular reviewing of an antibiotic prescription is essential. If the patient is clinically improving and infective markers are returning to normal, switching to oral antibiotics may be appropriate. The use of broad-spectrum antibiotics increases the risk of resistance developing and therefore, if culture results are now available, the one with the narrowest spectrum of activity should be used.

REFERENCES

1 Bochud PY *et al.* (2004). Antimicrobial therapy for patients with severe sepsis and septic shock: an evidence-based review. *Crit Care Med* 3211(Suppl): S495–S512.
2 Joint Formulary Committee (2014). *British National Formulary* (68th edn). London: BMJ Group and Pharmaceutical Press.

Antimicrobial allergy management

Allergy is an essential factor to consider when deciding upon the most appropriate antimicrobial for a patient. Obtaining a detailed accurate history from the patient is crucial to determine the exact nature of the allergic reaction. The main aim is to establish whether the patient describes any symptoms that are highly suggestive of an IgE-mediated allergic reaction. IgE-mediated reactions (also referred to as immediate-onset reactions) usually occur within 1 hour of administration and are life-threatening.

Clinical signs and symptoms include diffuse urticarial rash, pruritus, bronchospasm, angioedema, hypotension and anaphylaxis. The choice of antimicrobial can often be limited by a doubtful or unconfirmed allergy history. As the most commonly reported allergic reactions are to beta-lactam antibiotics, the focus of this section will be on the appropriate management of those patients with penicillin allergy.

About 10% of the general population will claim to have a penicillin allergy; of these, only 10% will have a genuine allergy.[1] True anaphylaxis to penicillin occurs in less than 0.05% of patients receiving treatment.[2] A number of studies have shown that patients allergic to penicillin are more likely to receive alternatives that are more costly and broader-spectrum and can therefore select for *C. difficile* and the induction of antimicrobial resistance.[3]

Those patients with a clear history suggestive of anaphylaxis or a severe reaction (e.g. angioedema, immediate-onset urticarial rash) should not receive a penicillin. A patient with an immediate hypersensitivity reaction may also react to cephalosporins and carbapenems and these too should be avoided (see section below).[2] Those patients reporting a history of minor rash (i.e. non-confluent, non-pruritic rash restricted to one area of the body) or a rash occurring more than 72 hours after administration of a penicillin are most probably not allergic. In the event of serious infections, a penicillin should not be unnecessarily withheld; however, the patient should be closely monitored for signs of an allergic reaction.[2] For those patients where the history is suggestive of side effects only, e.g. gastrointestinal upset, a penicillin can be given.

Cross-reactivity with cephalosporins

The reported cross-over risk between cephalosporins and penicillins is 0.5–6.5%[2]; the true rate of cross-reaction is dependent upon the generation of cephalosporin. The risk of cross-reactivity is higher with first-generation cephalosporins (e.g. cefalexin, cefradine) compared to second- and third-generation cephalosporins, which are less likely to be associated with cross-reactivity due to differences in chemical structure. If a cephalosporin is deemed essential in those patients with an immediate hypersensitivity reaction to penicillin, then cefotaxime, ceftazidime, cefuroxime or ceftriaxone can be used with caution and cefaclor, cefadroxil, cefradine and cefalexin should be avoided.[2]

Cross-reactivity with carbapenems and monobactams

In a review, penicillin-allergic patients (identified by skin testing) were then skin-tested for reaction to a carbapenem. The reported cross-sensitivity was 1% between penicillins and a carbapenem.[4] Aztreonam is a monobactam that may be administered to those with a penicillin allergy; there have been no significant reports in the literature of cross-reactivity. Aztreonam possesses a similar side chain to ceftazidime; therefore, those patients with an IgE-mediated reaction to ceftazidime should avoid aztreonam.

A

NICE guidelines recommend that those patients requiring treatment for an infection, which can only be treated by beta-lactam antibiotics (penicillins, cephalosporins, carbapenems) or have a high likelihood for future need for beta-lactam antibiotics should be referred to a specialist drug allergy service.[5]

It is recommended that a patient's drug allergy status should be determined before the prescription, dispensing or administration of any drug. The name of the drug, nature of the reaction and date the reaction occurred should be documented on patient records (including general practitioner referral letters, hospital discharge letters and on all prescriptions issued in any healthcare setting).[5]

REFERENCES

1 Yates AB (2008). Management of patients with a history of allergy to beta lactam antibiotics. *Am J Med* 121: 572–576.

2 *British National Formulary* 67 (2014). London: BMA and Pharmaceutical Press.

3 MacLaughlin EJ (2000). Costs of beta-lactam allergies: Selection and costs of antibiotics for patients with a reported beta-lactam allergy. *Arch Fam Med* 9: 722–726.

4 Frumin J, Gallagher JC (2009). Allergic cross-sensitivity between penicillin, carbapenem, and monobactam antibiotics: what are the chances? *Ann Pharmacother* 43: 304–315.

5 NICE (2014). *Drug Allergy: Diagnosis and Management of Drug Allergy in Adults, Children and Young People.* Draft for consultation.

Antiphospholipid syndrome

Antiphospholipid syndrome (APS) or antiphospholipid antibody syndrome (APLS) is an acquired autoimmune condition. Patients usually present with a venous thrombosis such as a deep-vein thrombosis (DVT) or pulmonary embolism (PE) or arterial thrombosis (transient ischaemic attack, stroke or, more rarely, myocardial infarction). Another manifestation is pregnancy complications and pregnancy failure, in the form of recurrent miscarriages, late miscarriages, still or premature birth. Testing for APS should be done in patients with an unprovoked DVT or PE, as recurrence is higher in patients with APS. Patients under the age of 50 years who present with a stroke should also be tested for APS, as should women who have three or more miscarriages before 10 weeks.[1] The laboratory tests required are for anticardiolipin antibodies, anti-beta-2 glycoprotein antibodies and lupus anticoagulant. As these can all be transiently raised by infections or antibiotics the tests, if positive, must be repeated after 12 weeks to ensure the increases weren't just transient. If positive on both occasions, a diagnosis of APS can be made.[2] Note that lupus anticoagulant can give a false-positive result in patients on anticoagulants, so this test should not be done until the patient is off anticoagulation. In the case of warfarin, the test should be done no less than 4 weeks after stopping warfarin but with other anticoagulants 7 days is sufficient.[3]

Patients with an incidental finding of APS but with no history of venous or arterial thrombosis should not receive treatment. Patients who present with a stroke and are found to have APS should be treated with aspirin. Warfarin is the anticoagulant of choice in patients with previous venous thrombosis (DVT, PE). The INR should be kept in the range 2–3, with a target of 2.5. Bridging with some form of heparin will be required if warfarin needs to be stopped for surgery or procedures. For patients who have recurrent venous thrombosis while the INR is therapeutic, an INR range of 3–4 (target 3.5) is used. The NOACs have not been studied in APS, but could be used in patients with a history of DVT or PE if warfarin isn't tolerated or there is poor control. For women with APS who have had recurrent miscarriages, aspirin plus low-molecular-weight heparin are recommended throughout pregnancy. Aspirin alone is recommended in some women.[4] Prepregnancy counselling is advised and changing from warfarin to a low-molecular-weight heparin should be done due to the teratogenic effects of warfarin.

Pharmaceutical interventions

- Ensure prothrombotic drugs such as oestrogens are stopped, with counselling on appropriate contraception, such as progestogen only.
- Ensure the INR is kept in the appropriate target range both as an outpatient and inpatient.
- Advise on bridging therapies for patients undergoing surgery or procedures where there is a requirement for the INR to be below 2.
- Advise on restarting warfarin postoperatively and appropriate monitoring and advice on when to stop heparin.
- Ensure young women starting on warfarin understand the dangers around warfarin and pregnancy and information on prepregnancy counselling is available. During pregnancy ensure appropriate dosing of low-molecular-weight heparin, especially if there are large weight changes, and ensure low-molecular-weight heparin is extended postpartum.

Some patients with APS on warfarin, who have never had a DVT or PE, often have a high INR range. It is important these individuals are investigated to ensure they are on appropriate treatment and an appropriate INR range and have confirmed positive results for APS.

REFERENCES

1 Keeling D *et al.* (2012). Guidelines on the investigation and management of antiphospholipid syndrome. *Br J Haematol.* 157: 47–58.

2 NHS Choices (2013). *Antiphospholipid Syndrome (APS) – Causes.* http://www.nhs.uk/conditions/hughes-syndrome/pages/causes.aspx (accessed 24 January 2015).

3 NICE (2012). *Venous Thromboembolic Diseases: The management of venous thromboembolic diseases and the role of thrombophilia testing* (CG144). http://www.nice.org.uk/guidance/CG144 (accessed 24 January 2015).

4 Royal College of Obstetricians and Gynaecologists (2011). *Recurrent Miscar-riage, Investigation and Treatment of Couples* (Green-top Guideline No. 17). https://www.rcog.org.uk/en/guidelines-research-services/guidelines/gtg17/ (accessed 24 January 2015).

Antipsychotics: equivalent doses

Calculating antipsychotic equivalent doses can be important, most often clinically when switching from one antipsychotic to another or when antipsychotics are combined (Tables A5 and A6). Equivalent doses are also important for clinical trials undertaking active comparator studies in order to compare like with like.

TABLE A5
Oral antipsychotic dose equivalent

Approximate equivalent oral dose to 100 mg oral chlorpromazine[1,2,3,4]	
Antipsychotic	*Equivalent dose*
Amisulpride	100 mg (range 40–150 mg)
Aripiprazole	4 mg
Asenapine	4 mg
Clozapine	100 mg (range 30–150 mg)
Flupentixol	2–3 mg
Fluphenazine	2 mg (range 1.25–5 mg)
Haloperidol	2–3 mg (range 1–5 mg) or 1.5 mg IM/IV for doses up to 20 mg
Lurasidone	16 mg
Olanzapine	3 mg
Paliperidone	1.2 mg
Quetiapine	60 mg
Risperidone	0.5–1 mg (range 0.5–3 mg)
Sulpiride	200 mg (range 200–270 mg)
Trifluoperazine	5 mg (range 2–8 mg)
Zuclopenthixol	25 mg (range 25–60 mg)

Considerations

Antipsychotic equivalent dose calculations are inexact due to their heterogeneity and the different calculation methods used and this is reflected by the range of values quoted in the literature. Many authors will not estimate dose equivalences for the 'atypical' or 'second-generation' antipsychotics, so all data for these agents should be treated with additional caution. These equivalences solely concern the dopaminergic effects of these agents. Adverse effects caused via other neurotransmitter systems need to be considered separately based on the propensity of each agent to cause them.

Calculations may be complicated by the half-lives of the different agents, and the effect of first-pass metabolism on oral dose forms. Calculated doses should always be checked against the SPC so

TABLE A6
Depot and long-acting injection antipsychotic dose equivalents

Antipsychotic	Equivalent dose (mg/week)
Aripiprazole	Only to be used for those responding to oral aripiprazole. See the SPC for conversion details
Flupentixol decanoate	10 mg (range 8–20 mg)
Fluphenazine decanoate	5–10 mg (range 1–12.5 mg)
Haloperidol decanoate	15 mg (range 5–25 mg)
Olanzapine pamoate	Only to be used for those responding to oral olanzapine. See the SPC for conversion details
Paliperidone palmitate	12.5 mg (as roughly 50 mg every month)
Pipotiazine palmitate	10 mg (range 5–12.5 mg)
Risperidone	12.5 mg (as 25 mg every 2 weeks)
Zuclopenthixol decanoate	100 mg (range 40–100 mg)

Approximate equivalent intramuscular dose to 100 mg oral chlorpromazine daily[1,2,3]

unlicensed doses are not inadvertently used. Equivalent doses should not be extrapolated beyond maximum licensed doses.

Clinical presentation should always be closely monitored, and inform dose adjustments as indicated. Published equivalents may lag behind licensing changes and also new agents becoming available.

REFERENCES

1 Joint Formulary Committee (2014). *British National Formulary* (68th edn). London: BMJ Group and Pharmaceutical Press.
2 Bazire S (2014). *Psychotropic Drug Directory 2014: The professionals' pocket handbook and aide memoire*. Dorsington: Lloyd-Reinhold.
3 Taylor D (2012). *The Maudsley Prescribing Guidelines in Psychiatry*, 11th edn. Chichester: Wiley-Blackwell.
4 Leucht S *et al.* (2014). Dose equivalents for second-generation antipsychotics: the minimum effective dose method. *Schizophr Bull* 40: 314–326.

Apomorphine

Apomorphine is licensed for the treatment of motor fluctuations ('on-off' phenomena) in patients with Parkinson's disease, which are not sufficiently controlled by oral anti-Parkinson medication. It is a potent, non-selective, direct-acting dopamine receptor agonist.[1,2] It may be used for long-term treatment in advanced disease or as a palliative treatment near the end of life. It is also occasionally used in the acute management of advanced Parkinson's disease where no oral access is available, e.g. in critical care.

The rapid and reliable response to apomorphine can be an advantage when oral doses of levodopa combined with other dopaminergic drugs become progressively less effective and less predictable. These 'on-off' phenomena or dyskinesias can be particularly problematic in younger-onset patients.

A

Apomorphine can be used as intermittent injections for use at the onset of 'off periods' or via continuous infusion for patients whose overall response is unsatisfactory despite use of intermittent injections. The 'off' period is characterised by symptoms such as dystonia, depression, pain, sleep dysfunction, bladder dysfunction and swallowing difficulties. An 'off' period can occur suddenly and unpredictably, with little indication to the patient of its approach.

Apomorphine initiation

Apomorphine should be initiated in the controlled environment of a specialist clinic. The patient should be supervised by a physician experienced in the treatment of Parkinson's disease (e.g. neurologist).

Antiemetic treatment

Nausea and vomiting can be problematic in up to 10% of patients on apomorphine, particularly at initiation. Domperidone, started at least 2 days before apomorphine therapy begins, has been shown to be successful in controlling symptoms.[1,2] Caution should be used when prescribing domperidone and a full cardiac review is needed prior to initiation. It is contraindicated in patients:[3]

- with conditions where cardiac conduction is, or could be, impaired
- with underlying cardiac diseases such as congestive heart failure
- receiving other medications known to prolong QT interval or potent CYP3A4 inhibitors
- with severe hepatic impairment.

It is usually possible to reduce and withdraw domperidone altogether once apomorphine treatment has been established.

Apomorphine challenge

Apomorphine will not produce positive response in all patients.[4] In order to determine likely response to apomorphine treatment, the patient should have an apomorphine challenge.

1 The patient is premedicated with domperidone, as above.
2 Normal anti-Parkinson medication should be withheld for 4–6 hours to provide an 'off' period.
3 Record baseline 'off' state assessment. Record lying and standing blood pressure; take Unified Parkinson's Disease Rating Scale (UPDRS) III to provide a baseline score. A 12-metre walk is suggested, but not compulsory, and should not be done for someone with postural hypotension.
4 A 1-mg dose of apomorphine is given by subcutaneous injection, and the patient monitored for response and side effects for up to 30 minutes. The desired response is reversal of parkinsonian symptoms within 5–10 minutes following injection and for a duration of 45–60 minutes. A positive challenge is defined as a UPDRS score of 20% above baseline, and where available, more than a 25% improvement in walking time.

5 If there is no response or a poor response, a further dose of 3 mg is given, and the patient assessed again, or specific symptoms, e.g. pain, are alleviated.
6 This process is repeated if necessary, first with a 5-mg dose, then a 7-mg dose. If there is no response with a 7-mg dose, the patient is classed as a non-responder, and apomorphine will not be suitable. If the response at 7 mg is mild, then a maximum of 10 mg should be tried.

The effective dose that is individually determined for the patient will typically require no further adjustment once it has been established.

Administration

Apomorphine is given subcutaneously in one of two ways:

1 intermittent injection from a prefilled disposable pen
2 by continuous infusion using a syringe driver, or an APO-go pump.

Continuous infusions are considered for patients needing more than 10 injections per day, or who have shown a good 'on' period response during the initiation stage of apomorphine therapy, but whose overall control remains unsatisfactory using intermittent injections.

When given by continuous infusion via APO-go pump or syringe driver, the 5 mg/mL prefilled syringes should be used, or the 10 mg/mL injection diluted with an equal volume of sodium chloride 0.9% to make the final concentration 5 mg/mL. If given more concentrated, apomorphine may provoke local inflammatory reactions. Water for injections should not be used as a diluent, as this can increase the risk of nodule formation and ulceration.

Continuous infusions are normally given during the patient's waking hours, and unless severe nighttime problems are experienced, 24-hour infusions are not advised. The infusion site needs to be changed every 12 hours.

Practical considerations for patients on apomorphine therapy

Apomorphine injection is very irritant and stains clothes and bed clothes on contact.

Skin nodules and ulcers are common with apomorphine use. It is important to minimise the formation of nodules as it is thought they may reduce the absorption of apomorphine and thus reduce the efficacy of treatment.

Local reactions can be minimised by clean technique, daily rotation of injection sites and using thumb tack needles. Gentle massage of the injection sites can also be helpful. Silicone gel patches can also help to reduce nodule formation and relieve itchiness.[4]

Monitoring

Haemolytic anaemia and thrombocytopenia have been reported in patients taking apomorphine; therefore, regular full blood count monitoring is advised.[1,2]

A

Impulse control disorders, e.g. pathological gambling, increased libido, hypersexuality, compulsive spending/buying, binge eating and compulsive eating, have also been reported with apomorphine; therefore, counselling and regular monitoring are essential.

REFERENCES

1 SPC. *APO-go Pre-filled Syringes 5 mg/mL*. www.medicines.org.uk/emc (accessed 5 August 2014).

2 SPC. *APO-go Pen 10 mg/mL*. www.medicines.org.uk/emc (accessed 5 August 2014).

3 Kings College Hospital NHS Trust (2002). The Use of Apomorphine in Parkinson's Disease. Shared Care Guidelines London: Kings College Hospital NHS Trust.

4 MHRA Drug Safety Update (2014). *Domperidone: Risks of cardiac side effects – indication restricted to nausea and vomiting, new contraindications and reduced dose and duration of use*. http://www.mhra.gov.uk/Safetyinformation/DrugSafety Update/CON418518 (accessed 5 August 2014).

Appetite stimulation

Loss of appetite is a problem in many debilitating illnesses such as HIV/AIDS and cancer. Stimulation of a patient's appetite is important to improve the patient's nutritional status and sense of well-being. It is important to identify any medical cause for weight loss. The reason a patient may not be eating, or not maintaining weight, is often complex and there may be pathophysiological and psychological components.[1]

Dieticians and psychologists have an important role to play in managing the cause of the weight loss in a patient; however, prescribers will often seek advice on appetite-stimulating drug treatment. It is useful to know what products exist, or have been tried, for this purpose, even though the evidence base is weak.

Alcohol

Anecdotal evidence suggests that an alcoholic beverage may improve appetite before meals. Alcohol is known to depress glycogenolysis, and this may lead to a compensatory increase in appetite as the body 'thinks' it needs food. A 25-mL measure of sherry or whisky is sometimes prescribed, equivalent to a single measure (one unit) of alcohol. There is a major psychological benefit in serving alcohol in a glass rather than in a medicine pot.

Cyproheptadine (Periactin)

Cyproheptadine was licensed as an appetite stimulant until 1994, when this indication was removed from its product licence.[2] The previously licensed adult dose was 4 mg three to four times a day, and in children over 3 years the dose was 2 mg three times a day.[3,4] Although no longer licensed, and lacking strong evidence, it may still be considered as an option.

A

Bitters and tonics

Traditionally mixtures containing simple and aromatic bitters are remedies used for loss of appetite; however, there is no evidence to support their use.[5] In the case of the tonics the main ingredients are various vitamins and minerals. The rationale for their possible effect is that in patients deficient in these substances, loss of weight and appetite does occur.

Progestogens (megestrol acetate and medroxyprogesterone acetate)

Although licensed for use in the treatment of breast and endometrial cancer in the UK, a coincidental increase in appetite and weight gain has been observed in patients treated with the drug. In the USA, the Food and Drug Administration has approved the use of megestrol acetate for the treatment of anorexia, cachexia or an unexplained, significant weight loss in patients with a diagnosis of AIDS. The usual starting dose is 800 mg daily in divided doses, although clinical trials found daily doses of 400–800 mg to be effective.[6] Progestogens have been used in the treatment of weight loss associated with cancer (the cancer anorexia cachexia syndrome). Megestrol at doses of 160–320 mg each day and medroxyprogesterone at doses of 200 mg three times a day have been used. It may take up to 2 weeks for the benefit to be seen but, in comparison with corticosteroids, the progestogens have fewer side effects.[7]

Corticosteroids

In palliative care, corticosteroids have been used to improve appetite and enhance a sense of well-being. Dexamethasone has been used in the dose range 2–4 mg daily.[7]

Mirtazapine

Mirtazapine is licensed as an antidepressant medication. When used to treat depression in elderly patients, it has also been shown to promote weight gain and increase appetite.[8]

REFERENCES

1 Yeh S-S, Shuster MW (1999). Geriatric cachexia: the role of cytokines. *Am J Clin Nutr* 70: 183–197.

2 World Health Organization (WHO) (1994) *Drug Information*, volume 8 number 2. http://whqlibdoc.who.int/druginfo/DRUG_INFO_8_2_1994.pdf (accessed 12 October 2014).

3 Rahimtoola RJ *et al.* (1970). Clinical experience with children on Periactin (cyproheptadine). *Pak J Med Res* 9: 15–19.

4 Halmi KA *et al.* (1982). Cyproheptadine for anorexia nervosa. *Lancet* 1(8285): 1357–1358.

5 Joint Formulary Committee (2014). *British National Formulary* (68th edn). London: BMJ Group and Pharmaceutical Press.

6 US FDA. *Product Label Megace Oral Suspension*. http://www.accessdata.fda.gov/drugsatfda_docs/label/2012/020264s017lbl.pdf (accessed 12 October 2014).

7 Watson M *et al.* (2009). *Oxford Handbook of Palliative Care* (2nd edn.). Oxford: Oxford University Press.

8 Huffman GB (2002). Evaluating and treating intentional weight loss in the elderly. *Am Fam Physician* 65: 640–651.

Arterial blood gases and acid–base balance

Overview	
Definition	Arterial blood is collected to measure for the partial pressure of O_2 and CO_2. Arterial blood gases (ABG) are also collected for the interpretation of acid–base balance[1]
Risk	• Insertion of an arterial line can be painful • Most commonly taken from the brachial artery • In intensive care, continuous arterial lines are used routinely and can be a source of infection if not changed regularly
Reference values (all)	Partial pressure O_2: 11–13 kPa Partial pressure CO_2: 4–6 kPa pH: 7.35 Base excess/deficit: 0 Serum bicarbonate: 18–26 mmol/L Serum lactate: <1.5 mmol/L
Common terms: ABG	**Hypercapnic respiratory drive:** hypercapnia is where the CO_2 concentration is higher than the reference range. It is this raised CO_2 that stimulates gas exchange in the alveoli. **Hypoxic respiratory drive:** if one lives with a permanently high concentration of CO_2 then the hypercapnic respiratory drive is lost and the patient is dependent on a hypoxic respiratory drive. This is typically a patient with COPD. In this patient group it is the low O_2 that stimulates gas exchange. **O_2 dissociation curve:** free O_2 (pO_2) is bound to haemoglobin and transferred from the lungs to the tissues in the form of 2,4-diphosphoglycerate. It then dissociates to pO_2 and it is this partial pressure of oxygen that is the free O_2, available for anaerobic metabolism in the mitochondria
Common terms: acid–base balance	**Metabolic acidosis:** this literally means production of excess acid in the body. There are two acids: lactic (formed after anaerobic metabolism) and hydroxybutyric acid (formed after diabetic ketoacidosis). There are other forms of iatrogenic metabolic acidosis, e.g. hyperchloraemic metabolic acidosis, which may occur after administration of excess sodium chloride 0.9%. **Metabolic alkalosis:** this is retention of excess bicarbonate and can occur after overdose of tricyclic antidepressants. Compensation is respiratory acidosis through retention of CO_2. **Respiratory acidosis:** occurs due to the retention of CO_2 in the form of carbonic acid and due to the kidneys causing bicarbonate-compensatory metabolic alkalosis. It commonly presents in opioid toxicity

	Respiratory alkalosis: caused by exhaling an excess of CO_2 and can occur in hyperventilation. Compensation is in the form of metabolic acidosis (kidney excretes extra bicarbonate).
	Base excess or deficit: this hypothetical figure describes the number of moles of bicarbonate to be either added or removed from blood to attain physiological pH 7.35; a negative base excess is indicative of metabolic acidosis. It can be an early sign of sepsis.
	Anion gap: this represents the concentration of unmeasured ions in circulation. A large anion gap can signal the presence of metabolic acidosis; it can help differentiate type (a larger anion gap signals organic acidosis) and can be used to monitor the effect of treatment. A normal anion gap is between 8 and 16 mmol/L
Clinical application (ABG)	Type 1 respiratory failure • Main presentation is hypoxia (pO_2 <11 kPa) • Occurs commonly in lower respiratory tract infection and asthma Type 2 respiratory failure • Main presentation is hypercapnia (pCO_2 >6 kPa) • Occurs commonly in COPD
Clinical application (acid–base balance)	• Body pH is balanced at 7.35 • Enzymatic reactions only occur at specific pH • Any drift of pH up or down from 7.35 can have grave consequences • The two organs involved in maintaining pH are the lungs (for CO_2 exchange) and the kidneys (for bicarbonate buffering)

Pharmaceutical care

| Assess | • Oxygen therapy: caution in COPD as patients may have lost their hypercapnic respiratory drive
• Sodium bicarbonate 8.4% (given via a central line except in emergencies) treatment for life-threatening metabolic acidosis when kidneys cannot retain sufficient bicarbonate. Always administer over 30 minutes to prevent intracellular acidosis. Correction of acid–base disturbance in the ICU is most commonly undertaken by renal replacement therapy
• Arterial line: a common source of infection in the ICU: change every 10–14 days depending on local policy |

REFERENCE

1 Warrell DA et al. (eds) (2012) Oxford Textbook of Medicine, 5th edn. Oxford: Oxford University Press.

Artificial saliva

Dry mouth (xerostomia) can be managed by saliva stimulants or substitutes. Saliva is made of 99% water and the remaining 1% is a combination of electrolytes and molecules that are important for saliva's many functions: lubricating, cleansing, digestion, buffering, mineralisation of teeth, taste and antimicrobial properties.[1] Artificial saliva is a poor substitute for natural saliva; saliva stimulants are

A

TABLE A7
Saliva substitutes and preparations to treat dry mouth[4]

Products available (manufacturer)	Formulation	Prescribable on NHS?	pH	Contains fluoride?	Animal-derived ingredients?	Gluten-free?	Sugar-free?
AS Saliva Orthana (AS Pharma)	Oral spray 50 mL	Yes ACBS	Neutral	Yes	Yes Porcine	Yes	Yes
	Lozenges (30)	Yes ACBS	Neutral	No	Yes Porcine	Yes	Yes Contains sorbitol
Biotene Oralbalance (GSK)	Saliva replacement gel 50 g	Yes (dentist prescribing: may be prescribed as artificial saliva gel)	Acidic	No	Yes (manufacturer did not provide information on what these were)	Yes	Yes Contains glucose oxidase, an enzyme added to inhibit bacteria growth. This is not a sugar
BioXtra products for dry mouth (RIS Products)	Moisturising gel 40 mL	Yes ACBS	Neutral	No	Yes Proteins extracted from cow's milk	Yes	Yes
	Gel mouth spray 50 mL	Yes ACBS	Neutral	Yes	Yes Proteins extracted from cow's milk	Yes	Yes
Glandosane (Fresenius Kabi)	Aerosol spray 50 mL (lemon, neutral, peppermint)	Yes ACBS	Acidic	No	No	Yes	Yes Contains sorbitol
Saliveze (Wyvern)	Oral spray 50 mL	Yes ACBS	Neutral	No	No	Yes	Yes
Saliva Stimulating Tablets (SST) (Medac)	Tablets (100)	Yes	Acidic	No	No	Yes	Yes Contains sorbitol
Xerotin (SpePharm)	Oral spray 100 mL	Yes Dental prescribing May be prescribed as artificial saliva spray	Neutral	No	No	Yes	Yes Contains sorbitol

preferred unless a main salivary duct is blocked. Chewing gum stimulates saliva production and is as effective as, and preferred to, mucin-based artificial saliva.[2] Gum should be sugar-free and in patients with dentures, low-tack, e.g. Orbit, Freedent.

The ideal artificial saliva should be easy to use, pleasant, effective and well tolerated, have a neutral pH to prevent demineralisation of teeth and contain fluoride to enhance remineralisation of teeth. Acidic products should be avoided in patients with stomatitis/mucositis as the acidity will increase pain; and in dentate patients due to the risk of dental decay may cause oral candidosis. Mucin-based products are generally better-tolerated and more effective than cellulose-based ones; however, mucin is derived from the stomach of pigs and therefore maybe an issue with certain groups, e.g. Muslims, Jews and vegetarians (see *Pharmacocultural issues* entry).[1]

Artificial saliva products have a short duration of action due to swallowing and evaporation, and therefore use may need to be frequent: every 30–60 minutes, before and during meals.[1]

Aquoral, Biotène Oralbalance Biotène gel or Xerotin can be used for any condition giving rise to a dry mouth. BioXtra, Glandosane, Saliva Orthana and Saliveze have ACBS approval for dry mouth associated only with radiotherapy or sicca (Sjögren) syndrome. Salivix pastilles, which act locally as salivary stimulants, are available for any condition leading to a dry mouth. SST tablets may be prescribed for dry mouth in patients with salivary gland impairment.[3]

Table A7 summarises the saliva substitute products currently available in the UK.

REFERENCES

1 Twycross R, Wilcock A (2011). Artificial saliva and topical saliva stimulants. In: *Palliative Care Formulary* (4th edn). Nottingham: Palliativedrugs.com, pp. 570–572.
2 Davies AN (2000). A comparison of artificial saliva and chewing gum in the management of xerostomia in patients with advanced cancer. *Palliat Med* 14: 197–203.
3 Joint Formulary Committee (2014). *British National Formulary* (68th edn). London: BMJ Group and Pharmaceutical Press.
4 Henderson S (2013). UKMi Medicines Q&A 190.6. *Saliva Substitutes: Choosing and prescribing the right product*. Liverpool: North West Medicines Information Centre.

Asthma

Overview	
Definition	Asthma is defined as 'a chronic inflammatory disorder of the airways in which many cells and cellular elements play a role; in particular, mast cells, eosinophils, T lymphocytes, macrophages, neutrophils, and epithelial cells'. The chronic inflammation causes an associated increase in airway hyperresponsiveness that leads to recurrent episodes of symptoms of asthma. These episodes are usually associated with widespread but variable airflow obstruction that is often reversible either spontaneously or with treatment

Causes	There is no known single cause for asthma, but it is well recognised that there are genetic and environmental factors that contribute to developing the condition: • Family history of asthma (especially a parent or sibling) or other atopic conditions, e.g. eczema, hayfever • Bronchiolitis as a child (40% of children exposed to respiratory syncytial virus or parainfluenza virus will continue to wheeze or have asthma into later childhood) • Tobacco smoke, particularly if the mother smoked during pregnancy • Premature birth or low birth weight • Occupational exposure (e.g. to plastics, agricultural substances and volatile chemicals such as solvents) • Obesity, especially if body mass index $>30 \text{ kg/m}^2$ • Bottle feeding: evidence shows that if an infant is breast-fed there is a decreased risk of wheezing illness compared to infants fed formula or soya-based milk feeds
Classification	Asthma is classified in different ways depending on the level of control and treatment. In the *British Guideline on the Management of Asthma*,[1] classification is based on the level of the treatment that is needed to maintain asthma control, from step 1 increasing up to step 5. Recently asthma research has introduced a new approach to identify and classify asthma according to different subgroups of asthma, such as eosinophilic asthma, atopic, late-onset asthma
Signs and symptoms	The classic signs of asthma are wheezing (especially expiratory wheeze), breathlessness, coughing (typically early-morning or nighttime) and chest tightness. The wheezing that occurs as a result of airway bronchoconstriction and coughing is likely to be due to stimulation of sensory nerves in the airways. These episodes are usually reversible either spontaneously or with treatment. In a severe exacerbation, wheeze may be absent and the chest may be silent on auscultation due to such severe obstruction of the airway. In these cases, often other signs will be present, such as cyanosis, drowsiness and an inability to complete full sentences. These severe cases are medical emergencies and require immediate medical attention
Diagnostic tests	There is no 'gold standard' test that can be used to diagnose asthma. Therefore, asthma diagnosis is usually based on one or more typical features, including: respiratory symptoms; evidence of variable airflow obstruction using lung function tests; and the person's response to asthma medication. The diagnostic process is different in adults and children and also varies among adults and among children. Processes for diagnosis in adults and children are described in the BTS/SIGN guidance[1]

Treatment goals[1]	The goal of asthma management is control of the disease. Complete control of asthma is defined as:

- No daytime symptoms
- No nighttime awakening due to asthma
- No need for rescue medication
- No exacerbations
- No limitations on activity, including exercise
- Normal lung function (in practical terms: forced expiratory volume in 1 second and/or peak expiratory flow rate (PEFR) >80% predicted or best)
- Minimal side effects from medication

Treatment options	

- Avoidance of triggers (such as pollen, animal dander, aspirin or NSAIDs) is a key component of improving control and preventing asthma exacerbations
- Medications used to treat asthma are divided into two general classes: quick-relief medications (e.g. short-acting beta-2 agonists), used to treat acute symptoms; and long-term control medications (e.g. inhaled corticosteroids), used to prevent further exacerbation. The current BTS/SIGN algorithm for chronic asthma can be found here:

BTS/SIGN Guideline Algorithm[1]

- Healthy lifestyle advice should be offered to patients, including moderation of alcohol consumption, smoking cessation, regular exercise, dietary advice to help manage weight, vaccinations (annual influenza and one-off pneumococcal)
- People with asthma should be provided with a written personalised action plan given as part of structured education. Typically action plans contain specific advice as to how to recognise loss of asthma control based on either symptoms or PEFR and what action to take if asthma deteriorates (e.g. when PEFR <50% it is best to seek emergency help). An asthma action plan can be downloaded from the Asthma UK website (www.asthma.org.uk)
- These plans can improve outcomes, giving self-efficacy, knowledge and confidence for people with asthma to manage their disease

A

Medicines Optimisation

The medication treatment options here are from BTS/SIGN guidance

Inhaled corticosteroid (ICS)	• Most effective treatment to reduce inflammation in the lungs and prevent exacerbations • Start at a dose appropriate to the severity of the disease and then titrate to the lowest dose at which effective control of asthma is maintained • Discuss the importance of regular inhaled corticosteroids use even when feeling well. The risk of side effects from long-term ICS to maintain adequate asthma control is minimal when compared with repeated courses of oral corticosteroids for asthma exacerbations and periods of poor control • Optimise dose: most patients with asthma can achieve well-controlled disease with relatively low doses of inhaled corticosteroids ($\leq$800 micrograms beclometasone (non-extra-fine)/day or equivalent). The BTS/SIGN asthma guideline contains a table showing dose comparisons between inhaled corticosteroids • Risk of systemic side effects is low with doses $\leq$800 micrograms beclometasone (non-extra-fine)/day or equivalent • Rinse mouth after use to reduce incidence of local side effects, such as oral *Candida* and hoarseness • Issue steroid warning card to all patients receiving high-dose inhaled corticosteroids (>800 micrograms beclometasone (non-extra-fine)/day or equivalent)
Short-acting beta-2 agonist (SABA)	• Most effective treatment to relieve acute symptoms of asthma • Beta-2-agonists can mask symptoms and do not change the underlying inflammatory disease process • Should always be prescribed 'when required' at all stages of the disease • Good control is associated with little to no need for SABA use. Increased use is a marker of uncontrolled asthma • Side effects such as tremor, cramps and $\downarrow$K (monitor) and palpitations are dose-related
Long-acting beta-2 agonist (LABA)	• Should always be prescribed in conjunction with an inhaled corticosteroid in people with asthma due to the increased risk of death associated with use without an ICS (a combination inhaler is recommended) • Risk of $\downarrow$K, therefore monitor
Leukotriene antagonist (LTRA)	• LTRA may be of benefit in exercise-induced asthma, aspirin-intolerant asthmatics and those with concomitant rhinitis • Clinical response seen within 4 weeks, though not all patients benefit

Methylxanthine (theophylline, aminophylline)	• Narrow therapeutic window – appropriate dosing and monitoring are essential
	• Aim for a steady-state serum theophylline concentration of 10–20 micrograms/mL
	• If the theophylline level is subtherapeutic, confirm the blood sampling time was correct, assess adherence and check drug interactions before considering increasing the dose. Recheck levels after any dose increase
	• Measure drug levels: when treatment starts, if side effects occur, if expected therapeutic benefit is not achieved and if potential drug interactions are suspected. Monitor levels daily if intravenous aminophylline is prescribed (see *Theophylline* entry) act on results
	• Side effects occur commonly, such as tachycardia, palpitations, headache, insomnia, nausea and other gastrointestinal disturbances
	• If intravenous aminophylline is prescribed to manage acute severe exacerbations, ensure a loading dose is given only if the person is not taking an oral methylxanthine
	• Check for drug interactions with prescribed, herbal and OTC medicines and withhold/adjust these medicines as appropriate
	• Prescribe oral products by brand, as bioavailability may vary from one brand to another
Oral corticosteroid	• Short courses (5–7 days) are prescribed to manage an asthma exacerbation
	• If long-term treatment is required to manage severe asthma, use the lowest dose possible to maintain control. To reduce the dose or eliminate the steroid tablets, also prescribe maximum dose of ICS
	• For steroid courses longer than 3 weeks, provide a steroid warning card
	• Consider osteoporosis prophylaxis for people on $\geq$7.5 mg prednisolone and/or more than four courses of oral steroids in a year. Using a high-dose corticosteroid inhaler in the long term may also be a risk. Epidemiological studies examining the relationship between inhaled corticosteroids and osteoporosis give conflicting results and are difficult to interpret due to confounding factors. General measures to counteract osteoporosis (such as regular exercise, smoking cessation, adequate dietary calcium) are recommended in people who require high doses of inhaled corticosteroids for prolonged periods of time
Anti-IgE therapy (omalizumab)	• Consider for people with documented allergic asthma and raised IgE
	• NICE technology appraisal guides prescribing[2]
	• Administered every 2 or 4 weeks by subcutaneous injection – initially a 16-week trial to monitor response
Muscarinic antagonists	• If ipratropium is being nebulised, the mask must be fitted carefully or ideally a mouthpiece used to avoid the aerosol coming into contact with the eyes, as this could cause glaucoma. Other antimuscarinic medication via an inhaled device should be withheld whilst on nebulised ipratropium, due to increase in the risk of adverse effects and no increased efficacy

Drug administration	• Give specific training and assessment on inhaler technique before starting any new inhaler treatment. *Ask patients to show you how they use their inhalers; it is not sufficient just to ask them if they know how to use them* • Make sure the patient's spacer device is compatible with the inhaler device and that patients know how to use the spacer • The use of nebulisers in the day-to-day management of asthma is rarely appropriate or necessary and can be dangerous. There is a documented increased risk of dying associated with overuse of SABAs during an exacerbation.[3] Confirm that a nebuliser is required and the patient has been allocated or has access to one
Essential interventions	• Strongly advise patients not to smoke: smoking worsens asthma symptoms and reduces responsiveness to inhaled corticosteroids in asthma patients • Monitor asthma control (use a validated tool, such as RCP 3 questions[4]) and recommend stepping up or down treatments appropriately • Ensure the patient understands that asthma is a chronic condition, even though the symptoms may vary • Assess adherence to medicine (by asking patients, reviewing repeat prescription frequency, examining dates on dispensing labels) • Ensure patients understand the differences between reliever and preventer medication • Ensure patients are offered an annual vaccination against influenza and a one-off vaccination against pneumococcal disease
Secondary intervention	• Patient health beliefs – disarming myths, such as weight gain, dependence and intolerance, especially regarding inhaled corticosteroids • Make sure patients are aware how to follow their personalised asthma action plan in response to their symptoms and/or peak flow readings • Provide health messages about avoidance of allergens • Consider assessment and treatment of comorbidities (e.g. allergic rhinitis, anxiety)
Monitoring on hospital admission	• Assess severity of asthma exacerbation, observing respiratory rate, heart rate, blood pressure, state of consciousness and whether the patient is able to speak in full sentences • Assess airflow obstruction (peak expiratory flow measurement), blood gas measurement, pulse oximetry, accessory muscle use and chest sounds • Review medication regimen, adherence, including need for changes, and possible side effects

Further reading	Asthma UK: http://www.asthma.org.uk/.
	Global Initiative for Asthma (GINA) (2014). *Global Strategy for Asthma Management and Prevention*. http://www.ginasthma.org (accessed 26 April 2015).
	National Review of Asthma Deaths (NRAD) *Why Asthma Still Kills*. https://www.rcplondon.ac.uk/sites/default/files/why-asthma-still-kills-full-report.pdf (accessed 26 April 2015).
	NICE (2013) *Quality Standard for Asthma*. http://www.nice.org.uk/guidance/qs25/resources/guidance-quality-standard-for-asthma-pdf (accessed 26 April 2015).
	Royal Pharmaceutical Society (RPS) (2015) *Medicine Optimisation Briefing – Asthma*. http://www.rpharms.com/promoting-pharmacy-pdfs/mo-briefing—asthma.pdf (accessed 26 April 2015).

REFERENCES

1 Joint British Thoracic Society/Scottish Intercollegiate Guidelines Network (2012). *British Guideline on the Management of Asthma*. Clinical guideline 101 https://www.brit-thoracic.org.uk/document-library/clinical-information/asthma/btssign-guideline-on-the-management-of-asthma/ (accessed 4 May 2015).

2 NICE (2013). *NICE Technology Appraisals* (TA278). *Omalizumab for treating severe persistent allergic asthma*. http://www.nice.org.uk/guidance/TA278/chapter/1-guidance (accessed 1 October 2014).

3 Royal College of Physicians (2014). *Why Asthma Still Kills: The National Review of Asthma Deaths (NRAD); confidential enquiry report 2014*. https://www.rcplondon.ac.uk/sites/default/files/why-asthma-still-kills-full-report.pdf (accessed 27 January 2015).

4 Royal College of Physicians (1999). *Measuring Clinical Outcome in Asthma, A patient-focused approach*. https://www.rcplondon.ac.uk/publications/measuring-clinical-outcome-asthma (accessed 27 January 2015).

Atrial fibrillation

Overview

Definition	Atrial fibrillation (AF) is an arrhythmia caused by disorganised electrical activity in the atria, usually leading to a rapid and irregular ventricular rate. It is an important cause of morbidity and mortality due to heart failure, stroke and thromboembolism, and is the most common arrhythmia seen in clinical practice, with a prevalence approaching 2% of the general population, rising to almost 10% in those over 80 years.
	AF may be:
	• Acute onset: started in the last 24–48 hours
	• Paroxysmal: recurrent and usually self-limiting, usually lasting <7 days
	• Persistent: lasts longer than 48 hours and does not revert spontaneously to sinus rhythm
	• Permanent: long-standing and not amenable to cardioversion

A

Causes	• Cardiac: ischaemic heart disease (IHD), hypertension, rheumatic heart disease, cardiomyopathy, pericardial disease • Non-cardiac: thyrotoxicosis, acute infection, pulmonary disease (pneumonia, malignancy, effusion), excess alcohol (acute or chronic) and the perioperative period • Around 10% of cases have no obvious cause
Signs and symptoms	Common presenting symptoms are those of heart failure (breathlessness, fatigue, pulmonary or peripheral oedema), palpitations, stroke and systemic thromboembolism. The left atrial appendage is a common site for thrombus formation. Strokes associated with AF tend to be more severe (higher mortality and more debilitating). Some patients may be asymptomatic and AF is an incidental finding
Diagnostic tests	• ECG shows absent p-waves and irregular, narrow QRS complexes • Thyroid function tests to rule out thyrotoxicosis • LFTs (including GGT). If elevated, alcohol may be the cause • Chest X-ray for pulmonary oedema • Transthoracic echocardiogram (TTE), particularly if rhythm control is to be attempted or if there is a suspicion of structural or functional heart disease (valve disease or heart failure) • Transoesophageal echocardiogram (TOE) when TTE demonstrates an abnormality that requires further assessment or is inconclusive or when TOE-guided cardioversion is to be attempted (to rule out the presence of atrial thrombus)
Treatment goals	• Reduce the risk of stroke • Control related symptoms, especially those of heart failure • Control ventricular rate (rate control) in most patients • Cardiovert to (and maintain) sinus rhythm (rhythm control) in some patients
Treatment options	• Drug therapy is the commonest intervention to reduce stroke risk, reduce heart rate or maintain sinus rhythm • In patients with a high stroke risk who are not suitable for anticoagulants, left atrial appendage occlusion may be an option • For patients with paroxysmal or persistent AF that has not been controlled with drug treatment, left atrial catheter ablation (e.g. pulmonary vein isolation) may be considered • For patients with permanent AF whose symptoms persist due to a high ventricular rate despite drug treatment, consider ventricular pacing and AV node ablation

A

Medicines optimisation

Assess[1,2]   Stroke risk: assess every patient with a history of AF using the CHA_2DS_2VASc score:

Risk factor	Score
Congestive heart failure (CHF)	1
Hypertension	1
Age >75 years	2
Age 65–74 years	1
Diabetes mellitus	1
Stroke, transient ischaemic attack or thromboembolism	2
Vascular disease (previous MI, peripheral artery disease, aortic plaque)	1
Female	1

Use HAS-BLED score to identify any modifiable bleeding risks:

Risk factor	Score
Uncontrolled hypertension (systolic blood pressure >160 mmHg)	1
Abnormal liver function (cirrhosis or bilirubin >2 × normal or aspartate transaminase/alanine transaminase/alkaline phosphatase >3 × normal)	1
Abnormal renal function (dialysis, transplant, serum creatinine >200 micromol/L)	1
Previous history of stroke	1
Prior major bleed or predisposition to bleeding	1
Labile INR	1
Elderly (over 65 years)	1
Antiplatelets or NSAIDs	1
Alcohol use (>8 drinks per week)	1

A HAS-BLED score of >3 indicates a high bleeding risk. Where possible, address modifiable bleeding risks (hypertension, interacting drugs, alcohol intake).
- Rate control versus rhythm control strategy: for most patients, an initial rate control strategy will be appropriate. Patients presenting with haemodynamic instability should be cardioverted urgently
- Lifestyle advice and modification, especially alcohol intake
- Treat underlying reversible causes, such as thyrotoxicosis, pneumonia
- Stop ivabradine if prescribed in patients with AF

A

Stroke prevention[1]	• Offer oral anticoagulants to all patients with a CHA_2DS_2VASc score of >2, taking bleeding risk into account. Consider oral anticoagulants for men with a CHA_2DS_2VASc score of 1, again taking bleeding risk into account • Continue anticoagulants in all patients with a history of AF, even if they revert to sinus rhythm, taking bleeding risk into account • Do not offer stroke prevention to men with a CHA_2DS_2VASc score of 0 or women with a CHA_2DS_2VASc score of 1 (very low stroke risk) • Do not deny anticoagulants solely based on a history of falls • Do not use aspirin monotherapy solely for stroke prevention in AF Review all patients receiving suboptimal stroke prevention therapy and address where appropriate: • Replace aspirin monotherapy or no stroke prevention treatment with an oral anticoagulant if indicated • Replace warfarin with an NOAC if anticoagulation control is poor (see below)
Choice of oral anticoagulant	Treatment choice should be guided by local/national policies. NOACs are licensed for use in patients with non-valvular AF and at least one stroke risk factor; therefore in patients with valvular disease, warfarin would be the appropriate oral anticoagulant. NOACs are renally excreted and are contraindicated in patients with significant renal impairment (creatinine clearance <30 mL/min for dabigatran and <15 mL/min for apixaban and rivaroxaban). In England, warfarin or an NOAC would be suitable first-line options in most patients. The decision about whether to start treatment with warfarin or an NOAC should be made after an informed discussion between the patient and the clinician about the relative risks and benefits of each agent. All patients starting anticoagulants should receive an anticoagulant therapy card and be counselled fully on the use of the drug
Warfarin[1]	When warfarin is used for stroke prevention in atrial fibrillation (SPAF), the desirable INR range is 2–3. Most strokes occur when the INR is less than 2.0. After the initial 3 months of treatment, consider changing to an NOAC (if indicated) in patients with poor anticoagulant control (following a review of the cause), defined as: • Two INR values higher than 5.0 or one INR value higher than 8.0 within the last 6 months • Two INR values less than 1.5 within the past 6 months • Time in therapeutic range: less than 65%
Apixaban[3]	Usual dose for SPAF is 5 mg twice daily, reduced to 2.5 mg twice daily if two or more of the following are present: age >80 years, body weight <60 kg or serum creatinine >133 micromol/L. Patients with creatinine clearance between 15 and 29 mL/min should also have the dose reduced to 2.5 mg twice daily Contraindicated in patients taking ketoconazole, itraconazole, voriconazole, posaconazole and HIV protease inhibitors

A

Dabigatran[3]	Usual dose for SPAF is 150 mg twice daily, reduced to 110 mg twice daily in patients aged >80 years and in those taking verapamil. Dose reduction should also be considered when the thromboembolic risk is low and the bleeding risk is high, if the patient weighs <50 kg or in patients with gastritis, oesophagitis or gastroesophageal reflux.
	Contraindicated in patients taking ketoconazole, itraconazole, dronedarone, tacrolimus and ciclosporin
Rivaroxaban[3]	Usual dose for SPAF is 20 mg once daily, reduced to 15 mg daily in patients with a creatinine clearance between 15 and 49 mL/min.
	Contraindicated with ketoconazole, itraconazole, voriconazole, posaconazole, dronedarone and HIV protease inhibitors
Anticoagulant plus antiplatelet combination[4]	<ul><li>Avoid the combination of antiplatelet and anticoagulant in most patients due to increased bleeding risk</li><li>Consider combining warfarin and aspirin in patients who have had an MI and have had it managed medically, have undergone balloon angioplasty or have undergone coronary artery bypass graft surgery</li><li>Consider combining warfarin with clopidogrel in patients who have had an MI and have undergone percutaneous coronary intervention with bare metal or drug-eluting stents</li><li>After 12 months, review the continued need for antiplatelet therapy</li></ul>
Rate control[1,2]	<ul><li>Offer rate control as the first-line strategy for most patients presenting with AF (see rhythm control section below for exceptions)</li><li>Initial monotherapy should be with a standard beta-blocker (not sotalol) or a rate-limiting calcium-channel blocker (verapamil or diltiazem)</li><li>Only consider digoxin monotherapy in sedentary patients or those presenting with significant pulmonary oedema/acute heart failure symptoms</li></ul>If monotherapy does not control symptoms, and if continuing symptoms are thought to be due to poor ventricular rate control, combine any two of the following:<ul><li>beta-blocker</li><li>rate-limiting calcium-channel blocker (but not verapamil and beta-blocker due to the risk of heart block)</li><li>digoxin</li></ul>Avoid routine use of amiodarone for long-term rate control due to the risk of side effects

A

Rhythm control[1]	Consider rhythm control for patients: with a reversible cause for their AF (e.g. acute infection), heart failure thought to be primarily due to their AF, new-onset AF (less than 48 hours' duration), with atrial flutter suitable for ablation therapy or if a rhythm control strategy is the preferred clinical option.
	Cardioversion may be pharmacological (if AF is present for less than 48 hours) with intravenous flecainide (if no IHD, structural heart disease or CHF) or intravenous amiodarone, or electrical.
	In patients with AF greater than 48 hours' (or uncertain) duration, therapeutic anticoagulation (with warfarin or an NOAC) should be given for at least 3 weeks before cardioversion or TOE-guided cardioversion (to rule out the presence of thrombus). Continuation of anticoagulation postcardioversion depends on overall stroke risk but should be for at least 4 weeks.
	Amiodarone may be used for 4 weeks before elective cardioversion and continued for up to 1 year to increase the success rate.[1]
	Standard beta-blockers are the first-line choice for long-term rhythm control. If beta-blockers are contraindicated or unsuccessful, consider: • flecainide or propafenone if no IHD, structural heart disease or CHF • dronedarone if no left ventricular systolic dysfunction (LVSD) or CHF present • amiodarone if LVSD or CHF is present
Pill in the pocket[1,5]	May be suitable for some patients with a history of paroxysmal AF. The patient does not take regular antiarrhythmic therapy but is given a single dose to use if the AF recurs. Standard agents are flecainide (300 mg for patients over 70 kg, 200 mg if below 70 kg) and propafenone (600 mg for patients above 70 kg, 450 mg if below 70 kg). Consider for patients who have no history of LVSD, valvular disease or IHD and have a history of infrequent paroxysms of AF and are not haemodynamically compromised during an episode of AF.
	Advise the patient to take the drug if AF persists beyond 5 minutes and go to hospital if the AF does not revert within 6–8 hours or if they develop new symptoms such as dyspnoea or presyncope. They should be advised to take no more than one dose in 24 hours. Following an episode they should see their general practitioner for a cardiology referral.
Continued monitoring	• In those with a CHA_2DS_2VASc score of 0, reassess the need for anticoagulation periodically • For those on warfarin, assess level of anticoagulant control • For those on NOACs, check renal function annually • If using amiodarone, warn the patient about photosensitivity and possible effect on night vision. Advise patients to use high-ultraviolet sun blocks. Thyroid function tests should be made before commencing treatment, then every 6 months until off amiodarone for a year • Avoid hypokalaemia if antiarrhythmic drugs are used

REFERENCES

1 NICE (2014) *NICE Clinical Guideline 180. Atrial Fibrillation: The management of Atrial Fibrillation.* http://www.nice.org.uk/guidance/cg180 (accessed 11 November 2014).

2 Camm AJ *et al.* (2012). 2012 focussed update of the ESC Guidelines for the management of atrial fibrillation. *Eur Heart J* 33: 2719–2747.

3 eMC (2014). http://www.medicines.org.uk/emc/ (accessed 11 November 2014).

4 NICE (2013) *NICE Clinical Guideline 172. MI-secondary prevention: Secondary prevention in primary and secondary care for patients following a myocardial infarction.* http://www.nice.org.uk/guidance/cg172 (accessed 11 November 2014).

5 Alboni P *et al.* (2004). Outpatient treatment of recent-onset atrial fibrillation with the 'pill-in-the-pocket' approach. *N Engl J Med* 351: 2384–2391.

B

B

Bariatric surgery

Patients undergoing bariatric surgery are highly complex and require pharmacist input to ensure safety of medicines administration. Pharmacy has an important role to play in the care and management of bariatric patients both pre- and postoperatively in view of anatomical changes that occur as a result of this type of surgery, which can affect the absorption and metabolism of medication. Examples of bariatric surgery include:[1]

- gastric balloon: the placement of a balloon inside the stomach via endoscopy, reducing the overall stomach capacity
- gastric banding: an adjustable band is fitted around the top of the stomach, creating a small pouch, thus reducing the amount of food that may be consumed
- sleeve gastrectomy: the reduction of stomach size by approximately 75%
- Roux-en-Y bypass: a large section of the stomach and duodenum is bypassed. The remaining stomach is attached to the small intestine, creating a small pouch, reducing possible food consumption and fat absorption.

A member of the pharmacy team should complete medicines reconciliation at preoperative assessment; regular medication should be reviewed, taking into consideration any modified anatomy that may result in altered absorption and bioavailability of medication. To aid the healing process and encourage drug absorption, the formulation of medication will require amendment to sugar-free liquid preparations where possible, or crushing tablets/opening capsules for 6–8 weeks postsurgery.

Postsurgery, the patient's stomach pouch capacity is reduced to approximately 50–70 mL, which can cause problems when administering medication in a liquid form, as the patient will feel full. The altered anatomy also results in a change in pharmacokinetic and pharmacodynamic profiles of some medications; the patient will need close monitoring for symptoms of under- and overdosing. The patient should be clinically reviewed postoperatively and counselled prior to discharge, ensuring that the GP is aware of all pharmaceutical issues, both long- and short-term.

Cost implications

Bariatric surgery is a costly intervention; however, weight loss may improve comorbidities such as diabetes or hypertension, resulting in reduced polypharmacy and medication costs. Liquid preparations may need to be sourced from 'specials' manufacturers; this can be expensive, but these are not required long-term, and should be reviewed at the 6–8-week follow-up.

Pharmaceutical care and counselling

Medicines reconciliation	Complete at preassessment clinic to enable appropriate, timely advice and recommendations pre- and postoperatively. Counsel the patient regarding potential changes to regular medications, including information on what additional medications will be prescribed on discharge
Smoking status	If the patient is currently smoking the operation may be cancelled due to increased risks of complications
Medicines adherence	Additional counselling may be required if adherence is an issue, as postoperative supplements must be taken lifelong. Patients using a compliance aid will require extra support as they may struggle with crushing tablets and measuring liquid preparations. Involve families and carers in discussions where possible. A medication reminder chart will be required; consider pictures if necessary
Medication review preassessment clinic	Review regular medications for risk and withhold if appropriate as per local guidelines for surgical procedures. Review for necessity postoperatively and stop where appropriate, e.g. regular laxatives should be stopped as they are contraindicated immediately postoperatively in this group of patients
Liquid preparations	Where possible, liquids should be sugar-free to avoid dumping syndrome (a group of symptoms that occur when food is emptied too quickly from the stomach). Liquids containing fructose, glucose and sucrose are not classed as sugar-free; those containing mannitol, sorbitol and hydrogenated glucose syrup are sugar-free.[2] Consider total volume of any liquids required due to pouch capacity restrictions; administration times may need to be distributed throughout the day to reduce volume. On converting to liquid preparations, consider bioavailability differences between formulations that may require dosage adjustment. 'Specials' may need to be sourced if tablets/capsules cannot be crushed/opened; consider how future supplies may need to be obtained by the patient and whether the community pharmacist needs informing of supplier/formulation details
Crushed tablets/opened capsules	Prescribers should be aware that this is an unlicensed use. Use appropriate reference sources or contact manufacturer for advice. Consider any issues associated with medication once in powder form, such as stability of the drug and third-party contact

Modified-release preparations	Unsuitable postoperatively, due to altered gastrointestinal (GI) tract anatomy. Convert to immediate-release preparations or consider alternatives. Consultant may need to be involved in this process due to disease instability; for example, respiratory, psychiatry and gastroenterology
Chronic pain relief	Patients should see their GP for alternatives to modified-release preparations before the surgery date to ensure adequate pain control; options include converting morphine sulfate modified-release to an immediate-release preparation or fentanyl patches.
	Non-steroidal anti-inflammatory drugs are contraindicated in this group of patients due to site of absorption and increased risk of bleeding and ulceration.
	Consider involvement of specialist pain team for postoperative acute pain management
Soluble/effervescent medicines	Avoid due to the high salt content of soluble tablets and risk of stomach bloating with effervescent tablets
Management of diabetes	Specialist diabetes team must be involved postoperatively as dosing requirements will alter dramatically with changes to diet and the frequency of food intake. Blood glucose concentrations must be regularly monitored. • Type I: require close monitoring and adjustment of insulin once sliding scale has discontinued • Type II: diabetes medication should be stopped postoperatively; this may be represcribed at appropriately reviewed doses dependent on blood glucose concentration. Dipeptidyl peptidase-4 inhibitors and glucagon-like peptide-1 agonists should be used with caution due to satiety
Venous thromboembolism prophylaxis	As per local policy for venous thromboembolism prophylaxis. Consider duration of 7–10 days postoperatively due to increased risk factors
Gastroprotection	Prescribe an oro-dispersible proton pump inhibitor for 3 months (6 months for balloon patients, i.e. for the duration of the balloon's placement)
Supplements	Due to malabsorption, these patients will inevitably develop deficiencies in vitamins and minerals, such as calcium, vitamin D, vitamin B_{12} and iron. Lifelong supplementation is therefore recommended and should be given to all patients
Antiemetics	Gastric balloon patients require antiemetics – possibly a combination of two for the first few days postinsertion

REFERENCES

1 Dent M *et al.* (2010). *Bariatric Surgery for Obesity*. Oxford: National Obesity Observatory.
2 NICE (2013). *NICE Guideline PH47. Managing overweight and obesity among children and young people: lifestyle and weight management services*. http://www.nice.org.uk/guidance/ph47 (accessed 20 August 2014).

Benzodiazepines and 'z' hypnotics

Benzodiazepines are generally divided by half-life: short-half-life agents are anxiolytics, e.g. lorazepam, and longer half-life agents are hypnotics, e.g. temazepam. They and 'z' hypnotics (zaleplon, zolpidem and zopiclone) are usually effective, safe and well tolerated; however, long-term use can lead to dependence and withdrawal, especially with shorter-half-life agents.

Considerations

Classification under the Misuse of Drugs Act 1971 will dictate storage and documentation.[1] Legislation pertaining to driving whilst using these agents needs to be considered.[2]

They should only be used on a short-term (and ideally intermittent) basis, where function is significantly compromised despite identification and mitigation of any physical or psychological contributing factors.[3] Non-pharmacological measures (e.g. sleep hygiene[4] or cognitive behavioural therapy-type psychological education) should always be used concomitantly.[3,5]

There is little to differentiate between short-acting benzodiazepines and the 'z' hypnotics, so the lowest acquisition cost should drive choice.[6] Shorter-acting agents may be better for people who have difficulty initiating sleep and longer-acting agents for people who have difficulty staying asleep.[5] Switching between hypnotics should not occur due to lack of efficacy, but may occur if an agent-specific adverse effect occurs.

Withdrawal

Benzodiazepine withdrawal symptoms are unpleasant and potentially dangerous. They can start within a few hours, or be delayed for a few weeks, after benzodiazepine cessation. They may manifest as stiffness, weakness, gastrointestinal disturbances, insomnia, anxiety, depression, appetite loss, tremor, perspiration, tinnitus, confusion, psychosis, convulsions or a condition resembling delirium tremens.[1,5]

A withdrawal regimen from benzodiazepines usually consists of switching to an equivalent dose of diazepam, and then decreasing the total daily dose by roughly one-eighth every fortnight.[1]

Diazepam is the drug of choice due to its relatively long half-life (it can be given once daily if tolerated) and range of available forms and strengths.[5,6] The withdrawal regimen is normally negotiated and agreed in advance; the rate of withdrawal and dose decrease increments are determined by clinical presentation and the person's ability to cope with the withdrawal symptoms, or anticipation of those symptoms.

Concomitant psychological interventions (e.g. relaxation or cognitive behavioural therapy) increase the likelihood of successful withdrawal.[5,6] Withdrawal is less likely to succeed if previous attempts have failed, there is a lack of social support, there is a history of substance use, in the older adult, if there has been previous severe

B

TABLE B1

Oral benzodiazepine dose equivalents

Approximate equivalent oral dose to 5 mg oral diazepam[1,5,7,8]	
Benzodiazepine	Equivalent oral dose
Alprazolam	0.5 mg (range 0.25–0.5 mg)
Chlordiazepoxide	15 mg (range 10–25 mg)
Clobazam	10 mg
Clonazepam	0.5–1 mg (range 0.25–4 mg)
Loprazolam	0.5–1 mg
Lorazepam	0.5–1 mg
Lormetazepam	0.5–1 mg
Nitrazepam	5 mg (range 2.5–20 mg)
Oxazepam	15 mg (range 10–40 mg)
Temazepam	10 mg
Zaleplon	10 mg
Zolpidem	10 mg
Zopiclone	7.5 mg

withdrawal (including seizures), a concomitant severe physical or mental illness or previous higher-dose/longer-term use.[5,6]

Equivalent doses

Equivalent doses are approximate. Calculations may be complicated by the half-lives of the different agents and their sedative potential. Calculated doses should always be checked against the SPC so unlicensed doses are not inadvertently used.

REFERENCES

1 Joint Formulary Committee (2014). *British National Formulary* (68th edn). London: BMJ Group and Pharmaceutical Press.

2 *Guidance for Health Professionals on Drug Driving*. https://www.gov.uk/government/ uploads/system/uploads/attachment_data/file/325275/healthcare-profs-drug -driving.pdf (accessed on 17 August 2014).

3 NICE (2011). *Clinical Guidance 113. Generalised anxiety disorder and panic disorder (with or without agoraphobia) in adults*. http://www.nice.org.uk/guidance/cg113 (accessed 17 August 2014).

4 NHS Choices (2013). *Treating Insomnia*. http://www.nhs.uk/Conditions/Insomnia/ Pages/Treatment.aspx (accessed 17 August 2014).

5 Taylor D *et al.* (2012). *The Maudsley Prescribing Guidelines in Psychiatry*, 11th edn. Chichester: Wiley-Blackwell.

6 NICE (2004). *Technology Appraisal 77. Guidance on the use of zaleplon, zolpidem and zopiclone for the short-term management of insomnia*. http://www.nice.org.uk/guidance/ta77 (accessed 17 August 2014).

7 Bazire S (2014). *Psychotropic Drug Directory 2014: The professionals' pocket hand-book and aide memoire*. Dorsington: Lloyd-Reinhold.

8 Ashton C (2002). *Benzodiazepines: How they work and how to withdraw (aka The Ashton Manual)*. http://www.benzo.org.uk/manual/index.htm (accessed 17 August 2014).

Bicarbonate

Normal range for serum bicarbonate: 20–30 mmol/L

B

Local range . . . .

Sodium bicarbonate is a buffer which breaks down to water and carbon dioxide after combining with hydrogen ions. It is reabsorbed in the kidneys following glomerular filtration and this action is balanced by the excretion of hydrogen ions to maintain the systemic pH. A blood pH <7.35 is classified as acidosis and a blood pH >7.45 is classified as alkalosis. In acidosis there is an increase in hydrogen ions or a reduction in bicarbonate ions in circulation, and in alkalosis there is an increase in bicarbonate ions or a decrease in hydrogen ions in circulation.[1]

In metabolic disorders the primary abnormality is a change in the serum bicarbonate concentration.[2]

Causes of metabolic acidosis include:

- increased acid production, which occurs in lactic acidosis or diabetic ketoacidosis (DKA), and also in salicylic intoxication, methanol and ethylene glycol ingestion
- decreased acid excretion, which occurs in renal failure and distal renal tubular acidosis (type 1)
- loss of bicarbonate from the GI tract through severe diarrhoea or fistula or by renal loss (proximal renal tubular acidosis type 2).

Causes of metabolic alkalosis include:

- loss of hydrogen ions – either from the GI tract or by renal losses
- excessive alkali administration – occurs during ingestion of large amounts of alkali, e.g. milk alkali syndrome, or when large amounts of bicarbonate are given.[2]

In most cases of metabolic alkalosis or acidosis, the lungs compensate for the change in serum bicarbonate by increasing or decreasing respiratory drive to change the blood carbon dioxide concentration. Potassium is moved out of cells in an attempt to buffer the acidosis and so hyperkalaemia may occur.[1]

Treatment depends on the severity, underlying cause and speed of response to interventions.

Oral sodium bicarbonate[3]

Sodium bicarbonate is used orally in patients with chronic acidotic states such as uraemic acidosis or renal tubular acidosis. For the correction of metabolic acidosis, a starting dose of 500 mg to 1 g three times daily may be given, but doses of 4.8 g daily or more may be required based on the patient's response. Patients on long-term prescribed therapy are usually under the care of a specialist.

Oral sodium bicarbonate may be used to alkalinise the urine for the relief of discomfort in mild urinary-tract infections. The initial dose is 3 g in water every 2 hours until urinary pH exceeds 7; for the maintenance of alkaline urine, 5–10 g daily is sufficient.

Sodium bicarbonate alone is not routinely recommended for the treatment of dyspepsia but is still found in many antacid preparations. As such, many patients may self-medicate with considerable quantities and this should be borne in mind when taking a medication history. Common side effects include belching and there is a risk of alkalosis with prolonged use.[3]

Intravenous sodium bicarbonate

In mild metabolic acidosis associated with volume depletion the patient should be managed with appropriate fluid replacement. This normally allows the acidosis to resolve as tissue and renal perfusion is restored.

In severe metabolic acidosis (pH <7.1) or when the acidosis remains unresponsive to correction of anoxia or hypovolaemia, sodium bicarbonate 1.26% or 1.4% can be infused over 3–4 hours with plasma pH and electrolyte monitoring.[4] Because they are markedly hypertonic, concentrations exceeding 1.4% should always be given via a central line except in emergency situations.

Sodium bicarbonate 1.26% may be used as a hydration fluid when it is undesirable to give chloride, for example, in hyperchloraemic acidosis, but be aware that it is incompatible with calcium- or magnesium-containing solutions, e.g. Hartmann's or Ringer's.[4]

Sodium bicarbonate may also be used to induce forced alkaline diuresis.

Excess bicarbonate may result in metabolic alkalosis, hypokalaemia and hypocalcaemia.

Sodium bicarbonate and DKA

Sodium bicarbonate is not routinely recommended to treat acidosis in DKA as adequate fluid and insulin therapy will resolve the acidosis. Administration of excessive bicarbonate may lead to a paradoxical increase in CSF acidosis and delay the fall in blood lactate. There is also some evidence that bicarbonate treatment may be implicated in the development of cerebral oedema in children and young adults.[5]

Sodium bicarbonate in cardiac arrest

For acidosis in cardiac arrest, the best treatment is a combination of effective chest compression and ventilation. The routine use of sodium bicarbonate in cardiac arrest, cardiopulmonary resuscitation or after return of spontaneous circulation is not recommended. 50 mmol of sodium bicarbonate (50 mL of 8.4% solution) may be given if the cardiac arrest is associated with hyperkalaemia or tricyclic antidepressant overdose. The dose may be repeated according to the clinical condition of the patient and the results of repeated blood gas analysis.[6]

TABLE B2

Bicarbonate content of various preparations[1]

Product	Strength (%)	Strength (mmol/L)	Millimoles contained in this presentation
Sodium bicarbonate capsules 500 mg			≈6 mmol/capsule
Sodium bicarbonate tablets 600 mg			≈7 mmol/tablet
Sodium bicarbonate infusion bag (500 mL)	1.26%	150 mmol/L	75 mmol
Sodium bicarbonate infusion bag (1000 mL)	1.26%	150 mmol/L	150 mmol
Sodium bicarbonate Minijet 4.2% 10 mL	4.2%	500 mmol/L	5 mmol
Sodium bicarbonate Minijet 8.4% 10 mL	8.4%	1000 mmol/L	10 mmol
Sodium bicarbonate Minijet 8.4% 50 mL	8.4%	1000 mmol/L	50 mmol
Sodium bicarbonate Polyfusor 1.26% 500 mL	1.26%	150 mmol/L	75 mmol
Sodium bicarbonate Polyfusor 4.2% 500 mL	4.2%	500 mmol/L	250 mmol
Sodium bicarbonate Polyfusor 8.4% 200 mL	8.4%	1000 mmol/L	200 mmol

Urine alkalinisation and methotrexate therapy

See separate entry on *Methotrexate: calcium folinate rescue regimen*.

REFERENCES

1 Doughtery J, Lamb J (eds) (2009). *Intravenous Therapy in Nursing Practice*, 2nd edn. Oxford: Wiley-Blackwell.
2 Swaminathan R (2011). *Handbook of Clinical Biochemistry*. New Jersey: World Scientific.
3 Joint Formulary Committee (2014). *British National Formulary* (68th edn). London: BMJ Group and Pharmaceutical Press.
4 Gray A, Wright J, Goodey V, Bruce L (eds) (2011). *Injectable Drugs Guide*. London: Pharmaceutical Press.
5 Joint British Diabetic Society Inpatient Care Group (2013). *The Management of Diabetic Ketoacidosis in Adults*, 2nd edn. http://www.diabetes.org.uk/Documents/About%20Us/What%20we%20say/Management-of-DKA-241013.pdf (accessed 14 November 2014).
6 Resuscitation Council UK (2010) *Resuscitation Guidelines*. http://www.resus.org.uk/pages/gl2010.pdf (accessed 14 November 2014).

Body surface area calculation

Body surface area (BSA) is employed in some circumstances as a basis for calculation of drug doses on the premise that drug handling (renal/liver function) can be related to BSA.[1] The evidence for this relationship is based on old research methods[2] and more recent work throws doubt on this.[3]

B

TABLE B3

Body surface area based on the Mosteller formula

Height (cm)	Body surface area																				
200	0.53	0.75	0.91	1.05	1.18	1.29	1.39	1.49	1.58	1.67	1.75	1.83	1.90	1.97	2.04	2.11	2.17	2.24	2.30	2.36	2.42
195	0.52	0.74	0.90	1.04	1.16	1.27	1.38	1.47	1.56	1.65	1.73	1.80	1.88	1.95	2.02	2.08	2.15	2.21	2.27	2.33	2.38
190	0.51	0.73	0.89	1.03	1.15	1.26	1.36	1.45	1.54	1.62	1.70	1.78	1.85	1.92	1.99	2.05	2.12	2.18	2.24	2.30	2.35
185	0.51	0.72	0.88	1.01	1.13	1.24	1.34	1.43	1.52	1.60	1.68	1.76	1.83	1.90	1.96	2.03	2.09	2.15	2.21	2.27	2.32
180	0.50	0.71	0.87	1.00	1.12	1.22	1.32	1.41	1.50	1.58	1.66	1.73	1.80	1.87	1.94	2.00	2.06	2.12	2.18	2.24	2.29
175	0.49	0.70	0.85	0.99	1.10	1.21	1.30	1.39	1.48	1.56	1.64	1.71	1.78	1.84	1.91	1.97	2.03	2.09	2.15	2.20	2.26
170	0.49	0.69	0.84	0.97	1.09	1.19	1.29	1.37	1.46	1.54	1.61	1.68	1.75	1.82	1.88	1.94	2.00	2.06	2.12	2.17	2.23
165	0.48	0.68	0.83	0.96	1.07	1.17	1.27	1.35	1.44	1.51	1.59	1.66	1.73	1.79	1.85	1.91	1.97	2.03	2.09	2.14	2.19
160	0.47	0.67	0.82	0.94	1.05	1.15	1.25	1.33	1.41	1.49	1.56	1.63	1.70	1.76	1.83	1.89	1.94	2.00	2.05	2.11	2.16
155	0.46	0.66	0.80	0.93	1.04	1.14	1.23	1.31	1.39	1.47	1.54	1.61	1.67	1.74	1.80	1.86	1.91	1.97	2.02	2.07	2.13
150	0.46	0.65	0.79	0.91	1.02	1.12	1.21	1.29	1.37	1.44	1.51	1.58	1.65	1.71	1.77	1.83	1.88	1.94	1.99	2.04	2.09
145	0.45	0.63	0.78	0.90	1.00	1.10	1.19	1.27	1.35	1.42	1.49	1.55	1.62	1.68	1.74	1.80	1.85	1.90	1.96	2.01	2.06
140	0.44	0.62	0.76	0.88	0.99	1.08	1.17	1.25	1.32	1.39	1.46	1.53	1.59	1.65	1.71	1.76	1.82	1.87	1.92	1.97	2.02
135	0.43	0.61	0.75	0.87	0.97	1.06	1.15	1.22	1.30	1.37	1.44	1.50	1.56	1.62	1.68	1.73	1.79	1.84	1.89	1.94	1.98
130	0.42	0.60	0.74	0.85	0.95	1.04	1.12	1.20	1.27	1.34	1.41	1.47	1.53	1.59	1.65	1.70	1.75	1.80	1.85	1.90	1.95

	5	10	15	20	25	30	35	40	45	50	55	60	65	70	75	80	85	90	95	100	105
125	0.42	0.59	0.72	0.83	0.93	1.02	1.10	1.18	1.25	1.32	1.38	1.44	1.50	1.56	1.61	1.67	1.72	1.77	1.82	1.86	1.91
120	0.41	0.58	0.71	0.82	0.91	1.00	1.08	1.15	1.22	1.29	1.35	1.41	1.47	1.53	1.58	1.63	1.68	1.73	1.78	1.83	1.87
115	0.40	0.57	0.69	0.80	0.89	0.98	1.06	1.13	1.20	1.26	1.33	1.38	1.44	1.50	1.55	1.60	1.65	1.70	1.74	1.79	1.83
110	0.39	0.55	0.68	0.78	0.87	0.96	1.03	1.11	1.17	1.24	1.30	1.35	1.41	1.46	1.51	1.56	1.61	1.66	1.70	1.75	1.79
105	0.38	0.54	0.66	0.76	0.85	0.94	1.01	1.08	1.15	1.21	1.27	1.32	1.38	1.43	1.48	1.53	1.57	1.62	1.66	1.71	1.75
100	0.37	0.53	0.65	0.75	0.83	0.91	0.99	1.05	1.12	1.18	1.24	1.29	1.34	1.39	1.44	1.49	1.54	1.58	1.62	1.67	1.71
95	0.36	0.51	0.63	0.73	0.81	0.89	0.96	1.03	1.09	1.15	1.20	1.26	1.31	1.36	1.41	1.45	1.50	1.54	1.58	1.62	1.66
90	0.35	0.50	0.61	0.71	0.79	0.87	0.94	1.00	1.06	1.12	1.17	1.22	1.27	1.32	1.37	1.41	1.46	1.50	1.54	1.58	1.62
85	0.34	0.49	0.60	0.69	0.77	0.84	0.91	0.97	1.03	1.09	1.14	1.19	1.24	1.29	1.33	1.37	1.42	1.46	1.50	1.54	1.57
80	0.33	0.47	0.58	0.67	0.75	0.82	0.88	0.94	1.00	1.05	1.11	1.15	1.20	1.25	1.29	1.33	1.37	1.42	1.45	1.49	1.53
75	0.32	0.46	0.56	0.65	0.72	0.79	0.85	0.91	0.97	1.02	1.07	1.12	1.16	1.21	1.25	1.29	1.33	1.37	1.41	1.44	1.48
70	0.31	0.44	0.54	0.62	0.70	0.76	0.82	0.88	0.94	0.99	1.03	1.08	1.12	1.17	1.21	1.25	1.29	1.32	1.36	1.39	1.43
65	0.30	0.42	0.52	0.60	0.67	0.74	0.79	0.85	0.90	0.95	1.00	1.04	1.08	1.12	1.16	1.20	1.24	1.27	1.31	1.34	1.38
60	0.29	0.41	0.50	0.58	0.65	0.71	0.76	0.82	0.87	0.91	0.96	1.00	1.04	1.08	1.12	1.15	1.19	1.22	1.26	1.29	1.32
55	0.28	0.39	0.48	0.55	0.62	0.68	0.73	0.78	0.83	0.87	0.92	0.96	1.00	1.03	1.07	1.11	1.14	1.17	1.20	1.24	1.27
50	0.26	0.37	0.46	0.53	0.59	0.65	0.70	0.75	0.79	0.83	0.87	0.91	0.95	0.99	1.02	1.05	1.09	1.12	1.15	1.18	1.21
Weight (kg)	5	10	15	20	25	30	35	40	45	50	55	60	65	70	75	80	85	90	95	100	105

However, many drugs still require dosing based on BSA and several formulae exist. Always use the formula approved in your organisation. Probably the most frequently used is the Dubois formula, although the most accurate is the Mosteller formula, which is based on the Dubois formula (Table B3 provides a range of BSAs for reference, using the Mosteller formula). Below are alternative methods of calculating BSA supported by the identified websites.

The online *British National Formulary* uses a modified Dubois formula:[4]

$$BSA\ (m^2) = 0.007184 \times height\ (cm)^{0.725} \times weight\ (kg)^{0.425}$$

The Mosteller formula is:[5]

$$BSA\ (m^2) = ([height\ (cm) \times weight\ (kg)]/3600)^{1/2}$$

Other formulae include:

The Haycock formula:[6]

$$BSA\ (m^2) = 0.024265 \times height\ (cm)^{0.3964} \times weight\ (kg)^{0.5378}$$

The Gehan and George formula:[7]

$$BSA\ (m^2) = 0.0235 \times height\ (cm)^{0.42246} \times weight\ (kg)^{0.51456}$$

The Boyd formula:[8]

$$BSA(m^2) = 0.0003207 \times height\ (cm)^{0.3}$$
$$\times weight\ (grams)^{(0.7285 - (0.0188 \times log\ (grams)))}$$

REFERENCES

1 Vu TT (2002). Standardisation of body surface area calculations. *J Oncol Pharm Practice* 8: 49–54.
2 Macintosh JF *et al.* (1928). Studies of urea excretion: the influence of body size on urea output. *J Clin Invest* 6: 467.
3 Dooley MJ, Poole SJ (2000). Correlation between body surface area and glomerular filtration rate. *Cancer Chemo Pharmacol* 46: 523–526.
4 Wang Y *et al.* (1992). Predictors of body surface area. *J Clin Anesth* 4: 4–10.
5 Mosteller RD (1987). Simplified calculation of body surface area. *N Engl J Med* 317: 1098 (letter).
6 Haycock GB *et al.* (1978). Geometric method for measuring body surface area: A height weight formula validated in infants, children and adults. *J Pediatr* 93: 62–66.
7 Gehan EA, George SL (1970). Estimation of human body surface area from height and weight. *Cancer Chemother Rep* 54: 225–235.
8 Boyd E (1935). *The Growth of the Surface Area of the Human Body*. Minneapolis: University of Minnesota Press.

Bronchiectasis (non-cystic fibrosis)

B

Overview	
Definition	Bronchiectasis is the irreversible and abnormal dilation of one or more bronchi and/or bronchioles.[1-3] The abnormal pathology impairs normal mucociliary clearance, which sets up a vicious cycle of infection, inflammation and further airway damage. The affected airways can become ulcerated and haemoptysis, occasionally massive, may occur.
	Bronchiectasis occurs in cystic fibrosis (CF) but is often seen in other conditions. Where CF has been excluded, this is referred to as non-CF bronchiectasis.
	The presentation is typically one of chronic production of purulent sputum associated with cough and recurrent chest infections.
	As for CF, the usual order of infections is:
	• *Staphylococcus aureus* (including methicillin-resistant *Staphylococcus aureus*)
	• *Haemophilus influenzae*
	• *Moraxella catarrhalis*
	• *Pseudomonas* species
	Colonisation with *Pseudomonas* spp. is associated with accelerated decline in lung function and a worsening prognosis
Risk factors	• Recurrent respiratory infection • Childhood
Diagnostic tests	The diagnosis is made on clinical grounds with a high-resolution computed tomography (HRCT) of the lungs for confirmation (and to rule out malignancy in patients with haemoptysis).
	A number of disease processes may result in bronchiectasis and identifying the underlying aetiology may significantly alter the approach to management.
	• Bronchiectasis is hard to identify on a chest X-ray unless it is severe and an HRCT is generally required to confirm the diagnosis
	• CF should be ruled out. The BTS recommends screening sweat chloride and for genetic mutations in the CF transmembrane regular (CFTR) gene in all patients ≤40 years and in those older than this without an identifiable cause[1]
	• Congenital abnormalities of ciliary function (such as primary ciliary dyskinesia/Kartagener's syndrome) may be the underlying cause. This is often associated with recurrent upper respiratory tract infections and otitis media. Ciliary function can be assessed using the saccharin test (time taken for a sample of saccharin placed in the nose to be tasted) or exhaled nitric oxide test
	• Sputum samples should be sent to identify infectious organisms, including atypical organisms, *Mycobacteria* spp. (including non-tuberculous mycobacteria – NTM) and *Aspergillus* spp.
	• *Aspergillus* – specific IgE and IgG immunology screen for allergic bronchopulmonary aspergillosis (ABPA) as an underlying cause

B

- Antibody deficiency should be considered, and IgG, IgA and IgM
- Immunodeficiency secondary to HIV, haematological malignancy or nephrotic syndrome should be considered
- Pharmacological immunosuppression is a recognised cause of bronchiectasis, with mycophenolate and other agents increasingly recognised as a cause of bronchiectasis
- Airway damage due to gastro-oesophageal reflux and aspiration may have a role and should be considered in those with a history of reflux symptoms

Treatment goals	• Identify and manage underlying cause • Prevent and manage infections
Treatment options	• Patient should be taught airway clearance techniques (by respiratory physiotherapist) to mobilise and clear secretions • Regular vaccination against: influenza, pneumococcus and *H. influenzae*

Pharmaceutical care and counselling

Assess	• Are immunosuppressive treatments contributing to the development of the condition and if so, can an alternative regimen be considered?
Mucolytics	• The role of mucolytics to facilitate expectoration of secretions is unclear. Nebulised hypertonic NaCl (6% or 7%) and carbocisteine are commonly used in conjunction with regular airway clearance. Regular nebulised dornase alpha has been shown to be harmful in non-CF bronchiectasis (in contrast to that associated with CF) and should not routinely be used[4]
ABPA	• All patients with bronchiectasis should be assessed for evidence of ABPA using an appropriate immunological test, such as *Aspergillus*-specific IgE and IgG assay • ABPA is associated with an excessive immune response and can by managed with corticosteroids ± antifungals (itraconazole, voriconazole or posaconazole under specialist advice)
Primary immune deficiency	• Primary immunodeficiency should be managed in conjunction with an immunologist and patients may benefit from regular infusions of immunoglobulins • Patients with immunodeficiencies who receive vaccination against influenza, pneumococcus and *H. influenzae* should have their antibody response checked 21 days after vaccination
NTM	• Treatment as per BTS guidelines, generally involving a combination of active antibiotics[1]
Exacerbations	• Prompt identification and management of infections, typically with a minimum of 14 days' treatment, are recommended. Choice of antibiotic should be based on known or suspected organism, local resistance patterns and patient-specific factors, such as: allergy status, potential for interactions with current medications and renal/hepatic function • Patients having ≥3 exacerbations per year may benefit from antimicrobial prophylaxis. Azithromycin 250 mg daily or 500 mg three times weekly and twice-daily erythromycin have been evaluated in clinical trials (BAT[5], BLESS[6] and EMBRACE[7])

	• If considering long-term antibacterial prophylaxis, it is important to exclude NTM infection as use of a single-agent macrolide may result in resistance in the organism and further complicate subsequent treatment
	• Consider periodically checking QTc interval, audiometry and hepatic function in patients on long-term azithromycin
Pseudomonal infection	• In patients who have *Pseudomonas aeruginosa* isolated for the first time, an attempt at eradication should be considered. The BTS recommends an initial 2-week course of ciprofloxacin 750 mg twice daily and, if unsuccessful either: (i) 2 weeks of intravenous antipseudomonal antibiotics or (ii) 4 weeks of ciprofloxacin 750 mg twice daily + 3 months' nebulised colistimethate 2 mega units twice daily or (iii) 3 months' nebulised colistimethate 2 mega units twice daily • Where eradication of *P. aeruginosa* cannot be achieved, nebulised antipseudomonal antibiotics may be considered as prophylaxis – typically colistimethate, tobramycin or gentamicin • For patients experiencing an exacerbation due to *P. aeruginosa*, a 14-day course of intravenous antipseudomonal antibiotic is generally required. This often requires hospital admission, although Outpatient Parenteral Antibiotic Therapy (OPAT) services, if available and appropriate, may allow treatment outside of the hospital setting
Nebulised antibiotics	• A range of antibiotics may be administered for the treatment of infections in non-CF bronchiectasis. Nebulised antibiotics may cause bronchospasm and patients should have a supervised test dose with pre- and postdose spirometry

REFERENCES

1 Pasteur MC *et al.* (2010). British Thoracic Society guideline for non-CF bronchiectasis. *Thorax* 65(Suppl 1): i1–58.

2 McShane PJ *et al.* (2013). Non-cystic fibrosis bronchiectasis. *Am J Respir Crit Care Med* 188: 647–656.

3 Barker AF (2002). Bronchiectasis. *N Engl J Med* 346: 1383–1983.

4 O'Donnell AE *et al.* (1998). Treatment of idiopathic bronchiectasis with aerosolized recombinant DNAse I. *Chest* 113: 1329–1334.

5 Altenburg J *et al.* (2013). Effect of azithromycin maintenance treatment on infectious exacerbation among patients with non-cystic fibrosis bronchiectasis: the BAT randomised controlled trial. *JAMA* 309: 1251–1259.

6 Serisier DJ *et al.* (2013). Effect of long-term, low-dose erythromycin on pulmonary exacerbations among patients with non-cystic fibrosis bronchiectasis: the BLESS randomised controlled trial. *JAMA* 309: 1260–1267.

7 Wong C *et al.* (2012). Azithromycin for prevention of exacerbation in non-cystic fibrosis bronchiectasis (EMBRACE): a randomised, double-blind, placebo-controlled trial. *Lancet* 380: 660–667.

C

Calcium

Overview	
Normal range	Normal range ('corrected', if appropriate): 2.1–2.6mmol/L[1]
Local range	
Background	• Calcium is the most abundant mineral in the body. It is required for bone and tooth formation, and as an essential electrolyte
Reference nutrient intake[1]	17.5 mmol/day (700 mg)
Corrected calcium	Approximately 40–50% of calcium present in serum is bound to plasma proteins, particularly albumin. Since only free calcium ions are active, the total calcium measured in the serum is adjusted to account for the bound ions. This is called the corrected calcium. Commonly used formulae to calculate corrected calcium, in mmol/L, are: • If albumin is <40 g/L, Corrected calcium = serum calcium level $+ ((40 - \text{serum albumin level}) \times 0.02)$ • If albumin concentration is 40–45 g/L, no adjustment is necessary • If albumin is >45 g/L, Corrected calcium = serum calcium level $- ((\text{serum albumin level} - 45) \times 0.02)$

Hypercalcaemia	
Symptoms	• Symptoms include thirst, polyuria, anorexia, constipation, muscle weakness, fatigue and confusion. In severe cases there may be nausea and vomiting and, rarely, cardiac arrhythmias. Extreme hypercalcaemia may result in coma and death. Chronic hypercalcaemia can lead to interstitial nephritis and calcium renal calculi
Causes	• Primary hyperparathyroidism • Malignant disease • Less commonly: granulomatous diseases, e.g. sarcoidosis, familial benign hypercalcaemia and renal failure • Drug causes include vitamin D intoxication (N.B. the duration of action of ergocalciferol injection is about 2 months), calcium supplements (+/− vitamin D) and thiazide diuretics (by reducing urinary excretion of calcium). Check use of OTC osteoporosis supplements and antacids as a cause of milk-alkali syndrome

Treatment	• Mild hypercalcaemia is best corrected by increasing oral fluid intake, and then identifying and treating any underlying aetiology
	• Remember to stop implicated drugs
	• If hypercalcaemia is severe, the first step is to rehydrate the patient with NaCl 0.9% (avoid calcium-containing fluids) to maintain intravascular volume and promote calcium diuresis. N.B. Normal adult fluid requirements are generally about 40 mL/kg/24 hours
	• Furosemide may be used to increase urinary calcium excretion at doses of 80–100 mg intravenously. Give every 1–2 hours as required, taking care to maintain fluid balance
	• Bisphosphonates are usually an effective treatment for tumour-induced hypercalcaemia. A significant fall in serum Ca is generally seen within 24–48 hours of initial IV administration; the full effect may not be seen for 3–7 days so be guided by the individual product SPC and avoid dosing again too early[2]
	• As an adjunct to the treatment of hypercalcaemia, calcitonins can have a rapid effect, particularly in patients with an increased bone turnover.[1] If other measures fail, calcitonin (salmon) is licensed for the treatment of hypercalcaemia of malignancy given at an initial dose of 100 units every 6–8 hours by SC or IM injection, but nausea and vomiting can be problematic. If tolerated, the dose may be gradually increased after 1–2 days to a maximum dose of 400 units every 6–8 hours if necessary[3]
	• In the emergency treatment of hypercalcaemia, calcitonin (salmon) has also been used intravenously at a dose of up to 10 units/kg diluted in 500 mL of sodium chloride 0.9% and given by slow IV infusion over at least 6 hours[3]

Hypocalcaemia

Symptoms	• Increased neuromuscular excitability, e.g. paraesthesias, carpopedal spasm, muscle cramps, tetany and convulsions; ECG changes; and mental disturbances, e.g. irritability and depression
Causes	• Impaired or reduced absorption from the gastrointestinal tract, e.g. in vitamin D-deficiency disorders
	• Chronic renal failure
	• Deficient parathyroid hormone secretion
	• Post thyroid or parathyroid surgery
	• Excessive phosphate administration
Assessment	• Measure: urea U, Cr, CrCl (or eGFR), serum Ca, serum Mg
	• ECG
	• IV calcium should generally be avoided in patients receiving cardiac glycosides because of the risk of the development of potentially life-threatening digitalis-induced arrhythmias[4]
	• Do not use IV for hypocalcaemia caused by renal impairment
	• Do not use in conditions associated with hypercalcaemia and hypercalciuria (e.g. some forms of malignant disease) and in severe renal impairment
	• Use with caution in patients with mild-to-moderate renal impairment, cardiac disease, sarcoidosis, respiratory acidosis or respiratory failure
Treatment	• Any underlying disease should be identified and managed. Oral calcium supplements are commonly used
	• Vitamin D-deficiency disorders and hypoparathyroidism are corrected with vitamin D supplements, sometimes in combination with calcium salts

Parenteral treatment[1]	Calcium salts are irritant and may cause tissue necrosis and sloughing if given via the IM or SC route. Calcium chloride is more irritant than calcium gluconate when given IV, although both may cause irritation and should be given with care to avoid extravasation.
	Acute hypocalcaemia: 2.25 mmol (calcium gluconate 10% injection 10 mL) by slow IV injection over a minimum of 3 minutes.
	In tetany this should be followed by 9 mmol (calcium gluconate 10% injection 40 mL) in 500 mL sodium chloride 0.9% or glucose 5% by IV infusion daily over 8–24 hours with frequent monitoring of serum Ca and Mg. Smaller volumes may be used in fluid restriction.
	An alternative regimen is to give 22.5 mmol Ca (calcium gluconate 10% injection 100 mL) in 1 litre of sodium chloride 0.9% or glucose 5% solution by IV infusion at an initial rate of 50 mL/hour. Adjust the rate of infusion according to 4–6-hourly serum Ca and Mg measurements
Oral supplements	Calcium supplements should be taken 3–4 hours after the following drugs to avoid reduced gastrointestinal absorption:[5] • levothyroxine • bisphosphonates • iron supplements • sodium fluoride • quinolones and tetracyclines (apart from doxycycline) Calcium supplements should not be given within 1 hour of enteric-coated preparations. Calcium supplements are usually only required where dietary calcium intake is deficient.[5] Dietary requirement varies with age and is relatively greater in childhood, pregnancy and lactation, due to an increased demand, and in old age, due to impaired absorption. In osteoporosis, a calcium intake of approximately 1400 mg (which is double the recommended daily amount) is given in combination with vitamin D, which reduces the rate of bone loss. Flavour, dose volume and texture are important factors in patient acceptance and adherence with therapy

TABLE C1

Calcium content of various oral preparations

Product	Calcium content[5]
Calcium gluconate tablets	53.4 mg (1.35 mmol)
Calcium gluconate effervescent tablets	89 mg (2.25 mmol)
Calcium lactate tablets	39 mg (1 mmol)
Adcal tablets	600 mg (15 mmol)
Cacit tablets	500 mg (12.6 mmol)
Calcichew tablets	500 mg (12.6 mmol)
Calcichew Forte tablets	1 g (25 mmol)
Calcium-500 tablets	500 mg (12.6 mmol)
Calcium Sandoz syrup	108.3 mg/5 mL (2.7 mmol/5 mL)
Sandocal-1000 tablets	1 g (25 mmol)

TABLE C2
Calcium content of various parenteral preparations

Product	Calcium content[A]
Calcium gluconate 10% injection	8.9 mg/mL (225 micromol/mL)
Calcium chloride 10% injection	27.3 mg/mL (680 micromol/mL)
Calcium chloride 13.4% injection	36 mg/mL (910 micromol/mL)

TABLE C3
Calcium content of various oral calcium and vitamin D preparations

Product	Calcium content[A]
Calcium and ergocalciferol tablets	97 mg (2.4 mmol) + 400 IU ergocalciferol
Accrete D$_3$ tablets	600 mg (15 mmol) + 400 IU ergocalciferol
Adcal D$_3$ tablets	600 mg (15 mmol) + 400 IU colecalciferol
Adcal D$_3$ effervescent tablets	600 mg (15 mmol) + 400 IU colecalciferol
Adcal D$_3$ caplets	300 mg (7.5 mmol) + 200 IU colecalciferol
Cacit D$_3$ granules	500 mg (12.5 mmol) + 440 IU colecalciferol
Calceos tablets	500 mg (12.5 mmol) + 400 IU colecalciferol
Calcichew D$_3$ tablets	500 mg (12.5 mmol) + 200 IU colecalciferol
Calcichew D$_3$ Forte tablets	500 mg (12.5 mmol) + 400 IU colecalciferol
Calcichew D$_3$ 500/400 caplets	500 mg (12.5 mmol) + 400 IU colecalciferol
Calfovit D$_3$ powder	1.2 g (30 mmol)/sachet + 800 IU colecalciferol
Kalcipos-D tablets	500 mg (12.5 mmol) + 800 IU colecalciferol
Natecal D$_3$ tablets	600 mg (15 mmol) + 400 IU colecalciferol

REFERENCES
1 *Martindale: The Complete Drug Reference* (2014). www.medicinescomplete.com (accessed 13 January 2015).
2 Gray A, Wright J, Goodey V, Bruce L (eds) (2011). *Injectable Drugs Guide*. London: Pharmaceutical Press.
3 SPC (2013). *Miacalcic 400 IU/2ml Solution for Injection and Infusion*. www.medicines.org.uk (accessed 5 September 2015).
4 Baxter K (ed.) (2014). *Stockley's Drug Interactions*. London: Pharmaceutical Press. http://www.medicinescomplete.com/ (accessed 3 September 2014).
5 Joint Formulary Committee (2014). *British National Formulary* (68th edn). London: BMJ Group and Pharmaceutical Press.

Carbamazepine

Carbamazepine is licensed for use in the treatment of epilepsy (including generalised tonic-clonic and partial seizures), trigeminal neuralgia and the prophylaxis of bipolar disorders unresponsive to lithium.[1]

Pharmacokinetic overview

Carbamazepine is almost completely absorbed, albeit slowly from the gut, and metabolised in the liver.[2] Carbamazepine induces its own metabolism and the half-life is markedly reduced in the first few weeks

TABLE C4
Drug monitoring information

Half-life[2]	25–45 hours (single dose) 8–24 hours (chronic dosing)
Pretreatment measures	FBC, U&Es, LFTs Individuals of Han Chinese or Thai origin should be screened for the HLA-B*1502 allele before starting carbamazepine treatment because this increases their risk of developing severe Stevens–Johnson syndrome
Therapeutic range	4–12 mg/L (20–50 micromol/L)[1] In bipolar disorders, trough levels >7 mg/L (>29 micromol/L) are associated with a therapeutic response
Sampling time[2]	Blood samples should be taken pre-dose. Samples should not be taken until steady state is achieved, which takes 2–4 weeks after commencing therapy. Further samples can be taken 4 days after any subsequent dose changes. Blood should be taken in 'brown-top' sample tubes
Other monitoring[1]	FBC, U&Es, LFTs every 2 weeks for 2 months, then annually

of therapy. Towards the end of the first month of therapy, plasma concentration falls by about 25% and the dose may need to be increased to maintain anticonvulsant effect. It should therefore be initiated at a low dose, and gradually increased over 1 month to the optimal dose.

Rationale for monitoring

The serum concentration of carbamazepine should be checked:

- in epilepsy, if seizure control is poor
- when toxicity is suspected
- if non-compliance is suspected
- to monitor the effects of drug interactions
- to help avoid escalating dose to levels above the usual quoted range associated with more risk of toxicity.

Bioequivalence

Different brands of oral preparation may vary in bioavailability. The MHRA guidance[3] classifies carbamazepine as a category 1 antiepileptic drug: doctors are advised to ensure that their patient is maintained on a specific manufacturer's product in order to avoid reduced effect or excessive side effects. This does not apply to indications other than epilepsy.

The bioavailability of the different formulations varies. In the management of epilepsy the modified-release formulation is generally preferred. However, the dose of the controlled-release formulation needs to be slightly higher to achieve the same effect. One suggested rough guide when moving from one to another is that approximately 100 mg of standard-release carbamazepine is equivalent to about 120–125 mg of the controlled-release preparation. The bioavailability of the rectal formulation is also lower than the standard-release oral preparations (Table C5).[4]

TABLE C5
Carbamazepine dose form bioequivalence

Tablet	Liquid	Suppository
100 mg	100 mg	125 mg

Toxicity

Signs and symptoms of toxicity include ataxia, blurred vision, nausea and vomiting, respiratory depression, dizziness, hypotension or hypertension, cardiac rhythm disturbances, convulsions and hyponatraemia.

Treatment of overdose

There is no specific antidote, and management is guided by the patient's individual condition. Specialist advice should be sought from a poisons information service, e.g. Toxbase.[5]

Interactions with other antiepileptics[6]

Carbamazepine is metabolized by cytochrome P450 3A4, and therefore any drug that inhibits the action of this enzyme can raise the plasma concentration of carbamazepine, and any drug that induces the enzyme can decrease the serum concentration of carbamazepine. Discontinuing any of these drugs may lead to a rebound change in carbamazepine serum concentration.

Antiepileptic drugs that can decrease carbamazepine concentration are: phenytoin, phenobarbitone and primidone. Some reports suggest clonazepam and oxcarbazepine may have the same effect.

Valproic acid may either raise or lower carbamazepine serum concentration.

Phenytoin serum concentration has been reported to have been raised and lowered by concomitant carbamazepine administration.

Carbamazepine may lower the serum concentration of the following antiepileptics: clobazam, clonazepam, eslicarbazepine, ethosuximide, lacosamide, lamotrigine, levetiracetam, oxcarbazepine, perampanel, pregabalin, primidone, retigabine, tiagabine, topiramate, valproic acid and zonisamide.

REFERENCES

1 SPC. *Tegretol Tablets 100 mg, 200 mg, 400 mg*. http://emc.medicines.org.uk/ (accessed 5 August 2015).
2 Hallworth M, Capps N (1993). *Therapeutic Drug Monitoring and Clinical Biochemistry*. London: Association of Clinical Biochemists.
3 MHRA (2013). *Formulation Switching of Antiepileptic Drugs*. http://www.mhra.gov.uk/ (accessed 1 January 2015).
4 Joint Formulary Committee (2014). *British National Formulary* (68th edn). London: BMJ Group and Pharmaceutical Press.
5 National Poisons Information Service. *Toxbase*. http://www.toxbase.org (accessed 4 August 2014).
6 Baxter K, Preston C (eds) (2013). *Stockley's Drug Interactions*, 10th edn. London: Pharmaceutical Press.

Chemotherapy-induced nausea and vomiting

Chemotherapy-induced nausea and vomiting (CINV) is common, with an incidence of up to 70%,[1] and the likelihood is partly dependent on the drugs used in the regimen. These can be classified as high- (>90%), moderate- (30–90%), low- (10–30%) and minimal- (<10%) emetogenic risk.[1]

It is important to note that these are single-agent classifications. When combining drugs in regimens, the overall classification will be guided by the most emetogenic drug included. For lower levels of emetogenic drug, if two from the same class are used, the combination will be assigned the next level of emetogenic potential, e.g. a two-drug regimen with both drugs in 'low' level would be classified as 'moderate'.

CINV may be subdivided into three classifications: acute (within 24 hours), delayed (beyond 24 hours), commonly caused by cisplatin-containing regimens, and anticipatory (days or hours prior to chemotherapy administration).[2]

For patients not treated with prophylactic antiemetics, it is estimated that 60–80% of patients receiving chemotherapy experience CINV.[3] However, the individual risk of developing CINV is affected by both patient-related and treatment-related factors. Patient factors associated with a higher risk of CINV include female gender, age <50 years, lower chronic alcohol intake (teetotallers are at highest risk), no tobacco use, susceptibility to motion sickness and prior episodes of CINV.[4–6]

It is important to exclude other causes of nausea and vomiting when assessing CINV. Other causes include radiotherapy, infection, metabolic/electrolyte disturbances, constipation, gastrointestinal obstruction, cachexic syndrome, metastases, and other emetogenic medication (e.g. opioids, antibiotics).[7]

Table C6 shows the drug combinations of antiemetics commonly used for CINV. These are given for both the acute and delayed phases of CINV.

TABLE C6

Antiemetics used for chemotherapy-induced nausea and vomiting

High-emetic-risk regimen containing cisplatin	NK1 receptor antagonist plus 5-HT$_3$ receptor antagonist plus corticosteroid plus standard antiemetic (e.g. metoclopramide, prochlorperazine, cyclizine)
High emetic risk	5-HT$_3$ receptor antagonist plus corticosteroid plus standard antiemetic (e.g. metoclopramide, prochlorperazine, cyclizine)
Moderate emetic risk	Corticosteroid plus standard antiemetic
Low emetic risk	Standard antiemetic/none
Minimal emetic risk	No routine prophylaxis

Choice of antiemetic for CINV

Oral, intravenous, subcutaneous and rectal routes should all be considered. The best route for an individual will depend on the presence of vomiting and platelet count. Where vomiting or nausea is present the oral route should be avoided because of poor absorption and exacerbation of the feeling of nausea. Where a low platelet count is present, intravenous, subcutaneous and rectal routes should be avoided in order to reduce bleeding and bruising caused by trauma.

For the anxiety of anticipatory nausea and vomiting, a 1-mg oral dose of lorazepam 1 hour before chemotherapy is usually effective. In more resistant cases lorazepam can be given at a dose of 1–2 mg up to four times a day.[8]

Levomepromazine is commonly used for patients not controlled with combinations of the above. Doses from 6 to 25 mg daily can be used either orally or subcutaneously and the dose may be divided, although a single dose at night is often effective.[9]

REFERENCES

1 Basch E *et al.* (2011). Antiemetics: American Society of Clinical Oncology clinical practice guideline update. *J Clin Oncol* 29: 4189–4198.

2 Berger AM, Clark-Snow RA. Adverse effects of treatment. In: DeVita Jr VT, Helman S, Rosenberg S (eds) *Principles and Practice of Oncology*. Philadelphia: Lippincott Williams and Wilkins, pp. 2869–2880.

3 Jenns K (1994). Importance of nausea. *Cancer Nurs* 17: 488–493.

4 Osoba D *et al.* (1997). Determinants of postchemotherapy nausea and vomiting in patients with cancer. *J Clin Oncol* 15: 116–123.

5 Perez EA (1999). 5-HT3 antiemetic therapy for patients with breast cancer. *Breast Cancer Res Treat* 57: 207–214.

6 Dodd MJ *et al.* (1996). Differences in nausea, vomiting and retching between younger and older out-patients receiving cancer chemotherapy. *Cancer Nurs* 19: 155–161.

7 Bentley A, Boyd K (2001). Use of clinical pictures in the management of nausea and vomiting: a prospective audit. *Palliat Med* 15: 247–253.

8 Malik IA *et al.* (1995). Clinical efficacy of lorazepam in prophylaxis of anticipatory acute and delayed onset nausea and vomiting induced by high doses of cisplatin. A prospective randomised trial. *Am J Clin Oncol* 18: 170–175.

9 Mannix K (2002). Palliation of nausea and vomiting. *Cancer Med* 1: 18–22.

Child–Pugh score

Drugs metabolised or excreted by the liver may accumulate in the body if liver function is impaired. Doses should be adjusted or the drug avoided altogether if necessary. Determining the degree of hepatic impairment is much trickier than with renal function. Several methods exist, but the most commonly used is the Child–Pugh classification, which has been developed as a prognostic tool in chronic liver disease.[1] Many medicines' SPCs use this classification to determine dose adjustments.

For the Child–Pugh classification, five clinical measures of liver disease are given scores of 1, 2 or 3 points in increasing severity, as shown in Table C7. The scores for each parameter are added together

TABLE C7

Scoring system for Child–Pugh classification of hepatic impairment

Measure	Scores 1 point	Scores 2 points	Scores 3 points
Bilirubin, total (micromol/L or mg/dL)	<34* (<2)	34–50* (2–3)	>50 (>3)
Serum albumin (g/L)	>35	28–35	<28
INR or prothrombin time (seconds)	<1.7 1–3	1.7–2.3 4–6	>2.3 >6
Ascites	None	Moderate or suppressed with medication	Refractory
Hepatic encephalopathy	None	Grade I–II (or suppressed with medication)	Grade III–IV (or refractory)

*In primary sclerosing cholangitis and primary biliary cirrhosis, the bilirubin reference ranges are increased to <68 micromol/L (<4 mg/dL) for 1 point and 68–170 micromol/L for 2 points (4–10 mg/dL).

and the degree of hepatic impairment is categorised as Child–Pugh class A–C as follows:

- 5–6 points: class A
- 7–9 points: class B
- 10–15 points: class C.

REFERENCE

1 Pugh RNH *et al.* (1973). Transection of the oesophagus for bleeding oesophageal varices. *Br J Surg* 60: 646–649.

Chloramphenicol (systemic)

Chloramphenicol is a broad-spectrum antibiotic active against many Gram-positive and Gram-negative organisms. It acts by interfering with bacterial protein synthesis. Chloramphenicol is known to cause bone marrow depression. This can occur as a rare but often fatal aplastic anaemia or as a dose-related reversible bone marrow suppression, e.g. agranulocytosis, hypoplastic anaemia and thrombocytopenia. Aplastic anaemia is idiosyncratic, may occur at any dose and onset can occur after cessation of therapy. Only about 20% of cases occur during a treatment course. Consequently its use should be reserved for life-threatening infections, e.g. typhoid, meningitis and other serious infections caused by bacteria-susceptible chloramphenicol.

Pharmacokinetic overview

Chloramphenicol is widely distributed in body tissues and fluids, including cerebrospinal fluid.[1,2] It is predominantly metabolised in the liver and only small amounts are recovered in bile. In the liver it undergoes conjugation with glucuronic acid to inactive metabolites. Consequently, in patients with liver disease, serum levels should be monitored and the dose reduced as appropriate. It is principally

excreted in the urine but only 5–10% appears in the unchanged
active form. Active chloramphenicol does not accumulate in
renal failure and dose modification is not required. Inactive
chloramphenicol metabolites accumulate in renal failure, though they
are not associated with toxicity.[1] The manufacturer recommends
levels should be monitored in renal impairment and doses adjusted
accordingly.

Rationale for monitoring

Chloramphenicol has a narrow therapeutic range; therefore, levels
should be checked in the following circumstances:

- neonates
- children under 4 years of age
- elderly
- hepatic and renal impairment
- if there are drugs added known to affect chloramphenicol serum
  concentration (see section on drug interactions, below).

Once levels are taken, they can be repeated after 5–7 days (Table C8).

TABLE C8
Chloramphenicol monitoring information

Half-life	1.5–4 hours
Pretreatment measures	FBC, U&Es, LFTs prior to commencement
Therapeutic range[3]	Peak: 10–25 mg/L
	Trough: <15 mg/L
	(Toxic effects observed with peak concentrations >25 mg/L and trough concentrations >15 mg/L)
Sampling time	Trough: 0–30 minutes predose
	Peak: 2 hours post oral or intravenous administration
Other monitoring	FBC repeated every 2–3 days. Discontinue treatment if leucopenia, thrombocytopenia or anaemia occurs. U&Es, LFTs repeated after 1–3 days, then at least weekly

Dose

The adult dose for oral and intravenous administration is 12.5 mg/kg
every 6 hours. In exceptional cases, such as septicaemia and
meningitis, the dose may be doubled to 25 mg/kg every 6 hours. The
dose should be reduced as soon as clinically indicated.[3]

To prevent relapses, treatment should be continued after the
patient's temperature has returned to normal for 4 days in rickettsial
diseases, and for 8–10 days in typhoid fever.[3]

Administration

Chloramphenicol may be given orally as capsules, or intravenously.
The intramuscular route is licensed, but not recommended, because
absorption may be slow and unreliable; therefore, intravenous bolus
injection is preferred.[2] The injection is presented as a powder
containing 1.377 g chloramphenicol sodium succinate (equivalent to
1 g chloramphenicol base). It is reconstituted with water for
injections, sodium chloride 0.9% injection or glucose 5% injection.

It should be given at a concentration of 10% (100 mg/mL) or less.[2,4] Add 9.2 mL of diluent to a 1 g vial to make a 100 mg/mL solution. The required dose is withdrawn from the reconstituted vial and can be given as a bolus intravenous injection over at least 1 minute. It can be further diluted with a convenient volume (e.g. 100 mL) of sodium chloride 0.9% or glucose 5% and given as an intravenous infusion over 15–30 minutes.[4]

Overdose

Symptoms

Symptoms of overdose include abdominal distension, lethargy, nausea and vomiting, jaundice, respiratory distress, pale cyanotic skin, hypotension and metabolic acidosis followed by cardiovascular collapse.

In infants these symptoms are referred to as 'grey-baby syndrome'. The occurrence of the syndrome in this group is due to their immature metabolism and inability to conjugate the drug.

Antidote

Seek specialist medical advice. There is no specific antidote to chloramphenicol overdose. Activated charcoal may be considered, though the benefit is uncertain; optimal effects are within 1 hour. Asymptomatic patients should be observed for 6 hours after ingestion. For symptomatic patients, as well as stopping therapy, general supportive therapy is recommended, e.g. haemodynamic support, correction of metabolic acidosis. Haematology advice should be sought for patients where bone marrow toxicity is present.[5]

Drug interactions

Chloramphenicol inhibits several liver enzymes, including CYP2C9 and CYP3A4. It can increase the effects of coumarin anticoagulants, tolbutamide, sulphonylureas and phenytoin; dose reductions of these drugs may be required.[2]

Phenobarbital and rifampicin may reduce plasma concentrations of chloramphenicol. Concurrent use of phenytoin and chloramphenicol may result in toxic chloramphenicol serum concentrations. Dose adjustment may be necessary.

Chloramphenicol may increase the plasma concentration of ciclosporin and tacrolimus and may reduce the antiplatelet effect of clopidogrel. Concomitant use with clozapine should be avoided due to the increased risk of agranulocytosis.[3]

REFERENCES

1 Grayson M *et al.* (eds) (2010). *Kucers' The Use of Antibiotics*, 6th edn. London: Hodder Arnold.

2 eMC (2014). *SPC Kemicetine succinate injection*. http://www.medicines.org.uk/emc (accessed 3 August 2014).

3 Joint Formulary Committee (2014). *British National Formulary* (68th edn). London: BMJ Group and Pharmaceutical Press.

4 Gray A, Wright J, Goodey V, Bruce L (eds) (2011). *Injectable Drugs Guide*. London: Pharmaceutical Press.
5 National Poisons Information Service. *Toxbase*. http://www.toxbase.org (accessed 4 August 2014).

C

Chronic obstructive pulmonary disease

Overview	
Definition	Chronic obstructive pulmonary disease (COPD) is characterised by air flow obstruction that is not fully reversible. The air flow obstruction does not change markedly over several months and is usually progressive in the long term and not fully reversible. The following should be used as a definition of COPD: • Air flow obstruction is defined as a reduced FEV_1/FVC ratio (where FEV_1 is forced expired volume in 1 second and FVC is forced vital capacity), such that FEV_1/FVC is less than 0.7 • If FEV_1 is $\geq$80% of predicted normal, a diagnosis of COPD should only be made in the presence of respiratory symptoms, for example, breathlessness or cough COPD is now the preferred term for the condition in patients with air flow obstruction who were previously diagnosed as having chronic bronchitis or emphysema
Causes	• COPD is predominantly caused by smoking substances (approximately 90% of cases) • Other risk factors include chronic or intense exposure to occupational dusts or chemicals, and exposure to smoke from home cooking and heating fuels • Alpha-1 antitrypsin deficiency is a genetic risk factor for COPD, but it accounts for only about 2% of cases of severe COPD
Classification	COPD is classified according to the extent of air flow obstruction:

Post-bronchodilator FEV_1/FVC	FEV_1% predicted	Severity of air flow obstruction
<0.7	$\geq$80%	Stage 1 – mild[*]
<0.7	50–79%	Stage 2 – moderate
<0.7	30–49%	Stage 3 – severe
<0.7	<30%	Stage 4 – very severe[†]

[*]Symptoms should be present to diagnose COPD in people with mild air flow obstruction.
[†]Or FEV_1 < 50% with respiratory failure.
Although FEV_1 is the most common variable used to grade the severity of COPD, it is a poor guide to a patient's symptoms, quality of life and mortality

Signs and symptoms	At first, COPD may cause no symptoms or only mild symptoms. As the disease progresses, symptoms usually become more severe. Common signs and symptoms of COPD include: • chronic cough (often called 'smoker's cough') • regular sputum production • breathlessness on exertion • wheeze and chest tightness • frequent chest infections Systemic manifestations include: weight loss, impaired systemic muscle function, osteoporosis, depression, pulmonary hypertension and cor pulmonale
Diagnostic tests	There is no single diagnostic test for COPD. Making a diagnosis relies on clinical judgement based on a combination of history, physical examination and confirmation of the presence of air flow obstruction using post-bronchodilator spirometry. A diagnosis of COPD should be considered in patients over the age of 35 years who have a risk factor, are generally current or ex-smokers and who present with one or more of the classic COPD symptoms
Treatment goals	The goals of COPD treatment are to: • relieve symptoms with no or minimal side effects of treatment • slow the progress of the disease • improve the ability to stay active and exercise • prevent and treat any complications from the disease • improve health overall
Treatment options[1]	• Currently, no treatments have been shown to improve lung function or decrease mortality significantly • Stopping smoking is the only intervention that slows the progression of the disease. All COPD patients still smoking, regardless of age, should be encouraged to stop, and offered help to do so, at every opportunity • Pulmonary rehabilitation should be offered to all people disabled by their disease • Pneumococcal vaccination and an annual influenza vaccination should be offered to all patients • Medicines are used to reduce breathlessness, improve exercise tolerance, aid sputum clearance, improve health status, reduce exacerbation frequency and manage acute exacerbations

Medicines optimisation

The medication treatment options here are from NICE guidance:[1]

Short-acting beta-2 agonist (SABA)	• Should always be prescribed 'when required' to reduce breathlessness • The onset of action is slower than in patients with asthma • When patients are very short of breath, combining the inhaler with a spacer device may be helpful • Side effects such as tremor, anxiety, cramps, ↓K (monitor), palpitations are dose-related. There is little clinical benefit in terms of efficacy in giving more than 1 mg salbutamol at a time in patients with COPD. Low but frequent doses are more effective for SABAs

Muscarinic antagonists	• Short-acting muscarinic antagonists (SAMA), e.g. ipratropium, used to reduce intermittent breathlessness • Long-acting muscarinic antagonists (LAMA) should be offered in preference to four-times-daily SAMA to people with stable COPD who remain breathless or have exacerbations despite using short-acting bronchodilators • SAMA and LAMA should not be prescribed together due to an increased risk of adverse effects and no added benefit • Monitor outcomes, such as improvement in symptoms, activities of daily living, exercise capacity and rapidity of symptom relief • If ipratropium is being nebulised, the mask must be fitted carefully or ideally a mouthpiece used to avoid the aerosol coming into contact with the eyes, as this could cause glaucoma
Inhaled corticosteroid (ICS) and long-acting beta-2 agonist (LABA)	• None of the ICS currently available is licensed for use alone in the treatment of COPD • Inflammation present in the airways of stable COPD patients is mediated by neutrophils, which are relatively insensitive to the effects of steroids • Recommend an ICS/LABA combination for patients with $\leq FEV_1$ 50% predicted, who are having two or more exacerbations requiring treatment with antibiotics or oral corticosteroids in a 12-month period • Be aware of the potential risk of developing side effects, including non-fatal pneumonia, osteoporosis or diabetes in people with COPD treated with ICS • Issue a steroid warning card to all patients receiving high-dose ICS (>800 micrograms beclometasone (non-extra-fine)/day or equivalent)
LABA	• Unlike in people with asthma, there is no increased risk of death if used alone without an ICS • Monitor outcomes, such as improvement in symptoms, activities of daily living, exercise capacity and rapidity of symptom relief
Oral corticosteroid	• Short courses (7–14 days) are prescribed to manage a COPD exacerbation • For steroid courses longer than 3 weeks, provide a steroid warning card and taper dose down. There is no standard regimen for a reducing course of oral corticosteroid and it does vary depending on the patient, e.g. length of time of corticosteroid exposure, any previous courses of corticosteroid, previous maintenance treatment – and consultant preference! It is usually fine to drop down to physiological dose and then reduce the last phase slowly, previous caveats notwithstanding. In practice many patients are just reduced by 5 mg every 3 days to zero or their regular maintenance dose • Maintenance use of oral corticosteroid therapy in COPD is not normally recommended and carries considerable risks (i.e. osteoporosis, muscle wasting) • Consider osteroporosis prophylaxis for people on ≥ 7.5 mg prednisolone and/or >4 courses of oral steroids in a year

Methylxanthine (e.g. theophylline, aminophylline)	• Narrow therapeutic window – appropriate dosing and monitoring are essential • To reduce the adverse effects, introduce at low dose and gradually increase according to symptoms and plasma levels • Aim for a steady-state serum theophylline concentration of 10–20 micrograms/mL • Measure drug serum concentration: when treatment starts, if side effects occur, if expected therapeutic benefit is not achieved and if potential drug interactions are suspected. Monitor levels daily if intravenous aminophylline is prescribed (see *Theophylline* entry–act on results) • If intravenous aminophylline is being used to manage acute severe exacerbations, give a loading dose if not currently prescribed an oral theophylline preparation • Side effects occur commonly, such as tachycardia, palpitations, headache, insomnia, nausea and other gastrointestinal disturbances • Consider drug interactions with any prescribed, herbal and OTC medicines • Prescribe oral products by brand name, as bioavailability may vary from one brand to another
Mucolytics	• Monitor effect on sputum clearance and/or cough – stop if no benefit after 4–6 weeks
Antibiotics	• Patients with exacerbations without purulent sputum do not need antibiotic therapy unless there is consolidation on a chest radiograph or clinical signs of pneumonia • Initial empirical treatment should be an aminopenicillin, a macrolide or a tetracycline according to your local antimicrobial formulary
Oxygen	• Patients should receive a formal oxygen assessment before being prescribed home long-term oxygen therapy • Inappropriate oxygen therapy in people with COPD may cause respiratory depression • Oxygen is classed as a drug and should be prescribed • Patients should be warned about the risks of fire and explosion if they continue to smoke when prescribed oxygen
Drug administration	• Give specific training and assessment in inhaler technique before starting any new inhaler treatment • *Ask patients to show you how they use their inhalers; it is not sufficient just to ask them if they know how to use them* • Make sure the patient's spacer device is compatible with the inhaler device and that patients know how to use the spacer • The use of nebulisers in the day-to-day management of COPD is rarely appropriate. Confirm that a nebuliser is required and available
Essential interventions	• Strongly advise patients not to smoke and consider nicotine replacement therapy • Ensure patient is offered an annual vaccination against influenza and a one-off vaccination against pneumococcal disease • People should be encouraged to seek help early in an exacerbation and not wait until they are experiencing severe difficulty • Provide patients with a self-management plan • Refer patients to a pulmonary rehabilitation course if disabled by breathlessness

Secondary intervention	• Patients with COPD may suffer from anxiety and depression
	• Refer patients with a body mass index <19 for nutritional advice
	• Encourage exercise and healthy lifestyle
	• If in hospital, refer eligible patients to their community pharmacist for an appropriate postdischarge intervention
Monitoring on hospital admission	• Assessment of functional capacity, cognitive status and nutritional status
	• Obtain chest X-ray, ECG (to exclude comorbidities)
	• Review of medication regimen, including the need for any changes and possible side effects
	• Measure ABG tensions, FBC, theophylline level (in patients on theophylline at admission); if sputum is purulent, a sample should be sent for microscopy and culture; blood cultures if the patient is pyrexial; serum u&Es, creatinine and eGFR
Further reading	British Lung Foundation: www.blf.org.uk.
	Global Initiative for COPD: www.goldcopd.com.
	NICE (2011). *Chronic Obstructive Pulmonary Disease Quality Standards* for www.nice.org.uk/Guidance/qs10 (accessed 30 April 2015).

REFERENCE
1 NICE (2010). *Chronic Obstructive Pulmonary Disease: Management of chronic obstructive pulmonary disease in adults in primary and secondary care.* CG101. www.nice.org.uk/guidance/CG101/ (accessed 7 January 2015).

Ciclosporin: management and monitoring

Ciclosporin is a potent immunosuppressant, used for the treatment and prevention of transplant rejection.[1] It is also licensed for use in severe psoriasis and eczema (oral route only), rheumatoid arthritis and nephrotic syndrome.[2] Its immunosuppressant properties have also been used in an unlicensed capacity for the treatment of ulcerative colitis.[3−5]

Pharmacokinetic overview

The route of elimination is by hepatic metabolism and excretion into the bile. Consequently it should be used with caution in patients with hepatic impairment and the dose adjusted in response to serum concentrations.

Rationale for monitoring

Ciclosporin is nephrotoxic and has a narrow therapeutic range.
　Monitoring of ciclosporin serum concentration is considered:

- when treatment is initiated
- where toxicity or non-adherence is suspected
- when hepatic function deteriorates, or gastrointestinal disturbances develop
- when an interacting drug is prescribed, e.g. erythromycin
- when a dosage change is made
- following a change in formulation.

Therapeutic drug monitoring

The target therapeutic range for ciclosporin is variable and is dependent on the indication. The relationship between the ciclosporin serum concentration and the clinical and toxic effect is not clear, and in the case of autoimmune diseases, there is no evidence linking a particular concentration with the desired effect. Nevertheless, monitoring trough levels of ciclosporin is useful (Table C9).

TABLE C9
Drug monitoring information

Half-life	6–24 hours[6]
Pretreatment measures	FBC, LFTs, U&Es, serum creatinine, blood pressure, lipid profile
Therapeutic range	For transplantation: *seek guidance from transplant centre* For ulcerative colitis: 150–350 ng/mL (124–290 nmol/L)[4]
Sampling time	A trough sample of ciclosporin should be taken before the dose
Other monitoring	See below

Dose

Doses for licensed indications can be found in the BNF. An unlicensed dose for ulcerative colitis is 2–4 mg/kg/day, given intravenously.

Administration of intravenous ciclosporin

Intravenous ciclosporin is available as Sandimmun 50 mg/mL. The infusion should be prepared by diluting the required dose 1:20–1:100 with sodium chloride 0.9% or glucose 5%, and then administering over 2–6 hours. Care is required in the selection of infusion bags and giving sets to avoid incompatibilities with some polyvinyl chloride products.

Once the infusion is commenced, the patient should be observed for the first 30 minutes and at regular intervals thereafter until the infusion is completed. This is necessary because the infusion concentrate contains polyethoxylated castor oil, which has been associated with anaphylaxis.

The patient's blood pressure should also be monitored at regular intervals, as hypertension may occur.

Administration of oral ciclosporin

Oral ciclosporin is available as branded capsules and Neoral oral solution. These should be taken in two divided doses. Neoral oral solution should be diluted with water, orange juice or squash immediately before being taken.

Patients should be prescribed and stabilised on a particular brand of ciclosporin because switching formulations may cause clinically important changes in blood ciclosporin levels.

Grapefruit, or grapefruit juice, should be avoided when taking ciclosporin as grapefruit can affect the P450 enzyme system and lead to higher serum concentrations of ciclosporin.

Monitoring

FBC, LFTs and bilirubin should be monitored every 3 months.

Renal function – U&Es and serum creatinine

Ciclosporin may cause hyperkalaemia and impaired renal function. Monitoring schedules are specific to the product licence, as follows:

- psoriasis – monitor renal function on two occasions prior to commencing therapy, every 2 weeks for the first 3 months of treatment, then monthly
- rheumatoid arthritis – see *Rheumatoid arthritis – drugs suppressing the disease process* entry
- atopic dermatitis – monitor renal function on two occasions prior to commencing therapy, then every 2 weeks
- transplant – refer to specialist centre protocol
- nephrotic syndrome – refer to local protocol.

Blood pressure

Ciclosporin can cause hypertension; therefore blood pressure should be monitored every 2 weeks for the first 3 months after the dose is stable, and then monthly.

Lipid profile

This should be monitored every 6 months.

Overdose

Seek specialist advice. The adverse effects of ciclosporin are usually dose-dependent and include nephrotoxicity, hepatic dysfunction, gastrointestinal reactions, convulsions, headache, paraesthesia, hypertension and hyperlipidaemia.

These are managed by symptomatic treatment and general supportive measures.

Interactions

Many drugs interact with ciclosporin. Those with clinical implications include:

- drugs that decrease ciclosporin serum concentration: barbiturates, carbamazepine, phenytoin, rifampicin, octreotide, orlistat, St John's wort, ticlodipine
- drugs that increase ciclosporin serum concentration: allopurinol, amiodarone, danazol, diltiazem, fluconazole, itraconazole, ketoconazole, macrolide antibiotics, methylprednisolone (high doses), metoclopramide, nicardipine, oral contraceptives, protease inhibitors, ursodeoxycholic acid and verapamil.

Care should be taken when the following drugs are used concomitantly with ciclosporin, as they may all increase the risk of nephrotoxicity: aminoglycoside antibiotics, amphotericin, ciprofloxacin, melphalan, non-steroidal anti-inflammatory drugs, trimethoprim (and sulfamethoxazole) and vancomycin.

Vaccines may be less effective because of a blunted immune response. The use of live attenuated vaccines should be avoided because of the risk of infection.

Ciclosporin may also affect the serum concentration of digoxin, leading to digoxin toxicity. Prednisolone serum concentration may also be raised by ciclosporin.

Miscellany

Oral Sandimmun preparations are available on a named-patient basis for those patients unable to tolerate Neoral.

If intravenous ciclosporin is used in combination with high-dose corticosteroids, then consider the prescribing of oral co-trimoxazole 480 mg twice daily three times a week as prophylaxis against *Pneumocysitis jirovecii* pneumonia.[7]

REFERENCES

1 SPC (2014). *Sandimmun Injection*. www.medicines.org.uk (accessed 28 January 2015).
2 SPC (2014). *Neoral Soft Gelatin Capsules*. www.medicines.org.uk (accessed 28 January 2015).
3 Parry S, Wilkinson M (2004). Current management of inflammatory bowel disease. *Prescriber* 15: 50–60.
4 Van Assche G *et al.* (2003). Randomized, double-blind comparison of 4 mg/kg versus 2 mg/kg intravenous cyclosporine in severe ulcerative colitis. *Gastroenterology* 125: 1025–1031.
5 Lichtiger S *et al.* (1994). Cyclosporine in severe ulcerative colitis refractory to steroid therapy. *N Engl J Med* 330: 1841–1845.
6 Dollery C (ed.) (1999). *Therapeutic Drugs* (2nd edn). Edinburgh: Churchill Livingstone.
7 Quan VA *et al.* (1997). Ciclosporin treatment for ulcerative colitis complicated by fatal *Pneumocysitis carinii* pneumonia. *BMJ* 314: 363–364.

Cigarette smoking: calculation of pack-years

A pack-year is a measure used to calculate the amount of cigarettes smoked over a person's life. A single pack-year is 20 cigarettes smoked per day for 1 year (see *Nicotine replacement therapy (NRT)* entry).

Calculation

$$\text{Total pack-years}^1 = \frac{\left(\begin{array}{c}\text{number cigarettes smoked per day} \\ \times \text{ number of years smoked}\end{array}\right)}{20}$$

The use of pack-years

Pack-years can be used to estimate the risk a patient has of developing smoking-related illnesses such as COPD. The pack-years calculation uses manufactured cigarettes as a standard cigarette. Smoking cigars, pipes or roll-ups provides different levels of risk to the patient and the calculation should be adjusted to allow for this (Table C10).

TABLE C10
A guide to cigarette equivalences[2]

Alternative method of smoking	Cigarette equivalence
1 cigar	4 cigarettes
1 pipe	2.5 cigarettes
Roll-ups: 25 g	Approximately 50 cigarettes

REFERENCES
1 Antoniou S, Barnes N, Khachi H (2010). COPD clinical features and diagnosis. *Clin Pharmacist* 2: 382–389.
2 General Practice Notebook (2014). *Cigarette Smoking Equivalence to Rollups.* http://www.gpnotebook.co.uk/simplepage.cfm?ID=x20110420091937244716 (accessed 2 December 2014).

Cigarette smoking–drug interactions

The interactions between cigarette smoking and medication are complex. The majority of interactions are caused by tobacco rather than nicotine. Monitoring and adjustments of medication may be required when patients stop or start smoking due to the changes in metabolism that occur[1] (see *Nicotine replacement therapy* entry).

Interactions with nicotine

- Nicotine possibly enhances the effect of adenosine.[2]

Interactions with tobacco

- Tobacco smoking induces the hepatic metabolic enzyme CYP1A2, resulting in altered pharmacokinetics of many drugs.[3]
- Levels of clozapine can increase by up to 50% within 2–4 weeks of smoking cessation. Serum concentration levels should be monitored to guide dose adjustments.[1] Other antipsychotics that may be affected include olanzapine, chlorpromazine and haloperidol.[2]
- Theophylline requirements in heavy tobacco smokers or people who chew tobacco are much greater than in non-smokers. When a patient stops smoking a reduction of up to 25–33% of theophylline may be required within a week. Levels should be taken to guide dosing (see *Theophylline* entry).[1]
- Other medications affected in this manner by smoking include cinacalcet and ropinirole.[2]
- Smoking tobacco may also increase insulin resistance, resulting in higher insulin doses than in non-smokers.[1] Insulin requirements may alter if the patient stops smoking.

REFERENCES

1 Baxter K, Preston CL (eds) (2014). *Stockley's Drug Interactions*. www.medicines complete.com (accessed 2 December 2014).

2 Joint Formulary Committee (2014). *British National Formulary* (68th edn). London: BMJ Group and Pharmaceutical Press.

3 Brayfield A (ed.) (2014). *Martindale: The complete drug reference*. www.medicines complete.com (accessed 2 December 2014).

Clozapine

Background

Clozapine is an antipsychotic that should be offered to people with schizophrenia whose illness has not responded adequately to treatment despite the sequential use of adequate doses of at least two different antipsychotic drugs. At least one of the drugs should be a non-clozapine second-generation antipsychotic.[1] It is also used to treat psychosis associated with Parkinson's disease.

It must be initiated by a specialist, and the psychiatrist and the pharmacist must be registered with the company supplying the drug.

There are currently three manufacturers supplying clozapine in the UK:

1 Novartis Pharmaceuticals: Clozaril
2 Denfleet Pharma: Denzapine[2]
3 Ivax Pharmaceuticals UK: Zaponex.[2]

Baseline and regular blood monitoring must be carried out before medication is supplied. This is because neutropenia, leading to agranulocytosis, is a known adverse reaction to clozapine. Routine monitoring of white blood cell count and a differential count of neutrophils, eosinophils and platelets will identify patients at risk.[2] Blood should be taken in 'red-cap' sample bottles.

After the start of clozapine treatment, the following are measured: white blood cells, absolute neutrophils, eosinophils and platelets. The manufacturer's clozapine monitoring service will advise on the frequency of monitoring, which is at least:

- weekly for the first 18 weeks of treatment
- fortnightly for the next 34 weeks of treatment
- at 4-week intervals thereafter.

Monitoring must continue throughout treatment and for 4 weeks after complete discontinuation of clozapine or until haematological recovery has occurred. Patients should be reminded to contact their doctor immediately if any kind of infection, fever, sore throat or other flu-like symptoms develop. Differential blood counts must be performed immediately if any symptoms or signs of an infection occur.

A 'traffic light' system is used to clarify results as follows:

- green – continue treatment
- amber – caution, continue treatment, but extra blood samples will be needed as advised by the manufacturer's monitoring service
- red – stop treatment immediately and act on advice given by the monitoring service. A red result also means that the patient must never be re-exposed to clozapine. In this case the patient should be prescribed whichever therapy previously produced the best response.

The patient's pharmacy will only dispense sufficient clozapine to maintain therapy until confirmation of the patient's next blood result.

Admission to hospital

If a patient taking clozapine is admitted to hospital, the following will need to be determined:

- which brand of clozapine is the patient taking?
- where is the patient registered for clozapine? This information will enable liaison with the patient's registered pharmacist
- has the patient brought his or her own supply of clozapine into hospital? If not, ideally the patient's carer or relative should be asked to bring the supply into the ward in order to maintain synchronicity with blood tests.

Once this information is obtained, contact the patient's registered pharmacist to confirm when the next blood sample is due, and the patient's current clozapine dose.

It is important to note that, if there is a break in treatment of more than 48 hours, clozapine needs to be retitrated. If this happens, contact the registered pharmacist for advice, or the relevant monitoring service.

Contact details

To access the website of your monitoring service you will need a:

- user identity . . . .
- password . . . .

Out of hours, the monitoring services can be contacted by telephone, even by non-registered pharmacists.

Clozaril

Clozaril Patient Monitoring Service (CPMS) contacts for queries:

- Website: https://www.clozaril.co.uk/scrlogon.asp
- General: 0845 769 8269
- Urgent results: 0845 769 8357
- Forgotten passwords: 01276 698125

Denzapine

Denzapine Clozapine Monitoring Service (DCMS) contacts for queries:

- Website: https://www.denzapine.co.uk/
- Queries: Tel: 0333 2004141

Zaponex

Zaponex Treatment Access System (ZTAS) contacts for queries:

- Website: http://www.ztas.co.uk/
- Queries: Tel: 0207 365 5842

REFERENCES

1 NICE (2014). Clinical Guideline 178. *Psychosis and Schizophrenia in Adults: Treatment and management*. http://www.nice.org.uk/guidance/CG178 (accessed 14 January 2015).

2 eMC (2014). www.medicines.org.uk (accessed 13 January 2015).

Cognitive assessment tools

There is a wide range of tests available for cognitive assessment screening; each has its own advantages and disadvantages. The tests vary in the length of time taken to conduct and the amount of equipment needed to perform the test. The shorter tests are preferred in primary care and general practitioner settings.

When interpreting the scores of the cognitive assessment test, it is important to take into account any factors that may affect performance, e.g. educational level or language.

The Alzheimer's Society has produced a toolkit that provides guidance on available cognitive tests and how they may be used in clinical practice.[1] The toolkit also contains copies of many of the tests.

Some of the popular tests currently in use are as follows.

Abbreviated mental test score (AMTS)[2]

This tool was developed in 1972 for assessing cognition. It was validated in acute geriatric ward inpatients but is frequently used in primary care settings. This is a 10-question scale that looks at orientation, memory and concentration. It is simple to perform and score – the cut-off point for dementia is 6–8 out of 10.

6-Item cognitive impairment test (6CIT)[3]

This tool was developed in 1983 and is used in primary care and acute care settings. It consists of six questions looking at orientation, memory and concentration.

It takes less than 5 minutes to complete the test but has a complex scoring system – it is inversely scored and the cut-off point for dementia is a score of 8 or more out of 28.

Mini mental state examination (MMSE)[4]

This tool was developed in 1975; it has been widely used and is included in many dementia guidelines. It is used in the memory clinic setting to aid diagnosis of dementia and assess its progression.

It is an 11-item question scale that looks at cognitive functioning; the test takes less than 10 minutes to complete and the cut-off point for dementia is 24 out of 30. The cut-off point is not valid in different cultures and in particularly highly or uneducated people.

This test is subject to copyright restrictions and incurs a cost at each use.

Addenbrookes cognitive examination 111 (ACE-111)

This is a more detailed assessment of cognition; the ACE-111 version replaced earlier versions in November 2012. This test is used in memory clinics and examines five domains: attention and orientation, memory, verbal fluency, language and visuospatial.

The test takes 10–20 minutes to complete and the cut-off point for dementia is 82–88 out of 100.

Specific training on conducting the test and scoring the test is recommended (www.neura.edu.au/frontier/research/test-downloads).

Montreal cognitive assessment (MoCA)[5]

This test was devised in Canada in 1996 and has been prospectively validated in a UK memory clinic. This test is used in a memory clinic setting or care home (if a patient has a diagnosis of cognitive impairment or dementia).

The test looks at executive functioning and attention tasks, language, memory and visuospatial.

It takes 10 minutes to complete and the cut-off point for dementia is 26 out of 30.

Guidance and further information are available at www.mocatest.org.

REFERENCES

1 Alzheimer's Society (2013). *Helping You to Assess Cognition. A practical toolkit for clinicians*. www.alzheimers.org.uk (accessed 17 January 2015).
2 Hodgkinson HM (1972). Evaluation of a mental test score for assessment of mental impairment in the elderly. *Age Aging* 1: 233–238.
3 Brooke P, Bullock R (1999). Validation of a 6 item cognitive impairment test with a view to primary care usage. *Int J Geriatr Psychiatry* 14: 936–940.
4 Folstein MF *et al.* (1975). Mini-mental state. A practical method for grading the cognitive state of patients for the clinician. *J Psychiatr Res* 12: 189–198.
5 Nasreddine ZS *et al.* (2005). The Montreal Cognitive Assessment (MoCA): a brief screening tool for mild cognitive impairment. *J Am Geriatr Soc* 53: 695–699.

Constipation

C

Overview	
Definition	Defecation that is unsatisfactory because of infrequent stools, difficult stool passage or incomplete defecation[1]
Subtypes	• Faecal loading/impaction – where the retention of faeces is unlikely to result in spontaneous evacuation[1] • Overflow incontinence – leakage of loose stool around impacted faeces[1]
Risk factors	Drug causes (aluminium, antimuscarinics, antidepressants, calcium supplements, diuretics, iron supplements, opioids, verapamil), low-fibre or high-fat diet, reduced exercise, dehydration and psychological factors
Diagnosis	• Symptoms such as abdominal pain, urinary retention, nausea • Faecal mass palpable on examination • Rectal examination • X-ray
Treatment goals[1]	• To clear faecal loading/impaction • To relieve symptoms and achieve a normal stool pattern • To withdraw use of laxatives in chronic constipation where possible; laxatives should be continued for patients on constipating drugs that cannot be discontinued, e.g. an opioid or patients with a medical cause of constipation
Non-pharmaceutical advice	• To adjust any constipating medication • To increase dietary fibre and increase fluid intake • To increase mobility/exercise
Pharmaceutical management[1]	• If non-pharmaceutical measures do not relieve the constipation, oral laxatives should be used • Bulk-forming laxatives are recommended first-line • If stools remain hard then an osmotic laxative should be used as an alternative or in addition to the bulk-forming laxative • If stools are soft but difficult to pass, then a stimulant laxative should be used • If a rapid effect is required or oral laxatives fail to provide relief then suppositories or microenemas can be used. Phosphate or arachis oil retention enemas should be reserved for when all other interventions have failed • Constipation caused by opioid use should be treated with osmotic and stimulant laxatives, avoiding the use of bulk-forming laxatives
Discontinuing laxatives	Once regular bowel movement is achieved with soft stools, laxatives should be withdrawn slowly

Treatment options

Bulk-forming laxatives[2]	• Include ispaghula husk, methylcellulose, sterculia • Act to increase faecal mass by retaining fluid within the stool, and stimulate peristalsis • Effect can be seen in 2–3 days[1] • Must ensure that adequate fluid intake is maintained to avoid intestinal obstruction • Patients should be advised to take with water and should not be taken before bed
Osmotic laxatives[2]	• Include lactulose, macrogols, magnesium salts, rectal phosphates, rectal sodium citrate • Act to increase the amount of water in the large bowel by either retaining fluid or by drawing fluid from the body. This allows fluid accumulation, causing distension in the lower bowel, and stimulates peristalsis[1] • Lactulose is often used in hepatic encephalitis due to the osmotic effect lowering the pH and preventing the proliferation of ammonia-producing organisms • Effect can be seen in 2–3 days with oral preparations[1] N.B.: there is no rationale for 'doubling up' lactulose with a macrogol – use one or the other (possibly guided by patient preference), but not both at the same time • Effect can be seen in 2–5 minutes with rectal preparations[3] • Must ensure that adequate fluid intake is maintained to avoid intestinal obstruction • Phosphate enemas contain sodium phosphates, and therefore sodium and phosphate levels may be elevated and calcium and potassium levels may be reduced[3]
Stimulant laxatives[2]	• Include bisacodyl, danthron, docusate sodium, glycerol suppositories, senna, sodium picosulphate • Act to increase intestinal motility • Glycerol suppositories act as a mild irritant • Effect can be seen in 8–12 hours with oral preparations[1] • Effect can be seen in 15–20 minutes with rectal preparations[1] • Danthron is only indicated for use in the terminally ill due to its potential carcinogenicity and evidence of genotoxicity
Faecal softeners[2]	• Include arachis oil and liquid paraffin (avoid arachis oil in peanut allergy) • Act as a lubricant to promote bowel movement
Side effects	Common side effects of laxatives include flatulence, bloating, abdominal cramps, nausea and diarrhoea[1,2]

Prucalopride[2]	• A selective serotonin $5HT_4$-receptor agonist with prokinetic properties enhancing intestinal motility
	• Indicated for chronic constipation in women when other laxatives fail to produce an adequate response
	• NICE guidance recommends the use of 'prucalopride in women for whom treatment with at least two laxatives from different classes, at the highest tolerated recommended doses for at least 6 months, has failed and invasive treatment is being considered'.[4] It should only be initiated by clinicians experienced in the treatment of chronic constipation
	• Review needed after 4 weeks
	• Common side effects include headache and gastrointestinal symptoms, which are usually transient
Linaclotide[2]	• A guanylate cyclase-C receptor agonist that increases intestinal fluid secretion and transit and reduces visceral pain.
	• Indicated for moderate-to-severe irritable bowel syndrome with constipation

REFERENCES

1 NICE (2013). *Clinical Knowledge Summary. Constipation.* http://cks.nice.org.uk/constipation (accessed 5 February 2015).

2 Joint Formulary Committee (2014). *British National Formulary* (68th edn). London: BMJ Group and Pharmaceutical Press.

3 eMC (2014). http://www.medicines.org.uk/emc/ (accessed 5 February 2015).

4 NICE (2010). *Technology Appraisal 211. Prucalopride for the treatment of chronic constipation in women.* https://www.nice.org.uk/guidance/TA211/chapter/1-guidance (accessed 5 February 2015).

Corticosteroid oral/intravenous equivalence

Patients taking a maintenance dose of oral corticosteroids present a problem if the oral route is unavailable. For example, a patient who has been taking a maintenance dose of prednisolone requires temporary conversion to intravenous therapy, usually as hydrocortisone sodium succinate.

The oral bioavailability of prednisolone and other corticosteroids has a wide interpatient variability, and it is important to appreciate that it is not possible to provide absolute conversion figures.

When there is stress due to intercurrent illness or surgery, the exogenous corticosteroid requirement for an individual may be increased if there is hypothalamic-pituitary-adrenal (HPA) axis suppression. Even in instances where the corticosteroid has been discontinued up to 3 months previously, a latent HPA insufficiency may become important and such individuals should be considered for interim parenteral corticosteroid supplementation. The NHS Steroid Card emphasises this with the warning: '*For one year after you stop the treatment you must mention that you have taken steroids*'.[1]

The following information provides broader assistance in the management of such patients, whilst the BNF contains guidance for the management of patients undergoing surgery (see 'Nil-by-mouth' – *management of long-term medicines during surgery* entry). Table C11 contains relative data for the commonly encountered oral corticosteroids.

TABLE C11
Equivalent anti-inflammatory doses of corticosteroids

Oral corticosteroid	Equivalent dose (relative to prednisolone 5 mg)[1]
Prednisolone	5 mg
Betamethasone	750 micrograms
Deflazacort	6 mg
Dexamethasone (as base)	750 micrograms
Hydrocortisone	20 mg
Methylprednisolone	4 mg
Triamcinolone	4 mg

Factors in determining the parenteral dose

If converting to intravenous or intramuscular (rarely used) hydrocortisone sodium succinate, consideration should be given to the potency and pharmacokinetics of the usual oral drug relative to oral hydrocortisone. The exact dose of corticosteroid administered will vary depending upon the previous corticosteroid dose, duration of therapy and the function of the HPA axis. Doses of supplementary intravenous hydrocortisone sodium succinate range from 25 mg to 100 mg up to four times a day. Parenteral hydrocortisone is used until the patient is able to tolerate oral corticosteroid again.[2]

Bear in mind that doses chosen have to be measurable in the clinical setting, so round up as necessary.

Interactions with other drugs should be considered, since clearance of some corticosteroids is increased by enzyme-inducing drugs. For instance, bioavailability of dexamethasone is markedly decreased by phenytoin.

Use of a high dose of parenteral hydrocortisone, given for more than a few days, carries the risk of appreciable mineralocorticoid effects such as fluid retention.

Dexamethasone

Dexamethasone sodium phosphate injection is usually widely available and can be used to substitute for oral dexamethasone. Traditionally the parenteral dose used is the same as the oral dose, though this will in effect make more dexamethasone available systemically. Caution is advised when prescribing parenteral dexamethasone, taking care to differentiate between the base and the sodium phosphate descriptions. Intravenous dexamethasone should be prescribed as the dexamethasone base, i.e. 3.3 mg/mL.

C

Administration

It is preferable to administer hydrocortisone as an infusion (as opposed to bolus doses) to avoid large swings in plasma cortisol concentration.[2] Rapid injection of dexamethasone is also associated with perineal itching.

Intravenous doses of hydrocortisone sodium succinate and dexamethasone are commonly administered in 50 mL or 100 mL minibag infusions of sodium chloride 0.9%, over 20–30 minutes.

N.B.: 100 mL infusions are usually cheaper and are therefore more suitable for routine use unless the patient is volume- or sodium-restricted.

REFERENCES

1 Joint Formulary Committee (2014). *British National Formulary* (68th edn). London: BMJ Group and Pharmaceutical Press.

2 Rahman MH, Beattie J (2004). Medication in the peri-operative period. *Pharm J* 272: 287–289.

Corticosteroids (topical)

Topical corticosteroids (TCs) are used to suppress or relieve the signs and symptoms of a wide variety of inflammatory skin conditions. Common conditions include eczema, psoriasis, contact dermatitis and insect stings. They are not curative and may cause a rebound exacerbation when stopped. They are generally used with other measures, such as emollients, are not effective (see *Emollients* entry).

TCs may worsen several concomitant skin conditions; they are contraindicated in rosacea and are not recommended for acne. They should be used with caution in ulcerated or secondarily infected lesions unless combined with an appropriate anti-infective agent.[1]

Choice of preparation

There are many different TC preparations available and choice is according to patient preference, formulation and potency.

Formulation

Ointments produce a deeper, more prolonged emollient effect and are useful for dry, thick, scaly lesions. They also increase efficacy of the TC by occlusion so tend to be preferred to creams. However, patients may prefer to use creams on exposed areas such as the face. Creams may also be of benefit in producing a cooling effect or if the skin is moist or wet. Creams should be used in preference to ointments if the skin is infected, to avoid occluding the area. Lotions and gels are preferred for hairier areas of the body, especially the scalp.

Potency

TCs are divided into four potencies: mild, moderate, potent and very potent. The least potent corticosteroid to produce the required effect should be prescribed. Choice of preparation is based on several factors, shown in Table C12.

TABLE C12
Factors to consider in choice of topical corticosteroid preparations

Patient's age	Children are more susceptible to adverse effects and are usually prescribed milder preparations
Severity of the disease	A moderate or potent preparation may be required to treat a disease flare or where a flare has not responded to a milder preparation. This should be stepped down to a lower-potency preparation once the flare comes under control
Body site	A mild preparation should be used for areas where skin is thin, e.g. face, genitals, flexures. Potent preparations may be required for thick areas of the skin, e.g. scalp, palms of hands, soles of feet
Size of the affected area	A less potent preparation may be preferred for widespread use to reduce the risk of systemic absorption of the corticosteroid
Concomitant treatments	Bandaging therapy will increase the potency of the steroid, so a lower-potency preparation should be used

Dose and application

TCs should be applied once or twice daily. Recommendations to apply TCs sparingly often result in underdosing and ineffective treatment. The amount of steroid to be used to treat a particular area is most commonly expressed as the fingertip unit (FTU). The FTU is the amount of cream or ointment from a tube squeezed from the tip of an adult index finger to the first crease. One FTU is approximately 0.5 g and is enough to treat an area of skin equivalent to two adult hands. Table C13 shows dosing quantities for TCs using the FTU.

TABLE C13
Dosing quantities of topical corticosteroids[2, 3]

	Face and neck	Arm and hand	Leg and foot	Trunk – front	Trunk – back, including buttocks
Age	Number of fingertip units				
3–6 months	1	1	1$\frac{1}{2}$	1	1$\frac{1}{2}$
1–2 years	1$\frac{1}{2}$	1$\frac{1}{2}$	2	2	3
3–5 years	1$\frac{1}{2}$	2	3	3	3$\frac{1}{2}$
6–10 years	2	2$\frac{1}{2}$	4$\frac{1}{2}$	3$\frac{1}{2}$	5
Adult	2$\frac{1}{2}$	4	8	7	7

Course length

A course of 1–2 weeks should be adequate to bring a disease flare under control. Longer courses of treatment increase the risk of side effects and of a rebound flare once the steroid is discontinued. Once a disease flare has responded adequately, treatment should be tapered to less potent steroids and then to emollients.

There are concerns about overuse of TCs in psoriasis. They are of most value in acutely inflamed plaques, and the British Association of Dermatology has issued the following guidance:[4]

- Do not use regularly for more than 4 weeks without review.
- Do not use potent steroids regularly for more than 7 days.
- Review every 3 months.
- Do not apply more than 100 g per month of a moderately potent or higher-potency preparation.
- Attempt to rotate topical steroids with non-steroid preparations.

Pharmaceutical care and counselling points

- Steroid phobia due to perceived risks of the side effects of TCs is a common cause of patients undertreating their skin disease. Reassure patients that side effects are uncommon when mild or moderately potent steroids are used in short bursts.
- Ensure patients understand how much steroid to use, where and when to apply it and for how long. Some patients may have different-potency preparations for different areas of the body and will need to be clear which to use where.
- TCs should not be applied within 30 minutes of emollient. There is no consensus as to the order in which emollients and steroids should be applied and patients should be advised to choose a regimen that fits their lifestyle.
- Treatment failure with TCs may indicate infection.

REFERENCE

1 Joint Formulary Committee (2014). *British National Formulary* (68th edn). London: BMJ Group and Pharmaceutical Press.
2 Anonymous (1999). Using topical corticosteroids in general practice. *MeReC Bull* 10: 21–24.
3 Bewley A (2008). Expert consensus: Time for a change in the way we advise our patients to use topical corticosteroids. *Br J Dermatol* 158: 917–920.
4 British Association of Dermatologists (2015). *Psoriasis*. http://www.bad.org.uk/healthcare-professionals/psoriasis (accessed 4 May 2015).

CosmoFer

Overview[1]	
Form	Iron (III) (as iron (III)–hydroxide dextran complex)
Dose	Total dose required (mg iron) = [body weight (kg) × (target haemogloblin (Hb) – actual Hb (g/L)) × 0.24] + X
	X = 500 mg and is the milligrams of iron required to replace the body's iron stores (or depot iron) and is only applicable for patients >35 kg

Administration routes	Intravenous 'total dose' infusion	Intravenous instalments	Intramuscular (intravenous route is preferred route)
	Yes	Yes	Yes
Administration	• A dose of 20 mg/kg is the upper limit for a total dose infusion • Doses >20 mg/kg should be split • Dilute dose in adequate volume of sodium chloride 0.9% or glucose 5% (usually 500 mL) • The first 25 mg iron should be given over a period of 15 minutes (this dose is given from the prepared total dose infusion). • The patient should be observed closely for at least 60 minutes • If no adverse reactions are seen, the remainder of the infusion dose can be given, over 4–6 hours	• Doses of 100–200 mg iron (2–4 mL) preferably diluted in 10–20 mL sodium chloride 0.9% or glucose 5% solution • 25 mg of iron should be injected over 1–2 minutes • If no reaction occurs within 15 minutes the remainder of the injection may be given by slow intravenous injection (0.2 mL/min) • Another option is to give the dose in 100 mL sodium chloride 0.9% and infuse the 25 mg test dose over 15 minutes observing for adverse effects. If no reaction occurs, infuse the remainder or the dose over 30 minutes	• A series of undiluted injections of up to 100 mg iron each • Given by deep intramuscular (IM) injection using the z-track technique into the upper outer quadrant of the buttock • Initial test dose (prior to first dose only): withdraw 25 mg (0.5 mL) and give by IM injection. Observe the patient carefully for signs of allergic reaction for at least 60 minutes; if no adverse effects are seen, give the remainder of the dose • Daily injections into alternate buttocks may be given if the patient is moderately active • Inactive or bedridden patients: the frequency of injections should be reduced to once or twice weekly • Should be continued until an adequate haemoglobin level is attained or the calculated total dose has been reached
Specific contraindications	• Decompensate liver cirrhosis and hepatitis • Acute or chronic infection • Acute renal failure		
Monitoring	• A test dose must be given prior to the administration of every IV dose[1,2] • Patients should be monitored for signs and symptoms of hypersensitivity reactions during and following each administration by any route for at least 30 minutes[2] • If hypersensitivity reactions or signs of intolerance occur during administration, the treatment must be stopped immediately		

REFERENCES

1 eMC (2014). *Summary of Product Characteristics Cosmofer*. https://www.medicines. org.uk/emc/medicine/14139 (accessed 27 August 2014).

2 MHRA Drug Safety Update (2013). Intravenous iron and serious hypersensitivity reactions: strengthened recommendations. https://www.gov.uk/drug-safety-update/intravenous-iron-and-serious-hypersensitivity-reactions-strengthened-recommendations (accessed 29 August 2015).

C-reactive protein

C-reactive protein (CRP) is an acute-phase reactant protein used to diagnose and monitor inflammatory and infectious disease. It is named because of its ability to react with the C-polysaccharide of *Streptococcus pneumoniae*.[1] It is part of the innate immune response and influences multiple stages of inflammation by activation of the complement system.[2] Synthesis is primarily in the liver and initiated by antigen-immune complexes, bacteria, fungi and trauma.[3]

Advantages compared with the erythrocyte sedimentation rate (ESR) include an earlier, more intense response within a few hours, with concentration increases of 1000-fold possible. Changes also occur faster relative to the patient's condition. Disadvantages include non-specificity (i.e. cause and location of the inflammation or infection are not identified) and the use of sophisticated laboratory equipment.[2]

Reference range

Levels of <10 mg/L can be expected in healthy individuals but this can vary with age, sex and race.[2]
CRP can be raised in:[1,3]

- inflammatory disorders, e.g. Crohn's disease, inflammatory arthritis, vasculitis
- tissue injury, necrosis or rejection, e.g. in burns, myocardial infarction, pulmonary emboli, transplant rejection
- bacterial infections, e.g. postoperative wound infections
- malignancy.

Some studies suggest that CRP may be an indicator of cardiovascular events[3] and the development of type 2 diabetes.[1] However, conditions such as viral infections, osteoarthritis, leukaemia, anaemia, polycythaemia and pregnancy (although elevation may occur in later stages) cause little or no rise in CRP.[1]

REFERENCES

1 Patient.co.uk (2014). *Acute-phase Proteins, CRP, ESR and Viscosity*. http://www.patient.co.uk/doctor/acute-phase-proteins-crp-esr-and-viscosity (accessed 17 January 2015).

2 UpToDate (2014). *Acute Phase Reactants*. http://www.uptodate.com/contents/acute-phase-reactants?source=search_resultandsearch=crpandselectedTitle=2~150 (accessed 17 January 2015).

3 Pagana DK, Pagana TJ (2009). *Mosby's Manual of Diagnostic and Laboratory Tests*, 4th edn. St Louis: Mosby.

CURB-65

Background

All patients should have a CURB-65[1,2] score calculated when a diagnosis of community-acquired pneumonia is made. The scoring determines whether patients are at low, intermediate or high risk of death, whether patients should be admitted to hospital and the choice of empirical antibiotics to be commenced.

SCORING SYSTEM	
Clinical feature	Score
Confusion (new onset – place, time, person)	1
Urea (>7 mmol/L)[*]	1
Respiratory rate (>30 breaths/min)	1
Blood pressure (diastolic ≤60 mmHg or systolic <90 mmHg)	1
Age (>65 years)	1
*There is a 5-point scoring system for patients presenting at hospital and a 4-point scoring system for patients presenting in the community; in these patients the score for urea is removed.	

Interpretation

Score = 0–1
- Low risk (<3% mortality risk)
- Home-based care can be considered for those scoring 0 or 1
- Consider a 5-day course of a single antibiotic (e.g. amoxicillin) – choice will depend on local formulary

Score = 2
- Intermediate risk (3–15% mortality risk)
- Consider hospital-based care for those scoring 2 or more
- Consider a 7–10-day course of dual antibiotics (e.g. amoxicillin and a macrolide) – choice will depend on local formulary

Score = 3–5
- High risk (>15% mortality risk)
- Consider intensive care assessment for those scoring 3 or more
- Consider a 7–10-day course of dual antibiotics (e.g. beta-lactamase and macrolide) – choice will depend on local formulary

REFERENCES

1 Lim WS *et al.* (2003). Defining community-acquired pneumonia severity on presentation to hospital: an international derivation and validation study. *Thorax* 58: 377–382.

2 NICE (2014). *Pneumonia: Diagnosis and management of community and hospital acquired pneumonia in adults* (CG 191). https://www.nice.org.uk/guidance/cg191 (accessed 8 February 2015).

Cushing's syndrome

C

Overview	
Definition	Cushing's syndrome is caused by chronic exposure to excess levels of corticosteroids from either exogenous or endogenous sources[1,2]
Risk factors	Endogenous Cushing's (Cushing *disease*) is usually a result of a pituitary tumour (in 70% of cases)
Differential diagnosis	The symptoms of Cushing's are slowly progressive and non-specific, so can be easily missed or attributed to other common conditions, including depression and menopause. It may also mimic common metabolic conditions, such as obesity, poorly controlled diabetes and hypertension
Diagnostic tests	Diagnosis is based on a review of the patient's medical history, physical examination and laboratory tests: • X-ray examinations of the adrenal or pituitary glands to locate tumours • 24-hour urinary free cortisol (positive result if the value is at least as high as the upper limit of normal for the assay used) • Late-night salivary cortisol • 1 mg dexamethasone suppression test (09:00 serum cortisol (after dexamethasone); <50 nmol/L excludes the disease) • Plasma adrenocorticotrophic hormone (ACTH)
Treatment goals	• Reduction of glucocorticoid levels
Treatment options	Dependent on source of glucocorticoid excess: • Stop exogenous glucocorticoid • Surgery to remove pituitary adenoma • Radiotherapy to destroy pituitary adenoma • Medication to reduce effects of excess ACTH (usually in ectopic tumours)

Medicines optimisation	
Assess	Treatment of Cushing's syndrome depends on the cause of excess cortisol. If the cause is long-term use of glucocorticoid hormones to treat another disorder, the dosage must be gradually reduced to the lowest dose adequate for control of that disorder. Once control is established, the daily dose of glucocorticoid hormones may be doubled and given on alternate days to lessen side effects
Essential intervention	Surgical resection of the pituitary, adrenal or ACTH-producing tumour is the primary treatment of choice and is often curative
Secondary intervention	Medical therapy is used to inhibit synthesis and secretion in the adrenal gland. Originally the choices were restricted to unlicensed therapies, with inhibition as a known side effect. The three main drugs used were ketoconazole, metyrapone and mitotane. These drugs are not usually effective as the sole long-term treatment of the disorder, and are used mainly either in preparation for surgery or as adjunctive treatment after surgery, pituitary radiotherapy or both procedures. Frequently, control of hypercortisolism is lost with corticotropin oversecretion, known as escape[3]

Secondary intervention	There is now one licensed therapy for the treatment of Cushing's disease (endogenous) that is not suitable for surgery or where surgery has failed. Pasireotide (Signifor) is given as a 0.6 mg subcutaneous injection twice a day.[4] Ketoconazole HRA has just been recommended for a licence for the treatment of Cushing's by the EMA. This is so new to the market that there is currently very little detail about its cost and dosing regimen; however, it is likely to match the unlicensed use in practice[5]
Continued monitoring	Monitoring for signs of treatment effectiveness is required in Cushing's syndrome. The pituitary–adrenal axis must be evaluated 6–12 months after surgery. Patients who have achieved remission should also be screened every 6–12 months for recurrence of disease. One of the tests used for diagnosis should be performed to detect recurrence (see above). Standard testing, follow-up and management for associated conditions of hypertension, diabetes and osteoporosis should be undertaken, as these conditions may persist after effective treatment of hypercortisolism.
	Pasireotide has a number of monitoring requirements due to its possible side effects:[4]
	• Glycaemic status (FPG/HbA$_{1c}$) should be assessed prior to starting treatment. Self-monitoring of blood glucose and/or FPG assessments should be done weekly for the first 2–3 months and periodically thereafter, as clinically appropriate, as well as over the first 2–4 weeks after any dose increase. In addition, monitoring of FPG 4 weeks and HbA$_{1c}$ 3 months after the end of the treatment should be performed
	• Monitoring of liver function prior to treatment and after 1, 2, 4, 8 and 12 weeks during treatment. Thereafter, liver function should be monitored as clinically indicated
	• An ECG should be performed prior to the start of therapy, 1 week after the beginning of treatment and as clinically indicated thereafter.
	• Hypokalaemia and/or hypomagnesaemia must be corrected prior to administration of pasireotide and should be monitored periodically during therapy
	• Hypocortisolism is a risk with treatment. Patients should be warned of the signs and symptoms associated with hypocortisolism (e.g. weakness, fatigue, anorexia, nausea, vomiting, hypotension, hyperkalaemia, hyponatraemia and hypoglycaemia)

REFERENCES

1 Prague JK (2013). Cushing's syndrome. *BMJ* 346: f945.
2 Pluta RM *et al.* (2011). Cushing syndrome and Cushing disease. *JAMA* 306: 2742.
3 Newell-Price J *et al.* (2006). Cushing's syndrome. *Lancet* 367: 1605–1617.
4 SPC (2014). *Signifor*. www.emc.medicines.org.uk (accessed 16 August 2014).
5 European Medicines Agency (2014). *Press Release: Ketoconazole HRA recommended for approval in Cushing's syndrome*. http://www.ema.europa.eu/ema/index.jsp?curl=pages/news_and_events/news/2014/09/news_detail_002174.jspandmid=WC0b01ac058004d5c1 (accessed 9 October 2014).

Cytotoxic chemotherapy waste

The List of Wastes (England) Regulations 2005 specifies that cytotoxic waste should be considered to be hazardous.[1]

The Waste (England and Wales) Regulations 2011, The Special Waste Amendment (Scotland) Regulations 2004 and Special Waste Regulations (Northern Ireland) 1998 cover storage and disposal of cytotoxic waste.[2–4] It is important to note that the definition of cytotoxic and cytostatic used in waste classification is broader than the term 'cytotoxic' used by the BNF and as such the BNF should not be used to classify waste.[5]

All materials used in the preparation and administration of cytotoxic chemotherapy should be classed as cytotoxic waste. This includes syringes, gloves and needles. All waste should be placed in clearly marked sharps containers, bags or bins for disposal. They must be segregated from other types of waste.

Spillage of cytotoxic agents must be dealt with promptly. Staff should be familiar with local standard operating procedures and regularly trained to deal with cytotoxic spillages. Cytotoxic spill kits should be made available in all areas where cytotoxic drugs are used. These should comprise: ChemoSorb pads or absorbent granules, at least two pairs of gloves (e.g. Chemoprotect), protective gown, shoe coverings, head cover, masks, safety glasses, dilute alkali detergent solution, water, tweezers for broken glass and a sign to identify the spill. A respirator may be included, as may an eyebath.

The following principles should apply when dealing with cytotoxic waste/spillages:

- Safe handling, good practice and training should be adhered to in order to minimise the risk of spillages.
- Spillages should be treated using different procedures according to the size and type (dry or liquid).
- All equipment and materials used to deal with the spill should be treated as cytotoxic waste.
- COSHH data sheets for cytotoxic drugs should be available at all times.
- Ensure spillage is recorded in an accident reporting form. Note details of the day, date, drug, approximate volume, liquid or powder, and the name of the person/people and location involved.

Check with your local procedure for dealing with cytotoxic waste. A suggested procedure is given below.

Initial procedure for all small and large spills

1 Assess the spill for size, type (dry or liquid), drug involved and danger to others.
2 Call for assistance and warn others. Do not leave spill site unguarded. This is to prevent others from being exposed to cytotoxic material. If a 'Warning! Cytotoxic spill' sign is available, this should be placed at the site of the spillage.

3 Individuals should be protected by wearing gloves (double-glove), facemask, goggles, shoe protection and gowns. A respirator may be required for powder spills.
4 The spill area should be cordoned off to avoid further spread.

Procedure for managing small spills (<5 mL or 5 g)

1 Gently cover and absorb liquid spills with dry absorbent towels. Avoid splashing.
2 Pick up solids (powder) with a moistened towel (use water).
3 Pick up sharp/broken material, preferably with forceps or swab; otherwise always double-glove and ensure adequate thickness.
4 Place sharps in a sharps bin labelled 'Cytotoxic waste' and then in a heavy-duty yellow bag to await destruction.
5 Ensure that bags or bins are sealed and clearly marked as 'Cytotoxic waste'.
6 All packaging material contaminated with the drug should be similarly placed in a plastic bag or sharps container for incineration as appropriate.
7 Label and treat all waste from the spill as cytotoxic.
8 The spillage area should be cleaned at least three times using mild detergent followed by large amounts of clean water.
9 Wash hands thoroughly and record spill in a cytotoxic spill book.
10 Exposure to cytotoxic drugs should be recorded and notified to the occupational health department.

Large spills (>5 mL or 5 g)

1 Work from the outside in.
2 Use the cytotoxic spill kit.
3 Lay the ChemoSorb spill pad from the spill kit over the spill or sprinkle absorbent granules over the spill area.
4 The pad/granules will absorb the liquid and transform the spill into a gel, which can be handled more easily.
5 Gather up the gel and place in a plastic bag and seal. Ensure that this is labelled as 'Cytotoxic waste'.
6 Repeat these steps several times.
7 After removal of the cytotoxic agent, the area should be cleaned at least three times using a mild detergent and clean water.
8 Use the remaining spill pads to pick up the rinse water and fully dry the area using absorbent towels.
9 Discard all contaminated material in disposal bag, including gloves and shoe coverings, and then seal. Ensure the bag is labelled as 'Cytotoxic waste'.
10 Wash hands thoroughly and record spill.
11 Inform the occupational health department.

Additional information can be found on the HSE website (www.hse.gov.uk), where further information on conducting risk assessments can be found.[6]

Patient waste

Patients receiving cytotoxic chemotherapy will also produce cytotoxic waste. Their faeces, urine, sweat and expired gases may all contain cytotoxic drug, either as unchanged drug or active/inactive metabolite. As such, patient waste must be handled as cytotoxic waste for up to 14 days after administration. Urinals, bedpans and vomit bowls should be handled with gloves and disposed of in an appropriate manner. Hospital policies may vary and should be consulted. Contaminated bed linen should also be treated in an appropriate manner, e.g. in alginate bags marked with cytotoxic material tape.

REFERENCES

1　The List of Wastes (England) Regulations 2005. http://www.legislation.gov.uk/uksi/2005/895/made (accessed 15 December 2014).

2　The Waste (England and Wales) Regulations 2011. http://www.legislation.gov.uk/ukdsi/2011/9780111506462/pdfs/ukdsi_9780111506462_en.pdf (accessed 15 December 2014).

3　The Special Waste Amendment (Scotland) Regulations 2004. http://www.legislation.gov.uk/ssi/2004/112/pdfs/ssi_20040112_en.pdf (accessed 15 December 2014).

4　The Special Waste Regulations (Northern Ireland) 1998. http://www.legislation.gov.uk/nisr/1998/289/contents/made (accessed 15 December 2014).

5　Department of Health (2013). *Health Technical Memorandum 07-01: Safe management of healthcare waste*. https://www.gov.uk/government/uploads/system/uploads/attachment_data/file/167976/HTM_07-01_Final.pdf (accessed 15 December 2014).

6　HSE (2014). *Safe Handling of Cytotoxic Drugs in the Workplace*. http://hse.gov.uk/healthservices/safe-use-cytotoxic-drugs.htm (accessed 15 December 2014).

D

D-dimer

D-dimer levels are tested to help diagnose, exclude or monitor thrombotic or bleeding conditions, such as deep-vein thrombosis (DVT), pulmonary embolus and disseminated intravascular coagulation.[1] It is a fibrin degradation product and consists of adjacent fibrin monomers that have been cross-linked (d-dimerised) by activated factor XIII and subsequently cleaved by plasmin during the process of clotting and clot degradation.[2,3] It is usually undetectable in the blood.

Reference range

The reference range for a normal D-dimer will depend on the laboratory performing the test, but commonly a value of $<500\,\mu g/L$ is considered normal.[4]

Local range . . . .

However, the D-dimer test is non-specific and can be raised in many conditions that involve fibrin formation and degradation (Table D1). For this reason its main use in clinical practice is excluding venous thromboembolism and a normal result can rule out the possibility of DVT in up to 97% of cases.[4]

TABLE D1
Conditions and factors increasing D-dimer levels

Conditions increasing D-dimer levels[5]	Factors increasing D-dimer levels[5]
Severe infection	Pregnancy
Trauma	Age
Inflammatory conditions	Smoking
Unstable angina	Haemolysis of sample
Atrial fibrillation	Raised rheumatoid factor levels
Acute myocardial infarction	Raised bilirubin levels
Vasculitis	Presence of fats (from greasy meal)

Treatment with heparins and oral anticoagulants can lower D-dimer levels.[6]

REFERENCES
1 Lab Tests Online UK (2014). *D-dimer*. http://www.labtestsonline.org.uk/
understanding/analytes/d-dimer/tab/glance/ (accessed 17 January 2015).

2 UpToDate (2014). *Clinical Use of Coagulation Tests*. http://www.uptodate.com/
  contents/clinical-use-of-coagulation-tests?source=search_result&search=d+dimer&
  selectedTitle=1~114#H19 (accessed 17 January 2015).

3 Pagana DK, Pagana TJ (2009). *Mosby's Manual of Diagnostic and Laboratory Tests*,
  4th edn. St Louis: Mosby.

4 perinatology.com (2010). *Reference Values During Pregnancy*. http://
  www.perinatology.com/Reference/Reference%20Ranges/D-Dimer.htm
  (accessed 17 January 2015).

5 NHS Choices (2014). *Deep Vein Thrombosis*. http://www.nhs.uk/Conditions/
  Deep-vein-thrombosis/Pages/Diagnosis.aspx (accessed 17 January 2015).

6 GP notebook (2010). *D-dimer*. http://www.gpnotebook.co.uk/simplepage.cfm?ID=
  26869806 (accessed 17 January 2015).

Delirium

Overview	
Definition	An acute-onset mental disorder characterised by: • Change or fluctuating mentation, i.e. mental activity, state of mind • Inattention and either one or both of: • Disorganised thinking • Altered level of consciousness
Causes	Multiple potential causes include (not an exclusive list): • Drugs (often antimuscarinics, benzodiazepines) or drug withdrawal (alcohol, nicotine, illicit drugs or any prescription-only medicine) • Eyes, ears and other sensory deficits • Low oxygen states (hypoxia, MI, cerebrovascular accident (CVA), PE) • Infection or inflammatory states • Retention (urinary or constipation) • Ictal, postictal • Underhydration and/or undernutrition • Metabolic (diabetes, postoperative patients, hypernatraemia)
Classification	The *Diagnostic and Statistical Manual of Mental Disorders* (DSM-V)[1] recognises classification by aetiology as a result of: • A general medical condition • An intoxicating substance (inattention and cognitive effects predominate) • Substance withdrawal (inattention and cognitive effects predominate) • Medication-induced (temporal relationship predominates) • More than one cause Delirium is often further specified by motoric form. This system helps highlight that a large group of patients are delirious but not agitated (and therefore not drawing attention to themselves): • Hyperactive: agitated, restless, combative (1–2%) • Hypoactive: drowsy, withdrawn, non-communicative (40–45%) • Mixed: oscillates between hyperactive and hypoactive (45–50%) DSM-V recognises delirium can be acute (lasting a few days) or persistent (lasting weeks to months)

Signs and symptoms	Sudden changes (over hours or days) or fluctuations in behaviour, often more obvious to regular carers or family. Hypoactive behaviour is more difficult to pick up.[2] • Cognitive function, e.g. worsened concentration, slow responses, confusion • Perception, e.g. visual or auditory hallucinations • Physical function, e.g. reduced mobility, reduced movement, restlessness, agitation, changes in appetite, sleep disturbance (rule out other reasons for agitation, e.g. untreated pain, frustration) • Social behaviour, e.g. lack of cooperation with reasonable requests, withdrawal, or alterations in communication, mood and/or attitude
Diagnostic tests	Screening tools are available that look for the main points listed under the definition above. The most widely used tool is the Confusion Assessment Method (CAM). Patients are interviewed, often by applying another intervention (e.g. Mini Mental State Examination (MMSE)) in order to generate interaction. The screener then reflects on the patient interaction to evaluate systematically for delirium: evidence for acute mental change/fluctuation, inattention, disorganised thinking, altered level of consciousness
Goals	Prevent delirium; alleviate symptoms; control behavioural aspects if necessary to maintain safety
Prevention	A comprehensive intervention package that targets the main drivers for delirium reduces the incidence of new delirium: • Drugs: carry out a medication review, removing unnecessary treatments and reducing exposure to medications known to cause delirium. Anticipate and treat withdrawal syndromes • Eyes, ears and other sensory deficits: ensure spectacles and hearing aids are working and available • Low-oxygen states (hypoxia, MI, CVA, PE): assess for hypoxia and optimise O_2 saturation; treat underlying/causative conditions • Infection or inflammatory states: look for and treat infection, avoid unnecessary catheterisation, employ good infection control procedures • Retention (urinary or constipation): prescribe laxatives where necessary; manage urinary retention • Ictal, postictal: look for seizures and control precipitants • Underhydration and/or undernutrition: encourage the person to drink, have fluid management plans. Offer parenteral fluids where necessary; maintain fluid charts and monitor. Monitor for appropriate nutrition; ensure dentures fit if needed. Ensure tube feeding where required • Metabolic (diabetes, post-op, hypernatraemic): monitor appropriate biochemical markers • Monitor and correct underlying problems, manage comorbidities In addition, NICE Clinical Guideline 103[2] advises other sensible measures, such as promoting good sleep hygiene, managing pain appropriately and encouraging the person to mobilise/walk and carry out active range-of-motion exercises. Orientation is important: use clear signage, clocks and calendars. Reorientate the person by explaining who the patient is, where s/he is and who you are. Facilitate visits by family and friends and encourage interaction. Prophylactic antipsychotics are not recommended

Treatment options[2]	Prevention measures should be (re)visited and employed. In delirium superimposed upon dementia, treat the delirium as usual.
	Delirium treatment with medication has two aims: treating cognitive defect and maintaining safety. These should be kept clearly in mind, as targeting one outcome may make the other less achievable and an appropriate balance must be sought

Treat cognitive deficit

Antipsychotics are frequently used in an attempt to clear the mind of the individual afflicted with delirium. NICE Clinical Guideline 103[2] bases recommendations on one study and, although the treatments are randomised in that study, they are not blinded (i.e. oral olanzapine versus intramuscular haloperidol versus no drug therapy).

- Haloperidol: 1–5 mg enterally or parenterally, usually three to four times a day
- Olanzapine: 5–10 mg enterally or parenterally usually once, occasionally twice, a day

It is clear that the medication does not work immediately. In the study it took an average of 3 days for the delirium to clear (7 days in control group). Any acute resolution of behavioural symptoms (e.g. agitation) is likely due to sedative side effects.

Since NICE Clinical Guideline 103,[2] there have been other studies looking at quetiapine. The studies are well conducted, placebo-controlled, blinded, randomised, but small. However, they do show that the number of days in delirium is reduced.[3,4]

- Quetiapine: 25–100 mg enterally twice a day (larger doses rarely used)

Maintain safety

The dangerously agitated patient is likely to require sedation to maintain the safety of the patient, staff and visitors. Unfortunately sedatives further cloud the patient's consciousness, so although sedatives do help calm the patient and manage the danger in the situation, they can render the patient more delirious. An exception to this includes benzodiazepine administration in alcohol or benzodiazepine withdrawal delirium (depending on the quantity administered).

- Use the minimum dose necessary for effect

Choose the best drug for the situation (e.g. intramuscular midazolam for short-acting effect in Critical Care; diazepam for a longer-acting effect in a general ward area)

Medicines optimisation

Therapeutic review	Review the medication chart to reduce the burden from medications likely to cause delirium, particularly:
	- medications with strong anticholinergic drive (e.g. amitriptyline, hyoscine, cyclizine)
	- gamma-aminobutyric acid (GABA) agonists (e.g. temazepam, lorazepam)
	- other medications known to cause confusion (e.g. steroids, quinolones)
	- potential withdrawal (e.g. nicotine, opiates, antidepressants)
	Switch to medications with lower deliriogenic potential, or reduce the dose if possible. Avoid changing the therapeutic approach every day. Ensure any plan makes the longer-term goals explicit, with stepwise/short-term goals to measure and highlight progress

Antipsychotics	Antipsychotics are not likely to work immediately, and with florid delirium are not likely to work at all until the drivers are removed.
	• Monitor QTc interval
	• Start at an appropriate dose and route
	• Recognise that you may need a rescue option for rapid sedation
	• Monitor for extrapyramidal side effects and the rare possibility of neuroleptic malignant syndrome
	• Do not use in patients with Parkinson's disease — here consider reducing regular therapy temporarily
	• When stopping, reduce the dose/frequency over a few days, with the nighttime dose being the last to stop
	• Make it clear the antipsychotic is for delirium and is expected to cease in the short- to mid-term. Most prescriptions should stop within 7–14 days and all within 1 month (with the exception of a tiny minority of cases). Further underscore the short-term nature of antipsychotic therapy in patients with dementia
Sedatives	Used to make the patient safe; they are not to make the patient tidy/easy to manage.
	• They may make delirium worse
	• Use the smallest dose for the shortest possible time
	• May need repeating
Night sedation and sleep aid	Sleep is often fragmented in delirious patients and there is a temptation to use sleep aids. Avoid deliriogenic medicines such as GABA agonists (benzodiazepines, z-drugs) and tricyclic antidepressants.
	• Try a slightly larger dose of the regular antipsychotic late evening (e.g. haloperidol 1 mg three times daily and 2.5 mg at night)
	• Trazodone 50 mg at night, increasing to 100 mg late evening. May cause hypotension, although not normally at these doses. May very rarely cause priapism
	• Mirtazapine 15–30 mg late evening
	• Some centres use melatonin, no more than 5 mg late evening

REFERENCES

1 American Psychiatric Association (2013). *Diagnostic and Statistical Manual of Mental Disorders*, DSM-5 (5th edn). Arlington: American Psychiatric Association.
2 NICE (2010). Clinical Guideline 103. *Delirium: Diagnosis, prevention and management*. http://www.nice.org.uk/guidance/CG103 (accessed 10 October 2014).
3 Devlin JW *et al.* (2010). Efficacy and safety of quetiapine in critically ill patients with delirium: a prospective, multicenter, randomized, double-blind, placebo-controlled pilot study. *Crit Care Med* 38: 419–427.
4 Tahir TA *et al.* (2010). Randomized controlled trial of quetiapine versus placebo in the treatment of delirium. *J Psychosom Res* 69: 485–490.

Depression

Overview

Definition	Depression is a common and recurrent disorder characterised by persistent low mood and anhedonia (the inability to experience pleasure from activities usually found enjoyable). Depressive disorder is associated with significant morbidity and mortality
Classification	May be classified using either the *International Classification of Disease-10* (ICD-10)[1] ('depressive episode', further specified as mild, moderate or severe) or DSM[2] ('major depression', further specified as mild, moderate or severe). The current NICE guideline uses DSM-IV diagnostic criteria and definitions of severity[3]
Differential diagnoses	May include neurological conditions, other psychiatric conditions (including bipolar affective disorder, anxiety disorders, personality disorders and negative symptoms of schizophrenia), organic brain disorder, hypoglycaemia, anaemia, endocrine disorders (including hypothyroidism), bereavement, sleep apnoea and iatrogenic causes (e.g. antihypertensives, steroids, oestrogens and central nervous system depressants)
Diagnostic tests	There is no specific test for depression. Investigations are of importance in order to exclude possible causes
Treatment goals	Remission of symptoms of depression, prevention of relapse, reduction in morbidity and mortality and restoration of premorbid social and occupational functioning
Treatment options[3]	**Subthreshold symptoms and mild depression:** sleep hygiene and active monitoring. Do not use antidepressants unless there is a history of moderate or severe depression. Consider low-intensity psychological intervention. **Persistent subthreshold symptoms and those who have not benefited from low-intensity psychological intervention:** antidepressants or high-intensity psychological intervention. **Moderate or severe depression:** antidepressants, high-intensity psychological interventions and combined treatments (when two antidepressants are used together)
Choice	Patients should be supported to make informed decisions about their care and these should be considered during development of the care plan. In addition to patient choice, the following factors should be taken into account when making decisions regarding choice of medication: comorbidities and concurrent medication, other patient-specific factors (e.g. lifestyle, physical health and predominant symptoms), national and local guidelines/policies, likely adherence to medication, risk of accidental or deliberate overdose, previous response and potential adverse effects

Pharmaceutical care and counselling

The options presented here are from NICE guidance[3] and concern the treatment of people aged 18–60 years only. Note that the recommended treatment varies in the presence of a chronic physical health problem. Consult relevant guidelines in this case

Assess	• An accurate medication history will aid in decision making regarding an appropriate treatment plan
	• Explore any concerns the patient has regarding the pharmacological treatment of depression and provide relevant information[3]
	• Determine likely adherence and suicide risk
Selective serotonin reuptake inhibitors (SSRIs)	• SSRIs are usually the first-line choice due to tolerability and relative safety in comparison to TCAs[3,4]
	• Increase synaptic serotonin levels by inhibiting the serotonin reuptake transporter
	• Side effects: GI disturbance, sexual dysfunction, motor symptoms (particularly akathisia), anxiety, increased risk of GI bleeding, insomnia, serotonin syndrome (see *Serotonin syndrome* entry for further details)
	• Risk of GI bleeding is further increased in the presence of NSAIDs and aspirin. Consider gastroprotection
	• Fluoxetine ($t_{1/2} \approx 140$ hours): lower risk of discontinuation symptoms, higher propensity for drug interactions, associated with bruxism (grinding the teeth and clenching the jaw)
	• Paroxetine ($t_{1/2} \approx 24$ hours): higher risk of discontinuation symptoms, inhibits its own metabolism, possibly greater weight gain with long-term use[5]
	• Sertraline: Most cost-effective of the SSRIs.[6] Antidepressant of choice post-MI; few interactions but higher rates of diarrhoea than others.
	• Citalopram: very few interactions. Associated with dose-related QTc prolongation
	• Escitalopram is the S-enantiomer of racemic citalopram
	• Start with low doses where there is a significant anxiety component to the presentation and increase very slowly
Tricyclic antidepressants (TCAs)	• Increase synaptic levels of serotonin and noradrenaline by blocking the relevant reuptake transporters. Different TCAs block the two transporters to different degrees, leading to slightly different clinical and side effect profiles
	• Can be considered if switching from SSRIs following lack of response
	• Doses less than 100 mg daily are unlikely to be effective[7]
	• Greatest risk in overdose
	• Increased risk of discontinuation due to side effects compared to SSRIs
	• Dosulepin should not be prescribed due to cardiotoxicity[3]
	• TCAs are as effective as SSRIs but their use is limited by their side effects: sedation, central and peripheral antimuscarinic effects, hypotension, cardiac toxicity and behavioural toxicity (reduction in psychomotor activity or cognitive ability)
	• Contraindicated in heart block, recent MI and mania or hypomania
Venlafaxine	• Inhibits reuptake of both serotonin and noradrenaline but also dopamine at higher doses (i.e. >225 mg). At lower doses (i.e. 75 mg daily) the pharmacological effect is predominantly on serotonin reuptake, meaning it behaves similarly to an SSRI. At doses >150 mg daily, synaptic noradrenaline levels are also increased.
	• Clinical effect may therefore be superior at higher doses, but this is controversial.

	• Side effects and discontinuation rates are more problematic than with some SSRIs • Tachycardia, prolonged QTc and seizures can occur in overdose, but fatality is rare • Sustained-release formulations may be associated with fewer side effects, particularly nausea
Mirtazapine	• Most cost-effective antidepressant in a 2009 analysis[6] • 5-HT$_{2/3}$ antagonism means less nausea and sexual dysfunction than with SSRIs • Can be more sedating at lower doses, where alerting effect of increased noradrenergic transmission is dominated by the sedating effects of histamine receptor antagonism • In addition to sedation, weight gain can be problematic in some patients • Sometimes combined with venlafaxine (this combination is known as 'Californian rocket fuel') for a synergistic effect • May be preferred for patients on warfarin or heparin. International normalised ratio may increase slightly • Withdraw immediately and perform full blood count if blood dyscrasias suspected
Duloxetine	• May be useful for those with a significant somatic component to their depressive illness
Monoamine oxidase inhibitors (MAOIs)	• Associated with the 'cheese reaction' following dietary tyramine, which can result in hypertensive crisis and death • In addition to restrictions to diet, several significant drug–drug interactions exist • A 2-week wash-out period is necessary when switching between MAOIs and other antidepressants to reduce the risk of serotonin syndrome
Reboxetine	• Least efficacious and least acceptable antidepressant in a 2009 review[6]
Trazodone	• Serotonergic reuptake inhibition is not saturated at doses less than 150 mg daily and so antidepressant effect is lost
Agomelatine	• Monitor LFTs • Not associated with weight gain or sexual dysfunction
Combination and augmentation	• Antidepressants can be combined with other antidepressants or augmented using lithium or atypical antipsychotics • Where combinations of serotonergic agents are used, monitor for serotonin syndrome • With lithium, all the usual monitoring requirements apply (see *Lithium – management and monitoring* entry) • When augmenting with atypical antipsychotics, consider risk of weight gain and hyperglycaemia in addition to monitoring LFTs, lipids and electrocardiogram where indicated
Response	• Clinical response can be expected in the first 1–2 weeks of treatment • Check compliance if there is no improvement in the first 2–4 weeks • Absent or minimal effect at 3–4 weeks warrants a change in treatment

Patient counselling	• Antidepressants are effective • It is important to take antidepressant medication as prescribed and not to stop suddenly due to risk of discontinuation symptoms • Treatment will continue beyond symptom remission and the duration will depend on the risk of recurrence • Antidepressants are not addictive • Side effects are relevant to the specific treatment chosen along with suitable management/monitoring strategies
Continued monitoring	• In addition to monitoring for clinical and side effects relevant to the individual, be aware that most antidepressants have been associated with hyponatraemia. If symptoms occur, monitor serum sodium and consider fluid restriction and withdrawal of the antidepressant accordingly. If no other cause of hyponatraemia can be identified, stop the antidepressant immediately and if the patient has serum sodium below 125 mmol/L, treat medically for hyponatraemia. Antidepressant withdrawal symptoms should be anticipated, but are unlikely to occur if the hyponatraemia occurs soon after initiation of antidepressant treatment • Following hyponatraemia, use of an antidepressant from a different class is recommended.[7] Start at a low dose and increase slowly. Monitor serum sodium weekly initially • Those not deemed to be at increased risk of suicide should be reviewed 2 weeks after starting an antidepressant. For those under 30 years or considered to present a higher risk, review at 1 week and then frequently until risk is no longer clinically important[3]
Duration of treatment	The treatment dose of the effective antidepressant should be continued for a minimum of 6 months from the point of remission of symptoms, taking into account the number of previous episodes, any concurrent physical health or psychosocial difficulties and the existence of any residual symptoms
Withdrawing treatment	• Potentially severe discontinuation symptoms can occur when an antidepressant is stopped • Gradually withdraw over a period of at least 4 weeks, and consult a standard reference (Maudsley[7] or Bazire[8]) for more detail
Further reading	Bleakley S (2013). Review of the choice and use of antidepressant drugs. *Progr Neurol Psychiatry* 17: 18–26.

REFERENCES

1 WHO (2015). *International Classification of Diseases* (ICD). http://www.who.int/classifications/icd/en/ (accessed 8 May 2015).
2 American Psychiatric Association (2000). *Diagnostic and Statistical Manual of Mental Disorders* (4th text revision edn). Washington, 3. DC: American Psychiatric Association.
3 NICE (2009). Clinical Guideline 90. *Depression in Adults*. http://www.nice.org.uk/guidance/CG090 (accessed 27 April 2015).
4 Anderson IM *et al.* (2008). Evidence-based guidelines for treating depressive disorders with antidepressants: A revision of the 2000 British Association for Psychopharmacology guidelines. *J Psychopharm* 22: 243–296.
5 Deshmukh R, Franco K (2003). Managing weight gain as a side effect of antidepressant therapy. *Clevel Clin J Med* 70: 614–623.

6 Cipriani A et al. (2009). Comparative efficacy and acceptability of 12 new-generation antidepressants: a multiple-treatments meta-analysis. *Lancet* 373: 746–758.
7 Taylor D et al. (eds) (2012). *The Maudsley Prescribing Guidelines in Psychiatry*, 11th edn. Chichester: Wiley-Blackwell.
8 Bazire S (2013). *Psychotropic Drug Directory 2013/14: The professionals' pocket handbook and aide memoire*. Cheltenham: Lloyd-Reinhold Communications.

Diabetes insipidus (cranial)

Overview	
Definition	Diabetes insipidus (DI) is defined as the passage of large volumes (>3 L/24 hours) of dilute urine (<300 mOsmol/kg). Cranial DI (neurogenic, pituitary or neurohypophyseal) is characterised by decreased secretion of antidiuretic hormone (ADH). Another form (nephrogenic) is caused by malfunction of the kidneys[1–3]
Differential diagnosis	• Type 1 diabetes • Hypercalcaemia • Head trauma • Sickle cell anaemia
Diagnostic tests	• A 24-hour urine collection for determination of urine volume (>3 litres) • Serum electrolyte concentrations and glucose level • Urinary specific gravity (<1.005) • Simultaneous plasma (>287 mOsmol/kg) and urinary osmolality (<200 mOsmol/kg) • Plasma ADH level Tests should be carried out when the patient is maximally dehydrated to ensure highest possible ADH levels and concentration of urine
Treatment goals	• Maintain fluid balance • Maintain sodium levels
Treatment options	• Fluid replacement • Desmopressin
Pharmaceutical care and counselling	
Essential intervention	• Fluid replacement. Patients must be encouraged to maintain their fluid levels and most can drink enough fluid to replace their urine losses. When oral intake is inadequate and hypernatraemia is present, losses must be replaced with an intravenous fluid that is hypo-osmolar with respect to the patient's serum. To avoid volume overload and overly rapid correction of hypernatremia, fluid replacement should be provided at a rate no greater than 500–750 mL/hour
Essential intervention	• Desmopressin is a synthetic ADH analogue that is used to treat cranial diabetes insipidus. It is available in a variety of formulations, which can be used depending on patient preference or need
Continued monitoring	• Sodium levels – overtreatment can result in fluid retention and severe hyponatraemia

REFERENCES

1 Verbalis JG (2003). Diabetes insipidus. *Rev Endocri Metab Disord* 4: 177–185.

2 Medline Plus (2011). *Diabetes Insipidus*. http://www.nlm.nih.gov/medlineplus/ency/article/000377.htm (accessed 15 October 2014).

3 Khardori R (2014). *Diabetes Insipidus*. Medscape. http://emedicine.medscape.com/article/117648-overview (accessed 15 October 2014).

Diabetes mellitus

Definition of diabetes mellitus

The term diabetes mellitus (DM) describes a metabolic disorder resulting from defects in insulin secretion, insulin action, or both. It is characterised by chronic hyperglycaemia and disturbances of carbohydrate, fat and protein metabolism.[1] This metabolic disruption can lead to the development of retinopathy, nephropathy and neuropathy (microvascular complications).[2] People with DM are also at increased risk of cardiac, peripheral arterial and cerebrovascular disease (macrovascular complications).[3]

DM may present with characteristic symptoms such as thirst, polyuria, blurring of vision and weight loss, although it is increasingly being picked up by improved screening programmes. However, symptoms may not be severe, or may be absent, and metabolic changes may be present for a considerable time, resulting in the development of complications before a diagnosis has been made. If timely recognition does not occur, diabetic ketoacidosis (see *Diabetic ketoacidosis* entry) or hyperosmolar hyperglycaemic state (see *Hyperosmolar hyperglycaemic state* entry) may develop and lead to severe metabolic disturbance, altered consciousness and, in the absence of effective treatment, death.

Classification of DM[4]

- Type 1: absolute insulin deficiency, usually due to autoimmune destruction of pancreatic beta cells; dependent on exogenous insulin; prone to ketoacidosis; accounts for 5–10% of patients.
- Type 2: a combination of resistance to insulin action and inadequate compensatory insulin secretion; may be 'insulin requiring'.
- Gestational diabetes: first recognised in pregnancy, gestational diabetes disappears after birth; affects about 4% of all pregnant women; may precede development of (usually) type 2 DM.
- Maturity-onset diabetes of the young (MODY): impaired insulin secretion most often inherited in an autosomal-dominant manner
- Secondary diabetes: caused by pancreatic injury, e.g. chronic pancreatitis, pancreatectomy, pancreatic carcinoma, cystic fibrosis, haemochromatosis; accounts for only 1–2% of patients
- Endocrine: seen with Cushing's syndrome (see separate entry), acromegaly, thyrotoxicosis, phaeochromocytoma (see separate entry), glucagonoma (because cortisol, growth hormone,

thyroid hormones, glucagon and adrenaline antagonise insulin action).

- Drug-induced: often occurs in association with insulin resistance; implicated drugs include thiazide diuretics, glucocorticoids, beta-adrenergic agonists, atypical antipsychotics, antiretroviral protease inhibitors.

Diagnosis of DM[5-7]

1 In a patient presenting with DM symptoms (e.g. polyuria, polydipsia, unexplained weight loss (for type 1)), the diagnosis of DM is confirmed with *one* of the following:
    - random venous plasma glucose concentration ≥11.1 mmol/L
    - fasting plasma glucose concentration ≥7.0 mmol/L (whole blood ≥6.1 mmol/L)
    - plasma glucose concentration ≥11.1 mmol/L 2 hours after 75 g anhydrous glucose in an oral glucose tolerance test.

2 Where a patient has no symptoms of DM, diagnosis should not be based on a single glucose determination. At least one additional glucose test result on another day with a value in the diabetic range is essential, whether fasting, from a random sample or 2 hours post glucose load.

3 A laboratory venous haemoglobin A1c (HbA_{1c}) test may be used to diagnose DM, although only in certain circumstances. An HbA_{1c} of 48 mmol/mol is recommended as the cut-off point for diagnosing DM; however, a value of <48 mmol/mol does not exclude DM diagnosed using glucose tests. In asymptomatic patients, a laboratory venous HbA1c should be repeated to confirm diagnosis.

REFERENCES

1 WHO (1999). *Definition, Diagnosis and Classification of Diabetes Mellitus and its Complications Part 1: Diagnosis and classification of diabetes mellitus.* http://apps.who.int/iris/handle/10665/66040 (accessed 3 February 2015).

2 Hanssen KF *et al.* (1992). Blood glucose control and diabetic microvascular complications: long-term effects of near-normoglycaemia. *Diabet Med* 9: 697–705.

3 Fox CS *et al.* (2007). Increasing cardiovascular disease burden due to diabetes mellitus: the Framingham Heart Study. *Circulation* 115: 1544–1550.

4 American Diabetes Association (2004). Diagnosis and classification of diabetes mellitus. *Diabetes Care* 27: 5–10.

5 WHO (2006). *Definition and Diagnosis of Diabetes Mellitus and Intermediate Hyperglycemia.* http://www.who.int/diabetes/publications/diagnosis_diabetes2006/en/ (accessed 3 February 2015).

6 World Health Organization (2011). *Use of Glycated Haemoglobin in the Diagnosis of Diabetes Mellitus.* http://www.who.int/diabetes/publications/diagnosis_diabetes2011/en/ (accessed 3 February 2015).

7 Diabetes UK (2015). *Diagnostic Criteria for Diabetes.* http://www.diabetes.org.uk/About_us/What-we-say/Diagnosis-prevention/New_diagnostic_criteria_for_diabetes/ (accessed 1 February 2015).

Diabetes mellitus: management of hypoglycaemia ('hypo') in adults

Hypoglycaemia is a lower than normal level of blood glucose. It is considered 'mild' if the episode is self-treated and 'severe' if assistance is necessary.[1] For people with diabetes, a blood glucose of <4.0 mmol/L should be treated[2]; however, adults who have poor glycaemic control may experience symptoms at blood glucose levels above this.

Hypoglycaemia is particularly dangerous when symptom recognition is poor and in those unable to respond appropriately, e.g. young children, people with dementia.

Symptoms of hypoglycaemia

Symptoms of hypoglycaemia can provide an individual with a useful warning that blood glucose levels are falling. Symptoms vary between individuals but can be broadly divided between autonomic symptoms caused by the activation of the sympathoadrenal system, the neuroglycopenic symptoms resulting from cerebral glucose deprivation and symptoms caused by general malaise (Table D2).[3]

TABLE D2
Symptoms of hypoglycaemia

Autonomic symptoms (occur at approx. 3 mmol/L)	Neuroglycopenic symptoms (occur at approx. 2 mmol/L)	General malaise
Sweating	Confusion	Headache
Palpitations	Drowsiness	Nausea
Shaking	Odd behaviour	
Hunger	Speech difficulty	
	Incoordination	

Hypoglycaemia must be excluded in any person with diabetes who is acutely unwell, drowsy, unconscious, unable to cooperate or who presents with aggressive behaviour or seizures.

Patients who lose their autonomic symptoms (e.g. due to beta-blocker use) can be taught to recognise neuroglycopenic symptoms. However, these usually occur at lower blood glucose levels and thus the window for effective treatment is narrower.

Loss of 'hypo' awareness may be caused by maintaining a level of control that is too tight – if this is the case, a period of looser control may restore recognition.

Management of hypoglycaemia in adults (16 years and older)

See treatment algorithm (Figure D1) for brief guidance based on JBDS guidelines.[2] The quantity of carbohydrate given should be

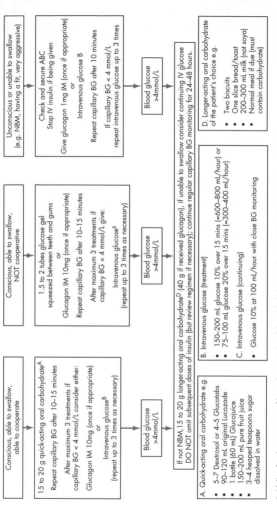

FIGURE D1   Guideline for the treatment of hypoglycaemia in adults with diabetes in hospital (blood glucose [BG] <4 mmol/L)
(if symptomatic but BG >4 mmol/L, give a small carbohydrate snack to relieve symptoms). NBM, nil-by-mouth; IM, intramuscularly; IV, intravenously

sufficient to treat the hypoglycaemic episode without substantially raising blood glucose levels after recovery.

Availability of 'hypo' treatments in clinical areas

- 15–20% of inpatients in England and Wales have known diabetes[4] and the prevalence of severe hypoglycaemia in hospital inpatients treated with insulin ranges from 5% to 32%.[5]
- The JBDS has recommended the availability of 'hypo' boxes in clinical areas.[2] These should contain quick-acting oral carbohydrate and also recommended concentrations of intravenous glucose.
- Intravenous glucose 10% or 20% should be available in all clinical areas in small-volume containers to avoid the risk of inadvertent administration of larger volumes: a glucose 20% 100 mL vial is available for this purpose.
- The use of glucose 50% intravenously is not recommended because of the higher risk of thrombophlebitis, extravasation injury and excessively raised posttreatment blood glucose levels.

Pharmaceutical care issues

- Fingers must be cleaned prior to capillary blood glucose testing. Contamination with glucose/sugar from self-treatment of a 'hypo' can mean essential treatment is withheld.
- Glucose 20% should ideally be given via central access but for emergency use peripheral administration via a large vein is acceptable. Glucose 10% must be given via central access only if the infusion continues for more than 24 hours. Give using an infusion pump if readily available but do not delay the infusion if not.
- All inpatients prescribed insulin or sulfonylureas should ideally also be prescribed an appropriate volume of intravenous glucose 10% or 20% to be given 'as required'. However, patients receiving metformin, pioglitazone, DPP-4 inhibitors, SLGT-2 inhibitors and GLP-1 analogues without insulin or sulfonylureas are unlikely to experience hypoglycaemia.
- Fruit juice is *not* an ideal 'hypo' treatment in patients following a low-potassium diet.
- In patients taking acarbose, hypoglycaemia (due to other agents) cannot be treated specifically with sugar in water because acarbose delays its absorption.
- Hypoglycaemia caused by sulfonylureas or long-acting insulin may recur: close monitoring is mandatory for 24–36 hours and a glucose infusion may be necessary.
- Intramuscular glucagon is only licensed for the treatment of insulin overdose. It works by mobilising liver glycogen and is less effective if patient is NBM, in malnutrition, in excessive alcohol intake, in severe liver disease, receiving sulfonylureas or experiencing repeated 'hypos'. Patients who have received glucagon require a

double portion of longer-acting carbohydrate to replenish glycogen
stores, but nausea may be an issue.
- After treating hypoglycaemia, *do not* omit insulin injection if due;
  however, the insulin regimen may require review.

'Pharmaceutical' risk factors for hypoglycaemia

- The most serious and common causes of inpatient hypoglycaemia
  are insulin prescribing errors, for example:
  - the use of abbreviations such as 'U' or 'IU' misread as a '0',
    resulting in a 10-fold overdose
  - confusing the insulin name with the dose, e.g. Humalog Mix50
    becoming Humalog 50 units
  - inappropriately timed insulin or oral hypoglycaemic therapy in
    relation to meals and inappropriate use of 'stat' doses
  - inadvertent restarting of previously stopped insulin or oral
    hypoglycaemic agents particularly at changes in care setting
  - transcription errors or unclear handwriting.
- Some drugs given in combination with insulin or sulfonylureas may
  increase the likelihood of hypoglycaemia, e.g. warfarin, quinine,
  salicylates, fibrates, sulfonamides (including co-trimoxazole),
  MAOIs, NSAIDs, probenecid, somatostatin analogues, SSRIs.
- Hypoglycaemia may be caused by sudden discontinuation of
  long-term glucocorticoid therapy.
- Whether acute or chronic, severe renal impairment may require
  reduction in insulin dose due to reduced insulin clearance and
  consequent increased insulin half-life.

REFERENCES

1 Diabetes Control and Complications Trial Research Group (1993). The effect of
  intensive treatment of diabetes on the development and progression of long-term
  complications in insulin-dependent diabetes mellitus. *N Engl J Med* 329: 977–986.
2 Joint British Diabetes In Patient Care Group (2010: revised 2013). *The Management
  of Hypoglycaemia in Adults with Diabetes Mellitus.* http://www.diabetes.org.uk/
  Documents/About%20Us/Our%20views/Care%20recs/JBDS%20hypoglycaemia%
  20position%20(2013).pdf (accessed 10 February 2014).
3 Deary IJ *et al.* (1993). Partitioning the symptoms of hypoglycaemia using multi-
  sample confirmatory factor analysis. *Diabetologia* 36: 771–777.
4 Sampson MJ *et al.* (2007). A national survey of in-patient diabetes services in the
  United Kingdom. *Diabet Med* 24: 643–649.
5 Farrokhi F *et al.* (2012). Hypoglycemia in the hospital setting. *Diabet Hypoglycemia*
  5: 3–8.

Diabetes mellitus: management of acute illness ('sick-day rules')

Illness can adversely affect diabetes control because of the increased
release of the counterregulatory hormones (cortisol, glucagon,
growth hormone and catecholamines) during stress. All patients with
diabetes mellitus should know what to do if they become acutely ill.

Specific guidance may be given to individuals by their own diabetes teams but the general principles of what to do if unwell are stated below:[1]

- Never stop insulin or tablets – illness usually increases the body's need for insulin.
- Test blood glucose level every 2 hours, day and night.
- Test urine for ketones every time you go to the toilet or test blood ketones every 2 hours if you have the equipment to do this.
- Try to drink at least 100 mL water or sugar-free fluid every hour – ideally you need at least 2.5 litres per day during illness (approximately 5 pints).
- Avoid strenuous exercise as this may increase your blood glucose level during illness.
- Eat as normally if possible. If you cannot eat or if you have a smaller appetite than normal during illness, replace solid food with one of the following: 400 mL milk, 200 mL carton fruit juice, 150–200 mL non-diet fizzy drink, 1 scoop ice cream.

Call your diabetes specialist nurse or general practitioner in the following circumstances:

- continuous diarrhoea and vomiting and/or high fever
- unable to keep down food for 4 hours or more
- high blood glucose levels with symptoms of illness (above 15 mmol/L). You may need an increased insulin dose[*]
- ketones at 2+ or 3+ in your urine or blood ketones 1.5 mmol/L or more. In this case, contact the person who normally looks after your diabetes immediately as you may need more insulin.[**]

REFERENCE

1 JBDS (2011). *Management of Adults with Diabetes Undergoing Surgery and Elective Procedures: Improving standards*. http://www.diabetes.org.uk/About_us/What -we-say/Improving-diabetes-healthcare/Management-of-adults-with-diabetes -undergoing-surgery-and-elective-procedures-improving-standards/ (accessed 13 February 2015).

Diabetes mellitus: monitoring and tests

The need for monitoring and control of diabetes mellitus (DM) is well established, although it is now recognised that raised blood glucose levels are merely an easily measurable surrogate for the underlying metabolic abnormalities occurring in uncontrolled DM.

[*]People with type 1 diabetes using the dose adjustment for normal eating (DAFNE) regimen are given detailed guidance on how to adjust their own insulin doses.

[**]Outside normal working hours contact the local out-of-hours service or attend your local hospital Emergency Department.

The Diabetes Control and Complications Trial (DCCT) (1993)[1] studied 1441 patients with type 1 DM and demonstrated that improved glycaemic control (and, by inference, other metabolic markers) decreased the likelihood of microvascular complications (retinopathy, neuropathy, nephropathy).

Similarly, the UK Prospective Diabetes Study Group (1998)[2] reported that improved glycaemic control and improved blood pressure control decreased complications associated with type 2 DM. Improved blood glucose control reduced the risk of major diabetic eye disease by a quarter and early kidney damage by a third. Improved blood pressure control reduced the risk of deaths from long-term complications of DM by a third, strokes by more than a third and serious deterioration of vision by more than a third.

Whilst tight blood glucose control produces the best results from the point of view of minimising complications, the risk of hypoglycaemia increases with tighter control, and inevitably has a negative impact on quality of life. All targets for control should be discussed and agreed with the patient.

Blood glucose monitoring

Generally the aim is to keep fasting and pre-meal capillary blood glucose levels at physiological concentrations, i.e. between 4 and 7 mmol/L. Tests performed 2 hours after meals should be no more than 8.5 mmol/L (type 2),[3] 9 mmol/L (type 1)[4] or 10 mmol/L (children).[4] These targets should be relaxed if there is a significant risk of disabling or unrecognised hypoglycaemia.

Frequency of testing for individual patients is determined by type of treatment and the ability of the patient or carers to respond to results. Insulin users and those starting new treatments should generally test more frequently, and blood glucose results should always be recorded and assessed so that appropriate action can be taken. N.B.: hypoglycaemic patients may recently have been handling glucose or sugar of some sort, which can affect capillary blood glucose results obtained by fingerprick.

Whilst mmol/L is the most common measurement unit used in the UK, mg/dL is the unit predominantly used in the USA and continental Europe (see Table D3 for conversions).

TABLE D3
Blood glucose conversions[5]

mmol/L	mg/dL	mmol/L	mg/dL	mmol/L	mg/dL	mmol/L	mg/dL
1	18	7	126	13	234	19	342
2	36	8	144	14	252	20	360
3	54	9	162	15	270	21	378
4	72	10	180	16	288	22	396
5	90	11	198	17	306	23	414
6	108	12	216	18	324	24	432

Urine glucose monitoring

In some patients urine glucose monitoring may be used. The urine only becomes positive for glucose once the patient's renal threshold for glucose excretion is exceeded. The renal threshold can vary widely between individuals, which can make urine testing unreliable. However, an individual's renal threshold should remain constant, thus enabling a judgement to be made about the patient's ongoing DM management. In most people the renal threshold for glucose is approximately 10 mmol/L, so a positive urine test indicates poor glycaemic control.

Urine tests lag behind blood glucose levels – these tests average what has happened to the patient's blood glucose level since s/he last passed urine. A patient may have a strongly positive urine glucose test and actually be hypoglycaemic.

Monitoring ketones

Ketones are a byproduct of lipid metabolism in the absence of insulin, so they are normally produced when patients with type 1 DM are severely insulin-deficient. They may also occur in severely stressed type 2 DM.

Previously it was only possible to monitor ketones using urine test strips, but now meters are increasingly available to check blood ketones (they measure 3-beta-hydroxybutyrate, the most significant of the three ketone bodies in blood).

Routine testing for ketones is not normally necessary but urine or blood testing may be used at home to assess severity of illness and to know when to seek medical help. During illness, ketones should be checked whenever urine is passed, or every 2 hours for blood ketones. Help should be sought from the diabetes team or general practitioner if urine ketones are 2+ or 3+ or blood ketones are ≥1.5 mmol/L (see *Diabetes mellitus – management of acute illness ('sick-day rules')* entry). Blood ketone monitoring is a significant part of the management of DKA and hyperosmolar hyperglycaemic state (see respective entries).

Clinic tests

Glycated haemoglobin (HbA$_{1c}$)

HbA$_{1c}$ is formed when glucose in the blood binds to haemoglobin in red blood cells: the higher the glucose, the higher the HbA$_{1c}$. HbA$_{1c}$ circulates for the lifespan of the red blood cell and so reflects the prevailing blood glucose levels over the 2–3 months prior to the test.

Generally, for an individual with DM, a target HbA$_{1c}$ of 48–58 mmol/mol should be agreed, taking into consideration the risk of severe hypoglycaemia, cardiovascular status and comorbidities.[3,4] Those at increased risk of arterial disease should ideally aim for >48 mmol/mol, whilst in children and those at risk from hypoglycaemia, 58 mmol/mol is acceptable.

HbA$_{1c}$ values were previously reported as a percentage (DCCT units), but now results are reported in mmol/mol (International

D

Federation of Clinical Chemistry (IFCC) units). See Table D4 for a comparison of these two types of result.

TABLE D4
HbA$_{1c}$ conversion[6]

IFCC (mmol/mol)	DCCT (%)	IFCC (mmol/mol)	DCCT (%)
36.6	5.5	63.9	8.0
42.1	6.0	69.4	8.5
47.5	6.5	74.9	9.0
53	7.0	80.3	9.5
58.5	7.5	85.8	10

IFCC, International Federation of Clinical Chemistry; DCCT, Diabetes Control and Complications Trial.

C-peptide

When insulin is synthesised by the beta cells of the pancreas it is produced as proinsulin. This molecule is then cleaved at two sites and the end segments are joined to form the active insulin molecule. The centre segment (C-peptide) is released with the insulin and the presence of C-peptide therefore indicates that an individual's pancreas is producing insulin. Injected insulin does not have a C-peptide component so the test can be used to distinguish between patients who have some residual pancreatic function and those who do not. In insulin resistance, C-peptide levels are raised because the patient may be hyperinsulinaemic despite being hyperglycaemic.

C-peptide was not previously thought to have any known function but recent research suggests that it may have a beneficial role in preventing microvascular complications.

Oral glucose tolerance test (OGTT)

This test may be used to distinguish between impaired glucose tolerance, impaired fasting glucose and DM.

The OGTT should not be performed during intercurrent illness or prolonged bed rest. For 24 hours prior to the test alcohol is avoided,

TABLE D5
Interpretation of oral glucose tolerance test results[7]

Diagnosis	Plasma glucose concentration	
Diabetes mellitus	Fasting	≥7.0 mmol/L or
	2 hours post glucose load	≥11.1 mmol/L
Impaired glucose tolerance	Fasting	<7.0 mmol/L and
	2 hours post glucose load	≥7.8 mmol/L and <11.1 mmol/L
Impaired fasting glucose	Fasting	6.1–6.9 mmol/L and (if measured)
	2 hours post glucose load	<7.8 mmol/L

and for 12 hours prior to the test no food should be taken. Water may be taken freely as required. Glucose (75 g) is consumed within 5 minutes and venous blood samples are taken immediately preceding and 2 hours after the glucose load. The interpretation of test results is shown in Table D5.

REFERENCES

1 Diabetes Control and Complications Trial Research Group (1993). The effect of intensive treatment of diabetes on the development and progression of long-term complications in insulin-dependent diabetes mellitus. *N Engl J Med* 329: 977–986.

2 UK Prospective Diabetes Study Group (1998). Intensive blood glucose control with sulphonylureas or insulin compared with conventional treatment and risk of complications in patients with type 2 diabetes (UKPDS 33). *Lancet* 352: 837–853.

3 NICE (2009). Clinical Guideline 87. *The Management of Type 2 Diabetes.* https://www.nice.org.uk/guidance/cg87 (accessed 23 February 2015).

4 NICE (2004). Clinical Guideline 15. *Type 1 Diabetes: Diagnosis and management of type 1 diabetes in children, young people and adults.* https://www.nice.org.uk/guidance/cg15 (accessed 23 February 2015).

5 Diabetes UK (2015). *Blood Sugar Converter.* http://www.diabetes.co.uk/blood-sugar-converter.html (accessed 21 February 2015).

6 Diabetes UK (2015). *HbA1c Units Converter.* http://www.diabetes.co.uk/hba1c-units-converter.html (accessed 21 February 2015).

7 WHO (2006). *Definition and Diagnosis of Diabetes Mellitus and Intermediate Hyperglycemia.* https://www.idf.org/webdata/docs/WHO_IDF_definition_diagnosis_of_diabetes.pdf (accessed 23 February 2015).

Diabetic ketoacidosis

Diabetic ketoacidosis (DKA) is a potentially life-threatening, complex disordered metabolic state characterised by ketonaemia, hyperglycaemia (although this may have been partially self-treated before admission) and acidaemia.

It usually occurs in people known to have type 1 diabetes mellitus (DM) (however, DKA may be the presenting condition in newly diagnosed patients), but type 2 DM patients can also develop DKA if sufficiently stressed (e.g. by surgery, severe infection or myocardial infarction (MI) and mortality remains high among non-hospitalised patients. Mortality has fallen in the last 20 years in patients receiving prompt and effective treatment: in this group cerebral oedema is the most common cause of death in children and adolescents, whereas the main causes of mortality in adults include severe hypokalaemia, adult respiratory distress syndrome and comorbid states, e.g. pneumonia, MI and sepsis[1] (see *Hyperosmolar hyperglycaemic state* entry).

Diagnosis of DKA[2]

The diagnosis of DKA is made if:

- blood ketones ≥ 3 mmol/L or there is significant ketonuria, i.e. 2+ or more on urine dipsticks
- blood glucose is > 11 mmol/L or known DM
- serum venous bicarbonate < 15 mmol/L and/or venous pH < 7.3.

Management of DKA in adults

In 2010 the JBDS Inpatient Care Group published guidance on treating DKA in adults,[2] so all Trusts should have a policy or care pathway in place. The main focus of treatment is now correction of the underlying metabolic abnormality rather than simply the normalisation of blood glucose levels. This has been facilitated by the easy availability of accurate bedside blood glucose and ketone meters, and rapid access to blood gas and blood electrolyte measurement. Early escalation to critical care should be considered in pregnant women, as well as patients with hypokalaemia at presentation, hypoxia, altered consciousness, hypotension, tachycardia or severe ketoacidosis (as indicated by blood ketones >6 mmol/L, venous bicarbonate <5 mmol/L or pH <7.1).

Separate guidelines exist for the treatment of children and adolescents.[3]

Fluid

Fluid and electrolyte deficits may be significant because of osmotic diuresis and vomiting (Table D6) and fluid replacement must be initiated promptly. For patients in whom judicious fluid replacement is required, e.g. elderly patients or those with impaired cardiac function, a central venous pressure (CVP) line may be inserted.

TABLE D6

Typical fluid and electrolyte deficits in diabetic ketoacidosia[2]

Water	100 mL/kg
Sodium	7–10 mmol/kg
Chloride	3–5 mmol/kg
Potassium	3–5 mmol/kg

Sodium chloride 0.9% is currently recommended as the fluid of choice because of lack of availability of licensed Hartmann's solution with adequate ready-mixed potassium.[4]

Table D7 gives an example of fluid replacement for a previously well 70-kg adult.[2] Slower infusion rates should be considered in young adults because of the increased risk of cerebral oedema.

TABLE D7

An example of fluid replacement for a previously well 70-kg adult

Sodium chloride 0.9% 1 L*	1000 mL over first hour
Sodium chloride 0.9% 1 L with potassium chloride	1000 mL over next 2 hours
Sodium chloride 0.9% 1 L with potassium chloride	1000 mL over next 2 hours
Sodium chloride 0.9% 1 L with potassium chloride	1000 mL over next 4 hours
Sodium chloride 0.9% 1 L with potassium chloride	1000 mL over next 4 hours
Sodium chloride 0.9% 1 L with potassium chloride	1000 mL over next 6 hours

Reassessment of cardiovascular status at 12 hours is mandatory; further fluid may be required

*Potassium chloride may be required if >1 L sodium chloride has already been given as fluid resuscitation.

If blood glucose falls below 14 mmol/L (usually 6–12 hours into treatment for DKA), commence 10% glucose at 125 mL/hour while continuing the sodium chloride 0.9% infusion, as further hydration is likely to be necessary. Giving glucose enables insulin administration to continue so that ketogenesis is suppressed.

After 12 hours, if DKA is resolved but patient is still unable to eat and drink, then convert to an intravenous variable-rate insulin infusion policy, as per local guidelines.

Potassium

Patients with DKA usually present with hyperkalaemia because of insulin deficiency; however, this represents a shift of potassium from the intracellular to the extracellular fluid and these patients actually have a total body potassium deficiency. A high initial potassium serum concentration should prompt cardiac monitoring until levels have returned to normal.

Once insulin is given, potassium levels can change rapidly: all patients require serum potassium measurement on admission and at least every 2 hours throughout treatment to assess requirements. Potassium is not usually added to the first litre of sodium chloride 0.9% but should be provided in subsequent bags to maintain normal serum potassium levels (Table D8).

TABLE D8
Suitable potassium replacement levels in diabetic ketoacidosis

Potassium level in first 24 hours	Potassium chloride to be added
<3.5 mmol/L	Senior review as additional potassium is essential (if necessary, via a central line in the High Dependency Unit)
3.5–5.5 mmol/L	40 mmol/L of fluid
>5.5 mmol/L	None

Intravenous insulin

1 A fixed-rate insulin infusion is recommended by the JBDS of 0.1 unit/kg/hour to suppress ketogenesis, reduce blood glucose and correct electrolyte imbalance. This is based on actual body weight: estimate if necessary.
2 Insulin may be infused in the same line as the intravenous replacement fluid, provided that a Y-connector with a one-way, antisyphon valve is used and a large-bore cannula has been placed.
3 A syringe pump should be set up containing 50 units of soluble insulin in 50 mL sodium chloride 0.9% and this should be infused at a starting rate of 0.1 unit/kg/hour.
4 Patients admitted on long-acting basal insulin analogues, e.g. glargine or Levemir, should continue on their usual dose while they are receiving the fixed-rate insulin infusion.

Monitoring

Measure blood ketones and capillary blood glucose every hour, ideally using quality-assured bedside meters. Measure venous blood gas for pH, bicarbonate and potassium at 60 minutes, at 2 hours and 2-hourly thereafter. Treatment targets are to:

- reduce blood ketone concentration by 0.5 mmol/L per hour
- increase venous bicarbonate by 3 mmol/L per hour
- reduce capillary blood glucose by 3 mmol/L per hour (but avoid hypoglycaemia)
- maintain serum potassium concentration between 4.0 and 5.0 mmol/L
- monitor fluid balance: aim for minimum urine output of 0.5 mL/kg per hour.

Further action

- If ketones and glucose are not falling as expected, always check that the insulin infusion pump is connected and working correctly.
- If blood ketones are not falling by at least 0.5 mmol/L per hour, call a prescribing clinician to increase insulin infusion rate by 1 unit/hour increments every hour until ketones fall at target rates (if blood ketone levels are not available, use either bicarbonate or plasma glucose as a surrogate and adjust insulin infusion rate accordingly).
- Resolution of DKA is defined as ketones <0.3 mmol/L, venous pH >7.3.

Additional pharmaceutical points

- All patients should receive low-molecular-weight heparin venous thromboembolism prophylaxis.[5]
- Intravenous bicarbonate is rarely indicated because adequate fluid and insulin therapy will resolve acidosis in DKA. If used, it should only be initiated on the instructions of a senior physician.[6,7]
- The patient's usual insulin regimen must be determined on admission so that any contributing factors can be highlighted and long-acting basal insulin analogues continued if appropriate.
- Subcutaneous insulin should be introduced or restarted as soon as the patient is biochemically stable and feels able to eat and drink. For all regimens the intravenous insulin infusion should be continued for at least 30–60 minutes after giving the subcutaneous dose in association with a meal.
- For patients not previously on insulin, the specialist diabetes team should be involved.

REFERENCES

1 Hamblin PS *et al.* (1989). Deaths associated with diabetic ketoacidosis and hyperosmolar coma, 1973–1988. *Med J Aust* 151: 439–444.
2 Joint British Diabetes Societies Inpatient Care Group (2010). *The Management of Diabetic Ketoacidosis in Adults.* London: Diabetes UK. http://www.diabetes.org.uk/About_us/Our_Views/Care_recommendations/The-Management-of-Diabetic-Ketoacidosis-in-Adults/ (accessed 14 September 2014).

3 BSPED (2009: minor review 2013). *Recommended DKA Guidelines*. http://www.bsped.org.uk/clinical/docs/DKAGuideline.pdf (accessed 3 February 2015).

4 NPSA (2002). *Potassium Chloride Concentrate Solutions – Patient safety alert*. http://www.nrls.npsa.nhs.uk/resources/?entryid45=59882 (accessed 17 January 2015).

5 NICE (2010). Clinical Guideline 92. *Venous Thromboembolism: Reducing the risk of venous thromboembolism (deep vein thrombosis and pulmonary embolism) in patients admitted to hospital*. http://www.nice.org.uk/guidance/cg92 (accessed 3 February 2015).

6 Morris LR *et al.* (1986). Bicarbonate therapy in severe diabetic ketoacidosis. *Ann Intern Med* 105: 836–840.

7 Hale PJ *et al.* (1984). Metabolic effects of bicarbonate in the treatment of diabetic ketoacidosis. *BMJ (Clin Res Ed)* 289: 1035–1038.

Digoxin

Digoxin is one of the oldest drugs in cardiovascular medicine, and traditionally used in patients with atrial fibrillation (AF) and heart failure (HF). In the last 20 years, the use of this drug has markedly declined and, in the most recent 2012 European Society of Cardiology (ESC) HF guidelines,[1] it is stated that for patients with HF and a left ventricular ejection fraction ≤40%, who are in sinus rhythm, 'digoxin may be used'. This recommendation is based on the Digitalis Investigation Group (DIG) trial,[2] in which the effect of digoxin on outcome was examined in 6800 patients with HF. For HF patients with AF, other drugs (in particular beta-blockers) should be preferred,[1] since they provide better rate control. Both the 2010 ESC AF Guidelines[3] and 2014 NICE AF guidance[4] state that digoxin is effective for long-term rate control at rest, but not during exercise. Prospective, randomised, placebo-controlled outcome studies examining the effect of digoxin in patients with AF (with or without HF) are not available.

Digoxin in heart failure

In the past, it was assumed that the beneficial effect of digoxin in HF was due to its (positive) inotropic properties, which are more pronounced at higher doses of the drug.[5] However, a large number of studies in patients with HF have shown that positive inotropic drugs lead to an unfavourable effect on outcome, and these drugs are now contraindicated in patients with chronic HF. In contrast to this inotropic effect, digoxin also exerts potentially favourable autonomic- or neurohormonal-inhibiting properties, which primarily occur at lower serum digoxin concentrations (SDCs).[6] This has been increasingly recognised in the last 25 years, and a post-hoc analysis of the DIG trial[7] showed that, in patients who received digoxin, low SDC (0.5–0.9 ng/mL) was associated with a lower all-cause mortality than in patients in the placebo group (29.3% vs 32.9%, adjusted hazard ratio 0.77, $P < 0.001$), while all-cause mortality in patients with SDC ≥1.0 was 41.7% (P = not significant for adjusted hazard ratio). However, no well-designed prospective trials have been conducted to confirm these findings.

More recently,[8] the effects of the sinus node inhibitor ivabradine in the Systolic Heart failure treatment with the *If* inhibitor Ivabradine Trial (SHIFT) were compared with the effect of digoxin in the DIG trial, and they showed a remarkable similarity. The composite morbidity–mortality outcome of cardiovascular death and HF hospitalisation (the most common endpoint in current HF trials) was reduced by 18% in SHIFT and by 15% in the DIG trial. In both trials, the main effect was on HF hospitalisations, which was −26% in SHIFT and −28% in DIG. However, it must be noted that in SHIFT this effect was against a background of other drugs, in particular beta-blockers, whereas in DIG no beta-blockers were used. Therefore, digoxin in patients with HF may still have a place, as a neurohormonal modulator, when given in low doses. Indeed, low-dose digoxin may still be useful, but trials examining this question are urgently needed.

Digoxin in atrial fibrillation

In a rate control strategy, the main goal of arrhythmia management becomes control of the ventricular rate. In patients with persistent and permanent AF, rate control applies continuously. In patients with paroxysmal AF, the objective of rate control is to limit ventricular response during an AF episode.

Poor control of the ventricular rate can be a major factor contributing to disability and symptom limitation in many patients with AF. Conduction through the atrioventricular node is under autonomic control and increases markedly with activity levels, so the goal of rate control is to avoid excessive rate increase with activity.[4] The primary effect of digoxin is slowing down atrioventricular conduction, leading to a reduction in ventricular response at rest, but much less so during exercise.[2] This effect of digoxin is due to enhancement of vagal tone and is less prominent during increased sympathetic activity, such as exercise, and it is for this reason that the NICE AF guidance states that digoxin should only be considered as monotherapy in sedentary patients.[4] Beta-blockers are more effective than digoxin in slowing heart rate during exercise in patients with AF, and beta-blockers now have a prominent place in AF patients, both with and without HF, and seem to have replaced digoxin in many patients. Digoxin should only be considered as monotherapy in sedentary patients, as it is less effective for rate control during exercise or in conditions of high sympathetic drive (e.g. infection or decompensated heart failure).

Formulations

Digoxin is available in three forms: tablet, liquid and injection. Each form has a different bioavailability (tablets 63%, liquid 75%, injection 100%) and, if changing between forms, the dose will need to be changed accordingly. It may be necessary to round a dose up or down to facilitate administration. Table D9 summarises practical dose equivalences of the formulations.

TABLE D9
Dose equivalence of digoxin formulations

Tablet (micrograms)	Liquid (micrograms)	Injection (micrograms)
62.5	50	50
125	100	75
250	200	150

Rationale for monitoring

Digoxin has a narrow therapeutic range, and therefore it may be necessary to check the serum concentration in the following circumstances:

- in suspected, or actual, overdose
- if the patient is showing signs of digoxin toxicity
- if the patient's renal function shows signs of deterioration
- if any drugs are added, or withdrawn, that are known to affect the serum concentration of digoxin or serum potassium concentration (see section on *Significant drug interactions*, below).

Therapeutic drug monitoring

During therapeutic drug monitoring, the target blood concentration will depend upon the indication (Table D10). For HF, a positive inotropic effect is needed and this is achieved at lower concentrations than the negative chronotropic effect needed to control AF.

TABLE D10
Drug monitoring information

Half-life	20–50 hours (in renal impairment it can be up to 100 hours)[10]
Pretreatment measures	(U&Es particularly potassium), creatinine, weight and age (and height if obese)[11] Thyroid function: digoxin sensitivity is enhanced when thyroid function is subnormal. In hyperthyroidism there is relative digoxin resistance and the dose may have to be increased
Therapeutic range	For heart failure: 0.9–1.5 microgram/L (1.2–1.9 nmol/L) For atrial fibrillation: 1.5–2.0 microgram/L (1.9–2.6 nmol/L) Toxic effects become frequent above 2.5 microgram/L (3.2 nmol/L)
Sampling time	At least 6 hours postdose. If monitoring is anticipated, the dose is best given in the evening and a sample taken the following morning. In some hospitals the digoxin dose is routinely given in the evening to facilitate this. Response to dose adjustment should be checked 7–10 days after the change (because of its long half-life). Blood should be taken in 'brown-top' sample tubes
Other monitoring	U&Es occasionally to monitor renal function. Thyroid function periodically (where thyrotoxicosis is being treated, digoxin dosage should be reduced as the thyrotoxicosis comes under control)

Potassium depletion increases the response of tissues to digoxin and can cause toxicity. A reduction in serum potassium concentration from 3.5 to 3.0 mmol/L is accompanied by an increase in sensitivity to digoxin of about 50% and digoxin toxicity may be present despite the serum digoxin concentration being in the apparent therapeutic range. To interpret a serum digoxin concentration, the serum potassium concentration must also be measured at the same time. In patients with hypokalaemia, the digoxin dose should be withheld (whatever the serum digoxin concentration) until the hypokalaemia is corrected.[9]

Dose

Loading dose (also known as 'digitalisation')

If a patient has not received cardiac glycosides in the preceding 2 weeks, a loading dose may be given. There are three approaches to loading digoxin: parenterally in an emergency situation, and rapid and slow oral loading. An assessment should be made of the patient's age, lean body weight and renal function to help determine the loading dose.

Emergency parenteral loading

For emergency parenteral loading (in patients who have not received cardiac glycosides within the preceding 2 weeks), the dose range is usually 500–1000 micrograms.[10] Approximately half the total anticipated dose should be given initially, and further fractions of the total dose given every 4–8 hours. The clinical response should be assessed after each additional dose to determine if the remainder of the loading dose is required.

The dose is given as a small-volume infusion. Digoxin injection must be diluted to at least four times its volume – in practice this will mean using a 50 mL or 100 mL mini-bag, containing either sodium chloride 0.9% or glucose 5%. The infusion should be given over at least 2 hours.

Digoxin should never be given as a bolus injection, as this can cause heart block and arrhythmia, possibly resulting in patient death.

Rapid oral loading

A dose of 750–1500 micrograms is given as a single dose. If there is less urgency, or the patient is at risk of toxicity (elderly, renal impairment), the dose should be given in divided doses 6 hours apart, with assessment of clinical response before giving each additional dose.

Slow oral loading

A daily dose of 250–500 micrograms is given daily for 1 week, followed by an appropriate maintenance dose.

Maintenance dose

In practice, prescribers often pick a dose intuitively; however, an appropriate digoxin dose for a given patient can be calculated using the steps described below. As interpatient variability can influence the digoxin concentration and therefore the patient's clinical response, the predicted values should only be used as a guide.

1 Calculate ideal body weight (IBW):

For men: IBW (kg) = 50 kg + 2.3 kg for each inch over 5 feet

For women: IBW (kg) = 49 kg + 1.7 kg for each inch over 5 feet

2 Calculate creatinine clearance (CrCl: mL/min):

$$\text{Male} = \frac{1.23 \times (140 - \text{age (years)}) \times \text{weight (kg)}}{\text{serum creatinine concentration (micromol/L)}}$$

$$\text{Female} = \frac{1.04 \times (140 - \text{age (years)}) \times \text{weight (kg)}}{\text{serum creatinine concentration (micromol/L)}}$$

If the patient's actual body weight (ABW) is within 20% of IBW, use the ABW in the above calculation and subsequent dosing.

3 Calculate digoxin clearance (DigCl: L/hour)

$$\text{DigCl} = (0.06 \times \text{CrCl}) + (0.05 \times \text{IBW weight (kg)})$$

Patients with HF require this modified calculation.

$$\text{DigCl (with HF)} = (0.053 \times \text{CrCl}) + (0.02 \times \text{weight (kg)})$$

4 Calculate predicted steady state level for a specific dose (C_{pss}: microgram/L):

$$C_{pss} = \frac{(F \times D)}{(\text{DigCl} \times \tau)}$$

F = bioavailability (tablets = 0.63; liquid = 0.75; injection = 1)

D = digoxin dose (micrograms), τ = dosage interval in hours.

The units the calculation produces for the predicted steady state of digoxin are in microgram/L. If a laboratory interprets results using nmol/L, the figures must be converted (nmol/L = microgram/L × 1.28).

The predicted steady-state figure should be increased if certain interacting drugs are present, or added to therapy (see below for details).

Significant drug interactions[12]

Amiodarone can approximately double the serum concentration of digoxin. The effect is evident after a few days and develops over 1–4 weeks. If amiodarone is stopped, the interaction can continue for several months due to its long half-life. If the two drugs are prescribed together, the dose of digoxin should be halved.[13]

Verapamil increases serum digoxin concentration by about 40% with a daily dose of 160 mg verapamil, and by about 70% with a daily dose of 240 mg verapamil. The digoxin dose should be reduced and serum digoxin concentration monitored if verapamil is added to therapy.

Spironolactone can increase serum digoxin concentration by 25%. Furthermore, many digoxin assays are affected by spironolactone and its metabolite, which makes monitoring difficult.

Potassium-depleting diuretics are thought to be implicated in increased digoxin toxicity. It is common practice in some hospitals to reduce this complication by co-prescribing potassium supplements or potassium-sparing diuretics.

Macrolide antibiotics (erythromycin, azithromycin and clarithromycin) can produce a two- to fourfold increase in digoxin serum concentration. The interaction is unpredictable, however, and is further complicated as one of the proposed mechanisms of the interaction may only affect up to 10% of the population. Patients should be monitored for signs of digoxin toxicity and the digoxin dose reduced if necessary (azithromycin has a 60-hour half-life so the interaction may persist for some time after the antibiotic course has finished).

Overdose – treatment with DigiFab

DigiFab is an immunoglobulin indicated for the treatment of known (or strongly suspected) life-threatening digoxin toxicity associated with ventricular arrhythmias or bradyarrhythmias unresponsive to atropine, where measures beyond withdrawal of digoxin and correction of serum electrolyte abnormalities are considered necessary.

There are several formulae for calculating the required dose of DigiFab depending on the clinical situation, and these should be consulted.[14] Each vial of DigiFab contains 40 mg of digoxin immune Fab and binds approximately 0.5 mg digoxin.

Administration

Each vial of DigiFab should be reconstituted with 4 mL water for injection and gently mixed, producing a solution of 10 mg/mL that should be used immediately. This may be added to a suitable volume of 0.9% sodium chloride (e.g. 50–100 mL mini-bag) and administered over at least 30 minutes. If infusion rate-related reactions occur, the infusion should be stopped and restarted at a slower rate. If cardiac arrest is imminent, DigiFab can be given by bolus injection, although there is an increased incidence of infusion-related reactions.[14]

DigiFab has a high affinity for digoxin that is greater than the affinity of digoxin for its sodium pump receptor, the presumed receptor for its therapeutic and toxic effects. When administered to the intoxicated patient, digoxin immune Fab binds to molecules of digoxin, reducing free digoxin levels; this results in a shift in the equilibrium away from binding to the receptors, thereby reducing cardiotoxic effects. Fab–digoxin complexes are then cleared by the kidney and reticuloendothelial system.[15]

Standard digoxin serum assays cannot be used to determine free, pharmacologically active digoxin after administration of DigiFab because these also detect Fab-bound digoxin. Total serum digoxin concentration may rise precipitously after DigiFab is given, but this will be almost entirely bound to Fab fragment and will not exert a pharmacological effect.[16]

REFERENCES

1 McMurray JJV et al. (2012). ESC guidelines for the diagnosis and treatment of acute and chronic heart failure 2012: the Task Force for the Diagnosis and Treatment of Acute and Chronic Heart Failure 2012 of the European Society of Cardiology. Developed in collaboration with the Heart Failure Association (HFA) of the ESC. Eur Heart J 33: 1787–1847.

2 The Digitalis Investigation Group (1997). The effect of digoxin on mortality and morbidity in patients with heart failure. N Engl J Med 336: 525–533.

3 Camm AJ et al. (2010). Guidelines for the management of atrial fibrillation. Eur Heart J 31: 2369–2429.

4 NICE (2014). Atrial Fibrillation: The management of atrial fibrillation (CG180). https://www.nice.org.uk/guidance/cg180 (accessed 24 January 2015).

5 Gheorghiade M et al. (2006). Contemporary use of digoxin in the management of cardiovascular disorders. Circulation 113: 2556–2564.

6 Van Veldhuisen DJ et al. (2013). Digoxin for patients with atrial fibrillation and heart failure: paradise lost or not? Eur Heart J 34: 1468–1470.

7 Ahmed A et al. (2006). Digoxin and reduction in mortality and hospitalization in heart failure: a comprehensive post hoc analysis of the DIG trial. Eur Heart J 27: 178–186.

8 Castagno D et al. (2012). Should we SHIFT our thinking about digoxin? Observations on ivabradine and heart rate reduction in heart failure. Eur Heart J 33: 1137–1141.

9 Aronson JK, Hardman M (1992). ABC of monitoring drug therapy: digoxin. BMJ 305: 1149–1152.

10 Dollery C (ed.) (1999). Therapeutic Drugs (2nd edn). Edinburgh: Churchill Livingstone.

11 eMC (2015). www.medicines.org.uk (accessed 24 January 2015).

12 Stockley's Drug Interactions (2015). www.medicinescomplete.com (accessed 24 January 2015).

13 Joint Formulary Committee (2014). British National Formulary (68th edn). London: BMJ Group and Pharmaceutical Press.

14 Resuscitation Council (UK) (2010). DigiFab. http://www.resus.org.uk/newsletr/nl12Wdf5.pdf (accessed 24 January 2015).

15 DigiFab, 40 mg/vial Digoxin Immune Fab, Powder for solution for infusion. http://www.mhra.gov.uk/home/groups/par/documents/websiteresources/con126289.pdf (accessed 5 December 2014).

16 National Poisons Information Service. Toxbase. http://www.toxbase.org (accessed 30 August 2015).

Dobutamine

Dobutamine is a positive inotrope which acts on β_1, β_2 and α receptors. Its predominant action on β_1 receptors causes increased force of cardiac contraction, therefore increasing cardiac output and stroke volume. At higher doses it will increase heart rate. It is also a potent vasodilator and as such will speed up the rewarming process following prolonged surgery.

The main use of dobutamine is in heart failure and cardiogenic shock, usually in combination with a low dose of dopamine. Hypovolaemia should be corrected prior to administration.[1]

The dose range for dobutamine is 2.5–10 microgram/kg/min (although up to 40 microgram/kg/min has occasionally been required).[2] It should be given as a continuous intravenous infusion.[3] A simple calculation and method for making a dobutamine infusion is as follows:

- body weight (kg) × 3 (mg) = dose (mg)
- dilute to 50 mL with sodium chloride 0.9% (or glucose 5%)
- each mL/hour is equivalent to 1 microgram/kg/min
- dose of dobutamine is usually 5–10 microgram/kg/min, i.e. 5–10 mL/hour.

Administration

Dobutamine infusions may be given at rates up to 5 microgram/kg/min without cardiac output monitoring. Higher doses require monitoring[4] and treatment should be stopped gradually.[2]

Dobutamine is compatible with sodium chloride 0.9% and glucose 5%.[5]

It is Y-site-compatible with adrenaline, amiodarone, atropine, calcium gluconate, dopamine, glyceryl trinitrate, hydralazine, isoprenaline, lidocaine, magnesium sulfate, noradrenaline, potassium chloride and sodium nitroprusside (in sodium chloride).

It is not compatible with aminophylline, digoxin, furosemide or sodium bicarbonate.[6]

REFERENCES

1 AHFS Drug Information (2014). *Dobutamine*. Medicines Complete: AHFS. https://www.medicinescomplete.com/mc/index.htm (accessed 15 July 2014).
2 Martindale (2014). *The Complete Drug Reference*. Medicines Complete: Martindale. https://www.medicinescomplete.com/mc/martindale/current/ (accessed 15 July 2014).
3 SPC (2014). *Dobutamine*. eMC. https://www.medicines.org.uk/emc/medicine/ 21491 (accessed 15 July 2014).
4 SPC (2004). *Posiject*. http://emc.medicines.org.uk/ (accessed 15 November 2004).
5 Welsh Intensive care website (2005). *Guidelines*. www.clinicalschool.swan.ac.uk/ wics/itugl/dop.htm (accessed 11 December 2004).
6 Shulman R *et al.* (eds) (2002). *Injectable Drug Administration Guide*. London: Blackwell Science.

Dopamine

Dopamine is a positive inotrope and its action relates to the dose administered. At low doses, i.e. 2 microgram/kg/min, dopamine stimulates the dopamine receptors in the kidneys, causing renal dilatation and increased urine output.[1]

At slightly higher doses, i.e. 2–10 microgram/kg/min, dopamine begins to stimulate the β_1 receptors in the heart, producing an increase in cardiac output. It is used in acute heart failure due to cardiogenic shock or myocardial infarction, renal failure, cardiac surgery and septic shock.[2] Do not offer low-dose dopamine to treat acute kidney injury.[3]

Once the dose is increased to more than 10 microgram/kg/min, dopamine also acts on α-receptors, causing vasoconstriction, which leads to impairment of renal perfusion. There is also an increased risk of arrhythmias.

Dose should be reduced gradually before discontinuation as stopping the infusion suddenly may cause hypotension.

It is given as an intravenous infusion using a pump, not a gravity-controlled intravenous set.[4]

Dose

- 2–5 microgram/kg/min increased gradually by increments of 5–10 microgram/kg/min until optimum dose for patient is reached.[5]
- Dilute with sodium chloride 0.9% (or glucose 5%). The usual dilution is 1600 micrograms per mL.[5]

Administration

Dopamine should be administered via a central line because of the risk of extravasation, which can be exacerbated by local vasoconstriction. If this is not possible, it may be given via the largest peripheral vein available, provided that the concentration does not exceed 1.6 mg/mL. If extravasation occurs, infiltration with phentolamine as soon as possible, and certainly within 12 hours, may relieve pain and prevent tissue necrosis.[6] Phentolamine 5 mg is mixed with 9 mL sodium chloride 0.9%, and a small amount is injected into the extravasated area; blanching should reverse immediately. If blanching should recur, additional injections of phentolamine may be needed.[7]

Dopamine is compatible with sodium chloride 0.9% and glucose 5%.[7–10]

It is Y-site-compatible with adrenaline, aminophylline, amiodarone, atracurium, dobutamine, doxapram, glyceryl trinitrate, heparin, insulin, labetalol, lidocaine, mannitol, noradrenaline, potassium chloride and sodium nitroprusside.

It is not compatible with alkaline agents, e.g. sodium bicarbonate and furosemide.[2]

Dopamine has significant interactions with MAOIs, α/β adrenergic blocking agents and general anaesthetics.[4]

Miscellany

Some hospitals do not use dopamine routinely because it is not renoprotective, and it is now known to suppress the output of the anterior pituitary gland (with the exception of adrenocorticotrophic hormone).[11]

REFERENCES

1 McCrory C, Cunningham AJ (1997). Low-dose dopamine: will there ever be a scientific rationale? *Br J Anaesth* 78: 350–351.

2 Martindale (2014). *Dopamine*. Medicines Complete: Martindale. https://www.medicinescomplete.com/mc/martindale/current/ (accessed 14 July 2014).

3 NICE (2013). *Acute Kidney Injury: Prevention, detection and management of acute kidney injury up to the point of renal replacement therapy*. NICE: CG169. http://www.nice.org.uk/guidance/CG169 (accessed 14 July 2014).

4 AHFS Drug Information (2014). *Dopamine*. Medicines Complete: AHFS. https://www.medicinescomplete.com/mc/index.htm (accessed 14 July 2014).

5 SPC (2014). *Dopamine 40mg/1mL Concentrate for Solution for Infusion*. www.medicines.org.uk (accessed 14 July 2014).

6 Martindale (2014). *The Complete Drug Reference*. Medicines Complete: Martindale. https://www.medicinescomplete.com/mc/martindale/current/ (accessed 15 July 2014).

7 Evanston Northwestern Healthcare (2005). *Dopamine Antidote*. http://www.enh.org/healthandwellness/bioterrorism/hf045600.asp?lid=1092/ (accessed 14 July 2014).

8 SPC (2014). *Dopamine Hydrochloride 800 mg in 5% Dextrose Injection*. www.medicines.org.uk (accessed 14 July 2014).

9 SPC (2014). *Dopamine 160 mg/mL Sterile Concentrate*. www.medicines.org.uk (accessed 14 July 2014).

10 SPC (2014). *Sterile Dopamine Concentrate BP Selectajet*. www.medicines.org.uk (accessed 14 July 2014).

11 Welsh Intensive care website (2005). *Guidelines*. www.clinicalschool.swan.ac.uk/wics/itugl/dop.htm (accessed 14 July 2014).

DVLA: advice concerning medication and medical conditions

Medical conditions

The UK Driver and Vehicle Licensing Agency (DVLA) specifies a set of notifiable conditions that may affect the ability to drive safely.[1] These can include:

- epilepsy
- stroke
- neurological and mental health conditions
- physical disability
- visual impairments.

Patients must inform the DVLA if they are diagnosed with any of these conditions or if their condition worsens since being issued with a licence. A full list of health conditions and advice is available on the DVLA website: https://www.gov.uk/health-conditions-and-driving.

Medication and driving

Section 4 of the Road Traffic Act 1988 identifies the offence to drive whilst impaired through drug use. The decision as to whether a person is impaired on any occasion is the responsibility of the driver.

Prescribers and suppliers of medicines must give sufficient clinical advice to patients. This might include:

- Alert patients that they may experience symptoms of sleepiness, poor coordination, impaired or slow thinking, dizziness or visual problems.
- Warn that the effects of a drug may be greatest at initiation or with dose changes.
- Consider drug interactions and disease interactions that may increase the risk of driving being impaired.

A new offence of driving came into force in March 2015, which refers to driving with a specified controlled drug in the body in excess of a specified limit.[2] A list of these drugs can be found in the guidance document. However, this legislation allows a patient to raise statutory medical defence if the drug was lawfully prescribed, supplied or bought over the counter and the drug was taken in accordance with advice given by the prescriber or supplier.[2]

REFERENCE

1 DVLA (2015). *Medical Conditions, Disabilities and Driving*. https://www.gov.uk/driving-medical-conditions (accessed 9 February 2015).

2 Department for Transport (2014). Drug driving and medicine: advice for healthcare professionals. http://www.gov.uk/government/publications/drug-driving-and-medicine-advice-for-healthcare-professionals (accessed 9 February 2015).

E

Early warning score

Early warning score (EWS)

Background	• It has been recognised that early recognition of deterioration in a patient's condition and appropriate escalation of care (a physiological 'track and trigger' system) improves treatment outcomes[1]
	• Hospital nursing and medical staff and also the emergency medical services use the EWS to assess degree of severity of illness in a patient. It is used at first presentation and also for ongoing monitoring while patients remain in hospital
	• The EWS is derived from the recording and scoring of various physiological parameters. These are monitored at least every 12 hours unless a decision has been made at senior level to increase or decrease frequency for an individual patient
	• Many different systems are in use across the NHS and the world and it has been recommended that use of a national early warning score (NEWS), as outlined below, would deliver a standardised approach across the UK[2]

National early warning score (NEWS)

Physiological parameter	Score 3	Score 2	Score 1	Score 0	Score 1	Score 2	Score 3
Respiration rate (breaths/min)	≤8		9–11	12–20		21–24	≥25
Oxygen saturations (%)	≤91	92–93	94–95	≥96			
Any supplemental oxygen		Yes		No			
Temperature (°C)	≤35.0		35.1–36.0	36.1–38.0	38.1–39.0	≥39.1	
Systolic blood pressure (mmHg)	≤90	91–100	101–110	111–219			≥220
Heart rate (beats/min)	≤40		41–50	51–90	91–110	111–130	≥131
Level of consciousness*				A			V, P or U

*Refers to the AVPU scale = alert, voice, pain, unresponsive.

Interpretation

NEWS total	Clinical risk	Frequency of monitoring	Response[2]
0	Low	Minimum 12-hourly	• Continue routine NEWS monitoring
1–4	Low	Minimum 4–6-hourly	• Inform registered nurse who must assess patient • Registered nurse to decide if increased frequency of monitoring and/or escalation of care is required
5–6 or 3 in one parameter	Medium	Increase frequency to a minimum of 1-hourly	• Registered nurse to inform medical team urgently • Urgent assessment by clinician competent to assess acutely ill patients • Clinical care in an environment with monitoring facilities
7 or more	High	Continuous monitoring of vital signs	• Registered nurse to inform medical team immediately (specialist registrar level or above) • Emergency assessment by, e.g., critical care outreach team • Consider transfer of care to level 2 or 3 care facility

E

REFERENCES

1 NICE (2007). Clinical Guideline 50. *Acutely Ill Patients in Hospital. Recognition of and response to acute illness in adults in hospital.* http://www.nice.org.uk/guidance/cg50 (accessed 17 February 2015).
2 Royal College of Physicians (2012). *National Early Warning Score (NEWS): Standardising the assessment of acute-illness severity in the NHS.* Report of a working party. London: RCP.

Emollients

Emollients are the mainstay of treatment for skin conditions such as eczema, psoriasis, contact dermatitis and dry skin resulting from a variety of other causes. They rehydrate the outermost layer of skin and reduce water loss, mimic the barrier effects of deficient lipids and restore the integrity of the skin barrier. When used correctly they help to maintain or restore suppleness and pliability of the skin, improve the cosmetic appearance, soothe and relieve skin irritation and reduce requirements for topical corticosteroids by helping to prevent disease flares.[1,2] In psoriasis, emollients also help to soften scaly, thickened plaques, making them more amenable to treatment.

Types of emollient

Emollient products include ointments, creams, lotions, soap substitutes and bath oils.

Ointments

Ointments are greasy semisolids. They have fatty, emulsifying, water-soluble or absorption bases. Ointments with fatty bases are not absorbed but form an occlusive layer on the skin surface and can be difficult to spread. Although they are effective emollients, their greasiness makes them cosmetically unattractive. Ointments with absorption bases spread more easily but are less occlusive than those with fatty bases. Water-soluble bases spread well and can be washed off easily.

Creams and lotions

Creams are semisolid emulsions. They are less occlusive than ointments and therefore less effective. However they feel less greasy, spread well and can be washed off easily, so are more cosmetically acceptable.

Emollient lotions are more dilute than creams and contain additives to increase their spreadability.

Soap substitutes and bath oils

Emollient wash products (or soap substitutes), e.g. aqueous cream or emulsifying ointment, cleanse the skin effectively, but do not lather like soap. They should be used in place of soaps, which otherwise may have a drying effect.

Bath oils are an alternative means of applying emollient by leaving a film of emollient after bathing. Some ointments can also be used as a bath additive by melting in hot water and adding to a warm, not hot, bath.

Choice of product

Inappropriate selection of product can result in emollient therapy being underused and dismissed as ineffective.[3] It is essential to find a product that matches a patient's needs and preferences. Emollient choice for an individual patient should involve consideration of the factors shown in Table E1.

Dosing and application

Emollients must be used in sufficient quantities to be effective. They should be applied as liberally and as frequently as possible. Table E2 gives approximate quantities for how much emollient an adult would expect to use over 1 week.

'Complete emollient therapy' is recommended in order to obtain the best effects from emollients (Table E3).

TABLE E1
Emollients – factors to consider

Patient needs or preference / lifestyle factors

- Different emollients may be used for different parts of the body, e.g. rich/more greasy emollients for limbs but a lighter product for the face
- Greasy products may be cosmetically unsuitable for daytime use but acceptable at night
- Richer products are required in winter to combat the drying effects of cold weather and central heating
- In psoriasis, heavier, greasy products are used to soften scaly, thickened plaques, making them more amenable to treatment

Consistency required

- Creams or lotions are more appropriate if skin is infected or oozing to avoid occlusion
- Ointments are more effective than lighter products on dry, scaly, thick areas of skin
- Creams may feel cooler and lighter on the skin than ointments, so may be preferred if itching is troublesome

Other ingredients / additives

- Some emollients contain potential allergens that may exacerbate the underlying skin condition. A patch test should be considered when starting new treatment
- Lanolin is widely considered to be a sensitiser; however, lanolin-sensitivity is uncommon. Lanolin-containing products are an appropriate option, with a patch test if necessary
- Some products, notably aqueous cream, contain sodium lauryl sulfate, which is a well-documented irritant. Products containing sodium lauryl sulfate are recommended as wash-off products and should not be used as a leave-on emollient

TABLE E2
How much emollient to use. These amounts are usually suitable for an adult for twice-daily application for 1 week

	Face	Scalp	Both hands	Both arms and legs	Trunk – front and back	Groin area
Amount of emollient to apply	15–30 g	50–100 g	25–50 g	100–200 g	400 g	15–25 g

TABLE E3
Complete emollient therapy[1,4]

Frequent application of emollient cream or ointment

Apply liberally with clean hands as frequently as possible – ideally, three to four times a day, but at least twice a day. Warming the emollient will make it easier to apply. If itching is a major problem, cool the emollient by storing it in a fridge

Emollient bath oil when bathing/showering

Baths should be warm but not hot to avoid exacerbating itching. Patients should be advised to use a bath mat to prevent slipping and to pat skin dry rather than rub

Routine use of emollient soap substitute

Use whenever washing hands and before getting into a bath or shower. Apply to dry skin and then rinse off with water

Avoidance of regular soaps/detergents/bubble baths

These remove lipids from the skin and may exacerbate dry-skin conditions

Pharmaceutical care and counselling points

- Ensure patients are aware of the importance of emollients as an active treatment and the need to apply even when the skin is clear.
- Apply emollient creams/ointments liberally with clean hands, ideally three to four times a day but at least twice a day.
- Apply in the direction of hair growth to prevent folliculitis.
- A sample pack containing a variety of products can help patients make choices on products that suit their needs and so aid compliance.
- Ensure patients are aware that other topical preparations, e.g. topical corticosteroids and vitamin D analogues, should not be used as emollients.
- Emollient use should generally outweigh topical corticosteroid use by 10:1 in terms of quantities used.
- Leave at least half an hour between emollient application and other topical preparations to avoid dilution or spread to unaffected areas.
- Use a high-temperature wash to remove grease from clothes and bedding and avoid biological washing powder and fabric softener. Run an empty cycle at high temperature with washing powder to clear greasy residue.
- Advise patients regarding the fire hazard with paraffin-based emollients. Emulsifying ointment or Liquid Paraffin 50%/White Soft Paraffin Ointment 50% in contact with dressings and clothing is easily ignited by a naked flame. This risk is greater when these preparations are applied to large areas of the body, where clothing or dressings become soaked with the ointment. Patients should be told to keep away from fire or flames, and not to smoke when using these preparations. The risk of fire should be considered when using large quantities of any paraffin-based emollient.[5]

REFERENCES

1 Clark C (2004). How to choose a suitable emollient. *Pharm J* 273: 351–353.
2 Anonymous (1998). The use of emollients in dry skin conditions. *MeReC Bull* 9: 45–48.
3 Tucker R (2011). What evidence is there for moisturisers? *Pharm J Online*. http://www.pharmaceutical-journal.com/files/rps-pjonline/pdf/pj20110416_cpd.pdf (accessed 29 January 2015).
4 Clark C (2001). Making the most of emollients. *Pharm J* 266: 227–229.
5 National Patient Safety Agency (2007). *Fire Hazard with Paraffin Based Products on Dressings and Clothing*. Rapid response report 4. http://www.npsa.nhs.uk/corporate/news/fire-hazard-with-paraffin-based-skin-products-on-dressings-and-clothing/ (accessed 29 January 2015).

Endocarditis

Overview	
Definition	Infective endocarditis (IE) is an infection of the inner lining of the heart cavity (endocardium), valves and adjacent structures
Causes/risk factors	It is caused by a range of bacteria and fungi. Bacterial endocarditis is most common; causative organisms include: staphylococci, streptococci, enterococci, HACEK group of Gram-negative bacteria, *Coxiella burnetii*, *Bartonella* species and a wide range of other Gram-negative pathogens, for example, *Pseudomonas aeruginosa*, Enterobacteriaceae, *Acinetobacter* species.
	Causative fungi include *Candida* species, *Aspergillus* species and a wide variety of others. Fungal endocarditis occurs most commonly in patients with prosthetic valves but can occur in those who are immunocompromised, intravenous drug users and neonates.[1]
	Endocarditis tends to occur following bacteraemia; the following patients are classed as having predisposing risk factors:[2]
	• valve replacement • acquired valvular heart disease with stenosis or regurgitation • structural congenital heart disease, including surgically corrected or palliated structural conditions, but excluding isolated atrial septal defect, fully repaired ventricular septal defect or fully repaired patent ductus arteriosus and closure devices that are judged to be endothelialised • previous IE • hypertrophic cardiomyopathy • intravenous drug use

Classification[3]	• Left-sided native valve endocarditis
	• Left-sided prosthetic valve endocarditis – this is usually split into 'early' and 'late'
	  • Early: occurring less than 1 year after valve surgery
	  • Late: occurring more than 1 year after valve surgery
	• Right-sided endocarditis
	• Device-related endocarditis (pacemaker or cardioverter-defibrillator)

Signs and symptoms	Some patients may present acutely unwell, displaying signs of sepsis; others may present with more indolent signs with a low-grade fever and non-specific symptoms. Common symptoms are fever, malaise, loss of appetite, night sweats and weight loss.
	Signs include: new murmur or a change in the nature of a pre-existing murmur, anaemia, splenomegaly, clubbing, presence of embolic phenomena, presence of petechiae, splinter haemorrhages, Janeway lesions, Osler's nodes and Roth spots, evidence of congestive heart failure and evidence of pulmonary embolism (right-sided IE)

E

Diagnostic tests	• Blood cultures: three sets taken at different times from different sites, prior to commencing antibiotic treatment • Transthoracic echocardiography (TTE). This is recommended as the first-line initial method of imaging • Transoesophageal echocardiography (TOE). This should be conducted in those patients with a negative TTE with a high clinical suspicion for IE, those with a positive or poor-quality TTE or those with a prosthetic valve or intracardiac device • ECG • Chest X-ray • Urinalysis (to check for microscopic haematuria) • Blood tests: FBC, U&E, LFTs, CRP • Serology: for those patients with blood culture-negative IE, serological testing should be performed for *Coxiella* and *Bartonella* • Modified Duke criteria:[4] these criteria are used to assist in the diagnosis of IE. Criteria for a definite diagnosis of IE require the presence of two major, or one major and three minor, or five minor criteria **Major criteria** • Evidence of endocardial involvement, identified as a positive echocardiogram (vegetation or abscess or new partial dehiscence of prosthetic valve) or new valvular regurgitation • Positive blood cultures for typical microorganisms consistent with IE from two separate blood cultures taken >12 hours apart or all three or a majority of four separate cultures of blood (with first and last sample drawn at least 1 hour apart) **Minor criteria** • Predisposing heart condition or intravenous drug use • Fever (>38°C) • Vascular phenomena (e.g. Janeway lesions, septic pulmonary emboli) • Immunological phenomena (e.g. Osler's nodes, Roth spots) • Microbiological phenomenon that does not meet major criteria • Polymerase chain reaction tests • Echocardiographic findings consistent with IE that do not meet major criteria
Treatment options[1]	• Intravenous antibacterial or antifungal treatment dependent upon the causative pathogen • Surgery: this can be helpful to remove infected material and drain any abscesses. Surgical review should be sought for all patients with intracardiac prosthetic material. Samples of the infected tissue or valve should be sent for microbiological and histological testing

Antibacterial treatment

All cases of suspected endocarditis should be discussed with a microbiologist. The choice of antibiotics may be empirical or targeted if there are positive blood cultures. If the patient is stable it is recommended to await blood culture results and then treat accordingly. Listed below are the empirical treatment options for those patients with suspected IE who have severe sepsis requiring treatment whilst awaiting blood culture results. Empirical treatment is directed towards the most common causative pathogens and should be based on the type of valve affected and risk factors for resistant pathogens. Targeted treatment recommendations for the various bacterial and fungal causes of endocarditis can be found within the British Society for Antimicrobial Chemotherapy endocarditis treatment guidelines.[1] Treatment duration is dependent upon the causative pathogen and the type of affected valve; it is usually for 4–6 weeks. In some cases, for example, IE due to *C. burnetti*, treatment is for 18 months to 4 years

Empirical treatment[1]	**Native valve and severe sepsis (no risk factors for Enterobacteriaceae, *Pseudomonas*)** • Vancomycin intravenous* (dosed in accordance with local guidelines) plus gentamicin* intravenous 1 mg/kg twice daily • If the patient is allergic to vancomycin, replace this with daptomycin* intravenous 6 mg/kg daily • If there are concerns about using gentamicin due to nephrotoxicity or acute kidney injury, then use ciprofloxacin (usual *British National Formulary* (BNF) doses) in place of gentamicin **Native valve and severe sepsis and risk factors for multiresistant Enterobacteriaceae, *Pseudomonas*** • Vancomycin intravenous* (dosed in accordance with local guidelines) plus meropenem* 2 g three times a day **Prosthetic valve awaiting blood cultures or with negative blood cultures** • Vancomycin intravenous* (dosed in accordance with local guidelines) plus gentamicin* intravenous 1 mg/kg twice daily plus rifampicin 300–600 mg twice daily intravenous or oral *Dose reduction required in renal impairment.
Therapeutic drug monitoring[1]	• Vancomycin monitoring should be undertaken in accordance with local protocols. Doses should be adjusted to achieve a pre-dose level of 15–20 mg/L • Gentamicin monitoring should be undertaken in accordance with local protocols. Doses should be adjusted to achieve a pre-dose level <1 mg/L and 1-hour post-dose levels of 3–5 mg/L

Essential interventions and monitoring	• Check for any drug allergies (see *Antimicrobial allergy management* entry) • Ensure patient is weighed: this is necessary for drug dosing and creatinine clearance calculation • Calculate creatinine clearance and recommend dosing according to renal function (see *Renal disease–assessment of renal function* entry) • Where gentamicin is required, dosing should be based on actual body weight unless the patient is obese (see *Gentamicin* entry). • Check for drug interactions. Rifampicin is a potent cytochrome P450 inducer and can interact with numerous medications, including warfarin. If daptomycin is used, withhold statins and fibrates • If rifampicin is used, counsel patients, as it can cause a reddish discolouration of sputum, urine, sweat and tears • Ensure therapeutic drug monitoring is undertaken and monitor urine output for those patients prescribed gentamicin and vancomycin • Regularly check U&Es, LFTs, FBC, weekly creatine kinase (if on daptomycin) • Monitor temperature and inflammatory markers for response to treatment • Ensure the indication and duration of antibiotic treatment are written on the prescription chart

REFERENCES

1 Gould FK *et al.* (2012). Guidelines for the diagnosis and antibiotic treatment of endocarditis in adults: a report of the Working Party of the British Society for Antimicrobial Chemotherapy. *J Antimicrob Chemother* 67: 269–289.

2 NICE (2014). Clinical Guideline 64. *Prophylaxis Against Infective Endocarditis: Antimicrobial prophylaxis against infective endocarditis in adults and children undergoing interventional procedures.* http://www.nice.org.uk/guidance/CG64 (accessed 11 August 2014).

3 The Task Force on the Prevention, Diagnosis, and Treatment of Infective Endocarditis of the European Society of Cardiology (ESC) (2009). Guidelines on the prevention, diagnosis, and treatment of infective endocarditis. *Eur Heart J* 30: 2369–2413.

4 Li JS *et al.* (2000). Proposed modifications to the Duke criteria for the diagnosis of infective endocarditis. *Clin Infect Dis* 3: 633–638.

Enoxaparin dosing in unstable angina

Enoxaparin is licensed in the UK for the treatment of unstable angina. The SPC for enoxaparin states that the dose is 1 mg/kg every 12 hours by subcutaneous injection, usually for 2–8 days until the patient is clinically stable; aspirin should be given concomitantly. Patients with a creatinine clearance <30 mL/min should have a reduced dose of 1 mg/kg once daily.[1]

The standard treatment for patients presenting with unstable angina is antiplatelet and antithrombotic agents. In the early management of unstable angina and non-ST-segment-elevation myocardial infarction (NSTEMI), the NICE Clinical Guideline

94 recommends fondaparinux as the antithrombotic of choice, with unfractionated heparin for patients with raised creatinine or likely to undergo urgent stenting where reversibility is required.[2] Fondaparinux is highly renally excreted and is not recommended in patients with a creatinine clearance <30 mL/min. NICE Clinical Guideline 94 does not discuss use of a low-molecular-weight heparin (LMWH), such as enoxaparin, as an option for unstable angina treatment, although many hospitals do use it either as first-line instead of fondaparinux or instead of unfractionated heparin for patients with poor renal function.[3]

The SIGN guideline 93 suggests enoxaparin as an alternative to heparin for non-ST elevation and ST-elevation acute coronary syndromes.[4] In both cases trials showed that LMWH plus aspirin reduced myocardial infarction and coronary revascularisation compared to unfractionated heparin plus aspirin, with no differences in mortality or major bleeding. The ExTRACT randomised controlled trial (enoxaparin versus unfractionated heparin for acute coronary syndromes) confirmed these findings.[5] SIGN therefore recommends fondaparinux or LMWH. Dalteparin is also licensed for unstable coronary artery disease at a dose of 120 units/kg, with a maximum dose of 10 000 units twice a day. The trials evaluating dalteparin were against placebo, where it showed superiority, and against unfractionated heparin, where it showed equivalence. Tinzaparin does not have a product licence for unstable angina.

The dose of enoxaparin must be checked against creatinine clearance, then accurately calculated for body weight, to avoid an increased risk of bleeding.

REFERENCES

1 SPC (2014). *Clexane Pre-filled Syringes*. www.medicines.org.uk (accessed 11 November 2014).

2 NICE (2013). Clinical Guidelines CG94. *Unstable Angina and NSTEMI: The early management of unstable angina and non-ST-segment-elevation myocardial infarction*. https://www.nice.org.uk/guidance/cg94 (accessed 11 November 2014).

3 SPC (2014). Arixtra Fondaparinux sodium solution for injection 2.5 mg/ 0.5 mL. www.medicines.org.uk (accessed 11 November 2014).

4 SIGN (2013). *Acute Coronary Syndromes*. http://www.sign.ac.uk/guidelines/ fulltext/93/ (accessed 11 November 2014).

5 Gabriel RS, White HD (2007). ExTRACT-TIMI 25 trial: clarifying the role of enoxaparin in patients with ST-elevation myocardial infarction receiving fibrinolysis. *Expert Rev Cardiovasc Ther* 5: 851–857.

Enteral feeding systems and drug administration

In the course of providing advice about the administration of medicines via enteral feeding tubes, knowledge of these feeding systems is of benefit.

Purpose of enteral feeding tubes

Enteral feeding tubes are used to provide nutritional support and hydration and to prevent or treat malnutrition. Providing nutrition enterally is preferable to parenteral feeding because feeding via the GI route is easier, safer, less expensive and more physiological.[1]

Selection of access device

Feeding tubes may be placed into the stomach or the small intestine either in the distal duodenum or proximal jejunum. The expected duration of feeding is the major determinant of method, but risk of aspiration, GI function, overall patient condition and placement technique are all factors.

Nasoenteric tubes are usually intended for short-term therapy and more commonly take the form of nasogastric (NG) tubes. Gastrostomy or jejunostomy tubes are devices intended for placements of 1 month or longer.

Nasoenteric tubes

These tubes are placed through the nose and are advanced to the point where the tip of the tube lies in the stomach or the small intestine. Such tubes can be placed at the bedside and cause a minimum of complications. For feeding purposes, fine-bore (e.g. 8–10 Fr) polyurethane or silicone tubes are used. Smaller tubes are less likely to lead to aspiration or swallowing difficulties, and are less irritant to the gut. Larger tubes can be used on critical care. All tubes used for NG feeding must be licensed for feeding, be radiopaque throughout their length and have externally visible length markings.[2]

The position of most nasoenteric tubes may be confirmed by the pH of aspirate. X-ray is used as a second-line test when no aspirate can be obtained or the pH paper has failed to confirm the position of the tube. NG tubes are more frequently used than nasoduodenal/jejunal tubes in the UK, though the latter have a role in critically ill patients at particular risk of pulmonary aspiration or delayed gastric emptying.

Complications of nasoenteric tube use may include nasal irritation, epistaxis, rupture of oesophageal varices, tracheobronchial injury or pulmonary compromise.

Gastrostomy and jejunostomy tubes

Where use of the nasal route for tube insertion is contraindicated, or when longer-term tube feeding is anticipated, an enterostomal device is preferred. In this scenario a tube is inserted percutaneously through a stoma created on the abdomen.

Percutaneous endoscopic gastrostomy (PEG) has become the most widely used approach for gastrostomy placement and the dual-access gastrostomy-jejunostomy (PEG/J) is a variation on this. These tubes are placed endoscopically under conscious sedation, pushing the tube

out from the stomach lumen through the stomach wall to emerge
through the skin of the abdomen.

A PEG tube is a single-lumen tube terminating in the stomach,
delivering feeds directly into the stomach. The PEG/J is a
double-lumen tube, one lumen terminating in the stomach and a
longer tube descending into the jejunum – the double-lumen system
allows feeding directly into the jejunum, and stomach decompression
via the stomach tube.

Both types of tube are held in place by an internal retainer
(a bumper or balloon) and an external retainer (disc, bumper or
cross-bar). The tubes are composed of silicone or polyurethane, which
are resistant to gastric secretions.

Once the placement of the tube has been confirmed by X-ray, tube
patency and patient tolerance are checked by giving a bolus or
infusion of sterile water. If tolerated, feeds can be started slowly with
full-strength formula according to hospital policy. To prevent
aspiration, the head of the bed should be elevated to at least $30-45°$
from the horizontal during feeds and for 1 hour after feeds. If patients
are asleep they should recline on their right side.

To avoid clogging feeding tubes, the tube should be flushed every
4–6 hours during feeds, after completion of a feeding session, and
before and after administration of medicines. Water is considered to
be the best liquid for flushing and maintenance of tube patency. Flush
volumes should be included in fluid balance calculations. In hospital
this should be sterile water but at home it can be tap water or cooled,
boiled water dependent on the health professional's risk assessment.

The stoma site should be cleaned daily using warm water
(or sterile sodium chloride 0.9% in a hospital setting) applied with a
sterile gauze swab. The area around the tube and under the flange
should then be gently dried with a sterile swab. The flange should be
left sitting lightly on the skin, allowing air circulation around it. After
4 weeks the tube should also be turned, clockwise and anticlockwise,
180° from its original position to keep the stoma healthy.

Feeding via enteral feeding tubes

The dietician will liaise with the patient, family and multidisciplinary
team to work out a feeding regimen that fits with the requirements of
the patient. This can include pump feeding, bolus feeding or a
mixture of both. Overnight feeding may be appropriate for patients
who are able to eat and drink small amounts.

Meticulous mouth care is of great importance in patients with
tube-feeding systems because of limited oral fluid intake. Ice chips,
mouth swabs, throat lozenges, throat sprays and chewing gum may
all have a role to play in this aspect of care.

Some hospitals recommend routine prescribing of proton pump
inhibitors (PPI) for patients who have PEGs as prophylaxis against the
inevitable gastro-oesophageal reflux that accompanies overnight
feeding and gastric distension.

Testing the pH of aspirate

pH testing using pH paper that is CE-marked and intended by the manufacturer to test gastric aspirate is the first-line method for confirming NG tube placement. A measured pH of <5.5 is indicative of gastric placement. The use of acid-suppressing drugs (e.g. PPIs, H_2-receptor antagonists) will increase gastric pH, leading to potentially misleading measurements. Whoosh tests, litmus paper (rather than pH paper) or assessing the appearance of aspirate must never be used to test the position of NG tubes.[2]

Problems with drug administration

A full medication review may reveal options for discontinuation of unnecessary drugs. Consider alternative administration routes such as transdermal, rectal, sublingual or parenteral. In some instances the patient may be able to continue to take medications by mouth. All medicines should be administered via a suitable oral / enteral syringe that is compatible with the enteral feeding system. These syringes are designed so that they do not fit with an intravenous system.[3]

In the choice of therapeutic agent for any given indication, an appropriate preparation for tube administration should be selected. However, the unavailability of many medications in a suitable liquid formulation is a barrier to effective administration of drugs via tubes. Some manufacturers have a range of unlicensed drugs available in liquid form, although cost may be a factor, since many of these products are relatively expensive and therapy may be of a long duration.

Many sugar-free oral liquids contain sorbitol, which can cause abdominal cramping and diarrhoea. Sorbitol doses of 7.5–30 g may cause adverse effects, with symptoms being particularly severe above 20 g,[4] and it is therefore important to minimise the intake of sorbitol where possible. The bore (internal diameter) of feeding tubes may be very small, and for this reason viscous fluids should be mixed with an equal amount of water immediately before administration. An injection formulation may be appropriate for the preparation of some liquid doses.

It is recommended to confirm the appropriateness of a medication for tube administration with a standard reference text[5,6] or with the manufacturer. General principles are explained below.

Crushing tablets

Solid oral dose forms have been widely crushed and mixed with water, but administration in this fashion is outside the product licence as it involves manipulation of the product. If this unlicensed method is chosen, the dose must be prepared immediately prior to administration. This will minimise drug degradation and reduces the risk of a drug administration error.

Crushing may be accomplished between two spoons, with a pestle and mortar, or a proprietary crushing device, and the resulting powder is then mixed with a small volume of water and transferred to the tube using a syringe. Any equipment used must be thoroughly cleaned after use and tablet-crushing devices should be reserved for use with one patient only because of the difficulty in removing all traces of medication. Many tablets will soften and disperse in water (a process referred to as 'mungeing' in some quarters) without the need for grinding. Modified-release preparations and many enteric-coated products are not suitable for crushing.

Use of capsules

Capsules may be opened (unlicensed use) to reveal a powder that may be miscible with water, or they may contain beads or pellets, which can sometimes be flushed down tubes (e.g. Slo-phyllin). It must be borne in mind that pellets may block the tube due to a 'bridging' effect.

Blockage management

Tablets or capsules, when given as above, may cause the feeding tube to become blocked, and some products should not be given in this way because of the high risk of such an occurrence. The manufacturer is a source of information if the properties of the product are not already known. Inadequate tube flushing is the most common cause of tube blockage. The consequence to the patient of a blocked tube that cannot be unblocked is potentially no food, fluid or medicine until a new tube is sited, which may take several days.

Some products manipulated for tube administration require special preparation or administration techniques. For instance, omeprazole (pellets from capsules) should be dispersed in a bicarbonate solution to remove the pellet coating but administration may still be unsuccessful. Losec MUPS should not be dispersed for tube administration because of the risk of tube blockage; Zoton FasTabs are a more suitable choice of PPI preparation.

Flushing

Feeding tubes should always be flushed with at least 30 mL of water before and after the administration of medications. You may have a local policy determining the quantity and grade of water to be used (i.e. tap water or sterile water).

Control of Substances Hazardous to Health (COSHH)

The powders liberated by the manipulation of tablets or capsules may present a hazard to staff preparing doses. Cytotoxic products and hormonal preparations should not be manipulated in this manner. Cyclophosphamide and busulfan may be obtained as 'specials' in a liquid form from some specialist manufacturers.

Interactions with feeds

Where possible, give medication doses during breaks in feeding to minimise the risk of interaction with feeds. To increase potential feeding time the number of medication doses per day should be reduced where possible. Medication should never be added directly to enteral feeds.

Some pharmaceuticals are known to be incompatible with feeds, and the standard advice regarding flushing of tubes is not adequate to prevent interaction. For example, the bioavailability of phenytoin suspension is reduced by the presence of enteral feed.[7] It is recommended that the feed should be stopped for 2 hours before administration of the drug and recommenced 2 hours after.[8] Therapeutic drug monitoring may be required to guide dose adjustment. This may be a consideration with many other drugs, and therefore it is essential that a full medication review is undertaken when a patient commences enteral feeding.

REFERENCES

1 Bowers S (2000). All about tubes. *Nursing* 30: 41–47.
2 NPSA (2011). *Reducing the Harm Caused by Misplaced Nasogastric Feeding Tubes in Adults, Children and Infants*. http://www.nrls.npsa.nhs.uk/resources/type/alerts/?entryid45=129640 (accessed 8 September 2014).
3 NPSA (2007), *Promoting Safer Measurement and Administration of Liquid Medicines via Oral and Other Enteral Routes*. http://www.nrls.npsa.nhs.uk/resources/type/alerts/?entryid45=59808&q=0%C2%ACsyringe%C2%AC (accessed 8 September 2014).
4 Duncan B et al. (1997). Medication-induced pneumatosis intestinalis. *Pediatrics* 99: 633–636.
5 Smyth JS (ed.) (2010). *The NEWT Guidelines for Administration of Medication to Patients with Enteral Feeding Tubes or Swallowing Difficulties* (2nd edn). Wrexham: North East Wales NHS Trust, 2010.
6 White R, Bradnam V (2010). *Drug Administration via Enteral Feeding Tubes* (2nd edn). London: Pharmaceutical Press.
7 BAPEN (2004). *Administering Drugs via Enteral Feeding Tubes, A Practical Guide*. http://www.bapen.org.uk/pdfs/d_and_e/de_pract_guide.pdf (accessed 8 September 2014).
8 SPC (2014). *Epanutin Suspension*. https://www.medicines.org.uk/emc/medicine/13289 (accessed 8 September 2014).

Epidural analgesia in the postoperative period

Continuous infusion of an analgesic solution (usually a mixture of local anaesthetic and opioid) into the epidural space close to the spinal cord via an indwelling catheter has become an increasingly popular method for postoperative pain relief. Epidural analgesia offers unique benefits in postoperative pain relief:[1]

- improved pain relief compared with other analgesic techniques
- reduction in postoperative and post-trauma morbidity, particularly in high-risk patients
- reduction in postoperative complications, e.g. preventing retention of secretions and development of pneumonia
- earlier discharge from hospital.

Epidural infusion solutions should be available in pre-prepared bags or syringes and they should be stored separately to other infusions. Preparation within the ward environment is discouraged.[2]

Medicines used in epidurals

Local anaesthetics

Almost all local anaesthetics can be given by epidural administration. Levobupivacaine and bupivacaine (0.1–0.25% (1–2.5 mg/mL)) are used most commonly as they have a longer duration of effect compared with lidocaine. Ropivacaine is a newer agent and may cause fewer side effects, most notably motor blockade, than bupivacaine.

Opioid analgesics

Lipophilic opioids, such as fentanyl and diamorphine, are preferred for epidural analgesia as they penetrate nerves more readily and result in less spread within cerebrospinal fluid. Fentanyl binds to the fat in the epidural space, which limits spread to other areas in the spinal cord where an effect may be undesirable. The usual strength of fentanyl in epidural solutions is 2–4 micrograms/mL.

Administration

Dedicated pumps should be used for epidural infusions and together with giving sets they should be clearly distinguishable from those used for other routes of administration.[2]

The epidural infusion rate is usually between 4 and 10 mL/hour. The continuous infusion can be supplemented by bolus doses given either by a healthcare professional, or by the patient using a patient-controlled epidural analgesia (PCEA) handset, typically 2–3 mL. As with intravenous patient-controlled analgesia (see *Patient-controlled analgesia* entry), for PCEA after a bolus dose there is a lock-out period, which prevents further doses being administered.

Contraindications

Epidurals should not be used where there is a lack of staff fully trained in the care of patients with epidurals.

Absolute contraindications to epidural analgesia include:

- lack of consent
- full anticoagulation (not venous thromboembolism prophylaxis)
- local or generalised sepsis.

Relative contraindications include:

- hypovolaemia or shock (increased risk of hypotension)
- coagulopathy
- thrombocytopenia (increases the risk of epidural haematoma)
- raised intracranial pressure.

Adverse effects

Potential adverse effects related to the route of administration include:[3]

- nerve injury
- epidural haematoma
- epidural abscess.

Monitoring

Epidural analgesia requires regular monitoring. Most hospitals have specific epidural prescription charts, which allow the recording of monitoring parameters, including:

- pain intensity
- respiratory rate
- sedation score
- blood pressure
- nausea or vomiting
- sensory and motor function
- observation of the infusion site.

REFERENCES

1 Wu CL *et al.* (2005). Efficacy of postoperative patient-controlled and continuous infusion epidural analgesia versus intravenous patient-controlled analgesia with opioids: a meta-analysis. *Anesthesiology* 103: 1079–1088.

2 National Patient Safety Agency (2007). *Epidural Injections and Infusions.* http://www.nrls.npsa.nhs.uk/resources/?EntryId45=59807 (accessed 22 November 2014).

3 Macintyre PE *et al.* (2010), *Acute Pain Management: Scientific Evidence* (3rd edn). Melbourne: ANZCA and FPM. http://www.anzca.edu.au/resources/college -publications/pdfs/Acute%20Pain%20Management/books-and-publications/ Acute%20pain%20management%20-%20scientific%20evidence%20-%20third% 20edition.pdf (accessed 27 November 2014).

Epilepsy: therapeutic drug monitoring of antiepileptics in adults

Routine blood monitoring of antiepileptic drug levels is not usually required if the dose is stable, seizure control is good and the patient is free of side effects. However, monitoring of serum concentrations is available for most antiepileptic drugs and may be useful if considered alongside the clinical presentation in the following circumstances:

- to check adherence
- in suspected toxicity
- to check the effect of a potential/suspected drug interaction
- in therapeutic failure
- after a dose change.

Drug interactions between antiepileptics can be complex. It is important to remember that adding or removing a drug to or from a given regimen can significantly affect levels of the other drugs, possibly resulting in toxicity or increased seizures. Therapeutic drug monitoring (TDM) can be a useful tool to add to clinical assessment in the management of these situations, although routine monitoring of the newer antiepileptic drugs is rarely necessary.

Suicidal ideation and behaviour have been reported in patients treated with antiepileptic agents in several indications. Therefore, all patients receiving antiepileptic drugs should be monitored for signs of this and appropriate treatment considered. Patients and carers should be advised to seek medical advice if signs of suicidal ideation or behaviour emerge.

Tables E4–E23 are summaries of antiepileptic drugs with details of TDM rationale. See *Carbamazepine* and *Phenytoin – management and monitoring* entries for details specific to these.

TABLE E4
Clobazam[1]

Half-life	• 36 hours for clobazam • 79 hours for the active metabolite N-desmethylclobazam
Pretreatment measures	Contraindicated in patients with: • history of drug/alcohol dependence • myasthenia gravis • sleep apnoea • severe hepatic insufficiencies
Therapeutic serum range	• 30–300 micrograms/mL • N-desmethylclobazam 300–3000 micrograms/mL[2]
Other monitoring	• For dependence (physical and psychological) • Tolerance
Interactions with other antiepileptics	• Interactions can occur but are not frequently recognised as a problem

TABLE E5
Clonazepam[1]

Half-life	• 20–60 hours (mean 30 hours)
Pretreatment measures	Contraindicated in: • severe respiratory deficiency • sleep apnoea • myasthenia gravis • severe hepatic insufficiency
Therapeutic serum range	• 20–70 micrograms/mL[2]
Other monitoring	• Concurrent use of other centrally acting agents can potentiate drug effects, e.g. sedation
Interactions with other antiepileptics	• Clonazepam serum concentration may be decreased by carbamazepine, phenobarbital, phenytoin and valproic acid • Clonazepam can increase or decrease the serum concentration of phenytoin and primidone

TABLE E6
Eslicarbazepine[1]

Half-life	• 13–20 hours
Pretreatment measures	• U&Es, ECG • For HLA-B*1502 allele in Han Chinese and HLA-A*3101 allele in European and Japanese population
Therapeutic serum range	• 3–35 mg/L
Interactions with other antiepileptics	• Eslicarbazepine serum concentration may be increased or decreased by lamotrigine • Eslicarbazepine serum concentration may be decreased by carbamazepine and phenytoin • Eslicarbazepine can increase the serum concentration of phenytoin • Eslicarbazepine can decrease the serum concentration of topiramate • Eslicarbazepine can increase or decrease lamotrigine serum concentration

TABLE E7
Ethosuximide[1]

Half-life	• 40–60 hours (adults), 30 hours (children)
Pretreatment measures	• FBC, U&Es, LFTs
Therapeutic serum range	• 300–700 micromol/L • 40–100 mg/L
Other monitoring	• Periodically check FBC, U&Es, LFTs
Interactions with other antiepileptics	• Ethosuximide serum concentration may be increased or decreased by valproic acid and phenytoin • Ethosuximide serum concentration may be decreased by carbamazepine, primidone, phenobarbital and lamotrigine • Ethosuximide can increase the serum concentration of phenytoin • Ethosuximide can decrease the serum concentration of valproic acid[1]

TABLE E8
Gabapentin[1]

Half-life	• 5–7 hours
Pretreatment measures	• U&Es
Therapeutic serum range	• There is much interpatient variability, and the serum concentration/therapeutic response is not well established. A putative range is 12–120 micromol/L (2–20 mg/L)[2]
Interactions with other antiepileptics	• No clinically significant interactions with other antiepileptics have been reported[3]

TABLE E9
Lacosamide[1]

Half-life	• 13 hours
Pretreatment measures	• U&Es • ECG (potential PR prolongation) • (Contraindicated in known second- or third-degree heart block)
Therapeutic serum range	• Not established
Interactions with other antiepileptics	• No clinically significant interactions with other antiepileptics have been reported

TABLE E10
Lamotrigine[1]

Half-life	• Range 14–103 hours (mean 33 hours) • Reduced to a mean of approximately 14 hours if enzyme inducers are present (see below) • Increased to a mean of approximately 70 hours if sodium valproate is present
Pretreatment measures	• LFTs
Therapeutic serum range	• Dosing is usually based on clinical response rather than a serum concentration, and concentration/therapeutic response is not well established. Aim for 12–64 micromol/L (3–15 mg/L)[4]
Interactions with other antiepileptics	• Lamotrigine serum concentration may be increased by valproic acid • Lamotrigine serum concentration may be decreased by carbamazepine, phenobarbital, phenytoin and primidone

TABLE E11
Levetiracetam[1]

Half-life	• 6–9 hours (elderly: 10–11 hours)
Pretreatment measures	• U&Es, LFTs
Therapeutic serum range	• The serum concentration/therapeutic response has not been well established. A putative range is 70–269 micromol/L (12–46 mg/L)[2] • N.B.: There is low intra- and intersubject variability and plasma levels can be predicted from the oral dose of levetiracetam as mg/kg body weight, reducing the need for monitoring levels[2]
Interactions with other antiepileptics	• No clinically significant interactions with other antiepileptics have been reported[3]

TABLE E12
Oxcarbazepine[1]

Half-life	• 1.3–2.3 hours for oxcarbazepine • 9.3 hours for 10-hydroxy-carbazepine (active metabolite)
Pretreatment measures	• U&Es, LFTs
Therapeutic serum range	• The serum concentration/therapeutic response has not been well established. A putative range for 10-hydroxy-carbazepine is 50–110 micromol/L (12–27 mg/L).[4] • Toxicity has been observed at 138–158 micromol/L (35–40 mg/L) • N.B.: pharmacokinetics of active metabolite are linear and show dose proportionality across the dose range of 300–2400 mg/day
Other monitoring	• Patients with renal impairment should have U&Es checked 2 weeks after commencement, and then monthly for the first 3 months • N.B.: In patients with cardiac insufficiency and secondary heart failure, regular weight measurements are needed to determine occurrence of fluid retention. In case of fluid retention or worsening cardiac condition, serum sodium should be checked
Interactions with other antiepileptics	• Oxcarbazepine serum concentration may be decreased by carbamazepine, phenytoin, phenobarbital and valproic acid • Oxcarbazepine can increase the serum concentration of phenytoin and phenobarbital • Oxcarbazepine can decrease the serum concentration of carbamazepine

TABLE E13
Perampanel[1]

Half-life	• 105 hours • Reduced to 25 hours in the presence of potent enzyme inducers
Therapeutic serum range	• No therapeutic serum concentration established
Interactions with other antiepileptics	• Perampanel serum concentration may be decreased by carbamazepine, oxcarbazepine, phenytoin and topiramate • Perampanel can decrease the serum concentration of carbamazepine, clobazam, lamotrigine, oxcarbazepine and valproic acid

TABLE E14
Phenobarbital[1]

Half-life	• Range: 75–136 hours (mean 100 hours)[4] • Shorter in children and with enzyme-inducing agents
Pretreatment measures	• FBC, U&Es
Therapeutic serum range	• 60–180 micromol/L (10–50 mg/L) • N.B.: Modified by development of tolerance
Sampling time	• Sampling time is not critical; however, it can take 3 weeks to achieve steady state[4]
Other monitoring	• FBC should be checked periodically as megaloblastic anaemia and blood dyscrasias occasionally occur[5]
Interactions with other antiepileptics	• Phenobarbital serum concentration may be increased by valproic acid, oxcarbazepine, phenytoin, felbamate and stiripentol • Phenobarbital serum concentration may be increased or decreased by phenytoin • Phenobarbital serum concentration may be decreased by vigabatrin • Phenobarbital can decrease the serum concentration of carbamazepine, phenytoin and valproic acid, ethosuximide, lacosamide, lamotrigine, clobazam and clonazepam, rufinamide, tiagabine, topiramate and zonisamide[3] Two other important interactions are with alcohol and coumarin anticoagulants. • Alcohol potentiates the CNS depression of barbiturates. • Phenobarbital stimulates the metabolism of coumarin anticoagulants, and because phenobarbital has such a long half-life, it can take 14 to 21 days for the liver enzymes to return to normal upon its withdrawal. This means close monitoring of the anticoagulation is necessary during this period to prevent haemorrhage

TABLE E15
Pregabalin[1]

Half-life	• 6.3 hours
Pretreatment measures	• ECG, U&Es
Therapeutic serum range	• 2–8 mg/L
Interactions with other antiepileptics	• No clinically significant interactions with other antiepileptics have been reported

TABLE E16
Primidone[1]

Half-life	• Range 4–22 hours[2] • Mean 10 hours • The principal metabolite of primidone is phenobarbital, so effect can persist much longer (see above)
Pretreatment measures	• FBC, U&Es, LFTs
Therapeutic serum range	• 23–55 micromol/L (5–12 mg/L)
Other monitoring	• FBC should be checked periodically as megaloblastic anaemia and blood dyscrasias occasionally occur
Interactions with other antiepileptics	• See phenobarbital above • Additionally carbamazepine and phenytoin can stimulate the conversion of primidone to phenobarbital

TABLE E17
Retigabine[1]

Half-life	• 6–10 hours
Pretreatment measures	• U&Es, LFTs, ophthalmology review, ECG, assessment of risk of urinary retention
Therapeutic serum range	• Not established
Other monitoring	• Six-monthly ophthalmology review
Interactions with other antiepileptics	• Retigabine serum concentration may be decreased by carbamazepine and phenytoin • Caution is advised in the concomitant prescribing of retigabine and lamotrigine as retigabine levels may increase and lamotrigine levels may decrease[3]

TABLE E18
Rufinamide[1]

Half-life	• 6–10 hours
Pretreatment measures	• LFTs • ECG (can shorten QT interval)
Therapeutic serum range	• 30–40 mg/L
Interactions with other antiepileptics	• Rufinamide serum concentration may be increased by valproic acid (most pronounced effects in patients with low body weight (<30 kg)

TABLE E19
Tiagabine[1]

Half-life	• 7–9 hours
	• (2–3 hours if enzyme induction occurs)
Pretreatment measures	• LFTs
Therapeutic serum range	• The serum concentration/therapeutic response has not been well established. A putative range is 200–1100 nmol/L (82–453 mg/L)[2]
Interactions with other antiepileptics	• Tiagabine serum concentration may be decreased by carbamazepine, phenobarbital, phenytoin and primidone
	• Tiagabine can decrease the serum concentration of valproic acid[3]

TABLE E20
Topiramate[1]

Half-life	• 21 hours
	• Reduced to 12–15 hours with enzyme inducers[4]
Pretreatment measures	• LFTs, U&Es
Therapeutic serum range	• The serum concentration/therapeutic response has not been well established. A putative range is 6–74 micromol/L (2–19 mg/L)[2]
Other monitoring	• Bicarbonate level may require monitoring if the patient shows signs of metabolic acidosis (although this side effect is rare)
Interactions with other antiepileptics	• Topiramate serum concentration may be decreased by phenytoin and carbamazepine
	• Topiramate can sometimes increase the serum concentration of phenytoin

TABLE E21
Valproic acid (sodium valproate)[1]

Half life	• Range 8–20 hours
	• Mean 12 hours
Pretreatment measures	• LFTs, U&Es
Therapeutic serum range	• 278–694 micromol/L (40–100 mg/L)
	• Toxic effects usually observed at >700 micromol/L (>100 mg/L)
Other monitoring	• LFTs before initiation, monthly for the first 6 months, and then annually
Interactions with other antiepileptics	• Valproic acid serum concentration may be increased by stiripentol
	• Valproic acid serum concentration may be decreased by carbamazepine, phenobarbital, phenytoin and tiagabine
	• Valproic acid can increase the serum concentration of ethosuximide, lamotrigine, phenobarbital, primidone and rufinamide
	• Valproic acid can decrease the plasma concentration of clonazepam and phenytoin (but increases the amount of free phenytoin, therefore if monitoring phenytoin measure the free form rather than the total phenytoin)

E

TABLE E22
Vigabatrin[1]

Half-life	• Range 5–8 hours
Pretreatment measures	• FBC, U&Es • An ophthalmological examination is required as vigabatrin can cause visual field defects
Therapeutic serum range	• The serum concentration/therapeutic response has not been well established. A putative range is 6–278 micromol/L (0.8–36 mg/L)[2]
Other monitoring	• Periodically monitor FBC and U&Es and carry out an ophthalmological examination
Interactions with other antiepileptics	• Vigabatrin can decrease the serum concentration of phenytoin, and may reduce phenobarbital and primidone levels[1,4]

TABLE E23
Zonisamide[1]

Half-life	• 60 hours; reducing in the presence of enzyme-inducing drugs
Pretreatment measures	• Exclude a personal or close family history of renal stones. Advise adequate hydration • Exclude hypersensitivity reactions to sulphonamides
Therapeutic serum range	• 20–30 micrograms/mL
Other monitoring	• FBC for aplastic anaemia
Interactions with other antiepileptics	• Zonisamide can gradually decrease the serum concentration of phenytoin

REFERENCES

1 eMC (2014). www.medicines.org.uk (accessed 11 November 2014).
2 Epilepsy Society (2014). *Guidelines for Therapeutic Drug Monitoring of Antiepileptic Drugs.* http://www.epilepsysociety.org.uk/sites/default/files/Therapeutic -Drug-Monitoring-of-Antiepileptic-Drugs-Table.pdf (accessed 19 November 2014).
3 Baxter K, Preston CL (2013). *Stockley's Drug Interactions: A source book of interactions, their mechanisms, clinical importance and management* (10th edn). London: Pharmaceutical Press.
4 Alarcon G *et al.* (2009). *Epilepsy* (Oxford Specialist Handbooks in Neurology). Oxford: OUP.
5 Dollery C (ed.) (1999). *Therapeutic Drugs* (2nd edn). Edinburgh: Churchill Livingstone.

Erythrocyte sedimentation rate

Erythrocyte sedimentation rate (ESR) is a widely used test to monitor inflammatory disease and infections. It is a non-protein acute-phase reactant where serum levels reflect plasma viscosity and indirectly measure acute-phase protein concentrations.[1]

It is defined as the rate (mm/hour) at which erythrocytes suspended in plasma in a vertical tube settle.

Advantages include the availability of abundant literature, and that it is inexpensive and easy to carry out. N.B.: samples require analysis within 4 hours.[2]

Disadvantages include non-specificity in that it doesn't identify the cause or location of inflammation, and changes occur slowly relative to the patient's condition. CRP concentrations generally change more rapidly.

Temporal arteritis and polymyalgia rheumatica are exceptions where a high ESR is used to diagnose and monitor disease activity.[1]

ESR can be raised in any inflammatory disorder and conditions such as tuberculosis, myocardial infarction, multiple myeloma, renal disease and anaemia.[3] Raised ESR may also be seen in menstruation and pregnancy.

Low ESR is seen in conditions such as congestive cardiac failure, sickle cells and some protein abnormalities.[3]

Predicted values

ESR increases with age and is higher in females (see formula below):[4]

- ESR in men = age in years divided by 2
- ESR in women = (age in years + 10) divided by 2.

Drugs such as methyldopa, oral contraceptives, theophylline and vitamin A can increase ESR; aspirin, steroids and quinine may decrease it.[1]

REFERENCES

1 UpToDate (2014). *Acute Phase Reactants*. http://www.uptodate.com/contents/acute-phase-reactants?source=search_result&search=crp&selectedTitle=2~150 (accessed 17 January 2015).

2 GP Notebook (2015). *Reference Range (ESR)*. http://www.gpnotebook.co.uk/simplepage.cfm?ID=389349443 (accessed 21 October 2014).

3 Patient.co.uk (2014). *Acute-phase Proteins, CRP, ESR and Viscosity*. http://www.patient.co.uk/doctor/acute-phase-proteins-crp-esr-and-viscosity (accessed 17 January 2015).

4 Miller A *et al.* (1983). Simple rule for calculating normal erythrocyte sedimentation rate. *Br Med J (Clin Res Ed)* 286: 266.

Eye drops: use and care

Key counselling points for patients administering eye drops are listed below.

Administration

1 With clean hands, unscrew the cap to expose the nozzle, or if the drops are in a glass bottle, draw up some of the solution into the glass dropper. Do not breathe on the eye drop nozzle or glass dropper.
2 Tilt the head back and look up towards the ceiling.
3 The lower eyelid should be gently pulled downwards and, without touching the eye with the nozzle or dropper, place one drop into the space between the lower lid and the eye (Figure E1).
4 Release the lid and close the eye for 30 seconds. Try not to blink more than usual; this removes the drops from the eye by drainage into the tear ducts.[1]
5 Replace the dropper or cap on the bottle securely.

Additional counselling points

- Avoid contamination of the eye drops during use.
- Date the bottle when first opened and discard 4 weeks after opening for multidose preservative eye drops (unless the manufacturer recommends a longer or shorter period). For ward use in some hospitals, this may be reduced to 1 or 2 weeks because of the greater risk of contamination. In section 11.2 of the BNF (control of microbial contamination) it is recommended to discard 1 week after opening, and to obtain a fresh supply on discharge from hospital.[2] Check your local policy.
- Never let any other person use your eye drops.
- It is generally inadvisable to wear contact lenses, particularly soft lenses, when using eye drops or ointment.
- Store the drops in a cool dry place out of reach of children. Some eye drops require refrigerated storage (2–8°C), e.g. chloramphenicol.

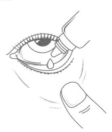

FIGURE E1   Instillation of an eye drop

- If using eye ointment at the same time of day as drops, use the drops first and wait 5 minutes before using the ointment.
- If using more than one kind of eye drop, wait 5 minutes between drops.

There are four types of eye drop preparations: multidose preserved eye drops, preserved eye drop gels, preservative-free single-unit dose eye drops (which should be used immediately after opening and then discarded immediately after use) and preservative-free multidose products such as Hylo-Forte. The contents of the Hylo range products are protected from contamination by the unique design of the delivery system, which is an airless, preservative-free multi-dose container.[3] Once a drop is delivered, the valve immediately closes and backflow is prevented. These products are sterile for 6 months once opened.[4]

Professional points

Flooding the eye with a number of drops from the same bottle is a common administration error. The eye can only accommodate one drop before overflow occurs. Instillation of more than one drop should be discouraged, as this may increase systemic side effects.[5] The volume of liquid contained in eye drop bottles is variable but for the calculation of likely number of doses available, each millilitre will provide about 15 drops.

Some patients demonstrate allergy to their eye drops, which is often related to the preservative rather than the active ingredient. Appropriate eye drops containing a different preservative may be prescribed, or alternatively single-use (preservative-free) eye drops may be used, which are more expensive. In the absence of infection it is generally acceptable to use one 'single-use' eye drop to treat both eyes if both require treatment. For patients requiring eye drops long-term, an ophthalmologist should properly diagnose any eye drop preservative allergy.

A large proportion of a typical eye drop will have drained from the conjunctival sac within 30 seconds under normal conditions; there will be no trace of the drop after 20 minutes.[1] Systemic side effects may arise from absorption of drugs into the general circulation from conjunctival vessels or from the nasal mucosa. Gently pressing on the inside corner of the closed eye (lacrimal punctum) for at least a minute reduces drainage into the nasolacrimal channel, therefore prolonging contact time of the drop in the eye and decreasing systemic absorption from the nasal mucosa.[2]

Several devices are also available to help with correct positioning of eye drop bottles. The Opticare range is available on NHS prescription, and can accommodate 2.5 mL to 20 mL dropper bottles. The Auto-Dropper is another example of this kind of device.

Postoperative treatments

When reviewing medications in patients after ophthalmic surgery, the continuing need for topical corticosteroids and antibacterial agents can be problematic. The following are examples of ophthalmic postoperative regimens for eye drops:

Glaucoma surgery (trabeculectomy)

- prednisolone acetate 1% eye drops 2-hourly
- atropine 1% eye drops three times a day
- ofloxacin 0.3% eye drops four times a day for 1 week.

Squint surgery

- dexamethasone, neomycin and polymyxin B (Maxitrol) eye drops four times a day for 4 weeks.

Cataract surgery – uncomplicated

- dexamethasone, neomycin and polymyxin B (Maxitrol) four times a day for 4 weeks.

Cataract surgery – for diabetic patients

- prednisolone acetate 1% eye drops four times a day for 4 weeks
- chloramphenicol 0.5% eye drops four times a day for 1 week.

A fresh supply of eye drops should be provided after any eye surgery and any used presurgery should be discarded.[2]

REFERENCES

1 Richards RME (2004). Ophthalmic products. In: Winfield AJ, Richards RME (eds) *Pharmaceutical Practice* (3rd edn). London: Churchill Livingstone, pp. 264–279.
2 Joint Formulary Committee (2014). *British National Formulary* (68th edn). London: BMJ Group and Pharmaceutical Press.
3 Titcomb L (2010). Are quality standards being reduced as eye drops are classed as devices? *Pharm J* 284: 633–638.
4 Scope Ophthalmics (2014). *Dry Eye Products*. http://www.scopeophthalmics.com/index.php?ECProduct=31&ec=dry-eye-products (accessed 25 October 2014).

Eye ointments: use and care

Eye ointments are available for a limited range of drugs, the most widely used product being chloramphenicol eye ointment.

The advantages of an ophthalmic ointment (compared with drops) is that a more sustained drug effect is achieved, which may allow less frequent administration whilst maintaining effective local drug concentrations. Use of ointments may also have the advantage of reducing nursing workload in the ward situation. Systemic side effects from nasal drainage of drugs applied to the eye are associated with eye drops much more often than with eye ointments.[1]

The disadvantages of ophthalmic ointment use are that patients may find the ointment less easy to apply and vision will be blurred for a few minutes after application.

Advice to patients: how to apply eye ointment

Key counselling points for patients administering eye ointment are listed below.

1 With clean hands, unscrew the cap from the tube and expel the first 0.5 cm.
2 Gently pull down the lower lid of the eye to be treated and squeeze a line of ointment about 0.5 cm (1/4 inch) along the inside of the eyelid (Figure E2).
3 Try to avoid touching the eye or eyelashes with the nozzle.
4 Close the eye for a few minutes. The ointment will melt rapidly; blinking will help to spread it.
5 Replace the cap on the tube.

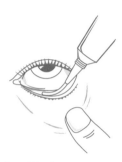

FIGURE E2 Application of eye ointment

Additional counselling points

- For a few minutes after application, vision may be blurred. It is advisable not to drive or operate machinery during this time.
- Avoid contamination of the eye ointment during use.
- Date the tube when first opened and discard 4 weeks after opening. For ward use in some hospitals this may be reduced to 1 or 2 weeks because of the greater risk of contamination. Check your local policy.
- Never let another person use your eye ointment.
- Eye ointments should not be used while wearing contact lenses.
- If using eye drops at the same time of day as an eye ointment, apply the drops 5 minutes before the ointment.

Dry-eye syndrome

Dry-eye syndrome (keratoconjunctivitis sicca) is a common chronic eye condition especially in older patients, as tear production decreases with increased age. It is also common in postmenopausal women and may be induced by hormone replacement therapy. Dry eyes can also be associated with Sjögren's syndrome and connective tissue disorders such as rheumatoid arthritis. Artificial tears preparations, such as simple eye ointment, VitaA-POS or Lacrilube, can be used to treat dry eyes. The advantage over eye drops is the prolonged retention time; the disadvantages of eye ointments are they are greasy and can produce stickiness and blurred vision. Eye ointments tend to be used as an adjuvant at night, with eye drops such as hypromellose used during the day. Patients usually start dry-eye treatment with a less viscous treatment such as hypromellose 0.3% eye drops or carbomers, e.g. Viscotears. These are gel-like and cling to the eye surface, which may reduce frequency of administration to four times a day. If a patient needs to use dry-eye preparations more than six times a day, preservative-free treatments should be used to reduce damage by benzalkonium chloride (preservative) as this disrupts the tear film. Suitable alternatives are Viscotears, Celluvisc single-dose unit or Hylo-Forte, Hylo-tear or Hylo-care preservative-free multidose.[2]

REFERENCES

1 Joint Formulary Committee (2014). *British National Formulary* (68th edn). London: BMJ Group and Pharmaceutical Press.

2 Morrissey EFR, Lloyd F (2013). *Pharmaceutical Care of the Eye, Continuing Professional Development*. NI Centre for Pharmacy Learning and Development. http://www.cppe.ac.uk/learning/Details.asp?TemplateID=EYE-P-01&Format=P&ID=115&EventID=43178 (accessed 18 August 2014).

Falls: pharmaceutical care

Defining falls and their importance

A fall is defined as 'an event which results in a person coming to rest inadvertently on the ground or floor or other lower level'[1] and may be accidental (such as a slip or trip) or the result of a predictable or unpredictable physiological factor (e.g. syncope). The chance of falling and sustaining an injury from a fall increases with age, with more than half of all reported injuries in older people being due to a fall.[2] A fall and its consequences can be life changing for an older person, damaging the person's physical health in the short term and adversely affecting the individual's mental health, independence and life span in the longer term.

Causes of falls

It's important to see falls as a symptom and not a diagnosis – people can fall for a wide variety of reasons, and any one fall is likely to have a multifactorial cause. Environmental hazards (e.g. poorly fitting footwear, thick rugs on the floor) are a significant risk, though an older person's physical ability to respond correctively to a slip or trip increases the chance and severity of a fall. Age-related physiological changes, such as impaired muscle strength and posture control, adversely affect gait and balance, whilst changes to visual acuity and hearing may alter environmental perception. There is increasingly robust evidence for a causal link between some medicines and the risk of falling,[3] but in practice it is often difficult to be certain one is a direct cause of a fall. It is also important to remember that reports of a fall may be a sign of abuse of an adult at risk.

Medicines as a cause of falls

It is known that falls risk increases with each additional medicine a patient takes beyond a four-drug regimen, regardless of the class of medicine added.[4] There are some classes of medicine that are more commonly associated with falling, although consideration must be given to the likelihood of increased side effects, duration of action and toxicity from inevitable age-related physiological changes for all medicines.

There is strong evidence linking antipsychotics, benzodiazepines (including the 'z-drugs') and antidepressants to increased falls risk, and in some cases fracture rates. It is believed they cause falls by reducing lower-limb muscle strength, reaction time and balance control. There is no robust evidence showing SSRIs or atypical antipsychotics carry less risk than more traditional choices, such as tricyclic antidepressants or typical antipsychotics, respectively. The evidence of a falls risk from opioids is inconsistent but cannot be discounted.[5]

The evidence linking falls risk and injury to medicines affecting the cardiovascular system is generally weak.[6] In theory, falls may be caused by postural hypotension, syncope or effects on rhythm, and the risk will increase with the use of multiple cardiac medicines. Most patients suffering symptoms related to these medicines often develop coping strategies, which limit the risk of falls (e.g. rising slowly), but as patients age the effects of these medicines may become more pronounced, so their compensatory measures can fail and regular monitoring becomes more important.

Anticholinergic effects may be contributory to the falls risk of some medicines (e.g. antipsychotics, antidepressants), although there is little evidence specifically linking falls risk with these effects as a defined class of medicines. Anticholinergic effects may include blurred vision, dry mouth and constipation, all of which may be a contributory factor of functional falls, including those linked to toileting.

Falls risk assessment and next steps

NICE recommends that older people presenting with falls injury or reporting recurrent falls should be offered a multifactorial falls risk assessment from a healthcare professional with appropriate skills and experience, which may include assessment of:[7]

- home hazards
- gait, balance and mobility, and muscle weakness
- perceived functional ability and fear of falling
- visual impairment
- cognitive impairment and neurological examination
- cardiovascular examination
- urinary incontinence
- osteoporosis risk
- current medication.

There is limited evidence that multifactorial falls prevention programmes reduce the number of fallers or fall-related injuries[8] and, despite various studies looking at how to reduce medicines-related falls risks, there is no clear evidence for an effective single intervention.[3] However, the following points are all considered part of good pharmaceutical care for patients following a fall.

1 Complete a full medicines reconciliation, including over-the-counter and complementary medicines (see *Medicines reconciliation* entry). A discussion should also be had on the patient's usual level of alcohol consumption.

2 Stop all potentially inappropriate medication either from adverse effects or interactions, or because of contraindications. The use of support tools may be useful, such as the STOPP/START[9,10] or Beers criteria,[11] or anticholinergic burden scales.

3 Reduce the dose of medicines linked to the fall where withdrawal is not desirable or possible: this is particularly important in psychoactive medication where rapid withdrawal or cessation is not possible, though challenges exist in maintaining reduction programmes when care is transferred (e.g. at hospital discharge).

4 Complete osteoporosis screening: confirm that the patient is receiving optimal bone protection therapy.

5 Further reduce polypharmacy and simplify the medication regimen: check all indications are valid, current and essential and that the medicines have an appropriate evidence base for effectiveness and acceptable risk profile.

6 Assess patient adherence to therapy and discuss the patient's understanding of the medication: falls may be due to inappropriate self-medication (e.g. taking double doses of an antihypertensive).

7 Explore the patient's ability to self-medicate effectively: practical strategies to support self-medication must be considered and employed wherever possible.

Medication changes made because of a falls risk must be clearly documented and communicated to the patient's general practitioner. Additional steps should also be taken to ensure ongoing support for patients at home. This may include referral to a local falls service, or to the patient's usual community pharmacy for medicines use review or new medicines service enrolment as necessary, particularly on discharge from hospital.

REFERENCES

1 WHO (2012). *Falls*. Factsheet No. 344. http://www.who.int/mediacentre/factsheets/fs344/en/ (accessed 4 June 2014).

2 McMahon CG *et al.* (2012). Diurnal variation in mortality in older nocturnal fallers. *Age Ageing* 41: 29–35.

3 Boyle N *et al.* (2010). Medication and falls: risk and optimization. *Clin Geriatr Med* 26: 583–605.

4 Deandrea S *et al.* (2012). Risk factors for falls in community-dwelling older people: a systematic review and meta-analysis. *Epidemiology* 21: 658–668.

5 Huang AR *et al.* (2012). Medication-related falls in the elderly. Causative factors and preventative strategies. *Drugs Ageing* 29: 359–376.

6 Zeimer H (2008). Medication and falls in older people. *J Pharm Pract Res* 38: 148–151.

7 NICE (2013). *Falls: Assessment and prevention of falls in older people*. Clinical guideline 161. http://www.nice.org.uk/nicemedia/live/14181/64088/64088.pdf (accessed 4 June 2014).

8 Gates S *et al.* (2008). Multifactorial assessment and targeted intervention for preventing falls and injuries among older people in community and emergency care settings: systematic review and meta-analysis. *BMJ* 336: 130.

9 Gallagher P *et al.* (2008). STOPP (Screening Tool of Older Persons' Prescriptions) and START (Screening Tool to Alert Doctors to Right Treatment): Consensus Validation. *Int J Clin Pharmacol Ther* 46: 72–83.

10 ELMMB (2013). *STOPP START toolkit*. http://www.elmmb.nhs.uk/guidelines/other-clinical-guidelines/?assetdetesctl522647=53110&p=2 (accessed 21 February 2015).

11 Fick D *et al.* (2012). American Geriatrics Society updated Beers Criteria for potentially inappropriate medication use in older adults. *J Am Geriatr Soc* 60: 616–631.

Ferinject

Overview[1]	
Form	Ferric carboxymaltose
Dose	• Calculated based on body weight and haemoglobin level (see table below for cumulative iron dose). • A single dose should not exceed 1000 mg of iron a day. • Do not administer more than 1000 mg once each week. • If total dose is greater than 1000 mg of iron, it should be divided and given over 2 weeks

	Body weight	
Haemoglobin	**35 kg to less than 70 kg**	**≥70 kg**
Less than 100 g/L	1500 mg	2000 mg
≥100 g/L	1000 mg	1500 mg

	• A cumulative dose of 500 mg of iron should not be exceeded for patients with a body weight <35 kg. • For haemoglobin values ≥140 g/L, an initial dose of 500 mg iron should be given and iron parameters should be checked prior to repeat dosing

Adminis- tration routes	**Intravenous infusion**	**Intravenous instalments**	**Intra- muscular**
	Yes	Yes	No

| Adminis-
tration | • Up to a maximum single dose of 1000 mg iron (up to a maximum of 20 mg/kg body weight)
• Dilute in sodium chloride 0.9% to a minimum of 2 mg/mL
• Observe for adverse effects for at least 30 minutes following each injection

The diluent volume and rate of administration are dependent on the dose required. | • Intravenous injection using undiluted injection
• Used for doses up to 1000 mg iron (up to a maximum 15 mg/kg body weight)
• Observe for adverse effects for at least 30 minutes following each injection

The administration time varies depending on the dose.
• Doses up to 200 mg: no prescribed administration time
• ≥200 mg up to 500 mg: iron should be administered at a rate of 100 mg/min
• >500 mg up to 1000 mg iron administered over 15 minutes | |

Dose of iron	Maximum sodium chloride 0.9% volume	Adminis-tration time
100–200 mg	50 mL	-
≥200–500 mg	100 mL	6 minutes
>500–1000 mg	250 mL	15 minutes

Monitoring	• Patients should be monitored for signs and symptoms of hypersensitivity reactions during and following each administration. • Observe patient for adverse effects for at least 30 minutes following each injection. • If hypersensitivity reactions or signs of intolerance occur during administration, the treatment must be stopped immediately

REFERENCE
1 eMC (2014). *SPC Ferinject*. https://www.medicines.org.uk/emc/medicine/24167 (accessed 27 August 2014).

Fluid balance

Fluid balance is more than estimating the input and output of fluid in the body. It must also account for redistribution of fluid and electrolytes outside the plasma volume (Figure F1).

In principle, all fluid into and out of the body should be measured and recorded on a fluid balance chart. In actual clinical practice it is more common to express an opinion about fluid status. Fluid inputs are estimated but fluid output is often unmeasured unless the patient is in intensive care. Fluid balance charts are notable for their omission of data and inaccuracy of the mathematics. Thus, medical staff tend to ignore them and this psychologically feeds back into poor attention to detail by the nursing staff. One of the first steps in managing a deteriorating patient is to contact the critical care outreach team whose actions include catheterising patients and starting an accurate fluid balance chart.

Fluid management

This includes the assessment of fluid status and the correction of any deficit or excess. In 2013 NICE published guidance on intravenous fluid therapy for patients on wards, although the data were limited and drawn from studies from intensive care and peri- and postoperative patients.[1] There is often a lack of understanding about fluid management with doctors and nurses as well as pharmacists. To many, fluids are boring, bulky and stored in the hospital dungeons. However, they are essential to the maintenance and homeostasis of life. Errors with fluid management are common and significant education and training are required.

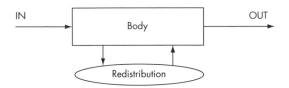

FIGURE F1   Fluid balance

Fluid physiology

Water comprises almost two-thirds of body weight and two-thirds of the water is within cells. Fluid manipulation occurs within the plasma volume that represents only one-twentieth of body weight; redistribution then occurs.

Assessment of fluid status

Consider:

- signs of pulmonary or peripheral oedema
- dry mucosa, sunken eye appearance or patient feeling thirsty
- poor urine output (<0.5 mL/kg/hour)
- slow capillary refill (more/less than 2 seconds)
- blood pressure – central venous or jugular or postural hypotension
- pulse and heart rate
- altered conscious state
- loss of weight over days (not weeks)
- concentration of biochemistry.

These data may be captured from simple clinical parameters (pulse, temperature and pressure charts) but have now been replaced by National Early Warning Scores (NEWS) charts, which also include urine output (see *Early Warning Score* entry). This comes from NICE guidance on the acutely deteriorating patient, where signs of hypovolaemia are a prelude to shock, and particularly that due to sepsis.[1,2]

Leg elevation

If a patient is lying horizontal in bed, raising one leg will move the blood volume into the central compartment and improve venous return to the heart, and therefore should increase cardiac output and blood pressure. If the patient's heart is failing the heart will become congested, pulmonary oedema will form and the patient will cough up pink sputum. In this latter case the leg can be lowered again and normality restored. This manoeuvre can be described as a reversible fluid challenge: a positive finding suggests the need for intravenous fluids and a negative finding indicates adequate fluid filling and possibly the need for diuretics. A similar (but reverse) test is to elevate the patient's head above the heart; if the patient feels dizzy or blood pressure falls, this shows the individual is hypovolaemic.

Fluid challenge

A fluid challenge is the administration of 500 mL of intravenous fluid over 15 minutes. A blood pressure rise, fall in heart rate or increase in urine output is a positive sign. If it remains at normal parameters then the challenge has corrected the condition and decisions about maintenance fluid can be considered. If the blood pressure does not change or starts to fall, then further fluid challenges can be given to resuscitate the patient.[3]

Five Rs of NICE fluid guidelines

Arguably, the most important activity is to review the decisions made as the patient's condition changes and responds to treatment. Repetition of the same plan without review is likely to be harmful.

TABLE F1
Five Rs with descriptions and actions

Component	Description	Action
Resuscitation with fluids	Acutely (1–4 hours), restoring normal fluid balance	500 mL of intravenous fluid (containing 130–154 mmol/L sodium)
Routine maintenance	Preferably delivered orally/enterally but may require intravenous support. It should be sufficient to maintain organ perfusion and kidney output	25–30 mL/kg/day water, 1 mmol/kg/day sodium chloride and potassium chloride and 50–100 g/day glucose (to avoid ketosis)
Replacement	Abnormal losses such as fistulas, surgical drains, diarrhoea, vomiting or nasogastric losses	Fluids that match the composition of losses
Redistribution	Water and electrolytes that have left the vascular space and moved into extracellular spaces (e.g. ascites) or into tissues (oedema)	Possibly hypertonic solution or colloids (albumin), but usually vasoconstrictors and diuretics to increase vascular osmotic pressure (Figure F2)
Review	Regularly reassess the fluid status and effects of treatments with a plan for the next 24 hours	Communication and education

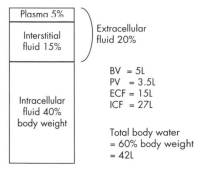

FIGURE F2   Fluid compartments. BV, blood volume; PV, plasma volume; ECF, extracellular fluid; ICF, intracellular fluid

Like any science experiment, outcomes of interventions should be regularly (sometimes frequently) reviewed. In practice this is one of the biggest failings and where pharmacists can contribute. Shift patterns and limits on working hours mean that often the same junior doctor will not review the same patient each day. This lack of continuity means that fluid balance is not assessed on a daily basis nor reviewed over several days or a week. Cumulative fluid overload can amount to 20 litres by the time a patient enters the intensive care unit. However, fluid and electrolyte undertreatment is the far more common phenomenon.

Patients should be weighed twice a week in hospital so that rapid weight changes can be detected and attributed to sudden changes in fluid balance.

In addition, significant education is required to restore understanding and enthusiasm about the importance of fluid management.

Vasoconstrictors and vasodilators

Use of vasoconstrictors is not an adequate substitute for poor fluid management but is used in the critically ill when a patient needs rescue. Vasoconstrictors effectively shrink the plasma volume so the fluid that is available can perfuse the vital organs. Similarly, vasodilators can produce a relative underfilling of the vascular compartment and produce tachycardia. Where there is insufficient blood in the vascular system, the heart tries to compensate by pushing it more quickly around the vital organs. Tachycardia is a precursor of arrhythmias and should be corrected by giving volume (Figure F3).

Postoperative fluids

Surgery and trauma produce a systemic inflammatory response syndrome (SIRS) that is not limited to a swelling up of injured tissues. In addition, a number of stress hormones are produced, including adrenaline and aldosterone. Adrenaline drives metabolic activity and

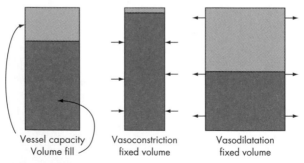

FIGURE F3   Vasodilation and volume

can produce tachycardia. Aldosterone causes sodium retention and potassium loss. During an operation, perfusion pathways may be altered, either because some anaesthetics are vasodilating (e.g. propofol) or because nitric oxide synthetase (NOS) is stimulated. NOS causes the release of nitric oxide that produces a profound vasodilatation. Reduced tissue oxygenation may produce acidosis. SIRS, anaesthetics and blood loss all produce a postoperative patient who is actually (or relatively) hypovolaemic, vasodilated, tachycardiac/arrhythmogenic and sodium-retentive or in acute renal failure. Whilst fluid resuscitation is required, consideration must be given to the sodium load, the potassium content and the temporary use of vasoconstrictors (such as phenylephrine).[4]

Anaesthetists often like to use compound sodium lactate (Hartmann's) because it contains a relatively low sodium content (131 mmol/L) and the buffer lactate (converted in the liver to bicarbonate). However, a combination of products may be needed to restore normal fluid balance.

Sodium chloride 0.9% is not physiologically normal and should not be referred to as 'normal'. It contains 154 mmol/L of sodium, whereas normal plasma contains 130–145 mmol/L sodium. It is a resuscitation fluid and should not be used for routine maintenance. It can be alternated with glucose 5% for postoperative patients if sufficient potassium is added – or preferably use a combined product of glucose 4% and sodium chloride 0.18% with potassium. As a rough guide, a patient who has lost a litre of blood may require 2–3 L of sodium chloride 0.9% for resuscitation, but progress must be regularly reviewed because of the SIRS response described above. The water and sodium ions will distribute into the extracellular fluid compartment, so may require repeat dosing to support intravascular volume.

Glucose 5% will quickly disperse from the vascular space. The water will be drawn osmotically into the extracellular and then intracellular compartments. Some glucose is needed to maintain blood sugar levels and avoid generation of ketones. However, this is not a substitute for proper nutrition (containing proteins, fats, vitamins and minerals as well as carbohydrates). In skilled hands it can be used to manage sodium distribution and balance as well as deliver potassium to the tissues.

Glucose 4% and sodium chloride 0.18% with 40 mmol potassium in 1 litre is not a resuscitation fluid because it only contains 30 mmol of sodium. However, 2 litres/day of this makes a useful maintenance fluid (60 mmol sodium, 80 mmol potassium, 88 mmol chloride and 80 g carbohydrate) in the postoperative phase. Fluid and electrolyte levels must be reviewed as, if used longer term, it will produce hyponatraemia.

There is much debate about the role of colloids containing macromolecules such as gelatines, starches and proteins (albumin). More research is clearly needed to clarify their potential role as blood substitutes or in septic resuscitation.

Mannitol (a non-reabsorbable sugar) may be given for head injuries or for patients with cerebral oedema. This will increase plasma oncotic pressure and redistribute water from tissues into vascular spaces. It also acts as an osmotic diuretic by a similar mechanism. Glucose should not be used in head-injury patients because it lowers plasma osmotic pressure and would worsen cerebral oedema.

REFERENCES

1 NICE (2013). *Intravenous Fluid Therapy in Adults in Hospital* (CG174). http://www.nice.org.uk/guidance/cg174 (accessed 17 July 2014).

2 NICE (2007). *Acutely Ill Patients in Hospital: Recognition of and response to acute illness in adults in hospital* (CG50). http://www.nice.org.uk/guidance/cg50 (accessed 17 July 2014).

3 Cecconi M *et al.* (2011). What is a fluid challenge? *Curr Opin Crit Care* 17: 290–295.

4 Cochrane JPS (1978). The aldosterone response to surgery and the relationship of this response to postoperative sodium retention. *Br J Surg* 65: 744–747.

Food–drug interactions

Many drugs undergo clinically significant food–drug interactions, where food may cause changes in the pharmacokinetic or pharmacodynamic properties of the drug. Interactions may be generic where the presence of any food will affect the drug. Food may aid the absorption of drugs such as saquinavir and griseofulvin and patients should be counselled to take the medication with or just after food; or food may delay or reduce the absorption of a drug – examples include flucloxacillin and trospium. In these cases, patients should be counselled to take the medication on an empty stomach, i.e. an hour before food or at least 2 hours after food. It may also be worth noting that it may be beneficial to take certain medication at the same time as food to reduce side effects such as nausea and vomiting, e.g. co-beneldopa and allopurinol; or to reduce GI disturbance, e.g. aspirin and NSAIDs.[1,2]

More specific food–drug interactions are listed in Table F2, and see also *Grapefruit juice–drug interactions* entry.

TABLE F2
Interactions with food and oral drugs[1,2,3]

Food	Example of interacting drugs	Mechanism
Alcohol	Antihypertensives, nicorandil, opiates, methyldopa	Increased hypotensive effect
	Opiates, tricyclic antidepressants, antihistamines	Increased sedative effect
	Oral antidiabetic drugs	Enhanced hypoglycaemic effect
	Disulfiram, metronidazole, procarbazine, levamisole	Disulfiram-like reactions-Prevents metabolism of ethanol, resulting in accumulation of acetaldehyde, characterised by flushing, sweating, vomiting and headaches

TABLE F2
(Continued)

Food	Example of interacting drugs	Mechanism
Caffeine	Theophylline	Drinks containing caffeine may increase theophylline levels
Cranberry juice	Coumarins	Unknown. May cause an increased or unstable international normalised ratio (INR). Do not consume while taking coumarins
Dairy products	Quinolones, tetracyclines, bisphosphonates, estramustine	The calcium ions present in dairy products can form complexes with certain drugs. These complexes are not easily absorbed from the GI tract, resulting in a lower drug concentration in the systemic circulation
Enteral feeds	Phenytoin (withhold feed 2 hours before dose; restart 2 hours after dose), ciprofloxacin	Some drugs may have a reduced absorption due to binding to some enteral feed ingredients
Tyramine-containing food and drink	MAOIs, linezolid (to a lesser extent)	Inhibition of the monoamine oxidase enzyme in the gut wall allowing tyramine to enter the systemic circulation and potentiate its pressor effect, possibly resulting in life-threatening hypertensive crisis
Vitamin K-rich foods	Coumarins	Coumarins are vitamin K antagonists. Change in the consumption of vitamin K-containing foods affects competition for the receptor site, increasing or decreasing anticoagulation

REFERENCES

1 Joint Formulary Committee (2014). *British National Formulary* (68th edn). London. BMJ Group and Pharmaceutical Press.
2 eMC (2014). http://www.medicines.org.uk/emc/ (accessed 3 September 2014).
3 Baxter K (ed.) (2014). *Stockley's Drug Interactions*. London: Pharmaceutical Press. http://www.medicinescomplete.com/ (accessed 3 September 2014).

Gastrointestinal bleeding risk management

Non-steroidal anti-inflammatory drugs (NSAIDs)

Use of NSAIDS increases the risk of gastrointestinal (GI) bleeding by approximately fourfold. The following groups are considered high-risk and should be offered gastroprotection with a proton pump inhibitor (PPI) if alternative analgesia is not suitable:[1]

- aged 65 years or older
- history of peptic ulcer disease, GI bleeding, or gastroduodenal perforation
- concomitant use of medicines known to increase risk of upper GI adverse events, e.g. anticoagulants, aspirin, corticosteroids, selective serotonin reuptake inhibitors
- serious comorbidity, such as cardiovascular disease, hepatic or renal impairment (including dehydration), diabetes or hypertension
- requirement for prolonged NSAID use, including people with:
  - osteoarthritis or rheumatoid arthritis, of any age
  - chronic low-back pain, age 45 years or older
- use of the maximum recommended dose of an NSAID.

Antiplatelets

Low-dose aspirin alone increases the risk of bleeding by approximately twofold, while dual antiplatelet therapy or use with anticoagulants increases this risk to approximately fourfold.[2] American consensus guidelines suggest use of a PPI in the following groups:[3]

- history of peptic ulcer disease or GI bleeding
- dual antiplatelet therapy
- concomitant anticoagulant therapy
- more than one of the following risk factors:
  - age 60 years or greater
  - corticosteroid use
  - dyspepsia or reflux symptoms.

In both NSAID and antiplatelet use, where there is a history of ulcer disease or upper GI bleeding, *Helicobacter pylori* should have been tested for and treated if present.

Scoring systems

There are no scoring systems for predicting risk of GI bleeding in the above groups; however, there are some scoring systems used to predict risk of bleeding in other scenarios:

- HAS-BLED – recommended by NICE[4] to predict the risk of bleeding on anticoagulation in patients with atrial fibrillation (see HAS-BLED score, under *Stroke and transient ischaemic attack* entry)
- Rockall score – prediction of mortality risk after upper GI bleeding (see *Rockall score for gastrointestinal bleed* entry)
- Glasgow-Blatchford score – prediction of the need for blood transfusion or endoscopic treatment in upper GI bleeding.

Both Rockall and Blatchford scores are recommended by NICE[5] in patients presenting with suspected GI bleeding.

REFERENCES

1 NICE (2013). Clinical Knowledge Summaries. *NSAID Prescribing Issues*. http://cks.nice.org.uk/nsaids-prescribing-issues (accessed 11 December 2014).

2 Garcia Rodriguez LA *et al.* (2011). Risk of upper gastrointestinal bleeding with low-dose acetylsalicylic acid alone and in combination with clopidogrel and other medications. *Circulation* 123: 1108–1115.

3 ACCF/ACG/AHA (2008). Expert consensus document on reducing the gastrointestinal risks of antiplatelet therapy and NSAID use. *Circulation* 118: 1894–1909.

4 NICE (2014). Clinical Guideline 180. *Atrial Fibrillation: The management of atrial fibrillation*. http://www.nice.org.uk/guidance/cg180 (accessed 11 December 2014).

5 NICE (2012). Clinical Guideline 141. Acute upper gastrointestinal bleeding: management. https://www.nice.org.uk/guidance/cg141 (accessed 11 December 2014).

Gentamicin

Gentamicin is classed as an aminoglycoside antibiotic and is a mixture of three naturally occurring aminoglycosides produced by *Micromonospora purpurea*. It has bactericidal activity against most strains of the following: *Escherichia coli*, *Klebsiella* spp., *Proteus* spp., *Pseudomonas aeruginosa*, *Enterobacter* spp., *Citrobacter* spp., *Providencia* spp. and staphylococci (including some MRSA strains).[1,2] It has no activity against anaerobic bacteria and is considered low-risk for selecting for *Clostridium difficile*. It inhibits protein synthesis by binding with the 30S ribosomal subunit of bacterial ribosomes, which results in bacterial cell death.

It is intrinsically resistant to streptococci and enterococci but it can be used synergistically with cell wall active agents (e.g. penicillins, vancomycin) in the treatment of infective endocarditis. It is contraindicated for use in those patients with myasthenia gravis.

Pharmacokinetic overview

Gentamicin exhibits concentration-dependent killing and produces a postantibiotic effect. It is excreted by glomerular filtration, appearing 90% unchanged in urine, and should be used with caution in those patients on concomitant nephrotoxic agents and those with existing renal impairment. It is poorly absorbed orally, so is given parenterally. As it has low protein binding and is water-soluble, it is freely distributed in the extravascular space and relatively freely in the interstitial spaces of most tissues.

G

Gentamicin has a narrow therapeutic range; it can cause nephrotoxicity that is dose-related and usually reversible.[1] Ototoxicity caused by gentamicin is independent of drug concentration; it may present as new tinnitus, hearing loss, poor balance, dizziness and oscillopsia. Auditory toxicity is usually due to the accumulation of gentamicin within the inner ear. Vestibular damage is more common than deafness, caused by damage to sensory hair cells, and effects are usually permanent.[1] Duration of treatment, age (>60 years) and repeated treatment courses are risk factors; healthcare professionals should be alert to monitoring for signs of vestibular toxicity and use the minimum duration possible.[3]

Gentamicin is not known to be harmful in pregnancy; however, it is recommended that it be used only in life-threatening situations where the benefits outweigh the possible risks. It is safe to use during breast-feeding.[2]

Adult dose

Gentamicin is given either as a multiple daily dosing regimen every 8 hours, or as a once-daily dosing regimen. Dosing regimens vary amongst hospitals, so follow your local policy. Low-dose gentamicin (1 mg/kg twice daily) is used for its synergistic effect in the treatment of infective endocarditis (see *Endocarditis* entry).

The calculation of the dose will depend upon the choice of once-daily (unlicensed) or multiple-daily dosing. Initial dosing is based on a patient's weight and renal function. Actual body weight is used, except in those patients who are obese (i.e. >20% above ideal body weight (IBW)), where a dose-determining weight (DDW) should be used. Creatinine clearance (CrCl), calculated using the Cockcroft and Gault equation, should be used to estimate renal function (see *Renal function – assessment* entry). It is important to note that, in patients who are anuric or have acute kidney injury, this calculation will not give a true reflection of CrCl.

Ideal body weight calculation

IBW: men (kg) = 50 + 2.3 × (height in inches above 5 feet)

IBW: women (kg) = 49 + 1.7 × (height in inches above 5 feet)

In obese patients, a DDW should be used; this is calculated as follows:

DDW = IBW + 0.4(actual body weight – IBW)

Creatinine clearance calculation

$$\text{CrCl(mL/min)} = \frac{F \times (140 - \text{age}) \times \text{weight (kg)}}{\text{serum Cr (micromol/L)}}$$

$F = 1.23$ for males; 1.04 for females.

Once-daily regimen

Once-daily administration enables effective bactericidal killing through achieving high peak drug concentrations and is generally considered to be less nephrotoxic (the effect on ototoxicity remains less clear).[1,3] The higher the initial concentrations, the more prolonged the postantibiotic effect. Once-daily dosing is not suitable for all patients due to lack of published data or due to risks of accumulation and toxicity. It is inappropriate for use in pregnancy, patients with major burns or ascites and those on dialysis. Initial doses usually range from 5 to 7 mg/kg once a day;[4] subsequent changes to dosing or frequency are made based upon the results of serum concentration monitoring. There are various approaches to once-daily dosing regimens, therefore ensure you follow your local policy. Two commonly used dosing options are described below.

Option 1: Hartford regimen

The Hartford once-daily dosing regimen[5] was originally developed by Hartford Hospital in Connecticut, USA. This regimen gives a fixed dose of 7 mg/kg once daily and the dosing interval is dependent upon estimated CrCl. The initial dose given should be as outlined in Table G1; doses should be rounded to the nearest 20 mg to aid administration.

TABLE G1
Hartford recommended dosing regimen[5]

Creatinine clearance	Recommended dose
≥60 mL/min	7 mg/kg every 24 hours
59–40 mL/min	7 mg/kg every 36 hours
39–20 mL/min	7 mg/kg every 48 hours
<20 mL/min	7 mg/kg single dose; only redose when levels <1 mg/L

With this regimen it is important that the time the dose is administered and the time the serum levels are taken are accurately recorded. After administration of the first dose a blood sample should be taken 6–14 hours after the start of the gentamicin infusion. The exact time when levels are taken should be recorded on the prescription chart and on the sample request form. Once the serum level is known, this should be plotted on the nomogram (Figure G1), which determines the frequency of future doses. If the result falls on a line, the longer interval should be chosen. If the level is above the 48-hourly line, therapy should be stopped and no further doses given until the level is <1 mg/L.

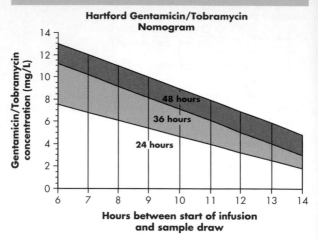

FIGURE G1   Hartford nomogram (reproduced with permission from Yorkshire Hartford prescription chart, based on the original Hartford nomogram)[6]

Option 2

Some hospitals follow a once-daily dosing regimen where the dosing interval is kept the same (every 24 hours) but the dose is reduced dependent upon estimated CrCl. The doses recommended in renal impairment are as listed in Table G2. Serum concentration should be taken before the second dose (Table G4) and subsequent doses altered accordingly. For those patients with a CrCl <10 mL/min, a single dose is given and the dose should only be repeated when serum concentrations are <1 mg/L.

TABLE G2
Recommended dose reductions in renal impairment[7]

Creatinine clearance (mL/min)	Recommended dose
>30–70 mL/min	3–5 mg/kg daily
10–30 mL/min	2–3 mg/kg daily
<10 mL/min	2 mg/kg single dose; only redose when levels <1 mg/L

Multiple daily dosing regimen

For those patients with normal renal function, a dose of 3–5 mg/kg in divided doses every 8 hours is given.[4] Doses should be rounded to the nearest 20 mg to aid administration. Dose reductions in renal impairment are outlined in Table G3.

Rationale for monitoring

Monitoring is essential to ensure that toxicity is avoided and in the case of multiple daily dosing to ensure that effective levels are

TABLE G3
Recommended dose reductions in renal failure[7]

Creatinine clearance	Recommended dose
>70 mL/min	80 mg* 8-hourly
>30–70 mL/min	80 mg* 12-hourly
10–30 mL/min	80 mg* daily
5–10 mL/min	80 mg* every 48 hours

*60 mg if body weight <60 kg.

G

achieved (Table G4). Serum concentrations should be monitored as follows:

- the first level should be taken before the second dose for once-daily dosing, or 6–14 hours after the first dose if using the Hartford regimen. For multiple daily dosing, levels should be taken before the third or fourth dose. Levels should be repeated every 2–3 days if renal function remains stable
- when there is a dose adjustment or change in renal function
- if drugs are added that are known to affect gentamicin serum concentration (see section on drug interactions, below).
- if a level comes back high, a decision is required on whether to withold the dose until a safe trough level is achieved and/or to reduce the prescribed dose. Gentamicin has first-order pharmacokinetics, i.e. reducing the dose by x% should reduce the serum concentration by x% also. A new trough level would need to be checked.

TABLE G4
Gentamicin monitoring information

Therapeutic range	• Once-daily dosing: pre-dose (trough) <1 mg/L • Multiple daily dosing: peak: 5–10 mg/L[4] (3–5 mg/L in endocarditis)[4] • Pre-dose (trough): <2 mg/L[2,4] (<1 mg/L in endocarditis)[4]
Sampling time	• Pre-dose (trough): 0–30 minutes pre-dose, or 6–14 hours after first dose (if following Hartford once-daily regimen) • Peak: 1 hour after an intravenous bolus or 1 hour after the start of an infusion (for multiple-dose regimens only) • In bacterial endocarditis trough concentrations should be performed twice weekly (more often in renal impairment)[4]
Other monitoring	• Urea and electrolytes, urine output; ask patient (if possible) about vestibular and auditory disturbances

Administration

For once-daily dosing, an intravenous infusion is the preferred method of administration. The dose should be added to 100 mL of sodium chloride 0.9%, or glucose 5%, and given over 30–60 minutes.[8] If a multiple daily dosing regimen is being used, then it can be made up to a convenient volume with the above diluents (e.g. 10–20 mL) and be given as a slow intravenous bolus injection over 3–5 minutes.[8]

Overdose

Ototoxicity, nephrotoxicity and neuromuscular blockade can occur. Neuromuscular blockade presenting as both acute muscle paralysis and apnoea can occur from rapid intravenous administration.[9] There is no specific antidote to gentamicin overdose. As well as stopping therapy, U&Es, FBC, LFTs and gentamicin serum concentration should be taken. Patients should be adequately hydrated and haemodialysis considered in those patients with acute kidney injury. Auditory and vestibular function should be checked and a referral made to an ear, nose and throat specialist if deemed necessary. The onset of ototoxicity and nephrotoxicity may be delayed and therefore follow-up is required at 48 hours and 1 week.[9]

Drug interactions

The risk of ototoxicity may be increased when given with loop diuretics, e.g. furosemide. The risk of nephrotoxicity is increased when gentamicin is coadministered with amphotericin, cisplatin, ciclosporin, tacrolimus, vancomycin, colistimethate and NSAIDs.[4] Neuromuscular blocking agents, e.g. suxamethonium, can enhance the potential neuromuscular blockade, causing persisting respiratory paralysis even after the blocking drug is stopped.[2]

Concurrent use with botulinum toxin is not recommended due to increased risk of neuromuscular block. Gentamicin will antagonise the effects of neostigmine and pyridostigmine. There is an increased risk of hypocalcaemia when given with bisphosphonates.

REFERENCES

1 Grayson M *et al.* (eds) (2010). *Kucers' The Use of Antibiotics* (6th edn). London: Hodder Arnold.
2 eMC (2014). *SPC Cidomycin Adult 80 mg/2 mL Solution for Injection.* http://www.medicines.org.uk/emc (accessed 17 August 2014).
3 Ariano R *et al.* (2008). Aminoglycoside induced vestibular injury: maintaining a sense of balance. *Ann Pharmacother* 42: 1282–1289.
4 Joint Formulary Committee (2014). *British National Formulary* (68th edn). London: BMJ Group and Pharmaceutical Press.
5 Nicolau DP *et al.* (1995). Experience with a once-daily aminoglycoside program administered to 2184 adult patients. *Antimicrob Agents Chemother* 39: 650–655.
6 The Leeds Teaching Hospitals NHS Trust (2009). *Gentamicin Prescription Chart (Yorkshire Hartford).* http://www.leedsformulary.nhs.uk/docs/RxGentamicin Hartford.pdf (accessed 4 May 2015).
7 Ashley C, Dunleavy A (2014). *Renal Drug Database.* https://www.renaldrug database.com (accessed 23 August 2014).
8 Gray A, Wright J, Goodey V, Bruce L (eds.) (2011). *Injectable Drugs Guide.* London: Pharmaceutical Press.
9 National Poisons Information Service (2014). *Toxbase.* http://www.toxbase.org (accessed 17 August 2014).

Glasgow Coma Scale

Background

- The Glasgow Coma Scale (GCS) is a commonly used scoring system for determining impaired consciousness.
- Initially a 14-point scale, the original 1974 version[1] has been widely replaced with a modified 15-point version that distinguishes between abnormal flexion and withdrawal to pain.

- Three behavioural aspects are independently measured and used alongside a composite score to rate a person's overall level of consciousness (see below).
- Although originally designed to assess the impact of head trauma, it is now applied to all acute medical and trauma patients and can help measure the impact of a variety of conditions, including acute brain damage from infection, vascular injury or metabolic disorder.
- It is not suitable for use when assessing children, especially those under 3 years old who are too young to have reliable language skills.[2]
- Although some clinical and operational aspects of the GCS have been challenged, alternatives such as the FOUR score tool have not been universally adopted.

G

SCORING SYSTEM

Clinical feature: eye-opening response (E)	Score
Spontaneous (open with blinking)	4
To verbal stimuli, command, speech	3
To pain only (not applied to face)	2
No response	1
Clinical feature: verbal response (V)	
Oriented	5
Confused conversation, but able to answer questions	4
Inappropriate words	3
Incomprehensible speech or sounds	2
No response	1
Clinical feature: motor response (M)	
Obeys commands for movement	6
Purposeful movement to painful stimulus	5
Withdraws in response to pain	4
Flexion in response to pain (decorticate posturing)	3
Extension response in response to pain (decerebrate posturing)	2
No response	1

Interpretation

A lower GCS score indicates a more severe loss of consciousness; the lowest score of 3 indicates a patient who is totally unresponsive.

- GCS score ≤8: severe brain injury (usually said to be in a coma)
- GCS score 9–12: moderate brain injury
- GCS score 13–15: mild (minor) brain injury

It is clinically important to provide the individual scores in addition to the total score e.g. 'GCS of 10 with E3, V3 and M4'.

Consideration should be given to non-traumatic factors that can alter a patient's level of consciousness, such as drug use, alcohol intoxication, shock or low blood oxygen.[3,4]

A GCS score should not be regarded as a static measure; regular repetition is necessary to monitor patient response to treatment or deterioration.

REFERENCES

1 Teasdale G, Jennett B (1974). Assessment of coma and impaired consciousness. A practical scale. *Lancet* 2: 81–84.
2 Simpson DA *et al.* (1991). Head injuries in infants and young children: the value of the Paediatric Coma Scale. *Childs Nerv Syst* 7: 183–190.

3 Jennett B, Teasdale G (1977). Aspects of coma after severe head injury. *Lancet* 23: 878–881.

4 Palmer R, Knight J (2006). Assessment of altered conscious level in clinical practice. *Br J Nurs* 15: 1255–1259.

Glucosamine

Glucosamine is indicated for symptomatic relief of mild to moderate osteoarthritis of the knee. It is a natural substance found in the body and an important component of cartilage. In the UK, it is available in two salt forms, glucosamine hydrochloride and glucosamine sulfate, which are not bioequivalent. Aside from the licensed products, the strength and quality of the active ingredient may vary between products of the same salt, so bioequivalence cannot be assumed.

Alateris (hydrochloride), Dolenio (sulfate) and Glusartel (sulfate) are the three licensed products in the UK for use in adults over 18 years old.

Evidence for effectiveness

The mechanism of action for glucosamine is not understood. Evidence from clinical trials to support its efficacy is mixed and many of the studies were of low quality and short duration.[1] However, studies using glucosamine sulfate resulted in a small reduction in pain as well as improvement in physical function, although the other salts failed to do so.

NICE[2] guidance does not recommend glucosamine for prescribing on the NHS and the BNF[3] classifies it as a drug less suitable for prescribing. There is insufficient evidence to support the efficacy of glucosamine hydrochloride as a disease-modifying agent.

Safety profile[4]

Glucosamine is generally well tolerated and the frequency of side effects is similar to placebo. Common side effects are mild gastrointestinal (GI) disturbances (nausea, abdominal pain, dyspepsia, flatulence, diarrhoea, constipation), drowsiness, headache, and, less commonly, flushing, rash and itching.

Due to the limited data available, causality has not been clearly established for many of the glucosamine–disease interactions. Therefore, the manufactures err on the side of safety with regard to the cautions and contraindications stated in the Summary of Product Characteristics.

Glucosamine is contraindicated in people with shellfish allergy; although it is derived from the shells of shellfish, it is the flesh that contains the antigens responsible for the allergy. Some studies show that glucosamine may interfere with blood glucose control; therefore, diabetic patients and those with impaired glucose tolerance are advised to monitor blood glucose levels closely at the start of treatment and periodically, particularly when they change doses or products. Isolated cases of asthma exacerbations, hypercholesterolaemia and renal impairment have been reported in patients taking glucosamine; therefore, asthma patients starting to take glucosamine must be advised to look out for signs of worsening symptoms and those with cardiovascular risk factors must have their lipid levels monitored. The drug should be used with caution in renal impairment or those taking nephrotoxic drugs and renal function monitored accordingly. The manufacturers advise to avoid in pregnancy and breast-feeding due to limited evidence in these circumstances.

G

Drug interactions

Glucosamine enhances the effects of warfarin and so should be avoided,[3] otherwise patients should be advised to look out for signs of bleeding and the INR should be monitored closely whenever either drug is started, discontinued[5-7] or the dose altered.

Key prescribing advice

It is important to rule out the presence of other joint diseases that may require other treatment before prescribing glucosamine. It is not indicated for the relief of acute pain and it may take several weeks for the benefits to be seen, particularly pain relief. If there is no pain relief after a 2–3-month trial, the ongoing need should be assessed and the drug discontinued. Agree with the patient the criteria and time period after which the drug will be discontinued if there are no benefits.

The recommended dose for the sulfate is 1500 mg daily or in three divided doses and the hydrochloride 1250 mg daily or in two divided doses. Each tablet should be swallowed whole. An oral solution and effervescent formulation are available for those who cannot, or prefer not to, swallow tablets.

The sulfate and effervescent formulations have high sodium content[5,6] so should be used with caution in patients on a reduced-salt diet.

Advice and counselling

Patients should be advised on how to evaluate or measure their pain before starting glucosamine so that any benefit resulting from its use can be assessed objectively. Advice on the common side effects, drug interactions and relevant monitoring required depends on the patient's pre-existing conditions and other drug therapy. Advise the patient to purchase a licensed product for consistency and to avoid over- or underdosing.

GI symptoms may be reduced if taken with or after food. Patients should be counselled on the value of weight loss and exercise as core treatments to be used alongside any pharmacological treatments in the management of osteoarthritis and to seek professional help if necessary.

Alternative pharmacological and non-pharmacological treatments[2]

All treatments should be offered in addition to core treatments of weight loss and exercise. Paracetamol is effective for pain relief and relatively safe, although regular dosing may be required. Topical NSAIDs or capsaicin can be offered in addition to paracetamol to provide pain relief to affected knees. The use of local heat or cold therapy as well as transcutaneous electrical nerve stimulation (TENS) can also be considered. Those who experience specific problems with functioning could be offered expert advice on assistive devices such as walking sticks.

REFERENCES

1 Towheed T *et al.* (2005). Glucosamine therapy for treating osteoarthritis. *Cochrane Datab Systemat Rev* Issue 2. Assessed as up to date: 12 November 2008.
2 NICE (2014). CG117. *Osteoarthritis: Care and management in adults.* http:// www.nice.org.uk/Guidance/CG177 (accessed 20 August 2014).
3 Joint Formulary Committee (2014). *British National Formulary* (68th edn). London: BMJ Group and Pharmaceutical Press.
4 UKMI (2012). *Medicines Q&As. Glucosamine – What are the adverse effects?* www.medicinesresources.nhs.uk/GetDocument.aspx?pageId=504032 (accessed 20 August 2014).
5 SPC (2011). *Dolenio 1500 mg film coated tablets.* Blue Bio Pharmaceuticals. Date of revision of text 20/9/2011. www.medicines.org.uk (accessed 6 May 2015).
6 SPC (2010). *Glusartel 1500 mg Powder for Oral Solution.* Rottapharm. Date of revision of text 22/10/10. www.medicines.org.uk (accessed 6 May 2015).
7 SPC (2010). *Alateris 625 mg Tablets.* Laboratories Expanscience. Date of revision of text 4/8/2010. www.medicines.org.uk (accessed 6 May 2015).

Grapefruit juice–drug interactions

Many drugs undergo oxidative metabolism by cytochrome P450 enzymes (CYP450) in the intestinal wall and liver. This may produce a first-pass effect that reduces bioavailability, or may increase bioavailability from a prodrug precursor. Both these effects can be significant and may be modified by the ingestion of grapefruit juice.

Mechanism of grapefruit interaction

Constituents of grapefruit juice (particularly flavonoids and furancoumarins) inhibit a number of CYP450 isoenzymes, primarily CYP3A4, resulting in reduced metabolism and therefore increased bioavailability of drugs affected. Enzyme recovery is delayed for up to 24 hours after as little as one glass of grapefruit juice; therefore, taking medicines at a different time to the juice is not a method for avoiding the interaction.[1] Regular consumption appears to increase the effect on drug pharmacokinetics.[2] Grapefruit also has an effect on drug pharmacokinetics by a second mechanism that involves inhibition of an influx transporter protein in the gut wall, leading to a reduced drug bioavailability and therefore reduced drug efficacy. This is competitive inhibition and the effect is therefore dependent on the volume consumed; the inhibition lasts around 4 hours, so ensuring a 4-hour gap is left between consumption and administration of medication avoids these interactions.

Most information sources refer only to grapefruit juice, although it seems wise to treat grapefruit flesh with the same caution.

Other problematic fruit

Sweet oranges, commercially available orange juices and tangerines do not cause these interactions. However, Seville oranges and pomelos manifest the interaction.[1]

Drugs affected by grapefruit

Common drugs known to be affected are listed in Table G5, although if a drug is not listed it does not mean that an interaction does not exist. It would be wise to be aware of the potential for interaction of drugs metabolised by the cytochrome CYP450 isoenzymes. The more significant and potentially toxic interactions are those with: amiodarone, carbamazepine, ciclosporin, sirolimus, tacrolimus, atorvastatin and simvastatin.

TABLE G5
Interactions with grapefruit juice and oral drugs [1,3,4,5]

Drug	Effect	Comments
Aliskiren	Reduced bioavailability	Avoid grapefruit juice
Amiodarone	Reduction of formation of major amiodarone metabolite	May be clinically significant – avoid grapefruit juice
Amlodipine	Modest increase in bioavailability	Probably subclinical
Atorvastatin	Increased bioavailability resulting in increased risk of myopathy	May be clinically significant
Carbamazepine	Increased bioavailability	May be clinically significant – avoid grapefruit juice
Ciclosporin	Significant increase in bioavailability	Serious – avoid grapefruit juice
Clomipramine	Increase in blood levels	Monitor for unexpected drug effects
Colchicine	Increased risk of toxicity due to increased absorption	Avoid grapefruit juice
Diazepam	Increased bioavailability	Avoid grapefruit juice
Dronedarone	Significant increase in blood levels	Avoid grapefruit juice
Felodipine	Increase in bioavailability	Avoid grapefruit juice
Fexofenadine	Possible decreased effect	Avoid grapefruit juice
Indinavir	Bioavailability may be reduced by about 25%	Clinical significance not established

(continued)

TABLE G5
(Continued)

Drug	Effect	Comments
Itraconazole	May decrease bioavailability with risk of treatment failure	Monitor response to treatment
Ivabradine	Increases exposure twofold	Restrict grapefruit juice consumption
Methylprednisolone	Increased bioavailability	Monitor therapeutic effect
Midazolam	Increased bioavailability and risk of excessive sedation	Avoid grapefruit juice
Nicardipine	Increased bioavailability	Little change in haemodynamic effect
Nifedipine	Increased bioavailability and risk of adverse effects	Avoid grapefruit juice
Nimodipine	Increased bioavailability	Avoid grapefruit juice
Omeprazole	Small increase in bioavailability	Not significant
Quetiapine	Possible reduced metabolism, therefore increased exposure	Avoid grapefruit juice
Ranolazine	Increased blood levels	Avoid grapefruit juice
Saquinavir	Increased bioavailability, effect similar to a doubled dose	Monitor for adverse effects/altered response
Sertraline	Moderate increase in blood levels	Avoid grapefruit juice
Sildenafil	Possible increase in blood levels	Avoid grapefruit juice
Simvastatin	Large increase in blood concentration	Avoid grapefruit juice
Sirolimus	Increased risk of toxicity from raised blood levels	Avoid grapefruit juice
Tacrolimus	Significantly increased risk of toxicity from raised blood levels	Avoid grapefruit juice
Terfenadine	Increased blood levels – fatality reported	Avoid grapefruit juice
Tolvaptan	Increased blood levels	Avoid grapefruit
Warfarin	May increase anticoagulant effect	Not well documented – monitor international normalised ratio (INR)

REFERENCES

1 Drug Data no. 56. (2004). Northern Ireland Regional Medicines and Poisons Information Service, The Royal Hospitals.
2 Pirmohamed M (2013). Drug–grapefruit juice interactions. *BMJ* 346: f1.
3 McNeece J (2002). Grapefruit juice interactions. *Aust Prescriber* 25: 2.
4 Joint Formulary Committee (2014). *British National Formulary* (68th edn). London: BMJ Group and Pharmaceutical Press.
5 Baxter K (ed.) (2014). *Stockley's Drug Interactions*. London: Pharmaceutical Press http://www.medicinescomplete.com/ (accessed 3 August 2014).

Human immunodeficiency virus treatment

The management of human immunodeficiency virus (HIV) is continually progressing and over the last decade has seen vast improvements in the drug options available to patients. These newer drugs are associated with significantly less toxicity than some of the older ones and are also associated with reduced tablet burden, which improves adherence and patient tolerability.

HIV is now managed as a chronic condition, with life expectancy significantly improved in recent years.[1] The main aim of treatment is to reduce the mortality and morbidity associated with the condition by:

- suppressing the virus – measured by checking the patients viral load (copies/mL) with a target of <50 copies/mL or 'undetectable'
- restoring and maintaining the patient's immune system – measured by the patient's CD4 count (cells/µL). In non-HIV patients this should be >500 cells/µL.

When treatment should be started

The WHO recommends starting treatment at CD4 counts <500 cells/μL.[2] The British HIV Association (BHIVA) recommends that treatment with antiretroviral therapy (ART) should be initiated in all HIV-positive patients with CD4 count <350 cells/μL.[3] To date there have been no published randomised trials that directly assess whether treatment-naïve people with higher CD4 cell counts should initiate ART immediately rather than defer to <350 cells/μL. In addition, BHIVA recommends starting treatment regardless of CD4 count if there is active hepatitis B virus (HBV) or hepatitis C virus (HCV) infection; a high risk for cardiovascular disease, in pregnant women, symptomatic primary HIV infection, HIV-associated nephropathy (HIVAN) and in serodiscordant couples.[3]

Antiretroviral therapy

There are six different classes of antiretroviral drugs that can be used in combination to treat HIV:

1　nucleoside reverse transcriptase inhibitors (NRTIs)
2　non-nucleoside reverse transcriptase inhibitors (NNRTIs)
3　protease inhibitors (PIs)
4　entry inhibitors
5　fusion inhibitors
6　integrase inhibitors.

Drug summaries, including information on adult doses and side effects, can be found in Tables H1–H5. The relevant product SPC should be consulted for further information and for guidance on dosing in children.

TABLE H1
Nucleoside reverse transcriptase inhibitors

Generic name	Trade name	Adult dose/dose adjustment in renal impairment	Counselling points/side effects
Abacavir	Ziagen[4] tablets and solution (abacavir) **Combination products** Trizivir[4] tablets (abacavir/ lamivudine /zidovudine) Kivexa[4] tablets (abacavir/ lamivudine) Triumeq[4] (lamivudine/ abacavir/ dolutegravir)	300 mg every 12 hours or 600 mg once daily Dose modification in renal impairment: none[5]	May be taken with or without food Contraindicated in patients positive for the human leukocyte antigen (HLA)-B*5701 allele, which is associated with increased risk of hypersensitivity reaction Lactic acidosis, hepatomegaly, hepatic steatosis, lipodystrophy, dyslipidaemia, hypersensitivity reactions
Emtricitabine	Emtriva[4] capsules and solution (emtricitabine) **Combination products** Atripla[4] (tenofovir/efavirenz/ emtricitabine) Eviplera[4] (tenofovir / emtricitabine/ rilpivirine) Stribild[4] (tenofovir/ emtricitabine, elvitegravir, cobicistat) Truvada[4] (tenofovir/emtricitabine)	200 mg daily (as oral solution: 240 mg daily) Dose modification in renal impairment[5] <table><tr><td>eGFR (mL/min)</td><td>Dose</td></tr><tr><td>30–50</td><td>200 mg every 48 hours</td></tr><tr><td>15–30</td><td>200 mg every 72 hours</td></tr><tr><td><15</td><td>200 mg every 96 hours</td></tr></table>	May be taken with or without food Lactic acidosis, hepatomegaly, hepatic steatosis, lipodystrophy, dyslipidaemia

(continued)

H

H

TABLE H1
(Continued)

Generic name	Trade name	Adult dose/dose adjustment in renal impairment		Counselling points/side effects
Lamivudine	Epivir[4] tablets and solution (lamivudine)	300 mg daily or 150 mg 12-hourly		May be taken with or without food
	N.B.: generic lamivudine products are now available	Dose modification in renal impairment in HIV[5]		Lactic acidosis, hepatomegaly, hepatic steatosis, lipodystrophy, dyslipidaemia
	Combination products	eGFR (mL/min)	Dose	
	Combivir[4] (lamivudine/zidovudine)	30–50	150 mg stat then 150 mg daily	
	Kivexa[4] (abacavir/ lamivudine)	15–30	150 mg stat then 100 mg daily	
	Triumeq[4] (lamivudine/ abacavir/ dolutegravir)	5–15	150 mg stat then 50 mg daily	
	Trizivir[4] (lamivudine, zidovudine, abacavir sulfate)	<5	50 mg stat then 25 mg daily[7] (SPC licensed dose) or 150 mg stat then 25–50 mg daily[1,6]	
Tenofovir	Viread[4] tablets and granules (tenofovir)	245 mg daily		To be taken with food
	Combination products	Dose modification in renal impairment:		Proximal renal tubulopathy, renal impairment, renal failure, lactic acidosis, hepatomegaly, hepatic steatosis, lipodystrophy, dyslipidaemia
	Atripla[4] (tenofovir/efavirenz/ emtricitabine)	eGFR (mL/min)	Dose	
	Eviplera[4] (tenofovir / emtricitabine/ rilpivirine)	30–50	245 mg every 48 hours	
	Stribild[4] (tenofovir/ emtricitabine, elvitegravir, cobicistat)	10–30	245 mg every 72–96 hours	
	Truvada[4] (tenofovir / emtricitabine)	<10	245 mg every 7 days	

TABLE H2
Non-nucleoside reverse transcriptase inhibitors

Generic name	Trade name	Adult dose/ dose adjustment in renal impairment	Counselling points/ side effects
Efavirenz	Sustiva[4] capsules, tablets and solution (efavirenz) **Combination products** Atripla[4] (tenofovir/efavirenz/ emtricitabine)	600 mg daily (as oral solution: 720 mg daily) Dose modification in renal impairment: none[5]	To be taken on an empty stomach, preferably at bedtime Rash, central nervous system effects – dizziness, depression. abnormal dreams, sleep disturbances, psychosis
Etravirine	Intelence[4] tablets (etravirine)	200 mg 12-hourly Dose modification in renal impairment: none[4]	To be taken with food Rash
Nevirapine	Viramune[4] tablets and suspension (nevirapine) N.B.: generic nevirapine products now also available	200 mg daily for 14 days, increased to 200 mg 12-hourly maintenance dose Dose modification in renal impairment: none[5]	2-week lead in recommended to reduce the incidence of rash May be taken with or without food Rash, allergic reactions, hepatitis, abnormal liver function tests
Rilpivirine	Edurant[4] (rilpivirine) **Combination products** Eviplera[4] (tenofovir / emtricitabine/ rilpivirine)	25 mg daily Dose modification in renal impairment: none[4]	Must be taken with food for maximum absorption Should only be used in patients with a viral load <100 000 copies/mL Dyslipidaemia, insomnia, raised amylase, raised transaminase

TABLE H3

Protease inhibitors

Generic name	Trade name	Adult dose/ dose adjustment in renal impairment	Counselling points/side effects
Atazanavir	Reyataz[4] tablets (atazanavir)	300 mg daily taken with ritonavir 100 mg daily Dose modification in renal impairment: none[5]	To be taken with food Jaundice, rash
Darunavir	Prezista[4] tablets and suspension (darunavir)	ART-naive patients – 800 mg daily with ritonavir 100 mg daily ART-experienced patients with no evidence of resistance/resistant mutations – 800 mg daily with ritonavir 100 mg daily ART-experienced patients – 600 mg 12-hourly with ritonavir 100 mg 12-hourly Dose modification in renal impairment: none[5]	To be taken with food Insomnia, rash, increased alanine aminotransferase, diabetes, dyslipidaemia, peripheral neuropathy
Lopinavir/ritonavir	Kaletra[4] tablets and suspension (lopinavir/ritonavir)	400/100 mg lopinavir/ritonavir 12-hourly Dose modification in renal impairment: none[5]	To be taken with food Dyslipidaemia, pancreatitis, diabetes, anxiety, hypertension, hepatitis, erectile dysfunction, menstrual disorders
Ritonavir	Norvir[4] tablets and solution (ritonavir) **Combination products** Kaletra[4] tablets and suspension (lopinavir/ritonavir)	Only to be used as a pharmacokinetic enhancer with other PIs – see information on previous PIs for dosing advice	To be taken with food Hypersensitivity, dyslipidaemia, dysgeusia, peripheral neuropathy, oral and peripheral paraesthesia, rash, pharyngitis, cough (refer also to side effects of the co-administered PI)

TABLE H4
Entry inhibitors

Generic name	Trade name	Adult dose/ dose adjustment in renal impairment	Counselling points/ side effects
Maraviroc	Celsentri[4] tablets (maraviroc)	300 mg 12-hourly – will need dose adjustment if on interacting medication: consult SPC Dose modification in renal impairment may be required if patient on potent CYP3A4 inhibitors: consult SPC[4]	Should only be used in patients with CCR5 tropic virus. May be taken with or without food Anaemia, anorexia, depression, rash, increases in alanine transaminase (ALT), increases in aspartate transaminase (AST)

TABLE H5
Integrase inhibitors

Generic name	Trade name	Adult dose/dose adjustment in renal impairment	Counselling points/ side effects
Dolutegravir	Tivicay[4] tablets (dolutegravir) **Combination products** Triumeq[4] (lamivudine/ abacavir/ dolutegravir)	No/not suspected integrase resistance – 50 mg daily Known/suspected integrase resistance – 50 mg 12-hourly Dose modification in renal impairment: none[5]	May be taken with or without food. In the presence of known integrase resistance, take with food to enhance exposure Insomnia, abnormal dreams, rash, pruritus, raised ALT, raised AST, raised creatine phosphokinase
Raltegravir	Isentress[4] tablets (raltegravir)	400 mg tablet 12-hourly (N.B. other formulations are not bioequivalent) Dose modification in renal impairment: none[5]	May be taken with or without food Decreased appetite, abnormal dreams, insomnia, depression, vertigo, rash, raised AST, raised ALT, hypertriglyceridaemia
Elvitegravir/ cobicistat	Stribild[4] (elvitegravir, cobicistat, emtricitabine, tenofovir)	Each tablet contains: elvitegravir 150 mg, cobicistat 150 mg, emtricitabine 200 mg, tenofovir 245 mg Dose: one tablet daily Dose modification in renal impairment[4]	To be taken with food Rash – but see also side effects of tenofovir and emtricitabine for combination tablet side effects

CrCl (mL/min)	Dose
70–90	Only use if other treatment options have been discussed and Stribild is still the preferred option
<70	Do not use

Which antiretrovirals should be used?

In treatment-naïve patients standard therapy should be initiated with a backbone of two NRTIs plus a third agent, which can be a ritonavir-boosted PI, an NNRTI or an integrase inhibitor[3] (Figure H1). The current BHIVA first-line treatment algorithms are also summarised in Figure H1.

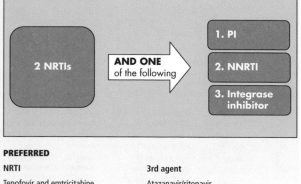

PREFERRED

NRTI	3rd agent
Tenofovir and emtricitabine	Atazanavir/ritonavir
	Darunavir/ritonavir
	Efavirenz
	Raltegravir
	Elvitegravir/cobicistat

ALTERNATIVE

NRTI	3rd agent
Abacavir (ABC)* and lamivudine (3TC)	Rilpivirine (RPV)**
	Lopinavir/ritonavir
	Fosamprenavir/ritonavir
	Nevirapine (NVP)***

*ABC is contraindicated if HLA-B*5701 positive
**Use recommended only if baseline viral load <100 000 copies/mL: RPV as a third agent, ABC/3TC as NRTI backbone.
***NVP is contraindicated if baseline CD4 cell count is greater than 250/400 cells/mL in women/men.

FIGURE H1 Standard antiretroviral therapy. NRTI, nucleoside reverse transcriptase inhibitor; PI, protease inhibitor; NNRTI, non-nucleoside reverse transcriptase inhibitor

Drug choice should be tailored to the individual patient, with considerations of:

- efficacy
- toxicity/side effect profile
- pill burden – both the number of tablets per day and the frequency with which they need to be taken
- comorbidities, that could contraindicate/caution some ART
- drug interactions
- patient preference.

Side effects

Minor side effects common to all antiretroviral drugs include nausea, vomiting, diarrhoea, headache and fatigue – these are generally worse in the first few weeks after initiation and usually subside with continued treatment. Important side effects specific to certain antiretrovirals are summarised below and in Tables H1–H5; consult the relevant SPC for a complete list of all side effects for each drug.

- Tenofovir is associated with renal impairment and osteoporosis.
- Zidovudine can cause macrocytic anaemia and lipodystrophy.
- Abacavir is associated with life-threatening hypersensitivity rash.
- NNRTIs, particularly efavirenz, may cause neuropsychiatric symptoms like dizziness and insomnia.
- Nevirapine has a risk of hepatotoxicity and Stevens–Johnson syndrome/toxic epidermal necrolysis.
- PIs are associated with a wide range of side effects, including hyperlipidaemia, hepatitis, diarrhoea and insulin resistance.
- Integrase inhibitors may cause headache and nausea, although this is rare.

Drug interactions

Antiretrovirals have the potential to interact with each other and with other medications. Before initiating ART, or introducing other medicines to patients already stable on ART, drug interactions should be checked, as some may be clinically significant. Interactions may be managed with dose modification or increased monitoring, or may even necessitate a change in therapy. The use of herbal remedies and 'recreational drugs' should also be considered as these often interact with antiretrovirals. The University of Liverpool has a comprehensive website that can be used to check interactions of HIV medicines (available at http://www.hiv-druginteractions.org, and also available to download as an app). Information on interactions is also available in the SPC for each drug.

Nucleoside reverse transcriptase inhibitors

(Abacavir, didanosine, emtricitabine, lamivudine (3TC), rilpivirine (RPV), stavudine, tenofovir, zidovudine)

NRTIs work by inhibiting the reverse transcriptase enzyme, preventing the formation of proviral DNA from the viral RNA. This is achieved by acting as nucleoside substrates during the formation of proviral DNA, resulting in termination of the DNA chain and therefore preventing replication. The most commonly used NRTIs are detailed in Table H1.

Non-nucleoside reverse transcriptase inhibitors

(Efavirenz, etravirine, nevirapine, rilpivirine)

NNRTIs also work by inhibiting the reverse transcriptase enzyme, preventing the formation of viral DNA. This is via a different mechanism – attaching directly to the reverse transcriptase enzyme, preventing it from working. The most commonly used NNRTIs are detailed in Table H2.

Protease inhibitors

(Atazanavir, darunavir, fosamprenavir, indinavir, lopinavir, ritonavir, saquinavir, tipranavir)

PIs work by blocking the protease enzyme that is needed to break large chains of viral protein into smaller building blocks that are used in the assembly of new HIV particles. This results in the production of an immature, less infectious HIV. The most commonly used PIs are detailed in Table H3. All PIs are used in combination with ritonavir, which acts as a booster to increase levels.

Entry inhibitors

(Maraviroc)

In order to fuse with the host cell the HIV virus must first bind to the CD4 receptor and a chemokine receptor 4 or 5 (CXCR4 or CCR5). The CCR5 inhibitor maraviroc is the only licensed drug in its class and works by binding to the CCR5 receptor. This prevents the virus from binding and fusing with the host cell. This will only work in patients who have CCR5 tropic virus, so tropism testing should be carried out before initiating maraviroc – dual tropic or CXCR4 tropic virus will not be successfully suppressed with maraviroc. More detail can be found in Table H4.

Fusion inhibitor

(Enfuvirtide)

This works by binding to a surface protein on the HIV particle, preventing fusion with and entry of the virus into the host cell. This drug is only available as an injection and has had limited use – it will not be discussed further in this chapter.

Integrase inhibitors

(Raltegravir, dolutegravir, elvitegravir/cobicistat)

Integrase inhibitors work by blocking the viral integrase enzyme, which is responsible for inserting and integrating viral DNA into the host DNA, preventing replication. Elvitegravir is the newest of the integrase inhibitors and must be co-administered with a pharmacokinetic enhancer (usually cobicistat), and is used as part of a single fixed-dose tablet regimen with tenofovir and emtricitabine – this is called Stribild or 'quad' because of its four drug components.

The most commonly used integrase inhibitors are detailed in Table H5.

H

REFERENCES

1 May M *et al.* (2011). Impact of late diagnosis and treatment on life expectancy in people with HIV-1: UK Collaborative HIV Cohort (UK CHIC) Study. *BMJ* 343: d61016.
2 WHO (2014). *Consolidated Guidelines on HIV Prevention, Diagnosis, Treatment and Care for Key Populations.* http://apps.who.int/iris/bitstream/10665/128048/1/9789241507431_eng.pdf?ua=1&ua=1 (accessed 13 December 2014).
3 Williams I *et al.* (2014). British HIV Association guidelines for the treatment of HIV-1-positive adults with antiretroviral therapy 2012 (2013 update). *HIV Med* 15(Suppl 1): 1–85.
4 eMC (2014). www.medicines.org.uk (accessed 20 October 2014).
5 Ashley C, Currie, A (eds) (2009). *The Renal Drug Handbook* (3rd edn). Oxford: Radcliffe Publishing.

Hyperosmolar hyperglycaemic state

Hyperosmolar hyperglycaemia state (HHS) is a medical emergency characterised by hypovolaemia, marked hyperglycaemia and raised serum osmolality.

HHS was formerly known as hyperosmolar non-ketotic syndrome (HONS or HONK).

HHS typically occurs in the elderly but, as the diabetes pandemic widens, HHS may now also be the initial presentation of type 2 diabetes mellitus in younger adults and teenagers.

A precise definition of HHS does not exist; it has different features to diabetic ketoacidosis (DKA) and it is therefore treated differently (see *Diabetic ketoacidosis* entry). Whilst DKA presents within hours of onset, HHS may develop over many days and consequently dehydration and metabolic disturbances are more extreme. HHS has a higher mortality than DKA and may be more complex, with vascular complications such as myocardial infarction, stroke or peripheral arterial thrombosis. Other uncommon complications of HHS include seizures, cerebral oedema and central pontine myelinolysis, the latter possibly being precipitated by rapid changes in osmolality during treatment. Some patients present a mixed picture of both DKA and HHS.

Diagnosis of HHS

The following are characteristic features of HHS:

- hypovolaemia
- marked hyperglycaemia (30 mmol/L or more) without significant blood ketones (<3 mmol/L) or acidosis (pH > 7.3; bicarbonate >15 mmol/L)
- serum osmolality – usually ≥320 mosmol/kg.

Management of HHS in adults

In 2012, the JBDS Inpatient Care Group published guidance on treating HHS in adults[1] so all trusts should aim to have a policy or care pathway in place. The main focus of treatment is to treat the underlying cause and gradually and safely to normalise osmolality, replace fluid and electrolyte losses and normalise blood glucose levels. Additionally clinicians should aim to prevent arterial or venous thrombosis, avoid complications such as cerebral oedema and prevent foot ulceration.

Early escalation to High Dependency Unit (HDU) should be considered if *one or more of the following is present:*

- osmolality >350 mosmol/kg
- sodium >160 mmol/L

- venous/arterial pH <7.1
- hypokalaemia <3.5 mmol/L *or* hyperkalaemia >6 mmol/L *on admission*
- hypoxia, (*oxygen saturation <92%, assuming normal baseline*)
- altered consciousness (*GCS <12 or abnormal AVPU*)
- systolic BP <90 mmHg *or*
- pulse outside 60–100 bpm.

For management in young people (<16 years), refer to published paediatric guidance.[2]

Fluid

These patients are severely dehydrated because of prolonged osmotic diuresis (Table H6) and fluid replacement is the first priority. Sodium chloride 0.9% with ready-mixed potassium as required is currently recommended as the fluid of choice because the majority of electrolyte losses are sodium, chloride and potassium.

TABLE H6
Typical fluid and electrolyte deficits in hyperosmolar hyperglycaemic state[3]

Water	100–220 mL/kg
Sodium	5–13 mmol/kg
Chloride	5–15 mmol/kg
Potassium	4–6 mmol/kg

Serum osmolality is a useful indicator of severity of illness, and also for monitoring rate of change with treatment. Because frequent measurement is not usually available in UK hospitals, calculated osmolality[1] is used to guide treatment, where:

$$\text{Osmolality} = 2Na^+ + \text{glucose} + \text{urea}$$

(normal range = 280–300 mosmol/kg)

- The rate of rehydration is determined by assessing initial severity plus any pre-existing comorbidities. Caution is needed, particularly in the elderly, where too rapid rehydration may precipitate heart failure but insufficient rehydration may fail to reverse acute kidney injury.
- Intravenous fluid replacement aims to achieve a positive balance, with 3–6 litres of fluid to be given over the first 12 hours and the remaining replacement of estimated fluid losses within the next 12 hours, although it may take up to 72 hours for complete normalisation of biochemistry.
- Calculate (or measure) osmolality every hour initially and adjust the rate of fluid replacement to ensure a positive fluid balance sufficient to promote a gradual decline in osmolality.

- Use intravenous sodium chloride 0.9% to reverse severe dehydration. The rate of fall of plasma sodium should not exceed 10 mmol/L in 24 hours. N.B.: fluid replacement (without insulin) will lower blood glucose and reduce osmolality, shifting water into the intracellular space. This inevitably results in a rise in serum sodium, which is not necessarily a reason to give hypotonic fluids. A fall in blood glucose of 5.5 mmol/L causes a 2.4 mmol/L rise in sodium; a greater rise than this indicates insufficient fluid replacement.
- Maintain an accurate fluid balance chart and aim for a minimum urine output of 0.5 mL/kg/hour.
- Only switch to sodium chloride 0.45% if the osmolality is not declining despite adequate positive fluid balance and an adequate rate of fall in blood glucose level.
- Patients should be allowed to take oral fluids as soon as they are able.

Intravenous insulin

A safe rate of fall in blood glucose should be between 4 and 6 mmol/L per hour to a target of 10–15 mmol/L in the first 24 hours.

- An intravenous insulin infusion should *only* be commenced once the blood glucose is no longer falling with fluid replacement alone *or* at the start of treatment for HHS if there is significant ketonaemia (blood ketones >1 mmol/L).
- Insulin may be infused in the same line as the intravenous replacement fluid, provided that a Y-connector with a one-way, antisyphon valve is used, and a large-bore cannula has been placed.
- A syringe pump should be set up containing 50 units of soluble insulin in 50 mL sodium chloride 0.9% (i.e. 1 unit/mL) and this should be infused at the lower starting rate of 0.05 unit/kg/hour because most patients with HHS are insulin-sensitive.
- Avoid hypoglycaemia: if blood glucose falls below 14 mmol/L, commence glucose 5% or 10% at 125 mL/hour while continuing the sodium chloride 0.9% infusion.
- Subcutaneous insulin is usually given to provide stability for a short time (weeks or months) following an episode of HHS. In the longer term most patients will be able to control their diabetes with either diet and oral therapy or diet alone.

Potassium

Patients with HHS are potassium-depleted but less acidotic than those with DKA, so potassium shifts are less pronounced. Patients with acute kidney injury may present with hyperkalaemia but patients on diuretics may be profoundly hypokalaemic. Potassium should be replaced or omitted as required (Table H7).

Anticoagulation

A major cause of death in HHS is thromboembolic disease. Prophylactic anticoagulation with low-molecular-weight heparin is

TABLE H7
Suitable potassium replacement levels in hyperosmolar hyperglycaemic state

Potassium level in first 24 hours	Potassium chloride to be added
<3.5 mmol/L	Senior review as additional potassium is essential (if necessary, via a central line in HDU)
3.5–5.5 mmol/L	40 mmol/L of fluid
>5.5 mmol/L	None

indicated for the full duration of admission, unless specifically contraindicated.[4]

Antibiotics

Infection is often difficult to exclude in patients with HHS. Antibiotics should be prescribed according to local guidelines when there are clinical or other signs to suggest infection.

Aftercare

- The underlying cause of HHS should be determined to minimise recurrence.
- The patient should have appropriate diabetes education and follow-up by the diabetes team.
- Prior to discharge there must be a plan in place for ongoing management and follow-up of diabetes depending on the patient's lifestyle and home circumstances.

REFERENCES

1 Joint British Diabetes Societies Inpatient Care Group (2012). *The Management of the Hyperosmolar Hyperglycaemic State (HHS) in Adults with Diabetes.* London: Diabetes UK. http://www.diabetologists-abcd.org.uk/JBDS/JBDS_IP_HHS_Adults.pdf (accessed 30 January 2015).
2 Zeitler P et al. (2011). Hyperglycaemic hyperosmolar syndrome in children: pathophysiological considerations and guidelines for treatment. *J Pediatr* 158: 9–14.
3 Kitabachi AE et al. (2009). Hyperglycaemic crises in adult patients with diabetes. *Diabetes Care* 32: 1335–1343.
4 NICE (2015). *Venous Thromboembolism: Reducing the risk of venous thromboembolism (deep vein thrombosis and pulmonary embolism) in patients admitted to hospital* (CG 92). http://www.nice.org.uk/guidance/cg92 (accessed 3 February 2015).

Hypodermoclysis

This is a technique used to administer fluids and electrolytes subcutaneously to achieve fluid maintenance or replacement in mildly dehydrated patients or in patients at risk of dehydration, when the oral or intravenous routes are not available. This might include patients in the first few days after a stroke, patients with poor venous access, palliative care patients or those who are agitated or confused and continually remove venous access devices.

It is not suitable for patients with severe dehydration, patients in shock, where more than 3 litres of fluid are required in a 24-hour period, or where precise control of the volume and rate of infusion is required.

Normally 500 mL of fluid is given over 8 hours, up to a maximum of 2 litres over a 24-hour period.

Solutions for hypodermoclysis

Solutions suitable for hypodermoclysis should ideally be isotonic (or close to isotonicity) with extracellular fluid. The suitability of a solution for subcutaneous administration must be established before use. Examples of solutions that have been used are:

- sodium chloride 0.9% or 0.45% solution
- glucose 5% solution (not more than 2 litres should be given in 24 hours, and the rate of administration should not exceed 2 mL/min. Higher rates or higher strengths have led to shock. The site should be inspected regularly for signs of irritation and inflammation due to the low pH of glucose solutions)
- sodium chloride 0.18% with glucose 4% solution
- potassium solutions up to 40 mmol/L (20 mmol/500mL) in isotonic glucose or saline (ulceration can sometimes occur due to low pH and high osmolarity, so regular observation of the infusion site is required).[1]

Solutions unsuitable for hypodermoclysis

The following solutions are *not* suitable for hypodermoclysis:

- colloids
- total parenteral nutrition
- potassium solutions greater than 40 mmol/L
- glucose solutions greater than 5%
- solutions containing ions other than sodium, potassium or chloride, unless the solution's physiological characteristics are completely understood, e.g. pH and tonicity.[2]

Administration

Solutions are administered using a standard giving set through a subcutaneous needle and should always be gravity-fed. The choice of site should be healthy, clean, non-oedematous and convenient for the patient's comfort. Commonly used sites are the abdomen, thigh, scapula, axillary and subclavicular chest wall.[3]

Care should be taken in young children and the elderly to control the speed and total volume of fluid administered and to avoid overhydration, especially in renal impairment.

Hyaluronidase may be used to increase the rate of absorption of subcutaneous fluids. In clinical practice, there are three strategies for its use in hypodermoclysis:

1 routinely every 24 hours
2 when required only, e.g. if an infusion is running very slowly, or there is swelling at the infusion site
3 at the start of the infusion only, and then only on resiting or as required.

The licensed dose of hyaluronidase is 1500 units per site every 24 hours.[4] This dose is dissolved in 1 mL of water for injections, or sodium chloride 0.9%, and is injected subcutaneously into the site before the infusion is set up. Alternatively, it can be injected into the tubing of the infusion set, about 2 cm back from the needle, at the start of the infusion. 1500 units is sufficient for administration of 500–1000 mL of most fluids.

Monitoring the infusion site

The infusion site should be checked when the bag is changed. More regular monitoring is required for solutions other than sodium chloride 0.9%. The site should be changed if pain is experienced at the infusion site, the site becomes inflamed, white or hard, or if blood is observed in the giving set.

REFERENCES

1 *Can potassium be given by subcutaneous infusion?* UKMI Q&A 45.6 (accessed via www.evidence.nhs.uk 19 August 2014).
2 *Can magnesium sulphate be given subcutaneously?* UKMI Q&A 14.5 (accessed via www.evidence.nhs.uk 19 August 2014).
3 Hypodermoclysis Working Group (1998). *Hypodermoclysis – Guidelines on the technique*. Wrexham: CP Pharmaceuticals.
4 SPC (2011). *Hyalase November 2011 revision*. http://emc.medicines.org.uk/ (accessed 19 August 2014).

Hypopituitarism

Overview	
Definition	Hypopituitarism is the complete or partial deficiency of one or more of the pituitary hormones and can occur in adults or children.
	Causes of pituitary insufficiency include:
	• pituitary tumours • radiotherapy or surgery • pituitary infarction • infection • head injury.
	The symptoms of hypopituitarism depend on the hormones involved and the degree of insufficiency[1,2]

Risk factors	Initially, a patient with any hormone deficiency may be asymptomatic. Individuals with the following deficiencies present with the indicated condition.
	- Adrenocorticotrophic hormone (ACTH) deficiency: adrenal (cortisol) insufficiency
	- Thyroid-stimulating hormone (TSH) deficiency: hypothyroidism
	- Gonadotrophin deficiency: hypogonadism
	- Growth hormone deficiency: failure to thrive and short stature in children; most adults are asymptomatic, but some may experience fatigue and weakness and decreased quality of life
	- Antidiuretic hormone deficiency (ADH) – polyuria and polydipsia
Differential diagnosis	Differential diagnosis depends on the hormones affected
Diagnostic tests	Hormonal studies should be performed in pairs of target gland and their respective stimulatory pituitary hormone for proper interpretation.[2]
	- Thyroid: TSH, thyroxine (T4), triiodothyronine (T3)
	- Adrenal function: ACTH stimulation test (or morning cortisol and ACTH)
	- Fertility: follicle-stimulating hormone (FSH), luteinising hormone (LH) and either oestradiol (if amenorrhoeic) or morning testosterone (as appropriate for sex)
	- Prolactin
	- Growth hormone-provocative testing
Treatment goals	- Replacement of affected hormones to physiological levels
Treatment options	- Pituitary hormone deficiencies are treated by replacing either the pituitary hormone itself, e.g. growth hormone, or the target hormone, e.g. levothyroxine, corticosteroids

Pharmaceutical care and counselling

Essential intervention	- Glucocorticoids are required if the ACTH–adrenal axis is impaired
	- Hypothyroidism is treated with levothyroxine
	- Gonadotrophin deficiency is treated with sex-appropriate hormones. Testosterone replacement is used in men and oestrogen replacement is used in women, with progesterone in women with an intact uterus
	- Growth hormone is replaced in children. It is not routinely replaced in adults unless the patient is symptomatic of growth hormone deficiency after all other pituitary hormones have been replaced. The use of growth hormone is advised by the National Institute of Health and Care Excellence via two technology appraisals for adults and children[3,4]
	- Diabetes insipidus is treated using desmopressin. See *Diabetes insipidus (cranial)* entry
Continued monitoring	Hormone levels should be monitored to determine complications of under- or overreplacement. Hormone treatment may need to be adjusted to physiological maintenance levels, using the lowest dose

REFERENCES

1 Jorn Schneider H (2007). Hypopituitarism. *Lancet* 369: 1461–1470.

2 Corenblum B (2013). *Hypopituitarism (panhypopituitarism)*. Medscape. http://emedicine.medscape.com/article/122287-overview (accessed 28 August 2014).

3 NICE (2010). *Human Growth Hormone (Somatropin) for the Treatment of Growth Failure in Children* (TA188). London: National Institute for Health and Care Excellence.

4 NICE (2003). *Human Growth Hormone (Somatropin) in Adults with Growth Hormone Deficiency* (TA64). London: National Institute for Health and Care Excellence.

H

I

Ideal body weight

Ideal body weight (IBW) may be useful for calculating creatinine clearance to assess renal function. It is also useful for dose calculations of drugs that are not highly lipid-bound and have narrow therapeutic ranges, e.g. digoxin, gentamicin.

Many formulae exist to calculate IBW and all have limitations, such as their unsuitability for children, small women and tall men. An internet resource gives much information on the history of measuring IBW, and suggests using the Devine formula for men and the Robinson formula for women, which represents the best compromise to the limitations of the formulae:[1]

- for men: IBW (kg) = 50 kg + 2.3 kg for each inch over 5 feet
- for women: IBW (kg) = 49 kg + 1.7 kg for each inch over 5 feet

These formulae are used throughout this book wherever an IBW calculation is required.

REFERENCE
1 Halls MD (2015). *Ideal Weight Formulas by Broca and Devine*. http://halls.md/ideal-weight-formulas-broca-devine/ (accessed 27 January 2015).

Immunoglobulin (normal) for intravenous administration

Normal immunoglobulin for intravenous administration is made from the pooled plasma of screened human blood donors, currently from outside the UK. It contains mainly immunoglobulin G (IgG), with a small amount of IgA, and has a broad spectrum of antibodies effective against various infective agents. Extensive guidance is available on the suitability of intravenous immunoglobulin therapy for various conditions.[1]

There are several brands available, with similar dosing regimens for the various indications, although there may be some variation from brand to brand. The main difference between brands is in their excipients, and this may be useful if a patient is sensitive to a particular ingredient.

All patients should be adequately hydrated prior to initiation of therapy in order to protect against potential renal dysfunction (the normal daily fluid intake for an adult is 1.5 litre). Urine output and creatinine clearance should be monitored, and loop diuretics should not be used concomitantly.

Immunoglobulins can precipitate acute renal failure. The products containing sucrose as a stabiliser have accounted for a disproportionate number of patients who have experienced renal dysfunction or acute renal failure, i.e. Vigam.[2] Patients with the following factors carry a higher risk of this occurring: pre-existing renal impairment, diabetes mellitus, hypovolaemia, overweight, concomitant nephrotoxic drugs and patients aged over 65 years.[3]

Intravenous therapy with immunoglobulins may impair the efficacy of live attenuated vaccines, and therefore, live virus vaccines should only be given at least 3 weeks before or 3 months after an injection of immunoglobulin.[4]

The following information summarising administration and dosing regimens (Table I1) is for Vigam, which has the widest range of licensed indications. A separate column has been left for insertion of local variations if a different brand is used.

Administration

Bring the product to room or body temperature before use. The liquid is given intravenously through a filter (a 15 micron filter is recommended), at an initial rate of 0.01–0.02 mL/kg/min for 30 minutes. If tolerated, the rate can gradually be increased to 0.04 mL/kg/min. The maximum rate of Vigam is 3 mL/min, although some brands allow a higher rate of infusion.

The product is preservative-free so administration should start immediately after piercing the cap. The patient should be observed for any adverse effects for at least 20 minutes after commencement of infusion, e.g. a drop in blood pressure or signs of allergy. If anaphylaxis occurs the patient should be treated as per local guidelines.

Undesirable effects

The most common side effects are chills, hypothermia, headaches, fever, flushing, urticaria, nausea and vomiting. In most cases adverse reactions can be avoided or reversed by using low infusion rates. If influenza-like symptoms recur and reducing the infusion rate does not prevent them, premedicating the patient with paracetamol may help, but the possibility of an underlying infection should be considered and treated if that is the case.

It should be noted that there are human normal immunoglobulin products available that are suitable for subcutaneous infusion or intramuscular injection. These may be useful for patients who are fluid-restricted or for treatment in the home. The appropriate SPC should be consulted if these products are to be used.

TABLE I1

Dosing regimens for Vigam[3]

Indication	Dose	Frequency	Local variations
Replacement therapy in primary immunodeficiency,	Starting dose: 0.4–0.8 g/kg Thereafter: 0.2–0.8 g/kg	Every 2–4 weeks to obtain IgG trough level of at least 4–6 g/L	
Replacement therapy in secondary immunodeficiency	0.2–0.4 g/kg	Every 2–4 weeks to obtain IgG trough level of at least 4–g/L	
Congenital AIDS	0.2–0.4 g/kg	Every 3–4 weeks	
Hypogammaglobulinaemia (<4 g/L) in patients after allogeneic haematopoietic stem cell transplantation	0.2–0.4 g/kg	Every 3–4 weeks to obtain 1 gG trough level above 5 g/L	
Immunomodulation in idiopathic thrombocytopenic purpura	0.8–1.0 g/kg or	On day 1, possibly repeated once within 3 days	
	0.4 g/kg/day	For 2–5 days	
Immunomodulation in Guillain–Barré syndrome	0.4 g/kg/day	For 5 days	
Immunomodulation in Kawasaki disease	2 g/kg	In one dose usually within 10 days of onset of symptoms, and with concomitant aspirin (dose as per BNFC)[5]	
Allogeneic bone marrow transplantation			
Treatment of graft-versus-host disease	0.5 g/kg	Weekly from 7 days prior to transplantation and for up to 3 months after transplantation	
Persistent lack of antibody production	0.5 g/kg	Monthly until antibody levels return to normal	

REFERENCES

1 *Clinical Guidelines for Immunoglobulin* Use (2008) https://www.gov.uk/government/publications/clinical-guidelines-for-immunoglobulin-use-second-edition-update (accessed 6 September 2015).

2 eMC (2014). www.medicines.org.uk (accessed 23 December 2014).

3 SPC (2015). *Vigam Liquid.* http://emc.medicines.org.uk (accessed 7 September 2015).

4 *Green Book*, Chapter 6 (2013). http://www.dh.gov.uk/ (accessed 23 December 2014).

5 Joint Formulary Committee (2015). *BNF for children* (online). London: BMJ Group and Pharmaceutical Press. www.medicinescomplete.com (accessed 6 September 2015).

Inflammatory bowel disease

Overview

Definition	Inflammatory bowel disease (IBD) is a chronic relapsing inflammatory condition of the gastrointestinal tract. It is a broad term for two diseases: • Crohn's disease (CD), which can affect any part of the gastrointestinal tract • ulcerative colitis (UC), which affects the rectum and colon
Causes	• Most likely a combination of genetic and environmental factors, resulting in an inappropriate immune-mediated response to indigenous flora and other antigens
Classification	Severity of disease is classified according to signs and symptoms. The most common tools used are the Truelove and Witts criteria for UC (Table I2)[1] and the Harvey–Bradshaw index for CD (Table I3)[2]

TABLE I2
Truelove and Witt's severity index

	Mild	Moderate	Severe
Number of bloody stools per day	<4	4–6	>6
Temperature (°C)	Afebrile	Intermediate	>37.8
Heart rate (beats/min)	Normal	Intermediate	>90
Haemoglobin (g/dL)	>11	10.5–11	<10.5
ESR (mm/hour)	<20	20–30	>30

TABLE I3
Harvey–Bradshaw index

General well-being (0 = very well, 1 = slightly below average, 2 = poor, 3 = very poor, 4 = terrible)
Abdominal pain (0 = none, 1 = mild, 2 = moderate, 3 = severe)
Number of liquid stools per day
Abdominal mass (0 = none, 1 = dubious, 2 = definite, 3 = tender)
Complications (score 1 per item): arthralgia, uveitis, erythema nodosum, aphthous ulcers, pyoderma gangrenosum, anal fissure, new fistula, abscess

Score <4 = remission, >8 = severe disease

Differential diagnosis	Irritable bowel disease, infection, coeliac disease, diverticular disease, bowel cancer

Signs and symptoms	Depending on the location of disease, both UC and CD can result in symptoms of diarrhoea with blood and mucus, abdominal pain, tenesmus, weight loss, malaise and fever. Signs may include: anaemia, raised inflammatory markers (e.g. CRP, ESR), and extraintestinal manifestations of IBD, which may affect joints (arthritis), skin (erythema nodosum or pyoderma gangrenosum), eyes (uveitis) or liver (primary sclerosing cholangitis). Fistulae and Intestinal strictures may also be present in CD
Diagnostic tests	• Stool culture – to rule out infection • Faecal calprotectin – can distinguish between inflammatory conditions such as IBD, and non-inflammatory conditions, e.g. irritable bowel syndrome • Flexible sigmoidoscopy and colonoscopy allow direct visualisation of the distribution and degree of inflammation; biopsies taken during investigation help differentiate between UC and CD • Radiological tests (e.g. abdominal X-ray, small-bowel meal, CT and MRI) also provide information on the location and degree of disease activity • FBC and CRP – inflammatory markers may be raised with more severe disease; thrombocytosis and anaemia may be seen
Treatment goals	• Minimise symptoms and improve quality of life • Induce and maintain remission • Promote mucosal healing • Reduce the need for surgery
Treatment options[2]	• Aminosalicylates, corticosteroids, enteral nutrition and immunomodulators are the main options for inducing and maintaining remission • Surgery to remove diseased bowel is normally reserved for when medical therapy has failed. For UC this is normally a colectomy which is curative; for CD, surgery is conservative, as disease may recur after resection and further surgery may be required in the future

Medicines optimisation

NICE has published guidance on the treatment of both CD[3] and UC[4]

Aminosali-cylates	• Main role for oral aminosalicylates (>2.4 g) is first-line for mild to moderate flares of UC. It may be considered in CD if patients decline steroids, but the evidence is poor. Lower doses (e.g. 1.2 g/day Asacol, Octasa) are sufficient for maintaining remission in UC. Although different brands may release in different parts of the gastrointestinal tract, there is no evidence to suggest any one brand is more effective than another • Once-daily mesalazine is as effective as multiple daily doses and may help adherence, though side effects may be increased • Rectal mesalazine (suppositories for proctitis, foams/enemas for more extensive disease) can be combined with oral therapy in UC and can improve remission rates, and is more effective than rectal steroids • Blood dyscrasias are rare, but patients should be advised to report any unexplained bleeding, bruising, sore throat, fever or malaise

	• Renal toxicity is possible; renal function should be checked – the British Society of Gastroenterology suggests annual creatinine serum concentration[5]
Corticosteroids	• Conventional steroids (oral prednisolone, intravenous hydrocortisone or intravenous methylprednisolone) are first-line for treating flares of CD and severe UC, and second-line for mild to moderate UC where there is insufficient response to aminosalicylates
	• In hospital patients on intravenous steroids, monitor for hypokalaemia (mineralocorticoid effects) and hyperglycaemia (glucocorticoid effect)
	• Steroid regimens should tapered to prevent relapse and adrenal insufficiency – a typical regimen is 40 mg prednisolone daily, reducing by 5 mg a week to zero
	• Budesonide is an option for ileal or right-sided colonic CD – it causes fewer side effects but is less effective than prednisolone
	• Enteric-coated beclometasone is another alternative in UC, although it has not been compared directly with oral prednisolone
	• British Society of Gastroenterology guidelines[5] suggest co-prescribing with calcium and vitamin D. Recent guidelines from the National Osteoporosis Guideline Group suggest using the Fracture Risk Assessment Tool (FRAX) osteoporosis risk assessment tool to quantify risk of fracture and the need to measure bone mineral density[6]
Thiopurines	• Main role is to maintain remission. Thiopurines can induce remission but onset of action is slow (8–12 weeks).
	• Started in UC in those with >2 flares year requiring steroids, in those that flare when steroids are reduced and after an acute severe flare.
	• For CD consider thiopurines to maintain remission, particularly for patients with poor prognostic factors (e.g. early onset, perianal disease, severe presentation or steroid use at presentation).
	• Dose is azathioprine 2–2.5 mg/kg/day or mercaptopurine 1–1.5 mg/kg/day.
	• Thiopurine methyltransferase (TAMT) should be measured before starting; avoid thiopurines if levels are low; consider lower doses if intermediate levels. Some centres measure azathioprine metabolite levels to guide dosing.
	• Up to 20% of patients do not tolerate thiopurines: early side effects of nausea, headache and flu-like symptoms may be reduced by splitting the dose or starting at a lower dose.
	• Leucopenia, hepatotoxicity and pancreatitis are rarer (<5%); patients should be advised to report any signs of infection, and of liver/pancreatic disease such as abdominal pain, yellow skin and dark urine.
	• There may be an increased risk of lymphoma and skin cancer. Advise patients to wear sun block and minimise sun exposure.
	• FBC/LFTs should be monitored, normally under shared care arrangements; typically at baseline, weekly for 1–2 months, followed by 3-monthly

Methotrexate	<ul><li>Alternative in CD if thiopurines are not tolerated, most commonly given subcutaneously or orally once weekly.</li><li>Side effects include bone marrow suppression, liver toxicity and pneumonitis. Patients should be advised to report signs of infection, liver disease, breathlessness or persistent cough.</li><li>FBC/LFTs/U&Es should be measured at: baseline, 1–2-weekly until stabilised and then every 2–3 months.</li><li>A National Patient Safety Agency (NPSA) alert gives advice on safe prescribing, dispensing and administration of oral methotrexate – patients should carry handheld records of current dose and test results[7]</li></ul>
'Biologics'	<ul><li>Infliximab (intravenous) and adalimumab (subcutaneous) 'are' approved by NICE for severe CD</li><li>Use in acute severe UC is approved where ciclosporin is considered clinically inappropriate; maintenance use is not currently approved by NICE</li><li>Exclude hepatitis B and tuberculosis prior to commencing (history, chest X-ray, QuantiFERON ± tuberculin testing)</li><li>Advise patients to report signs of infection</li></ul>
Ciclosporin	<ul><li>Used in acute severe colitis in those patients not responding to intravenous steroids, normally 2 mg/kg intravenously over 24 hours adjusted to achieve levels of 100–200 micrograms/L</li><li>Normally converted to oral (6 mg/kg/day) for 3 months in those that respond to allow bridging to azathioprine</li><li>Check magnesium and cholesterol pretreatment; low levels are associated with nephrotoxicity and neurotoxicity respectively</li><li>Risk of nephrotoxicity, hepatotoxicity and hypertension – monitor U&Es, LFTs and blood pressure. Dose reduction may be required</li></ul>
Other medicine-related issues	<ul><li>All patients admitted to hospital with active disease should receive thromboprophylaxis</li><li>Avoid antidiarrhoeals, opiates and antispasmodics in acute colitis, as they may increase the risk of toxic megacolon</li><li>Non-steroidal anti-inflammatory drugs should be avoided</li><li>Patients on immunosuppressants should receive annual influenza vaccine and pneumococcal vaccine, and avoid live vaccines – see Department of Health green book for up-to-date guidance[8]</li><li>Smoking cessation improves the course of CD – support and encourage patients to stop smoking</li></ul>

REFERENCES

1 Truelove SC, Witts LJ (1955). Cortisone in ulcerative colitis; final report on a therapeutic trial. *Br Med J* 2: 1041–1048.

2 Harvey RF, Bradshaw JM (1980). A simple index of Crohn's-disease activity. *Lancet* 1: 514.

3 NICE (2012). *Crohn's Disease. Management in adults, children and young people* (CG152). https://www.nice.org.uk/guidance/cg152 (accessed 15 December 2014).

4 NICE (2013). *Ulcerative Colitis. Management in adults, children and young people* (CG 166). https://www.nice.org.uk/guidance/CG166 (accessed 15 December 2014).

5 Mowat C *et al.* (2011). Guidelines for the management of inflammatory bowel disease in adults. *Gut* 60: 571–607.

6 National Osteoporosis Guideline Group (2013). *Osteoporosis Clinical Guideline for Prevention and Treatment*. http://www.shef.ac.uk/NOGG/NOGG_Executive_Summary.pdf (accessed 15 December 2014).

7 NPSA (2006). *Improving Compliance with Oral Methotrexate Guidelines*. http://www.nrls.npsa.nhs.uk/resources/?entryid45=59800 (accessed 15 December 2014).

8 Public Health England (2014). *Immunisation Against Infectious Disease*. https://www.gov.uk/government/collections/immunisation-against-infectious-disease-the-green-book (accessed 12 February 2015).

Inhaler devices in respiratory disease

Inhalers are fundamental to the management of asthma and chronic obstructive pulmonary disease (COPD), delivering medication to the lungs whilst minimising side effects. Unfortunately, evidence shows that many people cannot take their inhalers correctly,[1] and many healthcare professionals are unable to teach inhaler technique.[2] Suboptimal technique can lead to treatment failure, inappropriate escalation of treatments and adverse effects and waste valuable healthcare resources. Pharmacists have a responsibility to ensure that patients can use their inhaled medications effectively and safely.

Whatever the device, there are steps that all the devices have in common (Table I4).

TABLE I4

Seven steps to success to optimise inhaler technique[3]

1	Prepare the device (e.g. remove mouthpiece cover)
2	Prepare the dose (e.g. shake aerosol)
3	Breathe out gently as far as is comfortable, but not into the inhaler
4	Put the mouthpiece in the mouth and close the lips around it
5	Breathe in: <ul><li>Check coordination of breathing and actuation of metered dose inhaler</li><li>Encourage people to breathe in *slow and steady* for all aerosol devices (including through a spacer device) and *quick and deep* for all dry-powder devices</li></ul>
6	Remove inhaler from the mouth and hold the breath for up to 10 seconds
7	Repeat dose if required Replace mouthpiece cover or close device

Remember: patients should always be instructed to rinse their mouth and throat with water after inhaling corticosteroids.

Patient assessment

The following points are worth considering:

1 What device was the patient using previously?

2 Was the device being used effectively?

3 What problems with manual dexterity or coordination can be overcome?

REFERENCES

1 Broedersa MEAC *et al.* (2009). The ADMIT series – issues in inhalation therapy. 2) Improving technique and clinical effectiveness. *Primary Care Respir J* 18: 76–82.

2 Baverstock M *et al.* (2010). Do healthcare professionals have sufficient knowledge of inhaler techniques in order to educate their patients effectively in their use? *Thorax* 65: A117.

3 *Inhaler Device Technique Cards – Seven steps to success.* www.simplestepseducation .co.uk (accessed 2 November 2014).

Insulins

Routes of administration

Subcutaneous (SC) injection

This is the most common route for insulin used in routine treatment. Unmodified soluble insulin is fairly quickly absorbed from SC sites: initial blood glucose-lowering effects are seen within 20–30 minutes. Insulin then continues to be released from the injection site over the following 4–6 hours. However, the onset and duration of action of most insulin preparations are considerably longer than this because of their formulation. The anatomical site chosen for injection also influences the rate of absorption of insulins (see section on injection technique, below).

Intramuscular (IM) injection

Soluble insulin given by the IM route is slightly more rapidly absorbed than that given SC, but it is not routinely used.

Intravenous (IV) infusion

The half-life of soluble insulin given by IV infusion is only a few minutes. If using in type 1 patients, i.e. those who have no endogenous insulin secretion, the rate of infusion should *never* be reduced to zero, as the patient will rapidly become ketotic.

Inhaled insulin

The first inhaled insulin, Exubera, was taken off the UK market in 2007 after only a few months due to cost issues. However, Afrezza was launched in the USA in February 2015 and application has been made for licensing in the UK. It is a dry-powder formulation of ultra-short-acting insulin, which is licensed for preprandial administration in both type 1 and type 2 diabetes mellitus. Because of its route of administration, use is not recommended in asthma, chronic obstructive pulmonary disease or in those who smoke.

Prescribing insulins

Unmodified soluble insulin is fairly rapidly absorbed from SC injection sites, and insulin has therefore been produced in many different formulations and types aimed at increasing or decreasing rate of absorption following SC injection.

Mistakes in insulin prescribing and administration rank amongst the most frequent of all inpatient drug errors and have been associated with significant morbidity and mortality.[1] The National Patient Safety Agency identified 13 180 incidents in England and Wales in 2003–2009.[2] Errors typically involve omitted doses, incorrect doses and inaccurate transcription of the type, dose or timing of insulin. Key points are listed below.[2]

- Every effort should be made to continue a patient's usual type of insulin while in hospital if no change in regimen is deemed clinically necessary.
- Insulins should always be prescribed by brand name (specifying species if relevant) because release characteristics may vary even between insulins in the same category. Excipients such as preservatives may also differ between the brands and can result in local injection site reactions. A change in insulin brand requires more intensive monitoring until the effects of the change are fully appreciated.
- Insulin should be prescribed relative to meals rather than to set clock times and NBM orders should prompt urgent review of insulin therapy.
- Insulin prescriptions should always state the word 'units' in full: the use of abbreviations such as 'U' or 'IU' misread as a number 0 could cause a 10-fold overdose.
- Insulin should always be measured using insulin syringes designed for the purpose. The use of other syringes has resulted in fatal dosing errors.
- Incorrect prescription of insulin mixtures is a common source of insulin prescribing errors:
  - confusing the insulin name with the dose, e.g. Humalog Mix50 becoming Humalog 50 units
  - omission of part of the name, e.g. Humalog Mix50 becoming Humalog, resulting in the administration of a large dose of rapid-acting insulin.
- In 1983, all insulins available in the UK were standardised to a single strength: U100 insulin, i.e. insulin providing 100 units/mL. This massive task was undertaken to improve safety in dosing and reduce prescribing errors. However, new insulin products have recently become available containing higher insulin concentrations, e.g. Tresiba, Humalog and Toujeo. A biosimilar preparation (Abasaglar) and a new preparation containing insulin in combination with liraglutide (Xultophy) have also recently been launched. The MHRA has issued a Drug Safety Update providing extensive guidance on minimising the risk associated with availability of these non-standard preparations.[3]

Types of insulin

Insulin is either directly extracted from animal pancreases (porcine or bovine) or synthesised (human sequence insulins or human insulin analogues). These broad groups of insulin differ in terms of exact amino acid sequence.

- Animal insulins are no longer commonly used in the UK. They are sometimes used in patients who have experienced troublesome hypoglycaemia with 'human' insulins.
- Human sequence insulins are produced semisynthetically by enzymatic modification of porcine insulin (emp) or biosynthetically by recombinant DNA technology using bacteria (crb, prb) or yeast (pyr).

- Analogue insulins are genetically modified insulins produced to enhance the properties of human insulin, e.g. to speed up absorption of insulins taken with meals or prolong and improve the uniformity of the action of the basal insulins. They are generally more expensive.

The main types of insulin are classified as rapid/short-acting, intermediate/long-acting and biphasic. The onset of action, peak activity and duration of action of each product differ and they are all subject to interpatient variability. The key points about these insulins are listed in Table I5: the Joint British Diabetes Societies have published a useful wall chart outlining the categories and types of insulin available with a more specific guide to their onset and duration of action.[4]

TABLE I5

Insulin categories with key points

Examples	Appearance	Licensed routes	Approximate onset and duration (SC)	Key points
Rapid-acting insulin analogues				
Humalog Novorapid Apidra	Clear	IV SC	Onset: 10–20 minutes Duration: 2–5 hours	• Licensed for IV use but relatively expensive and have no advantages by this route • May be used as the 'bolus' component of basal-bolus regimens • Inject just before (ideally), with or just after food • May be particularly helpful where eating patterns are unpredictable
Short-acting insulins				
Actrapid Humulin S Insuman Rapid Hypurin Bovine or Porcine Neutral	Clear	IV SC IM (not Actrapid, Insuman)	Onset: 30–60 minutes Duration: 4–6 hours	• Sometimes referred to as 'soluble' insulin (or 'regular' in the USA) • Insulins of choice for IV insulin infusions • May be used as the 'bolus' component of basal-bolus regimens • Inject 15–30 minutes before food to reduce raised postprandial blood glucose levels (must eat within 30 minutes to avoid hypoglycaemia). Usually need further carbohydrate 2–4 hours later to cover remaining insulin activity ('meal and snack' pattern of eating)

(continued)

TABLE 15
(Continued)

Examples	Appearance	Licensed routes	Approximate onset and duration (SC)	Key points
Intermediate- and long-acting insulins				
Insulatard Humulin I Insuman Basal Hypurin Bovine or Porcine Isophane Hypurin Bovine Lente	Cloudy	SC only	Vary widely between insulins Onset: 1.5–4 hours Duration: 15–36 hours	• Must *never* be used intravenously • Resuspend particulate matter before use (see section on injection technique, below) • Usually injected once or twice daily
Long-acting insulin analogues				
Lantus Levemir Tresiba	Clear	SC only	Prolonged half-life. Steady state is reached 2–4 days after first dose	• Not appropriate for IV use • Given once a day at about the same time (Levemir is licensed for twice-daily use – may be helpful for large daily doses) • Clear in appearance, so potential for confusion with rapid- or short-acting insulins
Biphasic insulins (i.e. insulin mixtures)				
Humulin M3 Novomix 30 Hypurin Porcine 30/70 mix Insuman Comb 15 or 25 or 50 Humalog Mix 25 or Mix 50	Cloudy	SC only	Combinations of short- or rapid-acting insulins with longer-acting component. Onset and duration vary with component insulins	• Must *never* be used intravenously • Resuspend particulate matter before use (see section on injection technique, below) • Usually injected twice daily • Administration must be associated with a meal because of the quick-acting component • The number in the insulin name gives an indication of the percentage of the short-acting component • High risk of prescribing errors – see section on prescribing insulins, above

Typical insulin regimens

All regimens are adjusted on the basis of capillary blood glucose results.

Once-daily insulin regimens

- used in type 2 diabetes if blood glucose control is inadequate with other therapy
- insulins used: intermediate- or long-acting insulins
- other types of therapy may be continued to treat insulin resistance and enhance the efficacy of injected insulin.

Twice-daily insulin regimens

- used in type 2 diabetes, but may be used in type 1 if more intensive insulin regimens are unsuitable
- insulins used: usually biphasic insulins
- regimens vary, but a commonly used starting dose is to give two-thirds of the total daily dose before breakfast and one-third before the evening meal.

Basal-bolus insulin regimens

- used in type 1 diabetes to mimic physiological insulin secretion more closely: insulin doses can be adjusted to reflect the patient's needs
- comprise a longer-acting insulin given once (or occasionally twice) daily to provide a background or 'basal' level of insulin secretion, plus quick-acting insulin given before meals
- regimens vary but a commonly used ratio is to give half the total daily insulin requirement as longer-acting insulin at bedtime, and then split the remainder into three doses of quick-acting insulin to be given before meals.

Although these intensive insulin regimens involve giving four or five injections per day, they have several advantages for patients:

- increased flexibility of lifestyle – eating can be more spontaneous, so patients can eat when they are hungry instead of when they have to
- increased patient involvement – the day-to-day monitoring and adjustment of doses help patients to understand their diabetes and how to control it
- the potential for improved glycaemic control – better understanding enables improved decision making, can improve control and reduce the likelihood of diabetic complications
- improved ability to deal with 'crises' – once patients have learnt how to adjust doses in response to blood glucose results, they are better able to deal with intercurrent illness and stress.

Dose adjustment for normal eating (DAFNE)[5]

DAFNE is considered by NICE as the gold-standard education programme for patients with type 1 diabetes.

The DAFNE programme involves a formal 5-day training programme. Participants learn together in groups with other patients with type 1 diabetes and specialist nurses and dietitians lead the sessions. The course covers:

- carbohydrate estimation
- blood glucose and ketone monitoring
- insulin regimens and how to adjust doses
- eating out
- reading food labels
- 'hypos'
- illness ('sick-day rules').

Continuous SC insulin infusion (CSII)

CSII should be initiated only by a trained specialist team.[6] The basic principle of CSII use is that the pump is set to deliver a basal level of insulin throughout the 24-hour period, and this is augmented by bolus doses delivered to coincide with food intake. Rapid-acting insulins are usually used in the pumps. Patients using pumps are highly trained and intervention is only usually necessary if the patient is unwell and an intravenous insulin infusion is more appropriate. Refer queries to the diabetes specialist team.

SC insulin injection

Injection technique

The basic principles of SC injection technique are listed below.

1 Wash hands and ensure injection site is clean (use of alcohol injection swabs is *not* recommended because they can cause skin hardening).
2 If using a 'cloudy' insulin, resuspend by rolling the vial, cartridge or pen gently between the palms or inverting several times. The insulin suspension should look uniformly milky.
3 If using an insulin pen, fit a new needle, dial up 2 units and perform an 'air shot' to check that there are no air bubbles and the pen mechanism is working correctly.
4 Withdraw the required dose using an insulin syringe, or dial up the correct dose according to the manufacturer's instructions if using an insulin pen.
5 Select an area on the abdomen or outer thigh. Ideally, use the same anatomical area at the same time each day – sites on the abdomen absorb fastest and are therefore best for insulins intended to be quick-acting; sites on the outer thigh are best for longer-acting insulins. The buttock or the upper outer arm may also be used but there is an increased risk of inadvertent IM injection using the arm, so additional monitoring may be necessary.[7]
6 Pinch up a skin fold between the thumb and forefinger and hold throughout the injection. If you are using a short needle (4 or 6 mm) you may not need to do this.

7 Insert the needle into the thick part of the skin fold at a 90° angle to the skin.
8 Inject the insulin and continue to hold the needle in place for several seconds before withdrawing the needle and discarding it safely.
9 Do not rub the injection site after administration. Rotate sites within an anatomical area so that individual sites are not reused within 1 month.

Injection site reactions

It is common to have injection site reactions when insulin is started but these usually lessen with time. True insulin allergy is rare.

Overuse of injection sites: lipoatrophy and lipohypertrophy

Repeated insulin injections in the same site can cause fat and scar tissue to accumulate, causing unsightly hard, fatty lumps. Poor rotation of injection sites interferes with insulin absorption and is a significant cause of unexpected variations in blood glucose levels.

Disposal of used needles and blood lancets

Sharps bins are available on FP10 prescription forms, as are needle clippers. Diabetes specialist nurses and clinical commissioning group pharmacists should be able to provide information concerning local policies and services.

General insulin counselling points

- Patients on insulin should always carry glucose or some other means of treating hypoglycaemia, e.g. 200 mL carton of fruit juice.
- Patients on insulin should always carry a card identifying them as having diabetes mellitus and ideally an insulin passport.[8]
- A patient's main supply of insulin should be stored in a fridge, but must not be allowed to freeze, because freezing denatures insulin and makes it unfit for use.
- Insulin that is in use should be stored at room temperature, because injections are more comfortable and pen mechanisms are less likely to jam. Higher temperatures also enhance the activity of preservatives.
- Insulin can be kept out of the fridge for 4–6 weeks (dependent on brand). For patients on small doses, for example children, the pen/vial should be clearly marked with the date use commenced so that it can be discarded after an appropriate interval.

REFERENCES

1 Department of Health (2004). *Building a Safer NHS for Patients. Improving medication safety.* http://webarchive.nationalarchives.gov.uk/+/www.dh.gov.uk/en/Publicationsandstatistics/Publications/PublicationsPolicyAndGuidance/DH_4071443 (accessed 12 February 2015).
2 NHS Evidence (2010). *Safe and Effective Use of Insulin in Hospitalised Patients.* http://www.diabetes.nhs.uk/document.php?o=1040 (accessed 9 February 2015).

3 MHRA Drug Safety Update (2015). *High strength, fixed combination and biosimilar insulin products: minimising the risk of medication error*. https://www.gov.uk/drug-safety-update/high-strength-fixed-combination-and-biosimilar-insulin-products-minimising-the-risk-of-medication-error (accessed 10 September 2015).

4 The Joint British Diabetes in Patient Care Group (2013). *The Management of Hypoglycaemia in Adults with Diabetes Mellitus* – Chart on page 26. http://www.diabetes.org.uk/Documents/About%20Us/Our%20views/Care%20recs/JBDS%20hypoglycaemia%20position%20(2013).pdf (accessed 12 February 2015).

5 DAFNE Study Group (2002). Training in flexible, intensive insulin management to enable dietary freedom in people with type 1 diabetes: dose adjustment for normal eating (DAFNE) randomised controlled trial. *BMJ* 325: 746–751.

6 NICE (2008). TA151. *Continuous Subcutaneous Insulin Infusion for the Treatment of Diabetes Mellitus*. www.nice.org.uk/guidance/ta151 (accessed 12 February 2015).

7 Diabetes UK (2015). *The Arm as an Injection Site*. www.diabetes.org.uk (accessed 9 February 2015).

8 NHS England (2014). *The Adult Patient's Passport to Safer Use of Insulin*. http://www.nrls.npsa.nhs.uk/resources/?EntryId45=130397 (accessed 12 February 2015).

Insulin: variable-rate intravenous insulin infusion

This entry does not include the treatment of diabetic ketoacidosis (DKA) or hyperosmolar hyperglycaemic state (HHS) – refer to these respective entries.

When patients with diabetes are nil-by-mouth (NBM), they will often require insulin to be administered IV and titrated to the capillary blood glucose (CBG). 'Sliding-scale insulin' is a phrase often used; however, it should be replaced by the term variable-rate intravenous insulin infusion (VRIII). Such infusions are used to maintain control of blood glucose levels in patients undergoing elective or emergency procedures. Many trusts have written policies, so it is important to check your own hospital's policy before commencing treatment. Glucose–potassium–insulin (GKI) infusions are still used in some parts of the UK.

VRIII is used in patients with diabetes who are expected to have a starvation period comprising two or more missed meals. For planned procedures, starvation times should be kept to a minimum. Patients who are only expected to miss one meal should be managed by modification of their usual diabetes medication unless preadmission blood glucose control is poor.[1] VRIII is also used in level 3 critical care patients if blood glucose is above 7 mmol/L.

The aim of VRIII is to achieve and maintain normoglycaemia: ideally, CBG levels of 6–10 mmol/L, although 4–12 mmol/L is acceptable.[1] Additionally, the correct use of VRIII ensures that the patient with type 1 diabetes has a constant presence of insulin and so does not become ketotic. Patients who are NBM also require maintenance of fluid and electrolyte balance and this governs the choice of IV fluid given.

Key points

- Patients admitted on long-acting basal insulin analogues, e.g. glargine or Levemir, should normally continue on their usual daily maintenance dose while they are receiving the VRIII.[1]
- Only insulin infusions containing 1 unit/mL should be prepared and used.[2]
  - Draw up 49.5 mL sodium chloride 0.9% into a syringe suitable for use in a syringe pump.
  - Measure 50 units (0.5 mL) soluble insulin (e.g. Actrapid, Humulin S) using an insulin syringe and add to the prepared syringe.
  - Cap the syringe and mix well to give a solution containing 1 unit/mL.
- A glucose-containing infusion *must* be administered alongside the insulin, so that hypoglycaemia is avoided. The fluid is given via a volumetric infusion pump, and the fluid of choice is considered to be sodium chloride 0.45% with glucose 5% plus potassium chloride 0.15%,[1] which should be supplied as a ready-prepared fluid.[3] Subsequent fluids are adjusted based on at least daily serum electrolyte evaluations.
- The delivery of the glucose-containing solution and the VRIII must both be via a single large-bore cannula with appropriate one-way or antisyphon valves.
- The fluid replacement rate is set to deliver the hourly fluid requirements of the individual patient and this rate should not be altered without senior advice.
- The rate of administration of the insulin infusion is then initiated and varied to keep the CBG within the target range (6–10 mmol/L, although 4–12 mmol/L is acceptable). CBG is monitored at least hourly initially and more frequently if the readings are outside the target range.
- Hypoglycaemia is a common side effect of an insulin infusion and a CBG less than 4 mmol/L should be treated (see *Diabetes mellitus – management of hypoglycaemia ('hypo') in adults* entry).
- Once the patient is able to eat and drink, s/he may be transferred back to usual diabetes therapy.

Adjustment of insulin dosage

An example of a VRIII prescription is shown in Table I6.

If increased doses of insulin are consistently being required (blood glucose above 15 mmol/L and not falling), first check patency of IV access and the pump for malfunction. If no mechanical cause is found, seek advice from the diabetes team.

Changing back to SC insulin

Once the patient is conscious and able to eat and drink, SC insulin can be reintroduced. For all regimens, the intravenous insulin infusion should be continued for at least 30–60 minutes after giving the SC dose in association with a meal.

TABLE 16

An example of a variable-rate intravenous insulin infusion prescription

Bedside capillary blood glucose (mmol/L)	Infusion rate of insulin solution (units/hour)
<4	0.5 (0.0 if a long-acting insulin analogue has been continued)
4.1–7.0	1
7.1–9.0	2
9.1–11.0	3
11.1–14.0	4
14.1–17.0	5
17.1–20	6
>20	Seek diabetes team or medical advice

Glucose–potassium–insulin (GKI)

Regimens used vary from hospital to hospital (check your local policy), but generally a single bag is used containing glucose 10% 500 mL plus potassium chloride 0.15% run at 100–125 mL/hour. Soluble insulin is added to the bag (5, 10, 15 or 20 units/500 mL). New infusions are prepared dependent on the patient's CBG. Maintaining an accurate fluid balance chart is challenging because of frequent fluid bag changes; additionally, sodium chloride 0.9% may be run alongside because of the risk of hyponatraemia. This regimen is most commonly used as a maintenance regimen for patients undergoing surgery.

REFERENCES

1 JBDS (2011) *Management of Adults with Diabetes Undergoing Surgery and Elective Procedures: Improving standards.* http://www.diabetes.org.uk/About_us/What-we-say/Improving-diabetes-healthcare/Management-of-adults-with-diabetes-undergoing-surgery-and-elective-procedures-improving-standards/ (accessed 13 February 2015).

2 NHS Evidence (2010). *Safe and Effective Use of Insulin in Hospitalised Patients.* http://www.diabetes.nhs.uk/document.php?o=1040 (accessed 9 February 2015).

3 NPSA (2002). *Potassium Chloride Concentrate Solutions – Patient safety alert.* http://www.nrls.npsa.nhs.uk/resources/?entryid45=59882 (accessed 17 January 2015).

Interstitial lung disease

Overview

Definition

The interstitial lung diseases (ILDs) are a heterogeneous group of respiratory conditions grouped together because they primarily affect the lung interstitium/parenchyma. For some, the airways and pulmonary vasculature may also be involved.

The pathogenesis, prognosis and management options across the ILDs are distinct and the terminology confusing, having been subject to inconsistencies and reclassification over recent years.

As a group the pathology is one of varying degrees of inflammation and fibrosis, with varying propensity for inflammation to progress to fibrosis.

The main ILDs are:[1,2]

- Hypersensitivity pneumonitis (HP: previously referred to as extrinsic allergic alveolitis)
- Those associated with connective tissue disease (CTD-ILD)
- Idiopathic interstitial pneumonias (IIPs), further subdivided into:
  - Idiopathic pulmonary fibrosis (IPF) (previously referred to as cryptogenic fibrosis alveolitis)
  - Non-specific interstitial pneumonia (NSIP): further classified as either cellular or fibrotic
  - Smoking-related IIPs; desquamative interstitial pneumonia (DIP) and respiratory bronchiolitis-associated (RB-ILD)
  - Acute/sub-acute IIPs; acute interstitial pneumonia (AIP) and Cryptogenic organising pneumonia (COP) (COP previously referred to as bronchiolitis obliterans organising pneumonia, or BOOP)
  - Rare IIPs; lymphoid interstitial pneumonia and pleuroparenchymal fibroelastosis
- Combined pulmonary fibrosis with emphysema
- Sarcoidosis (see *Sarcoidosis* entry)
- Rarer conditions, including:
  - Idiopathic pulmonary haemosiderosis
  - Lymphangioleiomyomatosis
  - Pulmonary alveolar proteinosis
  - Pulmonary Langerhans' cell histiocytosis (PLCH)

Numerous adverse drug reactions may involve the lung interstitium and progress to pulmonary fibrosis.[3] A comprehensive database is maintained at http://www.pneumotox.com/.

Pneumoconioses caused by toxic accumulation of dusts in the lung and progressive fibrosis (such as silicosis, coal worker's lung, asbestosis, berylliosis) also affect the lung interstitium and are important in the differential diagnosis of ILDs, but will not be discussed further in this entry

Risk factors	- The cause is unknown for the majority of ILDs (accounting for ≈65% of patients) - Smoking is the main risk factor for DIP, RB-ILD and PLCH, which generally only occur in patients with a significant smoking history - IPF has been associated with exposure to metal and wood dust - Gastro-oesophageal reflux disease (GORD) has also been associated with the development of IPF and may be asymptomatic in some patients - HP is an immunological reaction due to ongoing inhalation of an organic antigen or chemicals (such as isocyanates), which act as haptens (i.e. small molecules that elicit an immune response when attached to a carrier protein, but which would not be immunogenic themselves). A huge range of antigens are known, giving rise to a number of eponymous conditions, such as bird fancier's lung, farmer's lung, mushroom worker's lung, hot tub lung

Differential diagnosis	There is considerable overlap in the clinical, radiological and histopathological presentations of the ILDs.
	Diagnosis should be undertaken by a multidisciplinary team comprising a clinician, radiologist and histopathologist with experience in the diagnosis of the ILDs.
	Important differential diagnoses include: opportunistic infections (especially in immunosuppressed patients), pulmonary oedema and carcinomatosis
Diagnostic tests[4]	• Cough is common and may be either productive or non-productive. Cough lasting >3 weeks is a common referral criterion to investigate the possibility of lung cancer but ILD should also be considered. Chronic cough may also be caused by postnasal drip, GORD, ACE inhibitors (see *ACE inhibitor-induced cough* entry) or active inflammation in the lung. Chronic cough due to fibrosis is often difficult to manage and is frequently distressing and disabling for the patient
	• Patients typically present with breathlessness that is more severe on exertion and described using the Medical Research Council (MRC) or modified MRC dyspnoea scale (Table I7)
	• Type I respiratory failure with hypoxia is common in advanced disease. Oxygen saturation on pulse oximetry may be low and fall on exertion and there may be clinical signs of hypoxia and cyanosis
	• Spirometry will typically show a restrictive pattern (↓ FVC with normal FEV_1/FVC ratio as lungs are stiffer and volumes are reduced. This is an important differential from obstructive airways disease such as COPD, where the pattern is ↓FEV_1/FVC with normal (or slightly reduced) FVC
	• Additional pulmonary function tests such as plethysmography or helium dilution will show a reduced total lung capacity (TLC) with preserved residual volume (RV)/TLC ratio. In neuromuscular disorders or severe obesity there is also a restrictive pattern but with ↑RV/TLC
	• Diffusing capacity of the lung for carbon monoxide (DLCO) or transfer factor of the lung for carbon monoxide (TLCO) provides an estimate of the lungs' ability to diffuse gases. It is calculated as a percentage predicted and provides a better estimate of the functional impairment than FVC. DLCO can be corrected for the TLC to give the rate of uptake of CO from alveolar gas (kCO)
	• The DLCO may also be reduced when there is a ventilation/perfusion (V/Q) mismatch, such as in pulmonary hypertension or pulmonary embolism, impairing lung perfusion
	• There is a lack of consensus on the description of disease severity based on DLCO: generally a DLCO <40% is considered as severe, 40–60% moderate and >60% a mild impairment of gas transfer. The FVC, DLCO and clinical context should be considered when assessing disease severity
	• Squeaks, squawks and fine crackles on auscultation are suggestive, but not specific, for ILD
	• Finger clubbing with loss on nail bed angle (Schamroth's sign) is common in ILD, but non-specific, occurring in a number of non-pulmonary conditions and may be idiopathic. Given the association with a number of serious pathologies, finger clubbing should prompt investigation

- Chest X-ray may be relatively specific for some forms of ILD, such as cystic pattern in lymphangioleiomyomatosis or PLCH. In the majority a chest X-ray is non-specific. High-resolution computed tomography (HRCT) is required for differentiation of the majority of ILD. Two common patterns are: usual interstitial pneumonia (UIP), which is a honeycombed pattern seen in fibrosis and the endpoint in a number of fibrotic processes, and NSIP, with patchy ground-glass opacities associated with inflammation.
  - NSIP is both a pattern on radiology and a diagnosis. The NSIP pattern is seen in a number of ILDs, including CTD-ILD. Where an underlying cause cannot be found the condition is termed NSIP (increasingly, idiopathic NSIP is being used).
  - Similarly, UIP is seen in a number of conditions and may represent end-stage fibrotic changes. Where no other cause can be found, this is termed IPF (i.e. idiopathic UIP = IPF).
- Autoimmune screening – if positive, suggest CTD-ILD or vasculitis.
- Precipitants – IgGs to specific antigens, such as avian or mixed moulds. If positive suggests HP, but precipitants for a number of HP causes are not routinely available and may be positive in the absence of association.
- Bronchioalveolar lavage with collection and analysis of cells within the airways may help differentiate cause (but is neither very sensitive nor specific):[5]
  - Very high total white cells with a high percentage of pigmented macrophages in smoking-related ILD
  - High lymphocyte count in sarcoidosis (CD4/CD8 ratio >2) and HP (CD4/CD8 ratio <1)
  - High neutrophil count in infection or acute respiratory distress syndrome
  - High eosinophil count in eosinophilic pneumonia and adverse drug reactions
- In some patients where a confident diagnosis cannot be made based on the above, a lung biopsy may be needed

Treatment goals	- Depending on the ILD treatment may be directed at management of inflammation, slowing progression of fibrosis or managing symptoms[6]
Treatment options	- Oxygen therapy is often required to manage hypoxia. Vagal nerve stimulation (fan to face), opioids or benzodiazepines may reduce the sensation of breathlessness.
	- Consider reversible causes of cough, i.e. GORD, rhinitis causing postnasal drip. Opioid cough suppressants may be helpful, but frequently are suboptimal. The British Thoracic Society cough guidelines recommend dextromethorphan because of the lower incidence of adverse drug reactions, but it is still blacklisted in the *Drug Tariff*, although readily available in many over-the-counter cough mixtures.[7] All the opioids (morphine, codeine, pholcodine) seem to be equally effective but there is no evidence to support one over the other. There is limited evidence for prednisolone or thalidomide in the management of IPF-associated cough
	- In HP, avoidance of the antigen (if identifiable) may reverse inflammation. In others corticosteroids, with or without a steroid-sparing agent, may be required

- CTD-ILDs are managed as for connective tissue diseases with corticosteroids and immunosuppressive agents, such as azathioprine, mycophenolate mofetil or tacrolimus. There is limited evidence for cyclophosphamide (either oral or intravenously) and rituximab in some CTD-ILDs
- Corticosteroids or immunosuppressive agents may manage inflammation in other ILDs, but the evidence base is limited and there is no consensus on appropriate options
- Immunosuppression with azathioprine and prednisolone has been shown to be harmful in IPF; the risks associated with immunosuppression in other fibrotic ILDs is less clear
- N-acetylcysteine is often used in IPF but has recently been demonstrated to be of no benefit in preventing disease progression and may be associated with cardiovascular harm[8]
- Recent availability of therapies specifically targeting fibrotic pathways include nintedanib and pirfenidone (only licensed in IPF)

Pharmaceutical care and counselling

Assess	- It is important to recognise that ILDs represent a heterogeneous group of conditions with distinct management options - Adverse drug reactions may present as an ILD and should be considered - Serial measurements of lung function (FVC and DLCO) are useful and non-invasive means of assessing disease progression. Other non-invasive measures include the 6-minute walk test, but this tends not to be used in trials
Antifibrotic agents	- Nintedanib and pirfenidone are only licensed for the IPF type of ILD in the UK and funding is based on disease severity staged using FVC - Nintedanib is associated with impaired wound healing and increased bleeding risk and should be avoided in those at high risk (including treatment dose anticoagulants and high-dose antiplatelets). Diarrhoea and faecal urgency are common problems and may be managed with loperamide. Patients may experience disturbances in liver function and LFTs are recommended monthly for the first 3 months and then quarterly - Pirfenidone is associated with GI disturbances (nausea and anorexia) and should be slowly titrated to a target dose 3 × 267 mg capsules three times a day. Splitting the dose, spacing it out throughout a meal rather than taking all capsules at the same time, may help reduce gastrointestinal upset. Dose reduction may be required in some patients. Photosensitivity rash may occur and all patients should avoid sun exposure and use a sun cream with a sun protection factor >25 during treatment. Patients may experience disturbances in liver function and LFTs are recommended monthly for the first 6 months then quarterly. Omeprazole may reduce pirfenidone activity and, if required, an alternative PPI or gastric acid suppressant should be used. Due to the increased risk of phototoxicity, concomitant doxycycline should be avoided. Pirfenidone levels are increased by ciprofloxacin and the combination should be avoided. If this is not possible temporary dose reduction of pirfenidone may be required

TABLE I7

Medical Research Council (MRC) and modified MRC (mMRC) dyspnoea scale

Description	MRC scale	mMRC scale
Not troubled by breathlessness except on strenuous exercise	1	0
Short of breath when hurrying or walking up a slight hill	2	1
Walks slower than contemporaries on the level because of breathlessness, or has to stop for breath when walking at own pace	3	2
Stops for breath after about 100 metres or after a few minutes on the level	4	3
Too breathless to leave the house, or breathless when dressing or undressing	5	4

REFERENCES

1 American Thoracic Society/European Respiratory Society (2002). International Multidisciplinary Consensus Classification of the idiopathic interstitial pneumonias. *Am J Respir Crit Care Med* 165: 277–304.

2 American Thoracic Society and European Respiratory Society Committee on Idiopathic Interstitial Pneumonias (2013). An Official American Thoracic Society/European Reparatory Society statement: Update of the international multidisciplinary classification of the idiopathic interstitial pneumonias. *Am J Respir Crit Care Med* 188: 733–748.

3 Kubo K *et al.* (2013). Conensus statement for the diagnosis and treatment of drug-induced lung injuries. *Respir Investig* 51: 260–277.

4 Baughman RP *et al.* (2012). Monitoring of non-steroidal immunosuppressive drugs in patients with lung disease and lung transplant recipients: American College of Chest Physicians evidence-based clinical practice guidelines. *Chest* 142: e1S–e111S.

5 Meyer KC *et al.* (2012). An official American Thoracic Society clinical practice guideline: the clinical utility of bronchoalveolar lavage cellular analysis in interstitial lung disease. *Am J Respir Crit Care Med* 185: 1004–1014.

6 Bajwah S *et al.* (2013). Interventions to improve symptoms and quality of life of patients with fibrotic interstitial lung disease: a systematic review of the literature. *Thorax* 68: 867–879.

7 Morice AH *et al.* (2006). BTS guidelines recommendations for the management of cough in adults. *Thorax* 61: i1–i24.

8 Idiopathic Pulmonary Fibrosis Clinical Research Network (2014). Randomized trial of acetylcysteine in idiopathic pulmonary fibrosis. *N Engl J Med* 370(22): 2093–2101.

Iron: guidance on parenteral dosing and administration

Parenteral iron is available in several different forms, including iron dextran (CosmoFer), iron sucrose (Venofer), ferric carboxymaltose (Ferinject) and iron isomaltoside 1000 (Monofer). They are licensed for the treatment of iron-deficiency anaemia.

The use of parenteral iron is complex, requiring dose calculation and specified administration techniques. (See individual entries for each product for specific details). The added hazards posed to the fetus when these products are used in pregnancy further complicate the issue.

Therapeutic indications for iron-deficiency anaemia (for adult use only)[1]

- Demonstrated intolerance to oral iron preparations.
- Where there is a clinical need to deliver iron rapidly to iron stores.
- Demonstrated lack of effect of oral iron therapy, e.g. active inflammatory bowel disease.
- Patient non-adherence with oral iron therapy.

Contraindications[1]

- Non-iron-deficiency anaemia.
- Iron overload or disturbances in utilisation of iron.
- Hypersensitivity to parenteral iron products, including iron mono- or disaccharide complexes and dextran.

Adverse reactions[1]

Severe side effects are uncommon but include serious allergic reactions, e.g. life-threatening and fatal anaphylactic and anaphylactoid reactions. These reactions can occur even when a previous administration has been tolerated (including a negative test dose). Caution is therefore needed with every dose of IV iron, even if previously well tolerated. IV iron should only be given in an environment where the patient can be properly monitored and where resuscitation facilities exist.[2] These are characterised by sudden onset of respiratory difficulty and/or cardiovascular collapse; fatalities have been reported. Other less severe manifestations of immediate hypersensitivity are also uncommon and include rashes, itching, nausea and shivering.

Administration must be stopped immediately if signs of allergy are observed and appropriate treatment instituted.

Other undesirable effects include nausea, hypotension, dyspepsia, diarrhoea, flushing, headache and pains in joints and muscles. Exacerbation of joint pain in rheumatoid arthritis can occur. Soreness and inflammation at the site of the injection have also been reported.

In patients with known allergies, including drug allergies, a history of severe asthma, eczema or other atopic allergy and in patients with immune or inflammatory conditions, e.g. systemic lupus erythematosus and rheumatoid arthritis, the risk of hypersensitivity reactions is increased.

Pregnancy and lactation

Parenteral iron products are contraindicated during the first trimester of pregnancy but may be considered for use from the second trimester onwards where oral iron is ineffective or cannot be tolerated and anaemia is serious enough to pose a risk to the mother or fetus. Any benefits of using IV iron should be carefully weighed against the risks: anaphylactic or anaphylactoid reactions could have serious consequences for both mother and foetus.[2] The choice of drug is dependent on local practice. The dose should be calculated on the pre-pregnancy weight.[3]

The parenteral iron products are considered to be safe for administration during breastfeeding.[4]

REFERENCES

1 eMC (2014). http://www.medicines.org.uk/emc/ (accessed 27 August 2014).

2 MHRA Drug Safety Update (2013). Intravenous iron and serious hypersensitivity reactions: strengthened recommendations; https://www.gov.uk/drug-safety-update/intravenous-iron-and-serious-hypersensitivity-reactions-strengthened-recommendations (accessed 29 August 2015).

3 British Committee for Standards in Haematology (2011). *UK Guidelines on the Management of Iron Deficiency in Pregnancy*. http://www.bcshguidelines.com/documents/UK_Guidelines_iron_deficiency_in_pregnancy.pdf (accessed on 27 August 2014).

4 Midlands Medicines NHS (2014). *UK Drugs in Lactation Advisory Service*. http://www.midlandsmedicines.nhs.uk/apps/ukdilas/resultsBNFcat.asp?SubSectionRef=09.01.01.02 (accessed 27 August 2014).

Kidney stones (renal calculi)

Overview	
Definition	A solid crystal formation as a result of urine saturation with proteins, salts and minerals, such as oxalates, carbonates and phosphates
Epidemiology	5–10% of people are affected by kidney stones, with only 1–2% being symptomatic. Kidney stones are more prevalent in men and first presentation of symptoms is usually between the ages of 20 and 50 years.
	Kidney stones are responsible for more than 12 000 hospital admissions each year in the UK[1]
Risk factors	A combination of intrinsic factors (heredity, age, sex) and extrinsic factors (geography, climate, water intake, diet).
	Poor fluid intake combined with high-protein diet containing high proportion of refined sugars is associated with increased risk of stone formation
Classification	Calcium forming (e.g. calcium oxalate), cystine, strivite, uric acid
Causes	Anatomical abnormalities of the kidney, excess stone-forming substances in the urine, lack of stone inhibitors in the urine, chronic urinary tract infections (UTIs), idiopathic
Symptoms	Only become a medical issue when symptomatic. • Severe lower-back pain (renal colic) – caused when the stones become large enough to cause obstruction or move into the ureter • Increased urine frequency and pain or burning on micturition • Haematuria • Fever, signs of infection
Complications	Urine obstruction, renal failure, urinary sepsis
Differential diagnosis	UTI, pyelonephritis, bladder/kidney tumour
Diagnostic tests	U&Es to measure renal function, calcium levels, FBC (haemoglobin, white cell count), urine dipstick for traces of infection and haematuria, CT scan, intravenous urogram

Treatment	Options depend on symptoms, location and size of stone:[2] • Observation and monitoring • Medical therapy • Analgesia – NSAID first-line treatment if tolerated with paracetamol. Opioids can be used during severe painful episodes • Alpha-blocker – (off licence) relaxes urethra to facilitate stone passage • Antispasmodic – relieves symptoms of renal colic • Thiazide diuretics – reduce urinary calcium excretion and incidence of stone formation • Non-surgical intervention • Extracorporeal shockwave lithotripsy (ESWL): fragments the stone to allow easier passage • Ureteroscopy • Surgical interventions • Laparoscopic stone removal • Percutaneous antegrade ureteroscopy • Insertion of ureteric stent • Nephrostomy • Open surgery
Treatment goal	Reduce symptom frequency and severity, reduce likelihood of stone formation, prevent complications

Pharmaceutical care and counselling

Medicines optimisation	• Treatment • Optimise analgesia during acute flares, include hyoscine butylbromide to help alleviate spasmodic pain • Prevention • Allopurinol to reduce uric acid production (gout and chemotherapy-induced) • Thiazide diuretic • Long-term prophylactic antibiotics (for cystine-forming stones)
Lifestyle advice	Increase fluid intake (avoid dehydration), reduce intake of oxalate-rich foods (beetroot, asparagus, chocolate), do not reduce calcium intake

REFERENCES

1 British Association of Urological Surgeons (2015). *Kidney Stones*. www.baus.org.uk /patients/symptoms/calculi (accessed 10 October 2014).

2 Preminger G *et al.* (2007). Guideline for the management of ureteral calculi. *Eur Urol* 52: 1610–1631.

L

Lactose-free medicines

Some patients are lactose-intolerant due to a lack or reduced activity of the enzyme lactase, which is responsible for the hydrolysis of lactose to glucose and galactose in the small bowel. The undigested lactose in the colon draws in fluid and is fermented by enteric bacteria,[1] leading to unwanted GI symptoms of abdominal bloating, cramping, nausea and diarrhoea.[1,2]

Lactose is an ingredient widely used by the pharmaceutical industry in the formulation of tablets and capsules, as a diluent or filler.[1] It can also be used in lyophilised products, as a carrier in dry-powder inhalers, and can be found in liquid formulations.[1] The amount of lactose used in medicinal products is small in comparison to dairy products and the dose provided is usually less than 2 g/day;[1,2] as a result, GI symptoms may not be experienced by all lactose-intolerant patients.

For any medicinal product the list of ingredients (excipients) can be found in the manufacturer's SPC. The manufacturer may need to be contacted for the quantity of lactose in a product.

The eMC website (www.medicines.org.uk/emc/) can also be used to search for all lactose-free products and to find a lactose-free medicine for a specific condition.[3] This can be done as follows:

1 Click advanced search option and select 'by SPC section'.
2 Select section to search by: either section 4.1 (therapeutic indication) or 6.1 (excipients).
3 Select add.
4 When selecting excipients, change 'contains' to 'does not contain' and type in lactose.
5 Click search.

REFERENCES

1 Pickett K (2013). *What Factors Need to be Considered when Prescribing for Lactose Intolerant Adults?* https://www.evidence.nhs.uk/search?q=%22What+factors +need+to+be+considered+when+prescribing+for+lactose+intolerant +adults%22 (accessed 3 February 2015).

2 UK Medicines Information (2013). What to consider when prescribing for lactose-intolerant adults. *Clin Pharmacist* 5: 273.

3 Wills S (2009). Learning light: reacting to additives in medicine. *Clin Pharmacist* 1: 449–450.

Learning disability: caring for people with learning disability and other vulnerable patients

Accessing health services often presents challenges to people with cognitive difficulties. Learning disabilities and autism spectrum conditions (including Asperger syndrome) are used as examples, but the issues involved can be generalised to assist in understanding and supporting other vulnerable people.

Pharmacists and other healthcare professionals must ensure that their services comply with their legal obligations under the Equality Act 2010[1] and Mental Capacity Act 2005.[2] Briefly, reasonable adjustments must be made to service provision to enable a person with a disability to make use of the service, and to follow the law concerning consent as described in the Mental Capacity Act 2005 when issuing medication to anyone with cognitive disabilities. Non-compliance with either carries a risk of litigation.

Learning disability

Practical difficulties experienced by a person with learning disabilities include understanding new or complex information, learning new skills and coping independently. The disability can be mild, moderate or severe. In the UK approximately 350 000 people have severe disabilities.[3] The most disabled individuals have more than one disability and limited or no communication, i.e. profound and multiple learning disability.

Autism spectrum condition

Autism is a lifelong neurodevelopmental disability, which affects how individuals make sense of the world around them and how they understand and communicate with others. People with autism often experience under- or oversensitivity to sounds, touch, taste, smells, light or colours. Thus, health facilities, particularly hospitals, are exceptionally 'autism-unfriendly' environments and may present overwhelmingly challenging and frightening experiences for patients. This, if not understood and catered for, may adversely affect the care that they receive.

Asperger syndrome is a form of autism where the person, although often being of 'average' or 'above-average' intellectual ability and having few problems with speech, may still have enormous difficulties with understanding and processing language.[4]

Issues relating to the care of patients with a learning disability

These include:

- 'diagnostic overshadowing' – an incorrect assumption that other health problems are associated with the person's learning disability
- difficulties in communication, understanding the unique way in which a person indicates that s/he is in pain, understanding the person's behaviours and routines
- institutional practice, e.g. drug rounds always being at set times, which may not be suitable for the patient's regimen
- inadequate consent and discharge care planning.

People with additional needs may have a reduced ability to understand and use healthcare information in order to make informed decisions and follow treatment instructions. Some may have depressed pain responses and/or poor bodily awareness. Limited communication skills may impair their capacity to convey their symptoms to others. Carers, relatives and support workers may play key roles in identifying their health needs. However, if people with such needs do not communicate verbally, even people who know them well may struggle to recognise their needs or to understand their experience of pain.

It is well documented that people with learning disabilities experience significant health inequalities.[5,6] In 2013 the Confidential Inquiry into Premature Deaths of People with Learning Disabilities (CIPOLD)[7] reviewed the deaths of 247 people with learning disabilities over the 2-year period 2010–2012. Forty-two per cent were considered to be premature deaths, with just under half of these considered to be avoidable using the Office for National Statistics definition. Over a quarter were amenable to better-quality healthcare. Whilst 86% of the illnesses that led to death were promptly recognised and reported to health professionals, 29% experienced a significant difficulty or delay in receiving a diagnosis and 30% had problems with their treatment. The lack of reasonable adjustments to facilitate their healthcare was a contributory factor in a number of deaths. General practitioners commonly did not mention learning disabilities, and hospital 'flagging' systems to identify people who needed reasonable adjustments were limited.

Importantly, both health and social care professionals demonstrated a lack of understanding of, and adherence to, the Mental Capacity Act 2005, particularly regarding assessments of capacity, the processes involved in making 'best-interest' decisions and, crucially, when an Independent Mental Capacity Advocate (IMCA) should be appointed. A lack of recognition of approaching end of life commonly led to problems in coordination of end-of-life care for the person and family.

Issues for pharmacists arising from CIPOLD

Many of the people with learning disabilities who died prematurely were vulnerable in a variety of ways:

- The BMI was different from that of the general population; a significant proportion were underweight.
- People with learning disabilities had multiple medical conditions – the median number of conditions was five. The people who died had seven or more medical conditions. The most frequently reported long-term conditions were epilepsy, cardiovascular disease and hypertension.
- The median number of medications prescribed to each person was seven, although some had up to 21. The most common prescription was for epilepsy (39%), with more than half of these people on at least two types of medicine and 5% of them taking five to seven medicines for this condition alone.
- Although most of the people with learning disabilities had received an Annual Health Check in the previous year, this did not seem to ensure that they had a Health Action Plan. Of those who did, there was little evidence that it was used to link them to appropriate services or to share information about them effectively.
- Although a fifth of people had a type of Hospital Passport, there was no evidence to suggest that this had supported medical staff in coordinating the needs of those with multiple comorbidities.
- In almost all cases there was no evidence of use of a pain assessment tool, although more than a third had difficulty in identifying or verbally communicating experience of pain. There was a significant difference in the prescribing of opioid analgesics according to the severity of learning disability: people with mild learning disabilities (37%), moderate (16%), severe (17%), multiple (21%).

Pain management

The reporting of pain is more sophisticated in some people than others. Over a third of people with learning disabilities had difficulty in identifying or verbally communicating any pain that they had, although many of their parents/carers were able to describe what they believe to be indicators of pain. It is important to be aware that some people, but especially those with autism spectrum conditions, have hypo- or hypersensitivities to pain.

CIPOLD noted that 32% of people who could describe their pain were on opioid analgesics at time of death, compared with 12% who could not. This significant difference suggests that people with more severe learning disabilities may not have been having their pain optimally managed at the end of their lives. In the CIPOLD cohort, despite difficulties in the recognition of the manifestation of distress/pain for almost half the group, only four people (1.6%) had documented use of a pain assessment tool.

Examples of pain assessment tools for adults and children with cognitive impairment and other vulnerabilities:

- Disability Distress Assessment Tool (DisDAT)[8]
- Paediatric Pain Profile.

Health/Hospital Passport

The sensory issues experienced by many people with an autism spectrum condition can present barriers to them receiving optimal treatment. Their impact for some patients must not be underestimated. For example, the texture, taste and colour of some medication may be intolerable; smells and noises in the hospital may be overwhelming; the social 'rules' and styles of communication unique to hospitals may be confusing. Sensory overload can occur for some people and their resultant distress may present challenges.

A Health Passport provides a picture of the whole person. It may include descriptions of what the person likes/dislikes over a range of areas such as physical contact, food preferences, interests and form of communication, enabling staff to help the individual feel safe and comfortable and highlighting issues that may help/hinder treatment.

Increasingly, health services in the UK are creating documentation to be completed with the patient's carer or relative to assist staff in making reasonable adjustments to healthcare as required by law. Having a Health Passport is an aid to this process. Importantly, staff and carers sign and date the document on completion. There are many examples available to download from the internet. The most helpful have involved collaboration with the local Adult Learning Disability service (for paediatric equivalents, the Learning Disability Team from the local Child and Adolescent Mental Health Service). Many health passports utilise a recognisable 'traffic light' format customised to suit local requirements.

For example:

- red: things you must know about me immediately
- amber: things that are really important *for* me
- green: things that are really important *to* me.

Reasonable adjustments

The NHS Operating Framework 2012–13[9] states that 'All NHS organisations must comply with the Equality Act 2010 and its associated Public Sector Equality Duty 2011'. As the focus is on outcomes, alternative methods of service delivery and availability may need to be devised. This could include changing the way things are done, providing extra aids or staff, provision of more accessible/understandable information and altering physical features such as signs, toilets and stairs. Adjustments can be any method that is adapted to the need of the individual to ensure maximum understanding, e.g. use of pictures, social stories, visual timetables, clock faces, Easy Read transcriptions to facilitate understanding about routines and taking medicines.[10]

The most effective way to support people with additional needs is for continued collaboration between acute hospital staff and local learning disability professionals so as to develop appropriate documentation and mutual systems of advice, support and training.

REFERENCES

1   The National Archives 2010. Equality Act. www.legislation.gov.uk (accessed 16 August 2014).

2   The National Archives 2005. Mental Capacity Act. www.legislation.gov.uk (accessed 16 August 2014).

3   NHS Choices (2013). *What is a Learning Disability?* http://www.nhs.uk/livewell/childrenwithalearningdisability/pages/whatislearningdisability.aspx (accessed 16 August 2014).

4   National Autistic Society (2014). *What is Autism?* http://www.autism.org.uk/about-autism/autism-and-asperger-syndrome-an-introduction/what-is-autism.aspx (accessed 16 August 2014).

5   Mencap (2012). *Death by Indifference: 74 deaths and counting.* https://www.mencap.org.uk/news/article/74-deaths-and-counting (accessed 16 August 2014).

6   Department of Health (2012). *Transforming Care: A national response to Winterbourne View Hospital: Department of Health Review: Final report.* www.gov.uk (accessed 16 August 2014).

7   Norah Fry Research Centre, University of Bristol (2013). *The Confidential Inquiry into Premature Deaths of People with Learning Disabilities (CIPOLD).* http://www.bris.ac.uk/cipold/ (accessed 16 August 2014).

8   St Oswald's Hospice (2008). *Disability Distress Assessment Tool (DisDAT).* http://www.stoswaldsuk.org/media/14997/DisDAT-19.pdf (accessed 16 August 2014).

9   Department of Health (2011). *The Operating Framework for the NHS in England 2012–13.* https://www.gov.uk/government/publications/the-operating-framework-for-the-nhs-in-england-2012-13 (accessed 15 May 2015).

10 NHS Choices (2013). *Going into Hospital with a Learning Disability.* http://www.nhs.uk/Livewell/Childrenwithalearningdisability/Pages/Going-into-hospital-with-learning-disability.aspx (accessed 16 August 2014).

LipidRescue

The term LipidRescue refers to the use of a lipid emulsion infusion to treat a drug overdose. Because of the nature of the condition being treated, randomised trials to prove its efficacy are not possible, and the optimal place in treatment cannot be established other than by case reports. Nevertheless, guidelines for its use have been produced by many organisations.[1] It was first promoted as a treatment for local anaesthetic toxicity, but has subsequently found a role in the treatment of overdoses of other, mainly lipophilic, drugs.

Mode of action

The simple mode of action is thought to be through lipid-soluble molecules partitioning into the lipid, so reducing the amount of drug able to act at receptors. While this may be part of the story, it is probably not the only mode of action. Fatty acids are involved in many aspects of cellular function, so increasing the availability would be likely to change how cells behave, which may in turn mitigate against the effects of drugs. Research is continuing into these effects.

Administration

The current consensus is that a 20% lipid emulsion should be administered as a bolus of 1.5 mL/kg, followed by an infusion of 0.5 mL/kg/min for 30 minutes. The bolus may be repeated if asystole persists, and the infusion rate may be increased if the blood pressure falls.[1]

Place in therapy

Wherever large volumes of local anaesthetics are used (e.g. regional blockade), supplies of lipid infusion (with instructions for use) should be available in case of toxicity, and its use should be considered early after identification of a problem.

In cases of severe intoxication with a lipid-soluble drug, there may be a place for LipidRescue, generally on the recommendation of the National Poisons Information Service. There would appear to be little justification in using it for water-soluble drugs.

Follow-up

As noted above, it is extremely difficult to generate evidence of efficacy. It is therefore important that, in all cases where LipidRescue is used, the outcomes are reported to help construct a more solid picture of its efficacy. This can be done through the National Poisons Information Service (http://www.toxbase.org) or the LipidRescue website.[2]

REFERENCES

1 *AAGBI Safety Guideline* (2010). http://www.aagbi.org/sites/default/files/la_toxicity_2010_0.pdf (accessed 19 August 2014).

2 *LipidRescue Resuscitation* (2012). http://www.lipidrescue.org (accessed 19 August 2014).

Lithium: management and monitoring

Lithium salts are used in the treatment and prophylaxis of mania, bipolar disorder and recurrent depression. Lithium should only be initiated by a specialist, and treatment should be carefully monitored.[1] The mechanism of action of lithium as a mood-stabilising agent is unknown. Many theories have been suggested, but none have been proven.

Pharmacokinetic overview

Lithium is completely absorbed from the gut within approximately 8 hours from taking the dose. Peak concentrations will occur 2–4 hours after ingestion and it is excreted by the kidneys.

Lithium is commonly given as slow-release lithium carbonate tablets at night to facilitate drug monitoring so that samples can be taken the next morning. When a lithium level is required for a patient taking a twice-daily dose, the morning dose should be omitted until a sample has been taken.

Brands should not be switched because preparations vary widely in bioavailability; changing the preparation requires the same precautions as initiation of treatment.[2] If a liquid is required, Li-Liquid and Priadel liquid are available as lithium citrate, containing 5.4 mmol/5 mL ($\cong$ lithium carbonate 200 mg/5 mL), and these are given twice daily.

Rationale for monitoring

Lithium has a narrow therapeutic range and is very toxic in overdose. It is therefore important to ensure the serum concentration of lithium is kept within the normal range, and therapeutic drug monitoring is indicated in the following circumstances:

- 7 days after the drug was initiated or the dose changed
- if there is no evidence of a therapeutic response (consider non-adherence)
- toxic symptoms occur (e.g. tremor, ataxia, dysarthria, nystagmus, renal impairment or convulsions)
- suspected drug interaction
- routine monitoring
- consider checking lithium level (at the right time) in any lithium patient admitted to hospital acutely unwell.

Other monitoring

Thyroid function

A small number of patients on long-term lithium therapy will develop either hypothyroidism or hyperthyroidism. Thyroid function should be checked, and the patient should be euthyroid prior to commencing lithium therapy. Once lithium is established, thyroid function tests should be carried out every 6 months (more frequently if results are abnormal – see *Thyroid function* entry).

Renal function

A pretreatment assessment of renal function should be carried out and lithium therapy initiated only if renal function is within normal limits. Lithium may be used cautiously in patients with mild to moderate renal impairment (see *Renal function – assessment* entry).

Once therapy is established, the patient's renal function should be monitored when the lithium serum concentration is checked to ensure that renal function is not deteriorating as this could lead to lithium toxicity.

Cardiac function

Cardiovascular effects of lithium are rare; however, the patient's cardiac function should be checked prior to initiating therapy. In practice, blood pressure should be checked for all patients, and ECG performed in patients with cardiovascular disease or cardiovascular risk factors. Once lithium therapy is initiated, any sign of cardiac disturbance, e.g. arrhythmias, syncope, should be investigated.

TABLE L1

Drug monitoring information

Lithium half-life	10–35 hours[3]
Pretreatment measures	• FBC, U&Es, calcium, eGFR • Thyroid function tests • Weight or BMI • ECG for people with cardiovascular disease or cardiovascular risk factors
Therapeutic range	• 0.4–1 mmol/L (lower end of range for maintenance therapy and elderly patients) • Aim for 0.6–0.8 mmol/L for patients being prescribed lithium for the first time • Consider maintaining plasma level at 0.8–1 mmol/L for 6 months for patients who have relapsed on lithium in the past or have subsyndromal symptoms
Sampling time	• 12 hours post dose (for twice-daily dosing, omit morning dose until sample taken). • Blood should be taken in 'brown-top' sample tubes

Lithium level: routine monitoring	NICE clinical guidelines[4] recommend the following regimen:
	• Every 3 months for the first 12 months
	• Every 6 months after the first 12 months or continue with every 3 months if the patient falls into any of the following categories:
	  • Older age
	  • Is taking any medication that interacts with lithium
	  • Has a risk of impaired renal function or thyroid function, raised calcium levels or any other complications
	  • Has poor symptom control
	  • Has poor adherence
	  • Where the last plasma level >0.8 mmol/L

Other monitoring	• Thyroid function should be monitored every 6 months (see below) or more frequently if results are abnormal. • U&Es, eGFR and calcium should be monitored every 6 months or more frequently if results are abnormal. • Weight or body mass index every 6 months

Dose

Lithium is usually initiated at a low dose and titrated upwards to achieve a serum lithium concentration of 0.4–1 mmol/L. See individual SPCs for starting doses.

Overdose

Seek specialist advice from the National Poisons Information Service (http://www.toxbase.org). There is no antidote to lithium toxicity. The lithium should be stopped and the patient must be hydrated appropriately (dehydration leads to increased lithium serum concentrations). If the lithium has been taken recently, gastric lavage may be carried out. In some instances, it may be necessary to use peritoneal dialysis or haemodialysis to remove the lithium.

Interactions

- Drugs that increase the serum concentration of lithium include ACE inhibitors, ARBs, NSAIDs, diuretics and methyldopa. Particular care should be taken to avoid sodium-depleting diuretics, e.g. thiazides, as sodium depletion can precipitate lithium toxicity.
- SSRI antidepressants increase the risk of central nervous system side effects.
- Lithium increases the risk of extrapyramidal side effects, and possibly neurotoxicity, when it is given with clozapine, haloperidol or phenothiazines.
- Diltiazem, verapamil, carbamazepine and phenytoin can cause neurotoxicity in combination with lithium therapy.
- Metronidazole increases the risk of lithium toxicity.
- Theophylline and sodium chloride increase lithium excretion, which leads to a decrease in the serum concentration of lithium.

Counselling – lithium patient information booklet

All patients should be given a purple lithium patient information booklet which contains a lithium record booklet and a lithium alert card.[1] Patients should be requested to carry the card at all times and should record the brand of lithium they normally take, and the results of their lithium blood levels, renal function, thyroid function and weight in the record booklet.

On commencing lithium patients should be counselled on the information contained in the purple patient information booklet and advised on the following:

- poor adherence or stopping lithium suddenly can increase risk of relapse
- monitoring arrangements
- the need to seek medical attention if any signs of toxicity develop, i.e. diarrhoea, vomiting, severe tremor, muscle weakness
- the need to maintain their fluid intake to avoid dehydration
- potential side effects
- avoid NSAIDs, e.g. ibuprofen.
- check with doctor/pharmacist before buying any over-the-counter medication
- if you stop taking lithium suddenly, your original symptoms may come back. If you and your doctor decide that you are going to stop taking lithium, it will usually be reduced gradually over at least 4 weeks and preferably over 3 months.
- tell your doctor now if you are pregnant or are planning to become pregnant.

REFERENCES

1 NPSA Alert (2009). *Safer Lithium Therapy*. http://www.nrls.npsa.nhs.uk/alerts/
?entryid45=65426 (accessed 15 January 2015).

2 Joint Formulary Committee (2014). *British National Formulary* (68th edn). London:
BMJ Group and Pharmaceutical Press.

3 Dollery C (ed.) (1999). *Therapeutic Drugs* (2nd edn). Edinburgh: Churchill Livingstone.

4 NICE (2014). *Bipolar Disorder: The assessment and management of bipolar disorder in adults, children and young people in primary and secondary care* (CG185).
http://www.nice.org.uk/guidance/CG185 (accessed 15 January 2015).

Liver disease (chronic)

Liver disease is the fifth commonest cause of death in the UK, and the
UK is one of the few developed nations with an upward trend in
mortality from liver disease.[1] The most common forms of chronic
liver disease include: non-alcoholic fatty liver disease, alcoholic liver
disease and chronic hepatitis C. There are a number of classical
signs/symptoms of chronic liver disease and these include ascites,
spontaneous bacterial peritonitis (SBP), variceal bleeding and hepatic
encephalopathy (HE). The primary management of these
complications routinely involves pharmacological interventions.

Ascites

Ascites (an accumulation of fluid in the peritoneal cavity) is the most
common complication of chronic liver disease and 60% of patients
with compensated cirrhosis (i.e. where the liver retains its core
functional capacity) develop ascites.

Ascites occurs when portal hypertension, which results from
increased intrahepatic vascular resistance and portal–splanchnic
blood flow, has developed. The development of ascites is linked to an
inability to excrete an adequate amount of sodium into urine, leading
to a positive sodium balance.[2]

Patients with ascites will often present with distended abdomen,
hyponatraemia, low arterial pressure and an elevated serum
creatinine – all of which needs to be taken into account when new
medications are initiated.

Treatments

The primary treatment of ascites is aimed at counteracting renal
sodium retention and achieving a negative sodium balance. The latter
can be achieved by reducing dietary sodium intake to approximately
80–120 mmol/day and promoting renal sodium excretion by
administration of diuretics.

Fluid restriction may also be advised but is usually restricted to
patients with dilutional hyponatraemia.

Diuretics are commonly prescribed for patients who have not
responded to sodium and fluid restriction. The most commonly

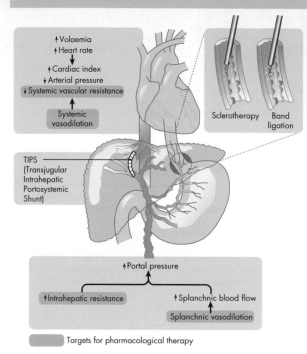

FIGURE L1   Pathophysiology of portal hypertension in cirrhosis[8]

prescribed is the aldosterone antagonist spironolactone and the loop diuretic furosemide.[3]

Frequent monitoring of serum creatinine, sodium and potassium concentrations should be performed while taking diuretics.

For patients with treatment-resistant or recurrent ascites, options include large-volume paracentesis (surgical removal of ascitic fluid), albumin infusion and insertion of transjugular intrahepatic portosystemic shunts (TIPS) (Figure L1). These procedures may be used to support a patient before liver transplantation.[4]

Spontaneous bacterial peritonitis

SBP is an infection of ascitic fluid without a definitive intra-abdominal source and is another common complication in patients with chronic liver disease.[5,6] The exact pathogenesis of SBP is somewhat unclear but it is thought it results from a combination of factors linked to cirrhosis and ascites, such as prolonged bacteraemia secondary to compromised host defences, intrahepatic shunting of colonised blood and defective bactericidal activity within the ascitic fluid.

The diagnosis of SBP is based primarily on a diagnostic paracentesis where a sample of ascitic fluid will be tested for pathogens. In approximately 40% of cases there will be growth of Gram-negative bacteria, usually *Escherichia coli* and Gram-positive cocci (mainly *Streptococcus* species and enterococci).[3] It is possible to have a culture-negative SBP that is identified when the ascitic fluid sample has a neutrophil count >250 cells/mm[3] but there is an absence of positive growth of bacteria.

Presenting signs and symptoms are typical of general sepsis and include fever, confusion and abdominal tenderness.

Treatments

Antibiotic treatment is increasingly recognised as standard practice postdiagnosis of SBP. There is a trend towards using piperacillin with tazobactam and co-amoxiclav as first-line antibiotics even though the evidence is currently unclear – check your local formulary. This probably reflects the underlying fear of *Clostridium difficile* infection associated with the use of quinolones and cephalosporins.

Long-term prophylaxis options still routinely involve the prescribing of quinolones, such as ciprofloxacin or norfloxacin. Co-trimoxazole may also be a suitable alternative if quinolones are not an option. Resistance may become an issue due to the long-term nature of the prophylaxis and therefore rotating antibiotics may be necessary.[7]

Variceal bleeding

Varices occur as a result of splanchic arterial vasodilation, which is common in chronic liver disease. This vasodilation leads to an increased portal blood flow and hence elevated portal hypertension. It is this increase in pressure that results in the formation of venous collaterals/varices. These can form in the oesophagus and the gastrointestinal tract.[8]

Approximately half of patients with cirrhosis have varices, and one-third of all patients with varices will at some point in their disease develop variceal haemorrhage, a major cause of morbidity and mortality in patients with cirrhosis. It is linked with mortality rates of at least 20%.[9]

Treatments

The primary aims of variceal treatments are to:

- decrease portal hypertension (with beta-blockers, surgical portal decompression or TIPS)
- treat the varices directly (with variceal banding or sclerotherapy).

Primary prophylaxis of varices that have not yet bled includes the use of non-selective beta-blockers, such as propranolol or carvedilol.

Secondary prophylaxis for patients who have experienced bleeding includes beta-blockers and endoscopic interventions, such as banding.[10]

In acute variceal bleeding vasoactive drugs, such as terlipressin or octreotide, used alongside broad-spectrum antibiotics and a high-dose proton pump inhibitor infusion (e.g. omeprazole) are recommended to be started as soon as possible.[11,12]

Hepatic encephalopathy

HE is a neuropsychiatric complication of chronic liver disease. Symptoms can range from mild confusion and delirium to coma. HE develops in up to 50% of patients with cirrhosis.[13]

Ammonia is thought to play a key role in the development of HE. Hyperammonaemia leads to the development of brain swelling, suggesting a link between ammonia and inflammation.[14] Other additional causes of HE include hyponatraemia and the presence of medications, such as benzodiazepines and sedatives.

Treatments

The primary management strategy of HE involves the identification of any precipitating factors and initiating a pharmacological approach targeted at reducing levels of ammonia and other gut-derived toxins.[15]

The osmotic laxative lactulose is routinely prescribed in HE. It is not absorbed from the digestive tract and helps to decrease the generation of ammonia by gut bacteria and renders any remaining ammonia to ammonium, which is not absorbable. Doses of 15–30 mL three times daily are usually sufficient, with the aim of achieving three to five soft stool motions per day. If oral administration is not possible then phosphate enemas are used, as they will relieve any constipation precipitating HE and increase bowel transit.

Rifaximin is a non-absorbable antibiotic from the rifamycin class. The rationale for its use is the fact that ammonia and other waste products are generated and converted by intestinal bacteria, and killing these bacteria would reduce the generation of these waste products. The landmark study examining the benefits of rifaximin in HE was published in 2010 and identified that, over a 6-month period, treatment with rifaximin maintained remission from HE more effectively than did placebo. However, it is worth noting that 91% of the study cohort was also on concomitant lactulose![16,17] NICE guidance recommends rifaximin, used within its marketing authorisation, as an option for reducing the recurrence of episodes of overt hepatic encephalopathy in people aged 18 years or older.[18]

L-Ornithine and L-aspartate (LOLA) are a combination of amino acids that play a role in the biochemical pathways that detoxify ammonia; they are unlicensed in the UK but are used in the EU. LOLA may be combined with lactulose and/or rifaximin if these alone are ineffective at controlling symptoms.

Pruritus

Pruritus is a common symptom in patients with chronic liver disease, particularly when cholestasis (impaired secretion of bile) is a prominent feature, such as in conditions like primary biliary cirrhosis. Pruritus associated with chronic liver disease is usually generalised and causes significant quality-of-life disruption for patients. It is often intractable and so can lead to sleep deprivation and suicidal ideation. It also leads to violent scratching, which can result in broken skin and infections.[19] Intractable pruritus from liver disease is an indication for liver transplantation even in the absence of liver failure.[20]

Treatments

The exact pathogenesis of pruritus in liver disease is not fully understood, making it challenging to identify efficacious treatments. The anion exchange resin colestyramine can bind to bile acids in the gastrointestinal tract to increase faecal excretion of bile acids. Colestyramine can interfere with the absorption of other prescribed drugs and so it is important to counsel patients to take the colestyramine an hour before, or 4 hours after, other medications.[21]

There is evidence to suggest that increased opioidergic neurotransmission in the brain appears to contribute to the pruritus. Opioid antagonists, such as naltrexone, have been shown to decrease scratching activity in patients with severe pruritus, with doses reported to show efficacy at 50 mg daily.[22] Caution should be used, however, as dependence can occur and a dose exceeding 50 mg twice daily should rarely be used.

It is also believed, although the evidence is not robust, that there is an interrelationship between the opioid and serotonin neurotransmitter systems. The serotonin antagonist ondansetron has been reported to alleviate pruritus induced by opioids and it may have a role to play in pruritus refractory to other therapeutic interventions.[23]

Pruritus in chronic liver disease has also been linked to a high concentration of serum bile acids. The antibiotic rifampicin is thought to inhibit the uptake of bile acids by hepatocytes and so has been used to treat pruritus.[24] It is important to note that rifampicin is a potent enzyme inducer and interacts with a multitude of medications and a drug–drug interaction screen should be completed before rifampicin is prescribed. This antibiotic is also hepatotoxic and so caution should be observed when prescribing it in cirrhotic patients. Starting dose for pruritus should be 150 mg twice daily, with maximum dose considered to be 300 mg twice daily.

REFERENCES

1   Moore KP, Aithal GP (2006). Guidelines on the management of ascites in cirrhosis. *Gut* 55: 1–12.

2   Fullwood D, Purushothaman A (2013). Managing ascites in patients with chronic liver disease. *Nurs Standard* 28: 51–58.

3　Runyon B (2012). *Management of Adult Patients with Ascites Due to Cirrhosis: Update 2012*. American Association of the Study of Liver Disease (AASLD). http://www.aasld.org/practiceguidelines (accessed 6 August 2014).

4　NICE (2014). *Subcutaneous Implantation of a Battery-powered Catheter Drainage System for Managing Refractory and Recurrent Ascites*. NICE interventional procedures guidance (IPG479). https://www.nice.org.uk/guidance/ipg479 (accessed 14 May 2015)

5　EASL (2010). *Management of Ascites, Spontaneous Bacterial Peritonitis, and Hepatorenal Syndrome in Cirrhosis*, Issue 4. http://www.easl.eu/_clinical-practice-guideline/issue-4-august-2010-management-of-ascites-spontaneous-bacterial-peritonitis-and-hepatorenal-syndrome-in-cirrhosis (accessed 6 August 2014).

6　Alaniz C, Regal R (2009). Spontaneous bacterial peritonitis – a review of treatment options. *Pharm Ther* 34: 201–210.

7　Goel A *et al.* (2014). Diagnosis and management of spontaneous bacterial peritonitis: is there a need for an urgent update of national guidelines? *Gut* 63 (Suppl 1): A215.

8　Dib N *et al.* (2006). Current management of the complications of portal hypertension: variceal bleeding and ascites. *CMAJ* 174: 1433–1443.

9　NICE (2012). *Acute Upper Gastrointestinal Bleeding: Management*. NICE guidelines (CG141) http://www.nice.org.uk/guidance/CG141 (accessed 6 August 2014).

10　Triantos C, Kalafateli M (2014). Primary prevention of bleeding from esophageal varices in patients with liver cirrhosis. *World J Hepatol* 6: 363–369.

11　Seo YS *et al.* (2014). Lack of difference among terlipressin, somatostatin, and octreotide in the control of acute gastroesophageal variceal hemorrhage. *Hepatology* http://www.ncbi.nlm.nih.gov/pubmed/24415445 (accessed 8 August 2014).

12　Kim SY *et al.* (2012). Management of non-variceal upper gastrointestinal bleeding. *Clin Endoscopy* 45: 220–223.

13　Leise M *et al.* (2014). Management of hepatic encephalopathy in the hospital. *Mayo Clin Proc* 89: 241–253.

14　Montagnese S *et al.* (2012). Encephalopathy or hepatic encephalopathy? *J Hepatol* 57: 928–929.

15　Waghray A *et al.* (2014). Optimal treatment of hepatic encephalopathy. *Minerva Dietol Gastroenterol* 60: 55–70.

16　Bass NM *et al.* (2010). Rifaximin treatment in hepatic encephalopathy. *N Engl J Med* 362: 1071–1081.

17　Patel V *et al.* (2014). Rifaximin is efficacious in the treatment of chronic overt hepatic encephalopathy: a UK liver multi-centre experience. *Gut* 63: A14–A15.

18　NICE (2015). Rifaximin for preventing episodes of overt hepatic encephalopathy (TA337). https://www.nice.org.uk/guidance/ta337 (accessed 11 September 2015).

19　Bergasa NV *et al.* (2014). *Frontiers in Neuroscience: Pruritus of Cholestasis*. http://www.ncbi.nlm.nih.gov/books/NBK200923 (accessed 8 August 2014).

20　Mela M *et al.* (2003). Review article: pruritus in cholestatic and other liver diseases. *Aliment Pharmacol Ther* 17: 857–870.

21　Scaldaferri F *et al.* (2013). Use and indications of cholestyramine and bile acid sequestrants. *Intern Emerg Med* 3: 205–210.

22　Jones EA *et al.* (2002). Opiate antagonist therapy for the pruritus of cholestasis: the avoidance of opioid withdrawal-like reactions. *Oxf J Med* 95: 547–552.

23　Jones EA *et al.* (2007). Ondansetron and pruritus in chronic liver disease: a controlled study. *Hepatogastroenterology* 54: 1196–1199.

24　Chen J, Raymond K (2006). Treatment effect of rifampicin on cholestasis. *Ann Clin Microbiol Antimicrob* 5: 3.

Liver function tests

Overview

Background	Liver function tests (LFTs) are a panel of laboratory results that can be helpful in diagnosing and assessing the extent of hepatic dysfunction. Since the liver performs a variety of functions, no single test is sufficient to provide a complete estimate of liver function.
	Effective interpretation of the hepatic function panel requires knowledge of underlying pathophysiology and the characteristics of panel tests. It is important to note that abnormal LFTs do not always indicate liver disease and equally they can be normal in patients with cirrhosis.
	The commonly used LFTs primarily assess liver injury rather than hepatic function. Indeed, these blood tests may reflect problems arising outside the liver, such as haemolysis (elevated bilirubin level) or bone disease (elevated alkaline phosphatase level).
	You should routinely consider the patient's clinical picture combined with abnormal LFT pattern when interpreting the level of dysfunction

L

LFTs – reference ranges[1] (but check your local laboratory reference ranges)	Measure	Range	Local
	Alanine aminotransferase (ALT)	5–35 units/L	
	Alkaline phosphatase (ALP) (will vary according to gender and age)	Adults: 30–150 units/L (adolescents have higher levels, particularly during growth spurts)	
	Aspartate transaminase (AST)	5–35 units/L	
	Bilirubin	3–17 micromol/L	
	Gamma-glutamyltranspeptidase (GGT)	Men: 11–51 units/L Women: 7–33 units/L	
	Albumin	35–50 g/L	
	INR	0.9–1.2	

Child–Pugh system	When assessing the severity/scale of hepatic dysfunction using LFTs then clinicians use a classification system called the Child–Pugh score.[2] This originated in the 1960s and was modified in the early 1970s. It is a useful predictor of outcomes and is also used by pharmaceutical companies in their SPCs to indicate at what level of hepatic impairment their product will require a dose adjustment (see *Child–Pugh Score* entry)

Amino transferases

These include alanine aminotransferase transaminase (ALT) and aspartate transaminase (AST).

Hepatocellular injury is the main trigger for release of these enzymes into the circulation

ALT	• ALT is an enzyme found in high concentrations in the liver and is therefore a sensitive marker for hepatocyte injury
AST	• AST is present in mitochondrial enzymes and is found in the liver, cardiac and skeletal muscle, kidneys, brain, pancreas and lungs. It is less sensitive and specific for the liver than ALT
Further information	• AST and ALT levels tend to be higher in cirrhotic patients with continuing inflammation or necrosis than in those without continuing liver injury. • As markers of hepatocellular injury, AST and ALT lack some specificity because they are found in skeletal muscle. Levels of these aminotransferases can rise to several times normal after severe muscular exertion, other muscle injury, or in the presence of hypothyroidism, which can cause mild muscle injury and the release of aminotransferases.[3] • Other common causes of elevated aminotransferases include: non-alcoholic fatty liver disease, alcohol, chronic hepatitis B and C and autoimmune liver disease
Drugs causing elevation	• Amiodarone, steroids, carbamazepine, phenytoin, isoniazid, antifungals, e.g. voriconazole, posaconazole, fluconazole When completing a drug history it is essential to enquire about prescribed medicines and also herbal or other 'alternative medicines', which have the potential to cause elevations in ALT and AST

Alkaline phosphatase (ALP)

ALP	• ALP originates mainly from two sources: liver and bone. The enzyme may also be found in a variety of other tissues, including the intestine, kidney and placenta. • Elevations can be seen in adolescents undergoing growth spurts and in the third trimester of pregnancy
Further information	• The most common causes of elevated ALP are linked to extrahepatic biliary obstructions (e.g. gallstones) and metastases, primary biliary cirrhosis (PBC), primary sclerosing cholangitis (PSC) (i.e. chronic inflammatory disorder of the small bile ducts). • Cholestasis (lack of bile flow) results from the blockage of bile ducts or from a disease that impairs bile formation in the liver itself. ALP levels typically rise to several times the normal level after several days of bile duct obstruction or intrahepatic cholestasis
Drugs causing elevation	• Anabolic steroids

Gamma-glutamyl transferase (GGT)

GGT	•	GGT is found in hepatocytes and biliary epithelial cells. It is a sensitive test of hepatobiliary disease, but its clinical usefulness is limited as it lacks specificity.[4] Raised levels may be seen in pancreatic disease, diabetes, myocardial infarction, renal failure, chronic obstructive pulmonary disease and alcoholism
Further information	•	The elevation of GGT alone, with no other LFT abnormalities, often results from enzyme induction by alcohol or medicines in the absence of liver disease. GGT level is often elevated in persons who take three or more alcoholic drinks (45 g of ethanol or more) per day; hence GGT is a useful marker for immoderate alcohol intake
Drugs causing GGT level changes	• •	Elevated GGT levels: alcohol, phenytoin, phenobarbital Lowered GGT levels: clofibrate, oral contraceptives

Bilirubin

Bilirubin	•	Bilirubin is formed from the lysis of the haem component of red blood cells. Serum bilirubin is usually classified as conjugated or unconjugated. Unconjugated is transported to liver and is loosely bound to albumin. It is water-insoluble and cannot therefore be excreted in the urine. Conjugated is water-soluble and can be excreted in the urine[4]
Further information	• • •	Serum bilirubin is normally predominantly in the unconjugated form, reflecting a balance between production and excretion. Conjugated bilirubin increases in haemolysis, muscle injury, PBC, PSC, extra- and intrahepatic obstruction. Unconjugated bilirubin increases when there is increased production in bilirubin as a result of haemolysis, blood transfusion or in defects in hepatic uptake or conjugation such as in Gilbert's syndrome. The latter is a common disorder characterised by unconjugated bilirubinaemia, which is exacerbated by fasting[3]
Drugs causing elevation	•	Allopurinol, carbamazepine, co-amoxiclav, diltiazem, total parenteral nutrition

Albumin

Albumin	Albumin production is an essential role of the liver. Albumin synthesis is immediately and severely depressed in inflammatory states, such as burns, trauma and sepsis, and is commonly depressed in patients with active rheumatic disorders or severe end-stage malnutrition. These factors should be taken into account when interpreting levels.
	In practice, patients with low serum albumin concentrations and no other LFT abnormalities are likely to have a non-hepatic cause for low albumin, such as proteinuria or an acute or chronic inflammatory state.
	Albumin has a plasma half-life of 3 weeks, and therefore serum albumin concentrations change slowly in response to alterations in synthesis

L

Prothrombin time (PT)

Prothrombin time	The liver synthesises blood-clotting factors II, V, VII, IX and X. PT measures the rate of conversion of prothrombin to thrombin, thus reflecting a vital function of the liver.
	PT does not become abnormal until more than 80% of liver synthetic capacity is lost. This makes PT a relatively insensitive marker of liver dysfunction; however, abnormal PT prolongation may be a sign of serious liver dysfunction. Because factor VII has a short half-life of only about 6 hours, it is sensitive to rapid changes in liver synthetic function, thus PT is very useful for following liver function in patients with acute liver failure.[3]
	Vitamin K is required for the carboxylation of the clotting factors outlined above and so an elevated PT can result from a vitamin K deficiency or indeed warfarin therapy. This deficiency usually occurs in patients with chronic cholestasis or fat malabsorption from diseases of the pancreas or small intestine. A trial of vitamin K injections (e.g. 5 mg daily administered subcutaneously for 3 days) is the most practical way to exclude vitamin K deficiency in such patients

REFERENCES

1 Longmore M *et al.* (2004). Oxford Handbook of Clinical Medicine (6th edn). Oxford: University Press.
2 Johnston D (1999). Special considerations in interpreting liver function tests. *Am Fam Phys* 59: 2223–2230.
3 Limdi JK, Hyde GM (2003). Evaluation of abnormal liver function tests. *Postgrad Med J* 79: 307–312.
4 Lewis-North P (2008). *Drugs and the Liver*. London: Pharmaceutical Press.

Low-molecular-weight heparin

Low-molecular-weight heparins (LMWH) are indirect factor Xa inhibitors. They activate antithrombin-like unfractionated heparin; the majority of their activity comes from inactivation of factor Xa. The three LMWHs with UK product licences – tinzaparin, enoxaparin and dalteparin – all have slightly different factor IIa (thrombin) to factor Xa activities and different molecular weights due to their method of preparation.[1]

In the preparations available, 25–50% of the molecules inhibit thrombin and factor Xa, with the remaining 50–75% only inhibiting factor Xa. Like any type of heparin, they are of porcine origin. This may not be acceptable to certain religious groups and it is important that patients are made aware of this.

All three agents are licensed for the treatment of venous thromboembolism (VTE) and for prophylaxis of VTE in certain patient groups. Their licences have slight differences and this should be borne in mind when selecting a suitable agent, although it is likely they will all have similar effects. They are less likely to cause heparin-induced thrombocytopenia (HIT) than unfractionated heparin and less osteoporosis. This is due to their shorter chain lengths. However, patients with a past history of HIT should not receive LMWH, and alternative agents such as fondaparinux, danaparoid or argatroban should be used.

All LMWHs are renally excreted to a certain extent, though enoxaparin is more renally excreted than the others. Dose adjustments must be made for patients with creatinine clearance <30 mL/min according to the enoxaparin product licence. Tinzaparin can be used at its normal recommended dose down to a creatinine clearance of 20 mL/min, but below this there is no evidence and a risk of accumulation. The dalteparin SPC does not discuss renal function or whether any dose reductions are required. Some hospitals advocate lower doses of dalteparin for patients with poor renal function. Antifactor Xa monitoring can be done and may be recommended in patients with poor renal function, very obese patients, in pregnancy and in children. A level of 0.5–1.0 units/mL 4 hours after a dose is a suitable treatment dose level; 0.2–0.5 unit/mL 4 hours after a dose is a suitable prophylactic dose level.

All agents can be used in pregnancy as LMWHs do not cross the placenta. These are therefore the most suitable agents for anticoagulated women wishing to become pregnant and for those who develop a VTE during pregnancy. The exception to this is the tinzaparin multidose vial; this contains benzyl alcohol, which should be avoided in pregnancy. The Royal College of Obstetricians and Gynaecologists' guideline on venous thromboembolism states that LMWH can be used safely in breastfeeding women, although this is unlicensed.[2]

REFERENCES

1 Hirsh J (1998). Low-molecular-weight heparin: a review of the results of recent studies of the treatment of venous thromboembolism and unstable angina. *Circulation* 98: 1575–1582.
2 Royal College of Obstetricians and Gynaecologists (2007) *Thrombosis and Embolism during Pregnancy and the Puerperium, the Acute Management of* (Green-top Guideline No. 37b) https://www.rcog.org.uk/en/guidelines-research-services/guidelines/gtg37b/ (accessed 17 November 2014).

Magnesium

Normal range: 0.7–1.0 mmol/L

Local range . . . .

Magnesium is the second most abundant cation in the intracellular fluid. It is an essential electrolyte and is a cofactor in many enzyme systems. Only about 1% of total body magnesium is present in the extracellular space, the majority being in bone (85%), muscle and soft tissue. Hypomagnesaemia in the general population is relatively common, with an estimated prevalence of 2.5–15% (prevalence may be as high as 65% in critical care settings) but this correlates poorly with total-body magnesium depletion.[1] The body is very effective at maintaining extracellular magnesium concentration through control of intestinal absorption and renal excretion and reabsorption, which makes it difficult to establish a daily requirement. However, there is a recommended nutrient intake for adults (Table M1).[2]

TABLE M1
Recommended nutrient intake of magnesium

Adult male	12.3 mmol/day (300 mg)
Adult female	10.9 mmol/day (270 mg)
	Additional 2.1 mmol (50 mg) required if breast-feeding

Magnesium deficiency

Hypomagnesaemia can be classified as follows:[1]

Mild hypomagnesaemia	0.5–0.7 mmol/L
Moderate to severe hypomagnesaemia	<0.5 mmol/L

Patients may be symptomatic or asymptomatic at either of these levels.

Causes of hypomagnesaemia[1]

Causes of hypomagnesaemia include:

- dietary deficiency
- excessive loss via the gastrointestinal tract, e.g. chronic diarrhoea, malabsorption syndromes, bypass surgery, vomiting or nasogastric suction, laxative abuse
- inadequate reabsorption via the kidneys, e.g. inherited renal tubular defects, effects of drugs

- drug causes include laxatives, proton pump inhibitors, diuretics (loop and thiazide), alcohol, antimicrobials (aminoglycosides, amphotericin, foscarnet, pentamidine), chemotherapy (cisplatin), immunosuppressants (ciclosporin, tacrolimus).[3]

Symptoms

Most patients with hypomagnesaemia are asymptomatic: symptoms are not usually seen until serum magnesium is <0.5 mmol/L. Symptomatic magnesium depletion is often associated with other biochemical abnormalities, such as hypokalaemia, hypocalcaemia and metabolic acidosis, so symptoms are not specific to hypomagnesaemia.

Symptoms may include muscle weakness, tremor, muscle fasciculations (small, local contractions), paraesthesiae, tetany and seizures. Atrial or ventricular arrhythmias may be seen and cardiac glycoside toxicity may be exacerbated.[4]

Treatment of magnesium depletion

Treatment route is determined by serum magnesium level and presenting symptoms, as shown in Table M2.

TABLE M2
Mode of treatment of hypomagnesaemia

Serum magnesium	Symptoms	Mode of treatment
0.5–7 mmol/L	Asymptomatic	No acute management is required. May consider oral supplementation with monitoring
0.5–0.7 mmol/L	Symptomatic	Oral magnesium replacement
<0.5 mmol/L	Asymptomatic	Oral magnesium replacement
<0.5 mmol/L	Symptomatic	Intravenous magnesium replacement

Oral magnesium replacement

In asymptomatic patients, oral replenishment may be sufficient; however, the oral route is of limited benefit because high doses will cause diarrhoea leading to further losses, and there may be poor gastrointestinal absorption.

Whilst several studies have looked at the bioavailability of various magnesium preparations, none has looked at clinical outcomes.[5] The usual starting dose in adults is about 24 mmol/day of magnesium[6] given using a preparation the patient finds acceptable. A number of different magnesium salts and products are available, including:

- magnesium aspartate – Magnaspartate (KoRa Healthcare) is classified as a food for special medical purposes and contains 10 mmol magnesium/sachet
- magnesium glycerophosphate – available as an unlicensed product from various suppliers, usually containing 4 mmol magnesium per tablet/capsule or 1 mmol/mL in liquid form
- magnesium hydroxide mixture – Phillips' Milk of Magnesia is licensed as an antacid and a laxative and contains magnesium 1.4 mmol/mL

- co-magaldrox – Maalox and Mucogel are licensed as antacids and contain aluminium hydroxide as well as magnesium hydroxide. Both contain magnesium 6.7 mmol/10 mL and a number of hospitals recommend their use unlicensed in hypomagnesaemia.[7,8]

The main side effect of all these products is diarrhoea, although the aluminium hydroxide component of co-magaldrox is constipating, and therefore diarrhoea may be reduced.

During oral replacement serum magnesium levels should be checked once or twice weekly; reversal of hypomagnesaemia may take 6–8 weeks. In some cases, long-term maintenance therapy may be necessary.

Intravenous magnesium treatment

For severe symptoms or if the oral route is unavailable, magnesium sulfate is given intravenously (by infusion unless symptoms are severe) (Table M3). Intramuscular injection can be very painful.

TABLE M3

Magnesium content of different strengths of magnesium sulfate injection

10% (100 mg/mL)	Approx. 0.4 mmol/mL
20% (200 mg/mL)	Approx. 0.8 mmol/mL
50% (500 mg/mL)	Approx. 2 mmol/mL

Patients with severe symptoms[9]

Note: rapid administration of magnesium sulfate can cause vasodilatation and hypotension.

- Haemodynamically unstable patients (e.g. arrhythmias consistent with torsade de pointes or hypomagnesaemic hypokalaemia) may require 4–8 mmol magnesium (1–2 g magnesium sulfate) over 2–15 minutes initially. Magnesium sulfate 10% and 20% injections may be given undiluted in these circumstances.
- Haemodynamically stable patients with severe symptoms (tetany, seizures) should be given 4–8 mmol magnesium (1–2 g magnesium sulfate) in 100 mL sodium chloride 0.9% or glucose 5% over 5–60 minutes followed by an infusion (see below).

Intravenous magnesium replacement

The magnesium deficit in symptomatic hypomagnesaemia may be 0.5–1 mmol/kg. Up to one-half of the intravenous magnesium dose will be excreted in the urine during replacement, so 1–2 mmol/kg will be required to replenish body stores. Body stores are replaced slowly and the process may take several days. Even if serum magnesium levels return to normal in 24 hours, it is important to recognise that body stores will probably not have been replenished in this time.

- In renal impairment (CrCl <30 mmol/L) the dose should be reduced by 50% to avoid the risk of severe hypermagnesaemia.[9] Magnesium levels should be monitored more frequently; consider giving lower doses or longer intervals between infusions.

- To give as an infusion, add the required dose to 250–1000 mL of sodium chloride 0.9% or glucose 5% (maximum concentration of 0.4 mmol/mL). Infuse at a rate of 4–8 mmol/hour.

Many regimens are in use and include:

- Giving 16–32 mmol magnesium over 12–24 hours, and repeating daily as necessary. Serum magnesium level should be checked at least daily.
- Giving 0.5 mmol/kg by infusion on day 1, then 0.25 mmol/kg by infusion on days 2–5, rounding the doses to conveniently measurable volumes. Serum magnesium level should be checked at least daily.

Hypermagnesaemia

Symptoms

Symptoms include nausea, flushing, headache, lethargy, diminished or absent deep tendon reflexes, hypotension, bradycardia, ECG changes, muscle paralysis, respiratory failure and cardiac arrest.

Causes of hypermagnesaemia

Causes include:

- excessive parenteral administration of magnesium salts
- patients with impaired renal function who have been taking large doses orally, for example as laxatives or antacids.

Treatment

In mild cases, restricting magnesium intake is sufficient to return the serum concentration to normal. In renal impairment administration of isotonic intravenous fluids plus a loop diuretic may be effective. Haemodialysis (using magnesium-free solutions) may be required.

In severe cases consult a poisons information service, e.g. Toxbase at www.toxbase.org (password and registration required) for full details of the management of magnesium toxicity. Ventilatory and circulatory support may be required and calcium gluconate 10% may be used to reverse the effect magnesium on the circulatory and respiratory systems.

REFERENCES

1 Ayuk J et al. (2011). How should hypomagnesaemia be investigated and treated? *Clin Endocrinol* 75: 743–746.

2 *Nutrient Intakes* (2014). www.gov.uk (accessed 13 February 2015).

3 al-Ghamdi SM et al. (1994). Magnesium deficiency: pathophysiologic and clinical overview. *Am J Kidney Dis* 24: 737–752.

4 Longmore M et al. (eds) (2004). *Oxford Handbook of Clinical Medicine* (6th edn). Oxford: Oxford University Press.

5 UKMI Q&A 111.1 (2013). *What Oral Magnesium Preparations are Available in the UK and Which Preparation is Preferred for the Treatment and Prevention of Hypomagnesaemia?* www.evidence.nhs.uk (accessed 17 February 2015).

6 Joint Formulary Committee (2014). *British National Formulary* (68th edn). London: BMJ Group and Pharmaceutical Press.

7 Southern Derbyshire (2012). *Shared Care Pathology Guidelines Hypomagnesaemia in Adults*. https://www.derbyhospitals.nhs.uk (accessed 17 February 2015).

8 NHS Grampian (2012). *Staff Policy for the Management of Hypomagnesaemia in Adults*. http://www.nhsgrampian.com (accessed 17 February 2015).

9 UpToDate (2013). *Evaluation and Treatment of Hypomagnesemia*. www.uptodate .com (accessed 17 February 2015).

Medicines reconciliation

There are more than 13 million hospital admissions in England alone each year. This number is growing and, with the average cost of a non-elective admission estimated to be £1739,[1] the pressure on health economies is great. It has been widely reported historically that 30–70% of patients have either an error or unintentional change to their medicines when their care is transferred.[2] More recent studies corroborate these findings and have demonstrated there are 1.3 unintended discrepancies for each medicines reconciliation completed by a non-pharmacy member of staff,[3] and two-thirds of discharge summary letters are inaccurate or incomplete prior to pharmacy screening.[4]

Medicines reconciliation (taking an accurate drug history and ensuring anomalies are investigated and appropriate action is taken to resolve these) is underpinned by NICE guidance.[2] It is important that information leaving the hospital is of high quality. Consistently ensuring that accurate information regarding medicines is included on the discharge letter starts with taking an accurate drug history on admission. This necessitates having mechanisms in place to ensure that any changes to medicines are easily identifiable, i.e. what has started, stopped, changed, and why, should be documented on charts, notes or the e-record. This makes completion of discharge documentation and also medicines reconciliation in the community postdischarge accurate, safer and easier for all parties.

The Royal Pharmaceutical Society transfer of care guidance[5] provides several examples of good practice that are potentially adoptable or adaptable to different hospital settings.[6] Below is an example of a medicines reconciliation checklist that can be adopted or adapted for local use. It contains core questions to ask the patient to elicit a drug history of consistent quality so nothing important is missed, and is intended as a prompt to underpin a standard operating procedure. Completed checklists can be inserted into the patient notes or form the basis of an e-form for hospitals using an electronic patient record. It should be noted that one of the questions asked at this first pharmacy encounter is 'which community pharmacy do you usually use?'; this information could prove useful for a later referral.

To find out more about checklists and how they can ensure quality is built into processes, read the excellent book by Atul Gawande: *The Checklist Manifesto*.[7]

Medicines reconciliation checklist (hospital admission)

Check each box (or leave blank if not appropriate or not possible to complete)

- ❑ **Insert** this checklist into drug history section of notes
- ❑ **Check** notes for drug history and likely diagnosis
- ❑ **Introduce yourself**: smile, make eye contact, **state** your name **and** role, and **ask**: *'Is it OK to talk about your medicines?'*

Can you communicate with patient? Yes No

- ❑ **Ask**: *'Who looks after your medicines at home?'*
- ❑ **Record** if and which regular community pharmacy
- ❑ **Ask**: *'Do you have any difficulties taking your medicines?'*
- ❑ **Ask**: *'Are they in separate boxes or one big pack?'*
- ❑ **Obtain** consent for GP summary/summary care record **or** GP fax
- ❑ **Document** drug intolerance/allergy, **including reaction** in notes, on chart etc.
- ❑ **Check/document** patient's own drugs (PODs): suitable? + document quantity
- ❑ **Check** medicine administration record (**and** note whether administered) or **contact** care home
- ❑ **Ask** about PODs at home; **document 'H'** on chart if PODs at home
- ❑ **Ask**: *'Any recent medication changes or hospital admission?'*
- ❑ **Ask**: *'Do you get medicines from anywhere other than your GP?'* e.g. home delivery, hospital, chemo (refer), clinical trial, community drug team
- ❑ **Ask** (where appropriate) if using any of the following:
  - ❑ If warfarin, where is yellow book? Refer to anticoagulant service
  - ❑ If diabetes mellitus – refer to diabetes specialist nurses
  - ❑ Other monitoring booklets, e.g. disease-modifying antirheumatic drugs, chemo
  - ❑ Once-weekly medication (state day of week)
  - ❑ Home oxygen
  - ❑ Over-the-counter, herbal, internet, 'recreational'
- ❑ **Check** if smoker: Cigarettes/day? Nicotine replacement therapy? Smoking cessation referral?
- ❑ **Complete** drug history on chart and notes (sign and date)

Take appropriate action to rectify discrepancies

REFERENCES

1 Kings Fund (2012). Data briefing. *Emergency Hospital Admissions for Ambulatory Care-sensitive Conditions: Identifying the potential for reductions* http://www.kingsfund.org.uk/sites/files/kf/field/field_publication_file/data-briefing-emergency-hospital-admissions-for-ambulatory-care-sensitive-conditions-apr-2012.pdf (accessed 30 August 2014).

2 NICE (2015). Medicines optimisation: the safe and effective use of medicines to enable the best possible outcomes. www.nice.org.uk/guidance/NG5 (accessed 20 August 2015).

3 Dodds LJ (2014). Optimising pharmacy input to medicines reconciliation at admission to hospital: lessons from a collaborative service evaluation of pharmacy-led medicines reconciliation services in 30 acute hospitals in England. *Eur J Hosp Pharm* 21: 95–101.

4 Dodds LJ (2013). Pharmacist contributions to ensuring safe and accurate transfer of written medicines-related discharge information: lessons from a collaborative audit and service evaluation involving 45 hospitals in England. *Eur J Hosp Pharm* doi:10.1136/ejhpharm-2013-000418.

5 Royal Pharmaceutical Society (2012). *Keeping Patients Safe when they Transfer Between Care Providers: Getting the medicines right.* http://www.rpharms.com/getting-the-medicines-right/keeping-patients-safe-report.asp (accessed 30 August 2014).

6 Gray A *et al.* (2013). Innovations in transfer of care. *Hosp Pharm Eur* 2013: 74.

7 Gawande A (2011). *The Checklist Manifesto: How to get things right.* London: Profile Books.

M

Methotrexate: calcium folinate rescue regimen

Calcium folinate (folinic acid, calcium leucovorin, tetrahydrofolate) can be used in the management of methotrexate overdose and to reduce the toxicity of high-dose methotrexate chemotherapy. Calcium folinate is a reduced form of folic acid, which bypasses the inhibition of dihydrofolate reductase by methotrexate. Calcium folinate also has a role in combination with fluorouracil in the treatment of bowel cancer, where its use enhances the effect of fluorouracil by inhibition of thymidilate synthase.[1]

Methotrexate serum concentration should be checked every 24 hours from 20 to 24 hours after administration in overdose, or from 24 hours after completion of therapeutic dosing.[2]

Calcium folinate should continue until the serum methotrexate concentration falls to below 0.1 micromol/L.[3] Administration of calcium folinate can be via the oral or intravenous route. This is given orally as calcium folinate 15 mg tablets every 3–6 hours depending on the methotrexate level and chemotherapy protocol. Intravenous administration is via an intravenous bolus given over 3–5 minutes or alternatively as a short infusion in sodium chloride 0.9% or glucose 5%.

There are a number of dosing schedules of calcium folinate rescue used for specific methotrexate regimens, with Table M4 being one example.[4]

It is sometimes necessary to convert methotrexate into different units and Table M5 shows equivalent values in moles, micrograms/L and micromol/L.

Urine must be alkalinised (pH > 7), usually with bicarbonate orally or intravenously. If using the intravenous route a commonly used

TABLE M4
Example of a folinate rescue remedy

Time after starting methotrexate	Methotrexate plasma concentration (micromol/L)				
	<0.1	0.1–<2	2–<20	20–100	>100
48 hours	None	15 mg/m² every 6 hours	15 mg/m² every 6 hours	10 mg/m² every 3 hours	100 mg/m² every 3 hours
72 hours	None	15 mg/m² every 6 hours	15 mg/m² every 3 hours	100 mg/m² every 3 hours	1000 mg/m² every 3 hours
96 hours	None	15 mg/m² every 6 hours	15 mg/m² every 3 hours	100 mg/m² every 3 hours	1000 mg/m² every 3 hours
120 hours	None	15 mg/m² every 6 hours	15 mg/m² every 3 hours	100 mg/m² every 3 hours	1000 mg/m² every 3 hours

TABLE M5
Conversion of serum methotrexate units

Molar (M)	micrograms/mL	micromol/L
1×10^{-3}	460	1013 (or 1.013×10^3)
1×10^{-4}	46	101 (or 1.01×10^2)
1×10^{-5}	4.6	10.1 (or 1.01×10^1)
1×10^{-6}	0.46	1.01
1×10^{-7}	0.046	0.1 (or 1×10^{-1})
1×10^{-8}	0.0046	0.01 (or 1×10^{-2})

To convert micrograms/mL to micromol/L, divide by 0.454.

M

schedule is 50 mmol bicarbonate in 1000 mL sodium chloride 0.9% given at a rate of 125 mL/m²/hour initially (this can be doubled to 100 mmol bicarbonate if urine pH is not maintained above 7). Oral dosing using tablets should be adjusted in response to urine pH to account for interpatient difference in absorption rates. Two 600-mg tablets every 4–6 hours would be a reasonable starting dose. The urine output should be maintained above 100 mL/m²/hour (average) until methotrexate level falls below 0.1 micromol/L.

Methotrexate and other medicines

Drugs that impair renal function should be avoided, e.g. aminoglycosides, non-steroidal anti-inflammatory drugs, salicylates, sulphonamides and high doses of penicillins.

Co-trimoxazole (and trimethoprim) should not be given concomitantly with methotrexate as both the sulfamethoxazole and trimethoprim components increase toxicity: sulfamethoxazole by displacement from protein-binding sites and trimethoprim by additive inhibition of dihydrofolate reductase. Pentamadine or dapsone may be a suitable alternative for prophylaxis of *Pneumocystis jiroveci* pneumonia in such patients.[5]

REFERENCES

1 Bleyer WA (1977). Methotrexate: clinical pharmacology, current status and thera-peutic guidelines. *Cancer Treat Rev* 4: 87–101.

2 SPC (2014). *Methotrexate Tablets, Injection.* www.medicines.org.uk (accessed 29 September 2014).

3 SPC (2014). *Calcium Folinate Tablets. Injection.* www.medicines.org.uk (accessed 29 September 2014).

4 Medical Research Council Working Party on Leukaemia in Adults (2006). *UKALL XIV Trial Protocol.* https://www.ctsu.ox.ac.uk/research/mega-trials/leukaemia-trials/adult-all/ukall-xii-ph-positive-patients/protocol-v5 (accessed 29 September 2014).

5 Dollery C (ed.) (1999). *Therapeutic Drugs* (2nd edn), vol. 2. Edinburgh: Churchill Livingstone, pp. M90–M96.

Monofer

M

Overview (see also *Iron: guidance on parenteral dosing and administration* entry)[1]			
Form	Iron (III) isomaltoside		
Dose	Total dose required (mg iron) $= $ [bodyweight (kg) $\times$ (target Hb $-$ actual Hb (g/L)) $\times$ 0.24] $+$ X $X = 500$ mg and is the milligrams of iron required to replace the body's iron stores (or depot iron) and is only applicable for patients >35 kg		
Administration routes	Intravenous infusion	Intravenous instalments	Intramuscular
	Yes	Yes	No
Administration	• Can be administered as a single infusion for cumulative doses up to 20 mg/kg/body weight or • As weekly infusions until the cumulative dose has been administered • Doses exceeding 20 mg/kg body weight should be split into two administrations with an interval of at least a week • Dilute in maximum volume of 500 mL sodium chloride 0.9% • Administer over 30 minutes for doses up to 1000 mg iron • Administer over 60 minutes for doses exceeding 1000 mg • Observe for adverse effects for at least 30 minutes following each injection	• Doses up to 500 mg iron may be given by intravenous bolus injection up to three times a week • Can be given as undiluted injection or diluted in a maximum 20 mL of sodium chloride 0.9% • The injection should be administered at a rate of up to 50 mg iron/minute • Observe for adverse effects for at least 30 minutes following each injection	

Specific contraindications	• Decompensated liver cirrhosis and hepatitis
Monitoring	• Patients should be monitored for signs and symptoms of hypersensitivity reactions during and following each administration[2]
	• Observe patient for adverse effects for at least 30 minutes following each injection
	• If hypersensitivity reactions or signs of intolerance occur during administration, the treatment must be stopped immediately

REFERENCE

1 eMC (2014). *Summary of Product Characteristics Monofer*. https://www.medicines. org.uk/emc/medicine/23669 (accessed 27 August 2014).

2 MHRA Drug Safety Update (2013). Intravenous iron and serious hypersensitivity reactions: strengthened recommendations. http://www.gov.uk/drug-safety- update/intravenous-iron-and-serious-hypersensitivity-reactions-strengthened- recommendations (accessed 29 August 2015).

M

Mouth ulcers and sore mouth

Mouth ulcers are sores that form in the oral cavity, commonly seen on the inside of the cheeks or lips. They typically present as painful, round (or oval) inflamed sores with circumscribed margins and erythematous haloes.[1] They are usually white, red, yellow or grey in colour[2] and are usually self-limiting, healing within 2 weeks. Those that are very painful, have lasted more than 3 weeks or are recurrent should be referred to a general practitioner.

Causes

Common causes include mechanical trauma (e.g. tongue or cheek biting) and thermal injury (i.e. contact with hot foods or liquid). Certain triggers such as stress, hormonal changes and smoking cessation as well as some foods, medications (e.g. aspirin and nicorandil) and underlying conditions (e.g. viral infections and vitamin B_{12} deficiency) can all increase the risk of mouth ulcers.[2]

Other common conditions that may also cause a sore mouth include gum disease such as gingivitis, fungal infections such as oral candidiasis, herpetic disease such as cold sores and oral mucositis occurring post-chemotherapy.

Treatment options

Self-management includes treating the cause, using a softer toothbrush, avoiding spicy or acidic foods and avoiding known triggers.

Medications should aim to protect the ulcerated area, reduce pain and inflammation and control secondary infection.[3] Options include:

- saline mouth wash – half a teaspoonful of salt in a glass of warm water used frequently and vigorously
- chlorhexidine gluconate 0.2% – use mouth wash 10 mL twice daily or apply gel to affected areas once or twice daily

- topical corticosteroids, e.g. hydrocortisone oromucosal tablets allowed to dissolve next to the ulcer; beclometasone dipropionate inhaler 50–100 micrograms sprayed twice daily on oral mucosa (unlicensed indication); betamethasone soluble tablets 500 micrograms dissolved in water and used as a mouth wash but not swallowed (unlicensed indication)
- local anaesthetics, e.g. lidocaine ointment 5% rubbed sparingly on the affected areas or lidocaine spray 10% (unlicensed indication). Proprietary products exist that are additionally mucoadhesive and form a physical barrier protecting the lesion as it heals[4]
- local anti-inflammatories, e.g. benzydamine mouth wash or spray
- low-dose doxycycline (20 mg twice daily) is also used for recurrent aphthous ulceration (unlicensed indication).

REFERENCES

1 Patient.co.uk (2013). *Oral Ulceration*. http://www.patient.co.uk/doctor/oral -ulceration (accessed 17 January 2015).
2 NHS Choices (2014). *Mouth Ulcers*. http://www.nhs.uk/conditions/Mouth -ulcer/Pages/Introduction.aspx (accessed 17 January 2015).
3 BNF Online (2015). https://www.medicinescomplete.com/mc/bnf/current/ PHP7340-drugs-for-oral-ulceration-and-inflammation.htm?q=mouth%20ulcers&t= search&ss=text&p=1#_hit (accessed 17 January 2015).
4 SPC (2010). *Iglü Gel*. http://www.medicines.org.uk/emc/medicine/20777 (accessed 10 February 2015).

Multiple sclerosis: symptomatic management

Multiple sclerosis (MS) is characterised by recurrent or chronically progressive neurological dysfunction. It is caused by perivenular inflammatory foci in the white matter of the central nervous system. Repeated episodes of inflammation result in characteristic widespread, demyelinated and sclerotic lesions (referred to as plaques) throughout the brain, optic nerves and spinal cord of affected individuals. An immune-mediated component is central to disease pathogenesis.[1,2]

The prevalence is about 100 cases per 100 000 people. The ratio of women to men with MS is approximately 2:1. The disease shows a geographic gradient of prevalence, with more cases found at the northern latitudes of Europe and North America and at the southern latitudes of New Zealand and Australia.[1]

To date there is no cure for MS. Disease-modifying therapies aim to reduce the number of relapses, although it is not clear if they have an effect on overall disease progression and disability. People with MS typically develop symptoms in their late 20s, experiencing visual and sensory disturbances, limb weakness, gait problems, bladder and bowel symptoms. They may initially have partial recovery, but over time develop progressive disability.[2] Symptomatic relief therefore forms a huge part of MS treatment, and is targeted around the most troublesome symptoms for individual patients.

Fatigue

Fatigue is one of the most common symptoms of MS and can be incredibly debilitating for patients. It is described as an overwhelming sense of tiredness with no obvious cause. Non-pharmacological treatments can be effective and include amending lifestyle to optimise, e.g. nutrition, relaxation techniques, sleep hygiene, physical activity and treating depression.[1,3]

Pharmacological treatments include amantadine, a low-affinity antagonist at the N-methyl-D-aspartate (NMDA) subtype of glutamate receptors.[2,4] It is not licensed in the management of MS; however, its use is recommended where pharmacological management of fatigue is necessary.

Spasticity

The degree of spasticity can vary from person to person, day to day and hour to hour. Posture is crucial in managing spasticity and pain; correct positioning combined with daily stretching and targeted exercises can provide effective relief. When managing spasticity it is also important to assess and offer treatment for factors that may aggravate spasticity, such as constipation, infections or pressure ulcers.[1–3]

The goal of treatment is to relieve the spasticity sufficiently to ensure comfort and prevent complications, without taking away rigidity needed to function. Baclofen or gabapentin are recommended for use first-line in the management of MS spasticity. Baclofen is a muscle relaxant, which works by simulating the gamma-aminobutyric acid-B ($GABA_B$) receptors; this stimulation in turn inhibits the release of the excitatory amino acids glutamate and aspartate. Common side effects include drowsiness, muscle weakness and hypotension that can limit tolerated doses.[5] Gabapentin also exhibits its activity via GABA receptors and is structurally related to the neurotransmitter GABA. Common side effects include drowsiness, dizziness and fatigue.[6] Doses should be optimised as tolerated. If dose escalation of one agent is not tolerated a combination of baclofen and gabapentin can be used.

Alternative agents include tizanidine and dantrolene (which requires careful monitoring of liver function). Benzodiazepines, e.g. clonazepam, are considered as a third-line option, but are limited by the risk of dependence and sedative effects. They can be useful in the management of nocturnal spasms.[2]

If oral preparations are unhelpful, where spasticity is disabling cannabinoid nasal spray or intrathecal baclofen could be considered. Botulinum type A is a potential treatment, but limited by quantity and frequency of administration required.

Bladder dysfunction

The most characteristic bladder complaint is of urgency and frequency, sometimes with incontinence, but also with hesitancy and poor stream. The NICE guidance on management of lower urinary tract dysfunction in neurological disease is a useful reference.[7] Non-pharmacological management, e.g. reducing caffeine intake and bladder retraining can be helpful.[3] Pharmacological management is often with antimuscarinic drugs for urge incontinence, including oxybutynin, propantheline or tolterodine. Use is often limited by antimuscarinic side effects, e.g. dry mouth. Desmopressin may be useful in nocturnal frequency and incontinence. Bladder dysfunction can lead to an increased risk of recurrent urinary tract infections, which should also be managed.[1]

Other MS symptoms and potential treatments are shown in Table M6.

TABLE M6

Overview of other multiple sclerosis symptoms and potential treatments

Symptom	Treatment options
Bowel dysfunction – constipation (most common) and faecal incontinence (relatively uncommon)	Pharmacological: laxatives, loperamide Non-pharmacological: increase dietary fibre, exercise and fluid intake
Sexual dysfunction – can be related to sensation but also erectile dysfunction	Pharmacological for erectile dysfunction: phosphodiesterase type 5 inhibitors, e.g. sildenafil
Ataxia and tremor	Pharmacological: propranolol, carbamazepine Non-pharmacological: thalamotomy, thalamic pacing, functional electrical stimulation (FES)
Cognitive decline	Pharmacological: disease-modifying drugs may help slow decline Non-pharmacological: psychological support, memory aids
Pain – neuropathic, e.g. trigeminal neuralgia and also musculoskeletal	Pharmacological: simple analgesia, neuropathic pain agents Non-pharmacological: mobility and posture
Depression and anxiety – lifetime prevalence of major depressive disorder in patients with MS is 50%[8]	Management as for depression in any other patient

The likelihood of a patient requiring therapy for more than one symptom is high. Therefore, it is important when managing symptoms of MS to consider the whole patient, rather than each problem individually. This helps to prevent polypharmacy and allows utilisation of one drug for management of multiple symptoms, e.g. gabapentin for spasticity and pain.

REFERENCES

1 Perkin GD, Wolinsky JS (2005). *Fast Facts: Multiple Sclerosis* (2nd edn). Oxford: Health Press.

2 NICE (2014). *Multiple Sclerosis: Management of multiple sclerosis in primary and secondary care* (CG 186). https://www.nice.org.uk/guidance/cg186 (accessed 28 January 2015).

3 Rashid W *et al.* (2013). *Guidelines: Symptomatic management of multiple sclerosis in primary care*. http://community.mssociety.org.uk/sites/default/files/resources/resource_files/Symptomatic%20management%20of%20MS%20in%20primary%20care%20-%20MGP%20guideline.pdf (accessed 28 January 2015).

4 SPC (2014). *Symmetrel Capsules*. www.medicines.org.uk (accessed 28 January 2015).

5 SPC (2013). *Lioresal Tablets 10 mg*. www.medicines.org.uk (accessed 28 January 2015).

6 SPC (2015). *Neurontin 100 mg. Hard Capsules*. www.medicines.org.uk (accessed 28 January 2015).

7 NICE (2012). *Urinary Incontinence in Neurological Disease: Management of lower urinary tract dysfunction in neurological disease* (CG 148). https://www.nice.org.uk/guidance/cg148 (accessed 28 January 2015).

8 Feinstein A (2011). Multiple sclerosis and depression. *Mult Scler* 17: 1276–1281.

M

N

Nausea and vomiting

Antiemetics are used to treat nausea and vomiting from many causes, e.g. in palliative care following chemotherapy (see *Chemotherapy-induced nausea and vomiting (CINV)* entry) and postoperatively (see *Postoperative nausea and vomiting (PONV)* entry).

To choose an antiemetic the following factors should be considered:

- mechanism of action
- ensuring no antagonism will occur if more than one antiemetic is chosen
- whether an antisecretory effect is sought
- side effects
- cost.

If more than one antiemetic is required, select ones with different mechanisms of actions (Table N1).

TABLE N1
Receptor site affinities of antiemetics[1]

Drug	Class	D_2	H_1	Muscarinic	$5HT_2$	$5HT_3$	$5HT_4$	NK1
Chlorpromazine		++	++	+				
Cyclizine	Histamine and acetylcholine antagonism		++	++				
Domperidone	Dopamine antagonist	++						
Haloperidol	Dopamine antagonist	+++						
Hyoscine hydrobromide				+++				
Levomepromazine	$5HT_2$, dopamine, acetylcholine and histamine antagonism	++	+++	++	+++			
Metoclopramide	Dopamine antagonism, $5HT_4$ agonism	++				+	++	
Ondansetron	$5HT_3$ antagonism					+++		
Prochlorperazine		++	+					
Aprepitant/fosaprepitant	Neurokinin 1 (NK1) antagonism							++

Pharmacological activity: + = slight; ++ = moderate; +++ = marked
Reproduced with the permission of the copyright holder.

REFERENCE
1 Twycross R *et al.* (2014). *Palliative Care Formulary* (5th edn). Oxford: Radcliffe Medical Press.

Neuroleptic malignant syndrome

Neuroleptic malignant syndrome (NMS) is a rare but potentially fatal idiosyncratic adverse drug reaction associated predominantly with the use of antidopaminergic agents, but also the withdrawal of dopaminergic agents. Other medicines have been implicated.[1] The syndrome can occur hours to months after the drug was initiated and can vary from a few signs and symptoms to an acute severe attack. Once the syndrome occurs the symptoms develop quickly over 24–72 hours. Symptoms last up to 14 days following discontinuation of oral drug therapy and up to three times as long after discontinuation of a long-acting medicine.[2]

Signs and symptoms

Signs and symptoms include:

- hyperthermia
- muscle rigidity (may include dysphagia and dyspnoea)
- altered consciousness
- autonomic instability, e.g. fluctuating blood pressure (BP), tachycardia, diaphoresis
- raised creatine kinase (CK)
- leukocytosis
- altered liver function.

Risk factors

Risk factors include:

- previous NMS
- organic brain disease
- Parkinson's disease
- high-potency typical antipsychotics, e.g. haloperidol
- high doses of antipsychotic drugs
- recent or rapid increase in dose
- dehydration/elevated ambient temperature
- agitation or catatonia
- abrupt withdrawal of antimuscarinics.

Management

Action and treatment will depend upon the severity of the syndrome, and include the following:

- Immediately withdraw antipsychotic medicines or reinitiate dopamine agonist.

- Correct dehydration and hyperthermia. Consider:
  - intravenous dantrolene
  - bromocriptine
  - benzodiazepines
  - cooling techniques and antipyretics.
- Monitor: temperature, pulse, BP, white cell count, CK (although this is controversial) and liver function tests.
- Benzodiazepines may be used to sedate patients if necessary (note that restraint and intramuscular injections can elevate CK).
- Electroconvulsive therapy (ECT) may be considered for treating psychosis.

Cautious reintroduction of antipsychotics may be considered 2 weeks after the resolution of NMS. Consider a structurally dissimilar drug, or one with a low affinity for dopamine, e.g. quetiapine or clozapine.[3] Depot injections are contraindicated. Start with a low dose and increase very slowly. Monitor temperature, pulse and BP.

REFERENCES

1 Bazire S (2012). *Psychotropic Drug Directory 2012.* Dorsington: Lloyd-Reinhold Communications.

2 Cowen C *et al.* (2012). *Shorter Oxford Textbook of Psychiatry* (6th edn). Oxford: Oxford University Press.

3 Taylor D *et al.* (eds) (2012). *The Maudsley Prescribing Guidelines in Psychiatry* (11th edn). Chichester: Wiley-Blackwell.

Neutropenic sepsis

Overview	
Definition	Systemic anticancer therapy can suppress the ability of the bone marrow to respond adequately to infection, potentially leading to neutropenic sepsis.
	Neutropenic sepsis is a medical emergency that requires prompt diagnosis and urgent treatment. Mortality rates of between 2% and 21% have been reported for this potentially fatal complication of chemotherapy treatment.[1] Delays often occur in recognising neutropenic sepsis and treating with antibiotics because of a lack of awareness or because patients may present feeling well
Diagnosis	A diagnosis of neutropenic sepsis should be considered in febrile (>38°C) patients who have recently received treatment with chemotherapy or radiotherapy and are unwell or have confirmed neutropenia.
	It is important to note that patients may also be afebrile in certain situations (e.g. if they have self-medicated with paracetamol)
Susceptibility	Increased susceptibility to infection is likely when the neutrophil count falls below 1×10^9/L, with increasing risk when the neutrophil count falls below 0.5×10^9/L. Duration of neutropenia is also important, with risk of infection increased especially if neutropenia lasts for more than 10 days[2]

Initial investigations	• FBC • CRP • U&Es • LFTs • Blood gases (including lactate) • Blood cultures (peripheral and also through intravenous catheter lumens if line is *in situ*) – these should be repeated if fever persists despite antibiotics

Pharmaceutical care and counselling

Assess	• Empirical antibiotic therapy should be given to all patients with suspected neutropenic sepsis.[2] • These should be administered as soon as possible after presentation and ideally within 60 minutes. • A typical regimen for a patient with no allergies may be beta-lactam monotherapy such as piperacillin with tazobactam 4.5 g four times a day given intravenously. Refer to local policy if penicillin-allergic
Essential intervention	• Multinational Association for Supportive Care in Cancer (MASCC) risk-scoring tool should be used to identify patients at low risk of complications from neutropenic sepsis. Patients should be assessed by a healthcare professional experienced in the management of oncological emergencies and patients deemed to be low risk may be suitable for early discharge with oral antibiotics. Patients who are not at low risk should receive intravenous antibiotics[3]
Essential intervention	• If patients remain febrile after 24–48 hours of antibiotics, consideration should be given to the possibility of invasive fungal infection and appropriate treatment and investigations commenced – discussion with microbiology is always advised
Patient information	• All patients receiving chemotherapy should be given information relating to their cancer treatment and potential side effects, including what to do and whom to contact if these occur. • Patients receiving chemotherapy should be advised to monitor their temperature regularly and to contact their cancer centre or accident and emergency if their temperature rises above 37.5°C. They should also avoid crowded places and contact with people who are known to have current infection
Neutropenic prophylaxis	• NICE recommends that prophylaxis with fluoroquinolones (e.g. ciprofloxacin 500 mg twice daily) should be offered to adult patients with acute leukaemias, stem cell transplants or solid tumours in whom significant neutropenia (neutrophil count 0.5×10^9/L or less) is an anticipated consequence of chemotherapy.[2] • Patients receiving chemotherapy for haematological malignancy may also require prophylaxis with antiviral and antifungal agents

REFERENCES

1 National Chemotherapy Advisory Group (2009). *Chemotherapy Services in England: Ensuring quality and safety*. http://webarchive.nationalarchives.gov.uk/+/www.dh.gov.uk/en/Consultations/Liveconsultations/DH_090150 (accessed 12 May 2015).

2 NICE (2012). *Neutropenic Sepsis: Prevention and management of neutropenic sepsis in cancer patients*. NICE Clinical Guideline CG151 http://www.nice.org.uk/guidance/cg151 (accessed 7 January 2015).

3 Klastersky J *et al.* (2000). The Multinational Association for Supportive Care in Cancer Risk Index: a multinational scoring system for identifying low-risk febrile neutropenic cancer patients. *J Clin Oncol* 18: 3038–3051.

Nicotine replacement therapy

All smokers should be advised to stop, unless there are exceptional circumstances. Health professionals should use patient interaction opportunities to provide brief interventions offering advice and help with follow-up or provide referrals to specialist smoking cessation services.[1,2]

Nicotine replacement therapy (NRT) is the most common form of support therapy used. There are a wide range of products available, which aim to reduce withdrawal symptoms associated with stopping smoking by replacing the nicotine from cigarettes. The use of NRT increases the chance of a person succeeding in smoking cessation.[3]

Options available

Patches that release nicotine transdermally over 16 or 24 hours provide a controlled prolonged method of preventing cravings from cigarettes. A 24-hour patch is beneficial in patients who experience strong nicotine cravings on waking, although higher-dose preparations may result in patients experiencing nightmares.[1]

Gums, lozenges, sublingual tablets, inhalators, nasal sprays and oral sprays are immediate-release nicotine preparations and are used to treat urges to smoke or prevent cravings.[1] Effectiveness of smoking cessation is more dependent on patient preference and tolerance of NRT than any differences between the products themselves.[3]

Combinations of a prolonged-release formulation and an immediate-release preparation have proved to be most successful, along with intensive behavioural support from a specialist smoking cessation service.[4]

Electronic cigarettes

The Royal Pharmaceutical Society supports the use of licensed products as an NRT option, but until the MHRA enforces this market (expected in 2016[5]) unlicensed products should not be recommended due to concerns of safety and efficacy.[6]

Pharmacokinetics

Nicotine is absorbed well through the skin and mucous membranes. Orally nicotine has very low bioavailability due to extensive first-pass metabolism.

Nicotine is well distributed, crossing the blood–brain barrier and placenta, and is found in breast milk. It is metabolised mainly in the liver via CYP450 isoenzyme CYP2A6. Nicotine and its metabolites are excreted in the urine.[7]

Cautions and side effects

Most risks associated with NRT also apply to cigarette smoking, but starting NRT when patients have acute cardiac changes should be done under specialist advice. Overall the benefits of smoking cessation with the use of NRT outweigh the risk of continuing smoking and should always be encouraged. Consideration should be given to the potential systemic and local effects of nicotine that vary in each preparation.[1]

Systemic side effects can occur with high-strength preparations; however, patients often confuse nicotine withdrawal symptoms with side effects from NRT. Common side effects of nicotine withdrawal include malaise, headache, dizziness, sleep disturbance, coughing, influenza-like symptoms, depression, irritability, increased appetite, weight gain, restlessness, anxiety, drowsiness and impaired concentration.[1]

Local side effects are common when NRT is commenced due to nicotine's irritant effect. Examples include skin irritation from patches, irritated throat from sprays and increased salivation from gum and lozenges. Gastrointestinal disturbances are also common due to the amount of swallowed nicotine.[1]

Other information

Nicotine is a highly addictive drug in every form. Patients should be encouraged to reduce their dosage of NRT over several months to prevent transferring dependence from one form of nicotine delivery to another.[5]

Tobacco smoking induces the metabolism of many different medicines.[1] When commencing NRT or advising patients to stop smoking, consider the need to alter doses of their medication to prevent toxicity. See entry on *Cigarette smoking – drug interactions,* for more detail.

REFERENCES

1 Joint Formulary Committee (2014). *British National Formulary* (68th edn). London: BMJ Group and Pharmaceutical Press.
2 National Institute for Health and Clinical Excellence (2006). N1014. *Brief Interventions and Referral for Smoking Cessation in Primary Care and Other Settings, Quick reference guide.* London: NICE.
3 Stead L *et al.* (2008). Nicotine replacement therapy for smoking cessation. *Cochrane Library* 3.
4 National Institute for Health and Clinical Excellence (2013). Public health guidance 48. *Smoking Cessation in Secondary Care: Acute, maternity and mental health services.* London: NICE.
5 MHRA (2013). *UK Moves Towards Safe and Effective Electronic Cigarettes and Other Nicotine-Containing Products.* http://www.mhra.gov.uk/home/groups/comms-po/documents/news/con286856.pdf (accessed 7 January 2015).
6 RPS (2013). *Guidance on Electronic Cigarettes.* http://www.rpharms.com/support-alerts/support-alert-article.asp?id=880 (accessed 7 January 2015).
7 Brayfield A (ed.) (2014). *Martindale: The Complete Drug Reference.* www.medicines complete.com (accessed on 4 December 2014).

'Nil-by-mouth': management of long-term medicines during surgery

'Doctors and nurses need to understand the difference between preoperative medication and the full English breakfast.' This is a quote taken from the National Clinical Enquiry into Perioperative Deaths.[1] The report stated that many patients had their routine medication omitted prior to surgery as they were 'nil-by-mouth' (NBM). The administration of medicines throughout the perioperative period should be considered in a timely fashion before surgery, as some medicines may need to be stopped with sufficient time to diminish their therapeutic actions or other effects. The administration and appropriateness of medicines after surgery should be considered if the NBM status is prolonged and the oral route is compromised.

Traditionally, patients were kept NBM from midnight the night before surgery. This led to poor nutritional intake and prolonged recovery, as vital oral medicines were unnecessarily omitted. With the introduction of enhanced recovery after surgery (ERAS)[2] principles, it is now standard practice to continue regular medication up to the point of surgery unless contraindicated. Evidence demonstrates that shortened periods of perioperative fasting do not increase the risk of harmful events for the patient, such as aspiration pneumonitis.[3] Oral medicines can be taken with clear fluids up to 2 hours prior to surgery without any detrimental effects.[4]

The decision whether to stop medication during the perioperative period or not should be based on the following:[5]

- consequences of not giving the medication
- indication for the drug
- risk of giving the medication – interactions, contraindications
- potential time scale of NBM and impact
- practicalities of administering the medication
- is replacement therapy indicated?
- administration via feeding tubes
- what are the effects of abrupt withdrawal?

The consequences of withholding certain medicines during the perioperative period could have detrimental effects on disease management, cause withdrawal or exacerbate a disease state. This should be weighed up against the potential risks associated with giving the drug – haemodynamic instability, bleeding risk, drug interactions or impaired healing.

There is not a definitive answer for every medicine a patient may be taking; however, there are numerous literature resources available. Examples of medicines that are contraindicated during surgery or that pose a risk if continued are given in Table N2.[6]

TABLE N2

Examples of groups of medicines and action during perioperative period

Medicine name/group	Action to be taken preoperatively	Additional comments
Antiplatelets	Usually stop 7–10 days prior to surgery depending on half-life of drug and accounts for platelet half-life	Indication of antiplatelet must be considered and risk of stopping versus risk of surgical bleeding, i.e. use of clopidogrel and aspirin post acute coronary syndrome within 12 months. Restart as soon as bleeding risk reduced
Anticoagulants	Stop 5–7 days prior to surgery. Require INR to be less than 1.5	May require LMWH as bridging therapy once INR less than therapeutic range. Indication of anticoagulant and risk of VTE determines whether treatment dose or prophylactic dose of LMWH is given
Lithium	Can discontinue 24–48 hours prior to surgery	Interacts with many anaesthetic agents, as can prolong neuromuscular blockade. Can continue lithium and use alternative anaesthetic agents to reduce risk. Avoid use of non-steroidal anti-inflammatory drugs. Avoid dehydration and monitor electrolytes closely
MAOIs	Stop 2 weeks before surgery. Newer MAOIs are reversible after 24–48 hours. Take psychiatric advice before stopping	Alternatively, continue and avoid interacting agents during surgery – discuss with anaesthetist
Hormone replacement therapy	If to be discontinued, stop 4 weeks prior to surgery	If stopped, there is risk of recurrence of menopausal symptoms but there is an increased risk of VTE if continued. Can reduce VTE risk through use of LMWH. This decision must be discussed with the patient and a plan decided preoperatively
Oestrogen-containing contraception	Patients can be given the option to discontinue 4–6 weeks prior to surgery but must ensure adequate contraceptive cover	If continued, risk of VTE can be reduced through use of LMWH and other mechanical precautions
Herbal medicines	Stop as far in advance before surgery as possible	Little evidence available about half-life of herbal medicines. Many interactions with perioperative medicines and effect on patient haemodynamics

N

Management of patients with diabetes

As a general principle, when patients who have diabetes require a surgical procedure, steps should be taken to minimise the period of fasting involved by ensuring the patient undergoes the procedure in the morning and is placed first on the surgical list. This is not always possible if the surgery is an emergency but being aware of which patients have diabetes mellitus is vital. A thorough medical and drug history of such patients is therefore very important, as this will influence the management throughout the perioperative period. Determining factors are:[5]

- timing of surgery
- usual treatment regimen:
  - insulin
  - oral hypoglycaemics
  - diet control
- how effectively the patient's diabetes is controlled prior to admission
- duration of starvation.

Type 1 or type 2 diabetes?

Patients who have type 1 diabetes are unable to produce insulin of their own and care must be taken to ensure that these patients do not become completely insulin-deficient at any time. The gold standard when treating these patients is use of the variable-rate intravenous insulin infusion (VRIII), previously known as 'sliding scale'. The use of VRIII is determined by the length of time the patient is expected to be NBM. If more than one meal is missed then an insulin infusion is indicated. Fewer than this, blood glucose levels can be managed with the patient's regular insulin regimen and intravenous fluids.

Patients who have type 2 diabetes can secrete their own insulin and are therefore much less likely to develop diabetic ketoacidosis. However, many type 2 patients do effectively become insulin-dependent during major surgery because of the physiological stress involved, and should be managed as such. Type 2 patients who are normally treated with diet alone will require much less aggressive treatment, particularly during minor surgical procedures, than those who require oral hypoglycaemic drugs to augment insulin secretion.

The patient's usual level of diabetes control

Well-controlled diabetic patients will not have to be in hospital for as long as those whose control is poor. Poorly controlled diabetics are known to be at increased risk of perioperative complications and mortality, and are prone to metabolic problems and poor wound healing. Patients whose HbA_{1c} indicates inadequate diabetic control will require to be admitted earlier for stabilisation of blood glucose levels prior to surgery or referred to a diabetes specialist nurse for drug therapy optimisation preoperatively. This demonstrates the importance of identification of such patients during the preoperative assessment or at the point of decision to operate.[5]

Duration of the surgical procedure and likely postoperative course

For procedures where the patient is expected to eat and drink within 4 hours of the operation, the relatively short duration of the fast involved for these procedures means that type 2 patients can often simply omit oral hypoglycaemics on the morning of surgery and restart therapy as soon as the first meal is eaten. Blood glucose levels require close monitoring and subcutaneous insulin may be required if they begin to rise. It is good practice for 'when required' short-acting insulin and glucose rescue therapy to be prescribed on the drug chart of patients with diabetes during this period.

Intravenous insulin replacement in patients with diabetes

The VRIII is a continuous infusion that is adjusted according to the patient's blood glucose concentrations.

- A glucose-containing infusion must be administered alongside the insulin, so that hypoglycaemia is avoided.
- Potassium-containing fluid must also run alongside to prevent insulin-induced hypokalaemia.
- Patients maintained on long-acting subcutaneous insulin should continue to receive it in order to reduce the risk of the development of ketonaemia and ketoacidosis.

VRIII should be withdrawn as soon as the patient is able to eat and drink. If the patient is usually treated with insulin, the VRIII should be continued for at least 30–60 minutes after giving the SC dose in association with a meal. For further information see *Insulin: variable-rate intravenous insulin infusion* entry.

Management of patients on corticosteroids[7]

Surgery causes an increase in plasma adrenocorticotrophic hormone and cortisol concentration. The magnitude of the increase is related to the amount of physical and psychological stress caused by surgery – major surgery tends to cause a greater increase compared to minor surgery. However, in a patient who either usually takes oral corticosteroids, or who has taken them recently, the hypothalamic–pituitary–adrenocortical (HPA) axis may be suppressed and so the natural stress response is impaired. Without an adequate cortisol replacement, the patient is at risk of hypoadrenal crisis (i.e. circulatory collapse and shock). The following factors must be taken into account when deciding on the level of corticosteroid replacement, and Table N3 gives further guidance:

- the dose of the steroid and the dosage regimen
- the duration of the steroid therapy
- the original adrenal status
- the type of surgery to be carried out
- if the patient has taken steroids in the past 3 months.

TABLE N3

Perioperative corticosteroid replacement therapy

Patients currently taking corticosteroids	<10 mg/day prednisolone or equivalent	Assume normal HPA response	Increased corticosteroid cover not required
	≥10 mg prednisolone or equivalent	Minor surgery	25 mg hydrocortisone sodium succinate at induction
		Moderate surgery	Usual preoperative corticosteroids, 25 mg hydrocortisone sodium succinate at induction and 100 mg/day for 24 hours (this can be given as divided doses or continuous infusion)
		Major surgery	Usual preoperative corticosteroids, 25 mg hydrocortisone sodium succinate at induction and 100 mg/day for 48–72 hours
	High-dose immuno-suppression	Give usual immunosuppressive doses during perioperative period	
Patients who have stopped taking corticosteroids	<3 months ago	Treat as if taking corticosteroids	
	>3 months ago	No additional perioperative corticosteroids	

Administration of hydrocortisone sodium succinate via infusion, rather than bolus injection, avoids large swings in plasma cortisol concentration and is therefore preferred.

Administration of medicines via feeding tubes

The administration of medicines via feeding tubes is one of the most common causes of tube blockage, and therefore it is extremely important to ensure the most appropriate formulation is used. To cover the administration of every medicine down a tube is beyond the scope of this book; however, there are several useful reference sources now available both on the internet (which are password-protected) for advice regarding individual drugs (subscription required)[8] or general advice (password-protected)[9] and now as a handbook[10] (see *Enteral feeding systems and drug administration* entry). The following basic principles should be remembered.

- Administration of many medicines via tubes is unlicensed.
- Do not crush enteric-coated, modified/slow-release (immediate release of high doses), cytotoxics and hormone preparations (risk to operator).
- Interactions may occur with the feed.
- Flushing with water before, after and between medicine administrations is essential to reduce the risk of blockage.

REFERENCES

1 National Confidential Enquiry into Perioperative Deaths (2002). *Functioning as a Team?* London: CEPOD.

2 Niranjan N *et al.* (2014). *Enhanced Recovery after Surgery – Current trend in peri-operative care.* Update in anaesthesia. www.anaesthesiology.org (accessed 7 October 2014).

3 Royal College of Nursing (2005). *Peri-operative Fasting in Adults and Children.* www.rcn.org.uk (accessed 7 October 2014).

4 AAGBI (2001) *Pre-operative Assessment. The role of the anaesthetist.* Association of Anaesthetists of Great Britain and Ireland. www.aagbi.org/pdf/pre-operative _ass.pdf (accessed 7 October 2014).

5 ASGBI (2012). *Issues in Professional Practice: Peri-operative management of the adult patient with diabetes.* www.asgbi.org.uk (accessed 13 May 2015).

6 Rahman MH, Beattie J (2004). Medication in the peri-operative period. *Pharm J* 272: 287–289.

7 Nicholson G *et al.* (1998). Perioperative steroid supplementation. *Anaesthesia* 53: 1091–1104.

8 White R and Bradnam V (2015). *Handbook of Drug Administration via Enteral Feeding Tubes.* www.medicinescomplete.com.

9 BAPEN (2014). http://www.bapen.org.uk/pdfs/drugs%26enteral/practical-guide -poster.pdf (accessed 7 October 2014).

10 The Royal Hospitals (2004). *Administering Medicines Through Enteral Feeding Tubes* (2 edn). Belfast: Pharmacy Department, Royal Hospitals.

N

Nutraceuticals for eye health

Age-related macular degeneration (AMD) affects the central area of the eye (macula) and causes central vision to become blurry/ distorted. Over time this progresses to a blank patch in the centre of vision.[1] Although the exact cause is unknown, there are several factors involved:

- age: more common in those over 65 years of age
- gender: more common in women
- family history of AMD
- smoking: increases the risk
- sunlight and diet.

Several dietary supplements claim to improve eye health; these supplements are available to buy from pharmacies, online and in health food shops.

The underlying cause of AMD is thought to be free-radical damage to the macula. A small percentage of free radicals are produced naturally by the body as it uses oxygen; however, cigarette smoking and exposure to ultraviolet radiation and visible blue light, which occurs naturally in sunlight, greatly increase free-radical generation. Antioxidants have the potential to combat free radicals, and therefore their use in protection from AMD has become popular.[2]

Vitamin C is used for growth and repair of tissues and supports healthy blood vessels. Vitamin E is a major antioxidant of all retinal cell membranes. Vitamin A comes in two forms in the human diet – preformed and provitamin. Preformed vitamin A (retinol) is in food from animal sources, e.g. fish and meat. Provitamin A carotenoids are mainly found in fruit and vegetables; beta-carotene is a provitamin A carotenoid that is converted to vitamin A in the body. Vitamin A is an essential component of rhodopsin, a protein that absorbs light in the cells of the eye.

Dietary xanthophylls lutein and zeaxanthin are found in high concentrations in the macula where they are called the macular pigment. The macular pigment protects the macula by interacting with free radicals and filtering out the damaging blue light.[3]

Evidence

In 2001 the Age-Related Eye Disease Study (AREDS), conducted in the USA by the National Institutes of Health, established that the AREDS formula (vitamin A (as beta-carotene) 15 mg, vitamin C 500 mg, vitamin E 400 IU, zinc 80 mg, copper 2 mg) can help slow the progression of AMD. In the AREDS trial, participants with AMD who took the AREDS formula were 25% less likely to progress to advanced AMD over the 5-year study period compared with placebo.[4]

Beta-carotene use has been linked to a heightened risk of lung cancer in smokers and ex-smokers. High zinc doses can cause minor side effects, such as stomach upset.[5]

A 5-year follow-up study began in 2006, called AREDS2 and conducted by the National Eye Institute. The second study aimed to find out if the original AREDS formulation could be improved by adding the carotenoid vitamins (lutein and zeaxanthin), omega-3 fatty acids, removing beta-carotene or reducing zinc. No overall additional benefit was gained from adding omega-3 fatty acid or a mixture of lutein and zeaxanthin to the AREDS formula. There was no apparent difference in effect when a lower zinc dose given. There was an 18% reduction in developing advanced AMD in the subgroup that received the AREDS formula plus lutein and zeaxanthin with no beta-carotene. Those with a low dietary intake of lutein and zeaxanthin who received the AREDS formula plus lutein and zeaxanthin were 25% less likely to develop advanced AMD compared to those with a similar dietary intake who did not receive lutein and zeaxanthin.[6] No matter which supplement was taken, after 5 years 30% of patients in AREDS2 progressed to advanced AMD.

Long-term use of the AREDS supplements appears safe and protective against advanced AMD. Zinc is an important component but it is unclear how much is necessary. Omega-3 fatty acids and beta-carotene do not reduce the risk, but adding lutein 10 mg and zeaxanthin 2 mg in place of beta-carotene may help.[7]

Products available in the UK

- Recommended daily dose of Viteyes 2 contains the AREDS2 formula (vitamin C 500 mg, vitamin E 400 IU, lutein 10 mg, zexanthin 2 mg, copper 2 mg, zinc 25 mg).
- Recommended daily dose of PreserVision AREDS2 is the same except it contains zinc 80 mg.

Diet

- Lutein is found in kale, red pepper, lettuce, leek, spinach, celery, broccoli, peas, sprouts and eggs.
- Zeaxanthin is found in corn, eggs, oranges and yellow fruit and vegetables.

REFERENCES

1 Royal College of Ophthalmologists and Royal National Institute of Blind People (2013). *Age Related Macular Degeneration*. http://www.rnib.org.uk/eye-health-eye-conditions-z-eye-conditions/age-related-macular-degeneration-amd (accessed 21 October 2014).

2 Macular Society (2015). *Antioxidant Vitamins*. http://www.macularsociety.org/about-macular-conditions/Nutrition/AntioxidantVitamins-A-C-E (accessed 25 January 2015).

3 Macular Society (2015). *Lutein and Zeaxanthin*. http://www.macularsociety.org/about-macular-conditions/Nutrition/Xanthophylls-Lutein-Zeaxanthin-Meso-zeaxanthin (accessed 28 January 2015).

4 The Royal College of Ophthalmologists (2013). Press release. *Diet Study Clarifies Optimal Nutrient Formula for Protecting Against AMD*. http://www.rcophth.ac.uk/news.asp?itemid=1369&itemTitle=Diet+study+clarifies+optimal+nutrient+formula+for+protecting+against+AMD&section=24&sectionTitle=News (accessed 21 October 2014).

5 National Institute of Health (2013). *NIH Study Provides Clarity on Supplements for Protection Against Blinding Eye Disease*. http://www.nih.gov/news/health/may2013/nei-05.htm (accessed 21 October 2014).

6 Macular Society (2014). *AREDS 2 Study Results Show Promise for Some*. http://www.macularsociety.org/How-we-help/About-us/Newsroom/Press-releases/areds-2-study-results-show-promise-for-some (accessed 21 October 2014).

7 Chew EY *et al.* (2013). Long-term effects of vitamins C, E, beta-carotene and zinc on age-related macular degeneration. *Ophthalmology* 120: 1604–1611.

Omeprazole: parenteral administration

40 mg dry-powder vials

- Omeprazole sodium is a proton pump inhibitor (PPI).
- It is used intravenously (IV) when the oral route is temporarily unavailable, to treat conditions where inhibition of gastric acid secretion may be beneficial: treatment and prevention of gastric and duodenal ulcers, in gastro-oesophageal reflux disease and Zollinger–Ellison syndrome.
- It is also used (unlicensed) for acute gastrointestinal bleeding and to prevent rebleeding following therapeutic endoscopy for acute bleeding gastric or duodenal ulcers.
- There are two preparations available: IV injection and IV infusion. The IV injection preparation is accompanied by 10 mL special solvent containing macrogol 400, citric acid and water for injection, and is not suitable for IV infusion.
- Doses are expressed in terms of omeprazole:

    Omeprazole 40 mg ≡ 42.6 mg omeprazole sodium.

Pretreatment checks

PPIs may mask symptoms of gastric cancer (and delay diagnosis); when a gastric ulcer is suspected, the possibility of malignancy should be excluded before treatment is instituted.

Biochemical and other tests

These include liver function tests (LFTs).

Dose[1,2]

- Prophylaxis of acid aspiration: 40 mg by IV injection or infusion completed 1 hour before surgery.
- Benign gastric ulcer, duodenal ulcer and gastro-oesophageal reflux: 40 mg by IV injection or infusion once daily, until oral administration is possible (recommended duration of treatment is up to 5 days).
- Zollinger–Ellison syndrome: 60 mg by IV injection or infusion twice daily.

- Gastrointestinal haemorrhage following successful haemostasis of bleeding peptic ulcers (unlicensed): 80 mg by IV injection followed by a continuous IV infusion of 8 mg/hour for 72 hours.[3]
- Dose in hepatic impairment: 20 mg daily by IV injection or infusion may be sufficient.

Intermittent intravenous infusion (using a preparation for IV infusion)

Preparation and administration

1 Add approximately 5 mL of compatible infusion fluid from a 100 mL bag to each omeprazole vial.
2 Mix thoroughly to dissolve and transfer the required dose to the infusion bag.
3 Repeat steps 1–2 to ensure the full dose is transferred or use a double-ended transfer needle device for the whole process.
4 The solution should be clear and colourless. Inspect visually for particulate matter or discolouration prior to administration and discard if present.
5 Give by IV infusion over 20–30 minutes.

Intravenous injection

Preparation and administration

1 Withdraw 10 mL of solvent from the ampoule provided and add approximately 5 mL to the omeprazole vial.
2 Immediately withdraw as much air as possible from the vial back into the syringe in order to reduce positive pressure and add the remaining solvent into the vial.
3 Rotate and shake the vial to ensure all the powder has dissolved.
4 The solution should be clear and colourless. Inspect visually for particulate matter or discoloration prior to administration and discard if present.
5 Give by IV injection over 5 minutes.

Continuous intravenous infusion (using a preparation for IV infusion)

Various (unlicensed) regimens are used. The one below produces a solution containing 200 mg/500 mL.

Preparation and administration

1 Reconstitute each of five vials (total 200 mg) with 5 mL of compatible infusion fluid taken from a 500 mL infusion bag and mix thoroughly to dissolve.
2 Withdraw the required dose (ensuring the entire vial contents are transferred) and add to the 500 mL bag, e.g. 5 × 40 mg vials added to 500 mL NaCl 0.9% gives a solution containing 400 micrograms/mL.

3 The solution should be clear and colourless. Inspect visually for particulate matter or discolouration prior to administration and discard if present.

4 Give by IV infusion at a rate of 8 mg/hour, i.e. 20 mL/hour of a 400 micrograms/mL solution. Prepare a fresh infusion bag every 24 hours.

Technical information[4]

Incompatible with:	Lorazepam, midazolam, tigecycline, vancomycin
Compatible with:	**Flush:** NaCl 0.9%
	Solutions: NaCl 0.9%, glucose 5%. Some generic brands state that only glucose 5% may be used as a diluent, but all preparations are similarly formulated.
	Y-site: No information, but likely to be unstable
pH	8.8–10.5
Sodium content	Negligible
Storage	Store below 25°C in original packaging
Stability after preparation	From a microbiological point of view, should be used immediately. However: • Reconstituted vials may be stored at room temperature and used within 4 hours. • Prepared infusions may be infused (at room temperature) within 24 hours

Monitoring

Measure	Frequency	Rationale
Signs of infection	Throughout treatment	• Use of antisecretory drugs may increase risk of infections, such as community-acquired pneumonia, *Salmonella*, *Campylobacter* and *Clostridium difficile*-associated disease
LFTs	Periodically	• Altered LFTs and hepatitis have been reported
Renal function		• Acute interstitial nephritis has been reported with PPIs. • ↓Na has been reported with PPIs
Vitamin B_{12}		• If on long-term therapy, malabsorption of vitamin B_{12} has been reported

Additional information

Common and serious undesirable effects	**Immediate:** hypersensitivity reactions, including anaphylaxis and bronchospasm, have been reported very rarely. **Injection/infusion-related** • Local: administration site reactions, particularly with prolonged infusion. **Other** • Common: nausea, vomiting, abdominal pain, flatulence, diarrhoea, constipation, headache, dry mouth, peripheral oedema, dizziness, sleep disturbances, fatigue, paraesthesia, arthralgia, myalgia, rash and pruritus. • Rare: taste disturbance, stomatitis, ↑liver enzymes, hepatitis, jaundice, fever, depression, hallucinations, confusion, gynaecomastia, interstitial nephritis, ↓Mg, ↓Na, blood disorders (including leucopenia, leucocytosis, pancytopenia and thrombocytopenia), visual disturbances, sweating, photosensitivity, alopecia, Stevens–Johnson syndrome and toxic epidermal necrolysis
Pharmacokinetics	Approximate plasma half-life is 0.5–3 hours. The IV infusion produces an immediate decrease in intragastric acidity and a mean decrease over 24 hours of approximately 90%[2]
Significant interactions[1]	*The following may ↓omeprazole levels or effect:* Tipranavir. *Omeprazole may ↑levels or effect of the following drugs (or ↑side effects):* Cilostazol (avoid combination), coumarins (monitor INR), raltegravir (avoid combination). *Omeprazole may ↓levels or effect of the following drugs:* Atazanavir (avoid combination), clopidogrel (avoid combination), nelfinavir (avoid combination). *Omeprazole may affect the following tests:* Antisecretory drug therapy may cause a false-negative urea breath test. May give false-positive tetrahydrocannabinol urine screening test results
Action in case of overdose	Stop administration and give supportive therapy as appropriate

REFERENCES

1 Joint Formulary Committee (2015). *British National Formulary* (online). London: BMJ Group and Pharmaceutical Press.

2 Electronic medicines compendium (2014). www.medicines.org.uk (accessed 14 September 2015).

3 Hasselgren G *et al.* Optimization of acid suppression for patients with peptic ulcer bleeding: an intragastric pH-metry study with omeprazole *Eur J Gastroenterol Hepatol* 1998; 10: 601–606.

4 Trissell LA (2012) *Handbook on Injectable Drugs* www.medicinescomplete.com (accessed 14 September 2015).

Oncological emergencies

Hypercalcaemia

Hypercalcaemia is an oncological emergency associated with advanced cancer. It can be life-threatening due to the effect of calcium on the kidneys, heart and brain. Ninety per cent of cases are caused by primary hyperparathyroidism or cancer.[1]

Hypercalcaemia may occur with or without bone metastases. It is caused by the release of parathyroid hormone-related peptide from cancer cells and most commonly occurs in squamous cell lung cancer, breast cancer and myeloma. Classification is shown in Table O1.

TABLE O1

Severity classification of hypercalcaemia

Severity	Adjusted calcium (mmol/L)
Mild	2.65–3.0
Moderate	3.01–3.4
Severe	>3.4

Symptoms are often non-specific and depend on the severity of hypercalcaemia and the rate of onset. Symptoms may include polyuria/polydipsia, nausea and vomiting, constipation, muscle weakness, confusion and drowsiness.

Rehydration is the first-line management of hypercalcaemia associated with malignancy. IV bisphosphonates (e.g. pamidronate or zoledronate) may also be given to reduce calcium resorption from bone. It is also important to stop any calcium-containing medicines and thiazide diuretics.

Metastatic spinal cord compression

Metastatic spinal cord compression occurs either through direct tumour compression of the spinal cord or via vertebral instability due to bony metastases. Back pain is almost always a feature and this may occur at any point along the vertebrae. Pain is usually the first sign of spinal cord compression and may be new or a significant change to long-standing pain.

Other symptoms caused by pressure on the spinal nerves may include motor deficits (e.g. muscle weakness, loss of coordination, paralysis), sensory deficits (e.g. paraesthesia, loss of sensation) or autonomic dysfunction (loss of control of bladder or bowel).

There are approximately 4000 new cases per year in England and Wales and 25% of patients may not have an established cancer diagnosis at the time of presentation.[2]

Treatment of metastatic spinal cord compression may include surgery, radiotherapy or corticosteroids (e.g. dexamethasone 16 mg/day with PPI).

Superior vena cava obstruction

Superior vena cava obstruction (SVCO) may be caused by external pressure, thrombus or direct tumour invasion. Ninety-five per cent of cases of SVCO are due to malignancy and 70–80% are in patients with lung cancer.[3]

Symptoms may be gradual or acute in onset and include: dyspnoea, elevated jugular venous pressure, face/arm swelling, chest pain, cough and dilated blood vessels over trunk/arms/neck.

Initial treatment of SVCO includes oxygen, corticosteroids (e.g. dexamethasone 16 mg/day with PPI) and sitting upright. Chemotherapy may be an effective treatment in chemosensitive cancers such as lymphoma, germ cell or small-cell lung cancers. If a clot is the cause for SVCO, anticoagulation should be considered.

Neutropenic sepsis

See *Neutropenic sepsis* entry.

REFERENCES
1 NICE (2014). *Clinical Knowledge Summaries. Hypercalcaemia.* http://cks.nice.org.uk/hypercalcaemia (accessed 7 January 2015).
2 NICE (2008). Metastatic spinal cord compression: Diagnosis and management of adults at risk of and with metastatic spinal cord compression. NICE Clinician Guideline CG75. https://www.nice.org.uk/guidance/cg75 (accessed 7 January 2015).
3 NICE (2004). Stent placement for vena cava obstruction. NICE interventional procedures guidance IPG79. https://www.nice.org.uk/guidance/ipg79 (accessed 7 January 2015).

Opioid comparative doses

Although morphine is still considered the first-choice opioid,[1] it is often necessary to consider converting or switching to an alternative opioid, perhaps because of lack of analgesic benefit or intolerable side effects.[2] In order to do this safely it is essential to have an understanding of the relative analgesic potency of different opioids. Table O2 shows the approximate analgesic potency of other commonly used oral opioids compared with morphine – this should not be confused with equivalent doses as some of these opioids have a ceiling effect.[3]

Conversion for different routes of morphine administration

If it is necessary to convert to subcutaneous or intramuscular morphine, the parenteral dose is half that of the oral morphine dose, e.g. 10 mg oral morphine ≡ 5 mg subcutaneous or intramuscular morphine.[2]

Converting between morphine and diamorphine

To convert from oral morphine to diamorphine, the dose is approximately one-third of the oral morphine dose, i.e. the total dose of morphine (mg) given during the previous 24 hours divided by 3, and this gives the dose of diamorphine to be administered over 24 hours by continuous infusion. A dose of approximately one-tenth

TABLE O2
Equianalgesic opioid potency

Opioid	Potency ratio with oral morphine
Buprenorphine	75–115
Codeine	1/10
Dihydrocodeine	1/10
Fentanyl	100–150
Hydromorphone	4–7.5
Methadone	5–10
Oxycodone	1.5–2
Pethidine	1/10
Tapentadol	2.5
Tramadol	1/10–1/5

to one-sixth of the total daily dose of diamorphine should be prescribed by subcutaneous injection for breakthrough pain. The patient should be monitored regularly and the dose of diamorphine given by continuous infusion and breakthrough pain adjusted according to the total requirement for the previous 24 hours.

It is essential to remember that great caution is always necessary when switching between different opioids or routes of administration: careful monitoring of the patient is essential as there is much interpatient variability. Subsequent dose adjustments may still be necessary. Conversion ratios are never more than an estimate and they should be used as a guide only, as they are based largely on single-dose studies in opioid-naive subjects and may not be as relevant when conversions are made after regular doses of an opioid have been given (either in the acute or chronic pain setting). Most studies have only considered opioid switching in one direction and, as the conversions do not account for incomplete cross-tolerance between opioids, it may be appropriate to reduce the calculated dose by 25–50%.

REFERENCES
1 NICE (2012). Clinical Guideline 140. Opioids in palliative care: safe and effective prescribing of strong opioids for pain in palliative care of adults. http://www.nice.org.uk/guidance/cg140 (accessed 27 November 2014).
2 Drewes AM *et al.* (2013). Differences between opioids: pharmacological, experimental, clinical and economical perspectives. *Br J Clin Pharmacol* 75: 60–78.
3 Twycross R, Wilcock A (2011). *Palliative Care Formulary* (4th edn). Nottingham: Palliativedrugs.com.

Opioid misuse management

Oral methadone and oral buprenorphine are recommended for the management of withdrawal syndrome from opioids.[1] If both drugs are equally suitable for a patient, then NICE recommends methadone as the drug of choice.

Methadone

Methadone is long-acting (half-life is 15 hours initially; 20–37 hours in a regular user), making stability from daily dosing easier to achieve. It is easy to titrate to achieve the correct dose and is less likely to be injected than other opioids.

Opioid withdrawal symptoms

Classic opioid withdrawal symptoms are: weakness, insomnia, yawning/sneezing, irritability/aggression, sweating, muscle spasms and jerking, diarrhoea, tremors, nausea and vomiting, goose bumps, loss of appetite, dilated pupils, high temperature but feeling cold, lacrimation and rhinorrhoea, abdominal cramps, tachycardia, hypertension and increased bowel sounds.[2]

If a patient is admitted to hospital who is on a managed opioid withdrawal regimen, or who is a substance misuser and is likely to exhibit withdrawal symptoms during admission, it is important to seek out and follow any local guidelines for your hospital. The following points should also be borne in mind.

Prior to prescribing methadone

The patient's consent should be obtained to contact the patient's usual prescriber or community pharmacist to confirm the dose. If this is not possible, and the patient has his or her own supply, it should only be used as a means of identifying the dose if the label has not been tampered with, and if it has been dispensed within the last 7 days.

The patient's community pharmacist and the local drug service will need to be informed as soon as possible to avoid potential diversion of the community supply to another individual.

The telephone number of the local drug service is:

. . . .

If it is necessary to contact a drug service outside of the locality, the UK National Drugs Helpline (0800 776600) may be of help. They provide 24-hour free and confidential advice, including information on local services.

Prescribing methadone without an established dose[3,4]

If a patient presents who is receiving methadone, or is in opioid withdrawal, and it is not possible to establish the patient's normal dose, s/he should be prescribed 10 mg or 20 mg of methadone mixture 1 mg/mL (depending on the severity of the patient's withdrawal symptoms) and observed for 2–4 hours to ensure s/he does not become intoxicated.

The aim is to provide an effective level of physical and psychological comfort, while minimising the likelihood of overdose.

Supplementary doses should only be considered where there is evidence of persistent opioid withdrawal. If a daily dose has been greater than 40 mg methadone, the patient should be closely monitored, as deaths have occurred with 40 mg commencement doses. The prescriber should consider the cumulative effect of administering methadone because of its long half-life.

If after 4 hours there are still withdrawal symptoms, another dose may be given depending on the severity of the symptoms:

- mild withdrawal symptoms: give no further methadone
- moderate withdrawal symptoms (muscle aches, dilated pupils, nausea, yawning): give 5–10 mg methadone
- severe withdrawal symptoms (vomiting, piloerection, tachycardia, elevated blood pressure): give 20 mg methadone.

Remember: methadone overdose can be fatal – withdrawal is not.

Once a whole 24 hours has passed, the total amount of methadone administered during that period should be prescribed thereafter as a single daily dose. There is an increased risk of death during commencement of methadone; toxicity may be delayed, as it takes five half-lives to reach steady state. Patients must be carefully monitored for signs of toxicity during this induction period.

Methadone equivalents

If a patient is not on a withdrawal programme, but is a known substance misuser and control of withdrawal symptoms is necessary, then the above advice should be followed. It is not possible to predict equivalent doses in most cases; purity of street drugs will vary and half-lives of different opioids are not the same.

If it is necessary to switch between oral and parenteral forms of methadone, there are a variety of views as to the appropriate equivalence. The Department of Health guidelines suggest using the same dose.[4] In cancer care it has been suggested that the oral dose should be halved for parenteral use.[5] The indications for prescribing in both cases are different, so dose comparisons may be inappropriate: a patient switched between forms for any reason should be monitored for signs of over- or underdosing, and the dose subsequently adjusted accordingly.

Adjuvant drugs for withdrawal symptoms

As well as methadone, it may be appropriate to control the physical symptoms of withdrawal with more conventional therapy, e.g. loperamide for diarrhoea, metoclopramide for nausea and vomiting, mebeverine for stomach cramps, paracetamol and NSAIDs for headaches and muscular pains.

Stabilisation and maintenance regimen

Where doses need to be increased during the first week, the increment should be no more than 5–10 mg on one day and the total increase should not exceed 30 mg above the starting dose. For subsequent weeks the dose of methadone is initially increased by not more than 10 mg weekly, usually over a period of 6 weeks, to between 60 mg and 120 mg daily. During this time the patient and carers should watch for signs of toxicity. ECG monitoring is recommended before the dose is increased above 100 mg daily and 1 week after, as cases of QT interval prolongation and torsade des pointes have been reported.[6]

The maintenance dose should continue until the patient is suitable for detoxification.

Missed doses

- If a patient misses 3 days or more of maintenance treatment with methadone, s/he is at risk of overdose because of loss of tolerance. In these cases consider reducing the dose of methadone.
- If a patient misses more than 5 days of maintenance treatment, an assessment of illicit drug use is recommended before recommencing methadone.

Detoxification

Once a patient is stable and is suitable for detoxification, and provided there is abstinence from heroin, the dose can be reduced. This will be by 5 mg every week or fortnight, which typically will result in zero after 12 weeks. During this period the patient should have appropriate psychosocial support and this should continue for at least 6 months after detoxification.

Some patients and prescribers may agree to reduce the dose slowly over a period of months or years to lead to a formal detoxification.

The overall goal is to maximise the patient's health, and this may actually mean continuing with maintenance treatment.

Buprenorphine

If methadone is not suitable, then buprenorphine is an appropriate choice of treatment. Some patients may prefer buprenorphine because it is less sedating than methadone.

Buprenorphine is a partial agonist/antagonist of the mu (μ) and kappa (κ) opioid receptors in the brain. It is used to treat opioid dependence, but because of the nature of its pharmacology it can precipitate withdrawal symptoms in opioid-dependent individuals. This is more likely with patients taking high doses of opioids (typically >30 mg methadone, or equivalent, daily).

Buprenorphine sublingual tablets are used for the management of opioid dependence. They have been misused by being crushed and injected; to prevent this misuse a formulation of buprenorphine plus naloxone (Suboxone) has been developed.

The SPC for buprenorphine[7] recommends an initiation dose from 0.8 to 4 mg is given as a single dose; in clinical practice, initiation doses may be 4–8 mg. The dose should be given at least 4 hours after the last dose of opioid (or 24–48 hours after the last methadone dose), or preferably when the first signs of opioid withdrawal occur. If the patient has been taking methadone, the dose of methadone should have been less than 30 mg daily (unless withdrawal is to be conducted by specialist drug services).

The dose is increased on subsequent days, usually by 2–4 mg (although 8-mg steps are sometimes used), according to clinical response, and to a maximum dose of 32 mg daily. It may take 1–2 weeks for the patient to feel comfortable with the buprenorphine, and lofexidine may be needed in the first 2 days to help with any withdrawal symptoms.

Lofexidine[1,8]

During sudden withdrawal of an opioid there is an increase in the amount of noradrenaline released, which results in an increased rate of neuronal firing, and this is seen in the patient as the symptoms of the withdrawal syndrome. Lofexidine is a presynaptic adrenergic alpha-2-receptor agonist. Its pharmacological effect is to decrease noradrenaline release and neuronal firing rate, thereby dampening down the withdrawal symptoms. It is used to relieve withdrawal symptoms in patients undergoing opioid detoxification and not to treat opioid dependence. It is useful for patients with only a short history of opioid abuse who have been taking up to a quarter of a gram of street heroin daily, or to complete methadone withdrawal, e.g. when the methadone dose falls to 15 mg/day.

Blood pressure should be measured before and during treatment, and if there is a clinically significant decrease in blood pressure, treatment with lofexidine should be discontinued. It is unsuitable for people with pre-existing low blood pressure or bradycardia.

The starting dose is 800 micrograms daily in divided doses, increasing in steps of 400–800 micrograms daily as necessary, to a maximum of 2.4 mg daily. The maximum single dose should not exceed 800 micrograms (4 × 200 microgram tablets). The duration of treatment is usually 7–10 days. It is withdrawn over 2–4 days, but a longer period may be needed if withdrawal symptoms manifest.

REFERENCES

1 NICE (2007). *Methadone and Buprenorphine for the Management of Opioid Dependence*. Technology Appraisal 114. http://nice.org.uk/guidance/TA114 (accessed 29 December 2014).

2 Department of Health (England) and the devolved administrations (2007). *Drug Misuse and Dependence: UK guidelines on clinical management*. London: Department of Health (England), the Scottish Government, Welsh Assembly Government and Northern Ireland Executive. http://www.nta.nhs.uk/uploads/clinical_guidelines _2007.pdf (accessed 22 December 2014).

3 East Lancashire Hospital NHS Trust (2012). *Guidelines for Prescribing of Methadone for Hospital In-patient Opiate Misusers*. Blackburn: ELHT.

4 Department of Health (2007). *Drug Misuse and Dependence: UK guidelines on clinical management*. http://www.nta.nhs.uk/uploads/clinical_guidelines_2007.pdf (accessed 12 May 2015).

5 Säwe J (1986). High-dose morphine and methadone in cancer patients: clinical pharmacokinetic considerations of oral treatment. *Clin Pharmacokinet* 11: 87–106.

6 SPC (2014). *Methadone 1 mg/mL oral solution*. www.medicines.org.uk (accessed 13 January 2015).

7 SPC (2015). *Subutex 2 mg sublingual tablets*. www.medicines.org.uk (accessed 13 January 2015).

8 SPC (2014). *BritLofex Tablets 0.2 mg*. www.medicines.org.uk (accessed 18 January 2015).

Opioid partial agonists

A partial agonist is a drug that binds to and activates a receptor but has only partial efficacy at the receptor compared with a full agonist. This means that it may have a ceiling effect and demonstrate both agonist and antagonist effects. When both a full agonist and partial agonist are given together, the partial agonist may act as a competitive antagonist, competing with the full agonist for receptor occupancy and overall producing less receptor activation than with the full agonist alone.

There are several opioid partial agonists, including buprenorphine, pentazocine and nalbuphine, used in clinical practice.

Buprenorphine

Buprenorphine is a partial agonist of the mu-opioid receptor that is experiencing resurgence in use for persistent pain following formulation for transdermal administration[1] and in the management of opioid dependence and addiction. In human studies using clinically relevant analgesic doses, buprenorphine does not have a ceiling effect to analgesia, hence, contrary to popular conception, it is possible to administer another opioid agonist such as morphine for the management of exacerbations of pain. However, buprenorphine does have a ceiling effect for respiratory depression[2] and it still can readily be reversed by naloxone, although often larger doses are required than for other opioids.

See the *Pain management* entry for the analgesic equivalence of transdermal buprenorphine compared with other commonly used opioids.

REFERENCES
1 Budd K, Collett BJ (2003). Old dog – new (ma)trix. *Br J Anaesth* 90: 722–724.
2 Dahan A *et al.* (2006). Buprenorphine induces ceiling in respiratory depression but not in analgesia. *Br J Anaesth* 96: 627–632.

Osteoporosis

Overview	
Definition	Osteoporosis is a degenerative disease characterised by low bone mass and microarchitectural deterioration of bone tissue, leading to increased bone fragility and susceptibility to fracture.[1,2] The World Health Organization defines osteoporosis as having a bone mineral density (BMD) of ≤ 2.5 standard deviations below peak BMD, as measured on dual-energy X-ray absorptiometry (DXA) applied to femoral neck.[3]
	Severe or established osteoporosis is having osteoporosis with one or more fragility fractures. A fragility fracture is defined as a fracture following a fall from standing height or less. A major osteoporotic fracture is one occurring at the spine, hip, forearm or proximal humerus. The most common fractures are hip, spine or wrist fractures.

Osteoporosis is caused by an increased rate of old bone loss or resorption (osteoclast activity) that is not matched by an increased rate of new bone formation (osteoblast activity) and results in reduced bone mass and structural deterioration, which eventually leads to osteoporosis. Ageing and low oestrogen levels associated with menopause, as well as secondary causes contribute significantly to this imbalance. Low calcium and vitamin D levels and hyperparathyroidism also increase bone loss

Risk factors	Increasing age (a 2% risk at 50 years to a 25% risk at 80 years), falls risk and low BMD are the strongest risk factors for an osteoporotic fracture, but other clinical risk factors also contribute, e.g. parental history of hip fracture, alcohol intake of 4 units or more per day, rheumatoid arthritis,[4,5] gender, previous fragility fracture(s), current oral corticosteroid treatment, current smoking and falls are partly independent of BMD. In contrast, low BMI and secondary causes of osteoporosis, such as prolonged immobility, drugs, untreated premature menopause, ankylosing spondylitis, endocrine and rheumatoid disorders, chronic obstructive pulmonary disease (COPD), chronic kidney disease and Crohn's disease are related to low BMD. SSRIs, PPIs and antiepileptic drugs also adversely affect bone strength through unknown mechanisms.

The National Osteoporosis Guidance Group and NICE make different recommendations on how to assess patients and the tools to be used. NICE recommendations are used in this section.

High-risk patients should be identified opportunistically and fracture risk should be assessed in the following groups:

- Women aged ≥65 years; men aged ≥75 years
- Women 50–65 years and men 50–75 years who have a risk factor for fragility fractures
- Anyone under 50 years if they have a major risk factor for fragility fractures, e.g. current or frequent use of oral corticosteroids, untreated premature menopause and previous or multiple osteoporotic fractures.

The Fracture Risk Assessment Tool (FRAX)[6] and QFracture[7] are tools recommended by NICE to calculate fracture risk. They predict the probability of a hip or major osteoporotic fracture over a 10-year period (expressed as a percentage). They do not include every risk factor, so may underestimate risks in certain situations, such as patients who have had multiple fractures. There are pros and cons to using either tool depending on the age of the patient and the availability of BMD measurement. QFracture is based on the UK population, incorporates more clinical risk factors than the FRAX tool and provides thresholds for which treatment is recommended. However, it does not utilise BMD measurements in risk calculation and so the FRAX tool *must* be used when BMD is available

Differential diagnosis	- Osteoarthritis - Degenerative disc disease - Osteomalacia - Skeletal metastases - Multiple myeloma

Diagnostic tests	Generally, osteoporosis is diagnosed by measurement of BMD using central (lumbar spine and proximal femur[1]) DXA scanning, and is expressed as the T-score. However, a diagnosis of osteoporosis may be assumed in women aged ≥ 75 years without the need for DXA confirmation if the responsible clinician thinks a scan is inappropriate or unfeasible.
	Biochemical markers and radiological X-rays have no role in the diagnosis of osteoporosis, but the latter may be used to confirm a suspected spinal fracture.[8]
Treatment goals	Treatment aims to preserve bone mass and reduce the risks of fractures. This involves modification of risk factors, falls prevention, calcium and vitamin D supplementation and drugs that reduce bone resorption or stimulate bone formation. It can also involve managing complications resulting from fractures, e.g. the use of analgesics and physiotherapy for acute and chronic pain

Pharmaceutical care and counselling

Assess	***Risk modification and falls prevention***
	All patients should be advised and supported to modify their risk factors where possible and make appropriate lifestyle changes, particularly smoking cessation, limiting alcohol intake and taking regular exercise. Useful exercises include low-impact, weight-bearing, strength-training, balance and gait-training exercises, which should be tailored to the individual's needs and abilities.
	Calcium and vitamin D status should be assessed and corrected as needed by increased dietary intake or pharmacological supplementation. A dietary calcium intake of 1000 mg daily should be maintained and can be estimated using the calcium calculator at http://www.sign.ac.uk/guidelines/fulltext/71/annex4.html.
	All older patients should be routinely asked about falls and associated risk factors should be identified and modified. Those at high risk should be referred to specialist falls teams. Multifaceted interventions recommended by NICE[9] to reduce frequency of falls include medication review, with modification or withdrawal of offending drugs
Calcium and vitamin D	Combination of both is more effective than either drug alone in fractures in patients over 60 years (hip) and those in a care home (hip and vertebral). Therefore, it should be prescribed routinely for care home patients with very few exceptions (unless adequate levels or contraindicated).
	The MHRA advises that patients at risk of developing osteopenia or osteoporosis who are taking long-term carbamazepine, phenytoin, primidone and sodium valproate should receive vitamin D supplementation. Therapeutic calcium alone has been associated with increased risks of myocardial infarction. Calcium levels should be checked prior to prescribing to avoid hypercalcaemia. Vitamin D supplementation alone can prevent falls in over-60-year-olds living in institutionalised settings or the community.
	Colecalciferol (vitamin D_3) oral preparations are available as single agents or in combination with calcium in various formulations. Non-adherence is common and the patient's preference is an important consideration when choosing the appropriate formulation

Anti-osteoporotic drugs	Once patients are identified and assessed, the decision to commence treatment will depend on the level of risk and therapeutic threshold. The therapeutic threshold is determined by a combination of the patient's age, BMD, clinical risk factors, indicators of low BMD and whether there has been previous fracture(s) or not.

NICE recommends that:

- Those at high risk and exceeding the therapeutic threshold should be treated without the need for BMD.
- Those at low risk should not be treated or referred for BMD.
- Those at intermediate risk should be referred for DXA to measure BMD. Then their risk should be recalculated using the FRAX tool. Those exceeding the therapeutic threshold should be treated and those below given lifestyle advice and reassessed after 5 years, or sooner as required. For those just below the treatment threshold, treatment should be considered if they have risk factors that are underestimated or unaccounted for in the FRAX tool.

Premenopausal women and those under 50 who have had an osteoporotic fracture should be referred for specialist management. The choice of drug will depend on cost-effectiveness, drug safety profile and patient factors, such as comorbidities, preferences, ability to comply with administration instructions and tolerance. All drugs available in the UK act primarily as antiresorptive agents, except for strontium (dual action) and teriparatide, which stimulate bone formation.

NICE recommends:

- Alendronate as first-line therapy based on cost-effectiveness and risks of adverse effects.
- Risedronate, if alendronate cannot be tolerated, adhered to or is contraindicated.
- Refer to secondary care for raloxifene, teriparatide or denosumab[10] according to criteria set by NICE, if alendronate or risedronate cannot be taken. The use of strontium ranelate is now restricted to severe osteoporosis when other drugs cannot be used and in those without cardiovascular contraindications.[11] Teriparatide is recommended as an alternative where there has been an unsatisfactory response to other drugs. Raloxifene and teriparatide are not recommended for primary prevention.

Poor adherence and persistence with oral bisphosphonates is a real problem, particularly within 3 months of initiation, as the risk of fractures increases when adherence falls below 50%.[12] Better education and intermittent dosing regimen given weekly; alternatively monthly (ibandronate oral), 3-monthly (ibandronate IV) and annually (zoledronate IV) preparations have been developed to assist with these problems

Patient counselling	- Check that the patient (or carer) understands the administration instructions, particularly for patients with cognitive impairment and patients whose medicines are dispensed in multicompartment compliance aids.

- For those on oral bisphosphonates, explain that these must be taken whole on an empty stomach with a full glass of water and the patient must remain upright for 30 minutes after taking the medication to improve absorption and reduce the risks of oesophageal reactions.
- Explain duration of treatment and that the outcome is only to reduce the risk, not completely eliminate fractures.

- Explain common and severe adverse drug effects, including what signs to look out for and actions to take.
- Explain the need to maintain good oral hygiene, regular dental check-ups and timing of dental procedures for those taking bisphosphonates.
- Ask for the presence of common and severe ADRs, e.g. heartburn, abdominal pain, muscle ache, groin pain with bisphosphonates; signs of cellulitis with denosumab; allergic rash with strontium.
- Explain complex dosing instructions clearly to reduce the risks of adverse effects, especially around the time the drug is initiated.
- Signpost patients for more information and support, e.g. the National Osteoporotic Society, NHS Choices, www.healthtalkonline.org, patient.co.uk

Continued monitoring	Review treatment within 3 months and regularly thereafter to check for adverse drug effects and adherence. Assess the continuing need for bisphosphonates after 3–5 years and continue if the patient is at high risk or refer for DXA. If fracture occurs, exclude secondary causes and refer to secondary care. Those taking regular corticosteroids should continue bisphosphonates until they stop, then have the fracture risk reassessed to determine the need for continuing treatment

REFERENCES

1 NICE (2012). CG146. *Osteoporosis: Assessing the risk of fragility fracture.* http://www.nice.org.uk/guidance/cg146 (accessed 23 August 2014).

2 NICE (2008). TA 161. *Alendronate, etidronate, risedronate, raloxifene, strontium ranelate and teriparatide for the secondary prevention of osteoporotic fragility fractures in postmenopausal women* (amended). https://www.nice.org.uk/guidance/ta161 (accessed 23 August 2014).

3 Kanis JA, on behalf of the World Health Organization Scientific Group (2007). *Assessment of Osteoporosis at the Primary Health Care Level.* WHO Collaborating Centre for Metabolic Bone Diseases, University of Sheffield. http://www.who.int/chp/topics/Osteoporosis.pdf (accessed 13 May 2015).

4 NICE (2008). TA 160. *Alendronate, etidronate, risedronate, raloxifene and strontium ranelate for the primary prevention of osteoporotic fragility fractures in postmenopausal women* (amended). Updated 2011. http://www.nice.org.uk/guidance/ta160 (accessed 23 August 2014).

5 NOGG (2014). *Guideline for the Diagnosis and Management of Osteoporosis.* Updated March 2014. http://www.shef.ac.uk/NOGG/NOGG_Pocket_Guide_for_Healthcare_Professionals.pdf (accessed 23 August 2014).

6 FRAX (2014). *WHO Fracture Risk Assessment Tool.* http://www.shef.ac.uk/FRAX/tool.aspx?country=1 (accessed 23 August 2014).

7 QFracture (2013). *Algorithm.* http://www.qfracture.org/index.php (accessed 23 August 2014).

8 NICE (2012). CKS. *Osteoporosis – Prevention of fragility fractures.* Updated September 2012. http://cks.nice.org.uk/osteoporosis-prevention-of-fragility-fractures#!topicsummary (accessed 23 August 2014).

9 NICE (2013). CG 161. *Falls: Assessment and prevention of falls in older people.* https://www.nice.org.uk/guidance/cg161 (accessed 23 August 2014).

10 NICE (2010). TA 204. *Denosumab for the Prevention of Osteoporotic Fractures in Postmenopausal Women.* http://www.nice.org.uk/guidance/ta204 (accessed 23 August 2014).

11 MHRA (2014). Strontium ranelate: cardiovascular risk – restricted indication and new monitoring requirements. *Drug Saf Update* 7: 8. http://www.mhra.gov.uk/Safetyinformation/DrugSafetyUpdate/CON392870 (accessed 23 August 2014).

12 Compston J, Seeman E (2006). Compliance with osteoporosis therapy is the weakest link. *Lancet* 368: 973–974.

Oxygen

Oxygen is regarded as a drug and must be prescribed. Various devices are used for the delivery of oxygen to the patient, usually via a pressure regulator and flow meter, which control the high pressure of oxygen delivered from the cylinder or other source.

- Nasal cannulae or simple facemasks generally deliver a higher concentration of oxygen as flow rate is increased. Nasal cannulae are generally preferred by patients as they are comfortable and allow patients to eat while *in situ*.
- Non-rebreathing or reservoir masks are used to deliver higher concentrations of oxygen (60–80% or above) in acute situations.
- Venturi masks deliver a constant oxygen concentration within and between breaths (increasing flow does not increase oxygen concentration). They are used in patients who require controlled oxygen therapy, e.g. COPD patients.

Oxygen therapy can be used in acute situations where there is hypoxia because of reduced ventilation or acute lung injury, when there is underlying chronic lung disease or when it is important to maintain oxygen delivery to tissues. A pulse oximeter is used to monitor oxygen saturation (or 'sats', i.e. the fraction of oxygen-saturated haemoglobin relative to total haemoglobin (unsaturated + saturated) in the blood). Oxygen should be prescribed to achieve a target saturation of 94–98% for most acutely ill patients or 88–92% for those at risk of hypercapnic (type 2) respiratory failure. Oxygen dosage is titrated up or down to maintain target oxygen saturation (Figure O1 gives a summary of available options for stepping dosage up or down).

Generally it is safe to use a high oxygen concentration empirically in acute situations as long as there is no risk that the patient has COPD. The main risk in some people with COPD is that CO_2 retention may occur. If COPD is suspected, the oxygen should be given via a 24% or 28% Venturi mask until arterial blood gases can be measured. Patients at risk of hypercapnic respiratory failure are advised to carry an oxygen alert card (Figure O2).[2]

Breathlessness in COPD is likely to increase on exertion, and simple everyday tasks such as washing, dressing or eating may cause problems. Some patients feel that a short burst of oxygen improves their symptoms. However, few patients benefit from this and such therapy should only be given if assessed formally.[3]

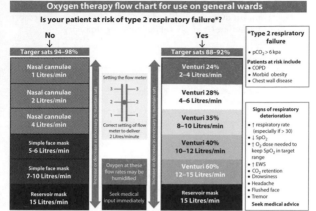

FIGURE O1   Oxygen therapy flow chart for use on general wards

---

Oxygen alert card

Name: _____

I am at risk of type II respiratory failure with a raised CO_2 level.

Please use my _____ % Venturi mask to achieve an oxygen saturation of _____ % to _____ % during exacerbations.

Use compressed air to drive nebulisers (with nasal oxygen at 2 litres/minute). If compressed air not available, limit oxygen-driven nebulisers to 6 minutes

FIGURE O2   Oxygen alert card

Chronic hypoxia

Chronic hypoxia produces a mixture of permanent and reversible structural changes in the lung. Reversal of the hypoxia in severe COPD has been found to reduce mortality if the oxygen is used for a minimum of 15 hours each day. Correction of hypoxia may have other benefits, such as reducing polycythaemia, and reducing or preventing progression of pulmonary hypertension.

Long-term oxygen therapy is indicated in patients with COPD who have a PaO_2 <7.3 kPa when stable or a PaO_2 >7.3 and <8 kPa when stable and one of: secondary polycythaemia, nocturnal hypoxaemia (oxygen saturation of arterial blood (SaO_2) is less than 90% for more than 30% of the time), peripheral oedema or pulmonary hypertension.[3]

REFERENCES

1 British Thoracic Society (BTS) (2008). Emergency Oxygen Guideline Group. Guideline for emergency oxygen use in adult patients. *Thorax* 2008; 63: Suppl VI. Available at: https://www.brit-thoracic.org.uk/document-library/clinical-information/oxygen/emergency-oxygen-use-in-adult-patients-guideline/emergency-oxygen-use-in-adult-patients-guideline/ (accessed 27 November 2014).

2 British Thoracic Society (2010). *Oxygen Alert Card.* https://www.brit-thoracic.org.uk/document-library/clinical-information/oxygen/emergency-oxygen-use-in-adult-patients-guideline/oxygen-alert-card-template/ (accessed 22 February 2015).

3 NICE (2010). CG101. *Chronic Obstructive Pulmonary Disease: Management of chronic obstructive pulmonary disease in adults in primary and secondary care* (partial update). http://www.nice.org.uk/guidance/CG101/ (accessed 27 November 2014).

O

P

Pain management

Pain is defined as 'an unpleasant sensory and emotional experience associated with actual or potential tissue damage, or described in terms of such damage'[1] and is a universal experience that has physical, psychological and social effects. The causes of pain vary considerably and can be acute (e.g. postoperative or acute injury), or persistent (e.g. lower-back pain or arthritis). Acute pain is usually associated with tissue damage and healing, whereas chronic (persistent) pain is continuous, long-term pain of more than 12 weeks, or persisting after the time that healing should have occurred.

Pain assessment

Reliable assessment of pain is essential for both clinical trials and effective pain management.[2] Unidimensional pain assessment tools only assess one aspect of pain, such as pain intensity, and are useful for acute pain. Chronic pain assessment requires assessment of the impact of pain on physical, emotional and social functions and requires multidimensional tools and health-related quality-of-life instruments.

Commonly used assessment tools for acute pain include the following:

- visual analogue score (VAS), where patients mark their pain intensity on a 10-cm line on a piece of paper, where one end of the line corresponds to no pain and the opposite end corresponds with their worst pain imaginable
- numerical rating scale (NRS), where patients rate their pain from 0 to 10, where 0 is no pain and 10 is their worst pain imaginable
- verbal rating scale (VRS), where patients are asked to rate their pain as words such as: no pain; mild; moderate; severe; excruciating.

Acute pain must be assessed both at rest (important for comfort) and during movement (important for function and risk of postoperative complications).

Many functional scales are used in persistent pain assessment. Some are disease-specific, such as the Western Ontario and MacMaster Universities for osteoarthritis, and others have more general application (e.g. the Brief Pain Inventory).

Pain rating scales specifically designed for use with children or patients with cognitive impairment or communication difficulties also exist.

Principles of pain management

In determining an initial treatment plan it is important to consider the likely cause of a patient's pain, the type of pain and its intensity, together with effectiveness of previous analgesics, which will determine drug options. Analgesic drugs may be prescribed regularly if the pain is continuous or when required if the pain is more variable. Regular reassessment is required to monitor effectiveness as analgesic requirements may change.

The management of both acute and chronic pain requires a multidisciplinary approach including anaesthetists, nurses and pharmacists. Pain management services are usually led by an experienced clinician, often with access to appropriate physiotherapy and psychological treatments.[3]

WHO analgesic ladder

The WHO analgesic ladder was introduced to improve pain control in patients with cancer pain.[4] It is a simple three-step model to guide initial selection and titration of analgesics to manage pain effectively; the pain intensity determines at which step to start.

Step 1	Step 2	Step 3
		Paracetamol and/or NSAID, plus a strong opioid, e.g. morphine, diamorphine, fentanyl
	Paracetamol and/or NSAID, plus a weak opioid, e.g. dihydrocodeine, codeine	
Paracetamol and/or NSAIDs		
Mild pain	Moderate pain	Severe pain

The principles behind the WHO analgesic ladder are:

- 'by the ladder' – according to pain intensity
- 'by the clock' – regular analgesia when required
- 'by the mouth' – the oral route is preferred
- 'by the individual' – doses should be individualised for each patient.

The principles of the WHO analgesic ladder have been applied to other types of pain, such as in the World Federation of Societies of Anaesthesiologists analgesic ladder for acute pain.[5]

Soluble analgesics may contain high sodium content, and this should be borne in mind for patients with high blood pressure and/or on a sodium-restricted diet (see *Sodium* entry).

Pharmacological treatment options for pain

Paracetamol

Despite much investigation and being used for over 50 years, the mechanism of action for paracetamol remains unclear. Paracetamol is used commonly in acute pain management; however, there is limited evidence for long-term effectiveness for persistent pain and NICE has highlighted concerns about potential harms. Paracetamol has a relatively narrow therapeutic window and it is important that the maximum dose is not exceeded (oral in adults: 1 g four times a day). The relatively recent introduction of an intravenous formulation has revolutionised surgical practice; a dose reduction is required for patients who weigh <50 kg (15 mg/kg 4–6-hourly with a maximum of 60 mg/kg/day) or who have risk factors for hepatotoxicity.

Non-steroidal anti-inflammatory drugs

NSAIDs have analgesic and anti-inflammatory effects by reducing prostaglandin synthesis by inhibiting the enzyme cyclooxygenase. However, as prostaglandins have wide-ranging physiological effects, side effects are relatively common. Well-documented side effects include GI disturbances, i.e. ulceration and bleeding, reduced kidney blood flow, prolongation of labour and bleeding. If a patient is at risk of GI side effects, e.g. elderly, history of GI ulceration, then a gastroprotective agent such as a proton pump inhibitor should be considered. The subsequent discovery of the COX-2 isoform led to design of drugs that had fewer GI adverse effects, but an increase in cardiovascular thrombotic events has become evident.[6]

Opioids

As a group, opioids have a broadly similar pharmacology, generally characterised by moderate to strong analgesia, euphoria (sometimes dysphoria), miosis, depression of the respiratory centre and cough reflex, constipation, postural hypotension, and nausea and vomiting.

Technically, an opiate refers to naturally occurring opium alkaloids, e.g. morphine, codeine and thebaine, while the term 'opioid' is properly used to describe semisynthetic or synthetic compounds acting on opiate receptors, e.g. dihydrocodeine, fentanyl.

Opioid side effects

All opioids may cause nausea, vomiting, constipation and drowsiness. It may be necessary to use other pharmacological interventions to alleviate these symptoms. Tolerance develops to some side effects (e.g. nausea and drowsiness) but not to others, particularly constipation.

Treatment with a combination of cyclizine (50 mg three times daily), metoclopramide (10 mg three times daily) or a 5-HT$_3$ receptor antagonist (e.g. ondansetron 4 mg three times daily) is usually effective for nausea and vomiting. Metoclopramide should be used for no longer than 5 days following guidance from the European

Medicines Agency to help minimise the risk of potentially serious neurological adverse effects.[7]

The combined use of a stimulant laxative (e.g. senna 15 mg at night) and a stool softener (e.g. docusate 200 mg twice daily) should be prescribed regularly for constipation.

Sedation may be most prevalent and pronounced during the first few days of therapy, and can also be related to other centrally acting drugs prescribed concomitantly, e.g. cyclizine.

Compound ('co-') analgesics

Compound preparations containing paracetamol or an NSAID and weak opioids sit at step 2 of the WHO analgesic ladder. Paracetamol in combination with low doses of a weak opioid (as in co-codamol 8/500, co-dydramol 10/500) is no more effective at controlling pain than paracetamol alone (although patient perception may differ). Only the higher-strength combinations (e.g. co-codamol 30/500) have an analgesic effect greater than paracetamol alone.[8]

Tramadol

In addition to an opioid receptor agonist, tramadol produces an analgesic effect, enhancing serotonin release and inhibiting neuronal reuptake of noradrenaline, meaning that it may be less likely to cause constipation and respiratory depression. However, it can produce convulsions and can precipitate serotonin syndrome, especially in combination with other commonly prescribed medicines, e.g. SSRIs (see *Serotonin syndrome* entry).

Morphine

Morphine is the prototypical opioid. When initiating oral morphine therapy (step 3), the usual starting dose is 5–10 mg of an immediate-release formulation every 2–4 hours when required. After dose titration to the minimum effective dose for pain control, the total amount of morphine given in the previous 24 hours may be prescribed as a modified-release formulation either once or twice daily: the first dose is given at the same time as the final dose of the immediate release form. It takes up to 5 hours to reach steady state with the modified-release formulations, making them unsuitable for 'when required' use.

The dose should be titrated to provide an adequate level of pain control *before* changing to once- or twice-daily dosing, and even then doses of immediate-release morphine should be prescribed for breakthrough pain.[9]

Exacerbations of pain (breakthrough pain)

The dose of 'when required' morphine for breakthrough pain relief should be equivalent to one-sixth of the total daily dose of morphine; or if still in the initial titration period, the dose is the same as the 4-hourly dose. If the patient has predictable movement-related pain, a dose of breakthrough analgesia may be given 30 minutes before movement, e.g. when 'turning' the patient, or before a dressing change.

Once a dose of breakthrough analgesia has been given, the patient's response should be observed after 30 minutes. If the pain has not been controlled, a further dose of breakthrough analgesic should be given, and the patient reassessed after a further 30 minutes. If there is still no relief there should be a full reassessment of the patient's analgesic requirements.

The dose of morphine for breakthrough pain should be kept constantly under review and increased in line with maintenance analgesia.

Diamorphine

Diamorphine is a lipophilic semisynthetic opioid but it has no advantages over morphine other than it has high water solubility, making it more suitable for parenteral use. Diamorphine is commonly given subcutaneously, although it may also be given using the parenteral or spinal routes.

Oxycodone

Oxycodone is another semisynthetic opioid that is available in oral, rectal and parenteral formulations. Although oxycodone does have a different receptor affinity to opioid receptor subtypes compared with morphine, its analgesic effect and side effects are still largely due to interaction with mu-opioid receptors. Oxycodone has fewer active metabolites than morphine but may still accumulate in severe renal impairment. It is considerably more expensive than morphine.

Opioid transdermal patches

Fentanyl and buprenorphine are both currently available for transdermal delivery and they may be useful when a patient cannot tolerate oral opioid administration.

Patches should be applied to a non-hairy, non-irritated and non-irradiated area of skin on a flat surface of the torso or upper arm. Areas with large areas of scar tissue should be avoided. If hair needs to be removed to create a site, it should be cut off with scissors and not shaved to avoid irritation and desquamation. If the site requires cleansing, plain water should be used (soaps, oils, lotions or any other product that might irritate the skin or affect adhesion of the patch should be avoided). The skin must be dry before application.

The patch is applied immediately after opening the outer pouch. It is peeled off from the backing film, pressed firmly to the selected site with the palm of the hand, and held in position for approximately 30 seconds. Upon removal, a new patch is applied to a different site and the previous site should not be used again for several applications.

The patient should be counselled to avoid excessive heat (e.g. heat lamps, heat pads, hot-water bottles, electric blankets, saunas or hot baths), as this may cause increases in drug release from the patch and increased systemic absorption. Similarly, patients who develop fever should be monitored for opioid side effects as an increase in body temperature may also potentially increase the release rate.[10]

Patches should never be divided or cut as this can lead to uncontrolled release of the drug. Any damaged, used or unwanted patches should be made unusable by folding the patch in half, adhesive side inwards, and discarding it safely (as clinical waste in secondary care). The hands should be washed after handling.

Fentanyl

The starting dose for a fentanyl patch is based on an assessment of the patient's clinical condition and recent opioid history. If the patient is opioid-naïve the maximum starting dose is 25 micrograms/hour. If the patient has previously received opioids, Table P1 may be used as a guide for initial selection of a suitable strength of fentanyl patch.[11]

TABLE P1
Fentanyl patch analgesic equivalence

Fentanyl patch (microgram/hour)	Oral 24-hour morphine (mg/day) (or equivalent)
25	<135
50	135–224
75	225–314
100	315–404
125	405–494
150	495–584
175	585–674
200	675–764
225	765–854
250	855–944
275	945–1034
300	1035–1124

It takes 24 hours to reach maximum analgesic effect, hence the analgesic effect should not be assessed until 24 hours after application of the first patch; previous analgesic therapy should be phased out over this period (e.g. if switching from morphine sulfate modified-release tablets to fentanyl patches, the first patch is applied when the final dose of morphine sulfate modified-release tablets is taken).

Patients may still require additional analgesia for breakthrough pain. In order to calculate the total morphine (or opioid equivalent) requirement for this, 25 micrograms/hour fentanyl patch ≈ 60 mg/day oral morphine, e.g. a patient with a 100 micrograms/hour fentanyl patch is receiving approximately 240 mg/day of oral morphine equivalence, so would require one-sixth of this dose for breakthrough pain, i.e. 40 mg oral morphine.

Buprenorphine

Buprenorphine is a highly lipophilic semisynthetic opioid with complex pharmacology (see *Opioid partial agonists* entry).

There are two different formulations that are intended for 7-day (5, 10 and 20 micrograms/hour) and twice-weekly (35, 52.5 and 70 micrograms/hour) application. Relative potency compared with other commonly used opioids is shown in Table P2.[9]

TABLE P2
Buprenorphine patch analgesic equivalence

	Strength of buprenorphine patch					
	5 micrograms/ hour	10 micrograms/ hour	20 micrograms/ hour	35 micrograms/ hour	52.5 micrograms/ hour	70 micrograms/ hour
Oral codeine	120 mg daily	240 mg daily				
Oral tramadol		100 mg daily	200 mg daily	400 mg daily		
Oral morphine	12 mg daily	24 mg daily	48 mg daily	84 mg daily	126 mg daily	168 mg daily

It takes at least 24 hours to achieve the full analgesic effect following the first application, so assessment of therapy should not be made until after this time.

P

Persistent pain

Persistent pain is a complex neurophysiological phenomenon with biopsychosocial contributing factors. A wide range of treatments, including medicines, stimulation (TENS, acupuncture, ultrasound, massage and spinal cord stimulation), nerve blocks and ablative neurosurgical techniques (e.g. sympathectomy or cordotomy) are used.

Neuropathic pain

Neuropathic pain is pain caused by damage or disease that affects the somatosensory system and does not respond well to conventional analgesics. Several antidepressants and antiepileptic drugs have been used to treat neuropathic pain.[12] Some of the drugs are licensed for this indication (e.g. duloxetine, carbamazepine, gabapentin and pregabalin); however, other drugs (e.g. amitriptyline and lamotrigine) are not and it is useful to know typical doses.

- Amitriptyline: usual starting doses are between 10 and 25 mg, taken in the evening (90 minutes to 2 hours before retiring to bed). Gradual dose titration to 50–75 mg daily may be required for maximum efficacy and tolerability.
- Lamotrigine: suggested dosing regimen starts at 25 mg daily for 1 week, then the dose is doubled at weekly intervals to a maximum of 400 mg daily in two divided doses. If analgesia is achieved using lower doses, then no further increase is necessary.

Neuropathic pain responds variably to strong opioids. It may be necessary to use several other medicines concurrently, necessitating polypharmacy, with its resulting problems with drug interactions and side effects.

Topical capsaicin (cream and patch) is licensed for neuropathic pain. Great care must be taken in its use to avoid inadvertent application to the eyes and broken or inflamed skin. An intense burning sensation may occur following initial application.

Adjuvant medicines for muscle spasticity

Skeletal muscle relaxants (e.g. baclofen, tizanidine) may be of use in spasticity and associated pain but usefulness is usually limited. Depending on the effects on the relative tone of extensor and flexor muscles, spasticity may be adversely affected by treatment.

REFERENCES

1 International Association for the Study of Pain (2014). http://www.iasp-pain.org/ Taxonomy?navItemNumber=576#Pain (accessed 23 November 2014).

2 Breivik H *et al.* (2008). Assessment of pain. *Br J Anaesth* 101: 17–24.

3 Royal College of Anaesthetists (2014). *Guidance on the Provision of Anaesthesia Services for Chronic Pain Management.* Available at https://www.rcoa.ac.uk/system /files/GPAS-2014-12-CHRONICPAIN.pdf (accessed 22 November 2014).

4 WHO (1986). *Cancer Pain Relief.* Geneva: WHO.

5 Charlton E (1997). The management of postoperative pain. *Update Anaesth* 7(2): 1–7.

6 Coxib and Traditional NSAID Trialists' (CNT) Collaboration (2013). Vascular and upper gastrointestinal effects of non-steroidal anti-inflammatory drugs: meta-analyses of individual participant data from randomised trials. *Lancet* 382: 769–779.

7 *Drug Safety Update* 2013; 7: issue 1 S2.

8 Moore SA *et al.*(1997). Paracetamol with or without codeine in acute pain: a quantitative, systematic review. *Pain* 70: 193–201.

9 NICE (2012). Clinical Guideline 140. *Opioids in Palliative Care: Safe and effective prescribing of strong opioids for pain in palliative care of adults.* http://www.nice.org.uk/guidance/cg140 (accessed 26 November 2014).

10 Joint Formulary Committee (2014). *British National Formulary* (68th edn). London: BMJ Group and Pharmaceutical Press.

11 Electronic Medicines Companion (2014). http://www.medicines.org.uk/emc/ (accessed 23 November 2014).

12 NICE (2013). Clinical Guideline 173. *Neuropathic Pain – Pharmacological management: The pharmacological management of neuropathic pain in adults in non-specialist settings.* http://www.nice.org.uk/guidance/cg173 (accessed 25 November 2014).

Palliative and end-of-life care

Palliative care is used to describe care that is given to patients with any advanced progressive disease that impacts on their physical, psychosocial and spiritual well-being. The aim of palliative care is to improve the quality of life of patients, their families and carers through preventing and relieving suffering, e.g. physical symptoms such as pain, by means of early identification, assessment and evidence-based treatments. Cancer patients remain one of the largest groups who receive palliative care; however, it is increasingly being provided to patients with other advanced progressive diseases, such as COPD, cardiovascular, renal or hepatic disease, HIV/AIDS and motor neurone disease.

End-of-life care encompasses the principles of palliative care and is provided to people who are likely to die within the next 12 months. This includes people whose death is imminent (expected within a few hours or days), e.g. as a result of disease progression or a life-threatening acute event such as head trauma.

Medications remain a significant part of the care given to relieve symptoms and will be the focus of this entry. Other therapies include radiotherapy, physiotherapy, and complementary therapies. For more information, see Further reading, below.

Pharmacy and palliative care

Pharmacy professionals in all sectors of healthcare are likely to come into contact with palliative care patients at some time. They are ideally placed to provide the following support:

- information about medications and their side effects; effective management can avoid unnecessary readmission, which is often not the wish of the dying patient or carers
- offering the patient and carer ways to keep their list of medications up to date to facilitate medicines reconciliation, for example when attending an outpatient appointment to review the dose of a strong opioid, or following admission to hospital with a syringe pump where urgent knowledge of the contents is required
- understand the importance of timely access to medications for end-of-life care, and may have processes in place that allow injectable medications for symptom control to be available in the place where the patient wishes to be cared for.

Pharmacy members of staff are encouraged to make contact with their local palliative care team. This will facilitate a multidisciplinary approach to care as well as shared learning concerning the issues above. Palliative care teams will often have a specialist pharmacist who can target support to pharmacy teams working in all healthcare settings.

Medication treatment of symptoms – overview

Table P3 lists the estimated prevalence of symptoms seen in cancer patients.[1]

This section will focus on three of the main symptoms: pain, constipation, and nausea and vomiting. For information on the treatment of other symptoms, for example, fatigue, delirium, shortness of breath, oral problems, confusion and the last hours and days, see Further reading, below.

Pain

The principles of managing chronic pain follow the recommendations of the WHO analgesic ladder (see *Pain management* entry). This

TABLE P3
Prevalence of symptoms in cancer patients

Symptom	Prevalence (%)
Pain	50–70
Weight loss	45–70
Fatigue	40–50
Anorexia	40–75
Insomnia	30–60
Constipation	25–50
Depression	20–30
Nausea and vomiting	15–45
Dyspnoea	20–50
Anxiety	10

stepwise approach to the use of analgesic medications allows optimal pain control with minimal side effects in up to 80% of cancer patients.

Not all pain is completely opioid-sensitive. Knowing the cause of the pain may determine a more logical choice and dosage of medication; for example, prescribing a tricyclic antidepressant can be helpful in neuropathic pain. These kinds of medication are known as 'adjuvant analgesics' and can be used at any stage of the analgesic ladder; they may not be primarily analgesic in their mechanism of action, but have analgesic effects in certain pain conditions.

This approach can allow the choice and dose of other analgesics the patient is taking to be reviewed; for example, a lower dose of opioid may be sufficient for the pain, avoid unnecessary side effects and help the patient to adhere to treatment. In some cases, adjuvant analgesics alone can provide adequate pain relief.

Table P4 lists different adjuvant analgesics and the pain conditions they may be considered for.

TABLE P4
Adjuvant analgesics in palliative care

Adjuvant analgesic	Type of pain	Examples of medication(s) and typical starting doses
Antidepressants and antiepileptics	Neuropathic (e.g. tumour infiltration, spinal cord compression, radio- or chemotherapy-induced damage)	• Amitriptyline 10 mg at night • Gabapentin 300 mg at night (in elderly/frail consider 100 mg) • Pregabalin 75 mg twice daily (in elderly/frail consider 25–50 mg twice daily)
Bisphosphonates	Metastatic bone pain persisting despite analgesics and radiotherapy	• Disodium pamidronate • Several regimens exist, for example, 90 mg every 3–4 weeks for as long as benefit is maintained

(Continued)

TABLE P4
(Continued)

Adjuvant analgesic	Type of pain	Examples of medication(s) and typical starting doses
Corticosteroids	Pain and weakness associated with: • Nerve root compression • Spinal cord compression	• Dexamethasone 4–8 mg/day • Dexamethasone 12–16 mg/day
N-methyl-D-aspartate (NMDA) receptor channel blockers	Neuropathic pain unresponsive to standard analgesics	• Ketamine and methadone given under specialist supervision
Skeletal muscle relaxants	Painful skeletal muscle spasm (e.g. tumour infiltration, cramp, myofascial pain)	• Baclofen 5 mg two to three times daily • Diazepam 2 mg at night
Smooth-muscle relaxants (antispasmodics)	Visceral distension pain and colic (e.g. tumour infiltration of an organ or the bowel wall, respectively)	• Hyoscine butylbromide 20 mg subcutaneous injection stat, then 20–60 mg/day as a continuous subcutaneous infusion • Avoid oral route due to poor oral bioavailability

The concept of 'total pain' has physical, psychological (e.g. anxiety and depression that affect the perception and intensity of pain), social (e.g. financial concerns or isolation) and spiritual (e.g. religious struggle as what is happening goes against the person's beliefs) components that require management in order to gain control of the patient's pain. It is important for the pharmacy team to understand this multidisciplinary approach to treating pain.

Starting a patient on a strong opioid

The term 'strong opioid' refers to medications on step 3 of the analgesic ladder and includes morphine, oxycodone, alfentanil and fentanyl in the treatment of severe pain. When starting a patient on a strong opioid it is important to consider choice of strong opioid, dose and route of administration.

Initial dose titration

First-line: use regular oral immediate-release morphine:

- 5 mg oral immediate-release morphine 4-hourly, and
- 5 mg oral immediate-release morphine 4-hourly when required for rescue doses during the titration phase.

Consider reducing the dose in elderly/frail patients, for example a 50% dose reduction.

Seek specialist advice when using strong opioids in patients with moderate to severe renal impairment (particularly if creatinine clearance is ≤30 mL/min). The patient should be reviewed regularly (e.g. daily) with regard to pain control and adverse effects.

Dose increments are not normally >30% of the previous dose. When the optimal balance of pain control and side effects has been reached the patient should be prescribed maintenance treatment. Specialist advice should be sought if this balance is not reached after a few dose adjustments.

Maintenance treatment

First-line: use oral modified-release morphine. Once pain is controlled the total amount of oral immediate-release morphine given in the last 24-hour period is added up, then divided into two 12-hour release morphine doses, for example:

- 5 mg oral immediate-release morphine 4-hourly = 30 mg oral morphine in 24 hours. This is converted to 15 mg oral modified-release morphine twice daily.

Management of breakthrough pain

First-line: use oral immediate-release morphine as rescue medication for breakthrough pain in patients on maintenance oral morphine. One-sixth of the total daily dose of morphine should be prescribed as the 'when required' dose (4-hourly as required).

Specialist advice should be sought if the breakthrough dose is not effective.

Communication

When patients are started on a strong opioid, aim to discuss any concerns regarding:

- side effects
- the idea that the introduction of opioids implies the final stages of life or hastens death (neither of these is correct)
- addiction and tolerance – both of which are rare and do not significantly affect pain management in the majority of patients.

Offer verbal and written information to patients and carers on strong opioids, including:

- when and why strong opioids are used to treat pain
- how to take strong opioids for background and breakthrough pain, and how long pain relief should last
- side effects and signs of toxicity and what to do if they appear
- safe storage and disposal of unwanted medication.

Check the patient and carer have information on out-of-hours contacts and planned follow-up by their specialist.

Treatment if oral opioids are not suitable

Oral opioids may be unsuitable:

- for people with swallowing difficulties
- when oral absorption is impaired
- when pain is unstable
- for 'tablet phobia' or poor adherence with oral medication.

If oral opioids are not suitable, consideration should be given to alternative routes, including transdermal, transmucosal and subcutaneous.

Transdermal opioid patches

Caution should be used when calculating the opioid equivalence for transdermal opioid patches, e.g. a fentanyl 12 micrograms/hour patch equates to approximately 45 mg oral morphine daily.

It is important to remember that opioid conversion charts are an approximate guide only.

It can take up to 2 days after starting a transdermal opioid patch, or changing the dose, for the full effect to be seen. Switching between opioid preparations should be timed correctly so that pain remains controlled and side effects are avoided. Patients should always be reviewed regularly following a change from one opioid to another.

Table P5 details the main safety facts to consider when using transdermal opioid patches.

TABLE P5
Safety considerations of opioid patches

Fentanyl transdermal patches
- Remove the patch and replace every 3 days
- A range of generic products is available; no clinical difference exists between products

Buprenorphine transdermal patches
- Remove and replace patches once a week (7-day patch: BuTrans), or twice a week (4-day patch: Transtec)
- The 4-day patch can be replaced on fixed days in the week, i.e. after 3 and 4 days

Patches have a long duration of action
- Clinically significant levels of opioid can remain in the blood for up to 30 hours after patch removal

Do not cut patches in half
- Absorption may not be uniform across the surface area of the patch once cut

Factors affecting drug absorption from patches
- Pyrexia or external heat can increase absorption
- Absorption may be reduced in cachectic patients

Old patches still contain medication
- Dispose of carefully; fold in two with the medication side of the plaster facing inwards

Switching to an alternative strong opioid

Morphine remains the first-line strong opioid of choice. Patients who are unable to tolerate morphine or where adequate pain relief is not achieved may be considered for an alternative strong opioid, e.g. oxycodone. Specialist advice should be sought in these cases and a clear record of the reason(s) for switching made in the patient's clinical notes.

Management of the side effects of strong opioids
Constipation

All patients starting a strong opioid medication should be considered for a regular laxative. See section below on constipation.

Nausea

Transient nausea may occur when starting strong opioid treatment or when the dose is increased. A 'when required' antiemetic should be considered in these situations. Optimise antiemetic treatment before considering switching opioids.

Drowsiness

Transient and mild drowsiness or impaired concentration may occur when opioid treatment is started or when the dose is increased.

Patients should be warned that impaired concentration may affect their ability to drive and undertake manual tasks safely. The Driver and Vehicle Licensing Agency has produced guidance addressing medications and fitness to drive.[2] Check with your local palliative care team for a patient information leaflet on driving with strong opioids (see *DVLA: advice concerning medication and medical conditions* entry).

In patients with either persistent or moderate to severe central nervous system side effects consideration should be given to:

- reducing the dose of the opioid if the pain is controlled.
- switching to an alternative opioid if the pain is not controlled.

If adverse effects remain uncontrolled despite optimising treatment, the patient should be referred to the palliative care team.

Constipation

Palliative care patients are particularly susceptible to constipation due to a variety of causes. Table P6 lists some of these.

TABLE P6
Factors influencing constipation in palliative patients

Organic factors	Functional factors
- **Pharmacological:** antacids, antimuscarinics, antidepressants, antidiarrhoeals, antiemetics ($5HT_3$ antagonists), opioids, antiepileptics, antihypertensives, antiparkinsonians, antitussives, chemotherapy (vinca alkaloids and platinum-based chemotherapy), proton pump inhibitors, diuretics and neuroleptics - **Metabolic:** dehydration, hypercalcaemia, hypokalaemia, hypothyroidism, uraemia and diabetes - **Neurological:** cerebral tumours, spinal cord involvement, sacral nerve pathology and autonomic failure - **Structural:** pelvic tumour mass, radiation fibrosis, painful anorectum (haemorrhoids, anal fissure or perianal abscess) and uncontrolled pain of any cause	- **Diet:** reduced food/ fibre/fluid intake - **Environmental:** lack of privacy, comfort or assistance with going to the toilet - **Other:** reduced physical activity, dyspnoea preventing effective straining, depression and sedation

The aims of treatment are:

- re-establish comfortable bowel habits the patient is satisfied with
- relieve pain and discomfort
- restore independence in relation to bowel habits
- prevent or reduce related symptoms: nausea and vomiting, abdominal bloating and pain.

Most cases of constipation in palliative care, including opioid-induced constipation, are best treated with a combination of a stimulant laxative and softening laxative, for example:

- stimulant: senna tablets 7.5–15 mg orally twice daily or senna syrup (7.5 mg/5 mL) 10–20 mL twice daily
- softener: docusate 100–200 mg orally twice daily or macrogol oral powder 1–3 sachets daily in divided doses. Macrogol oral powder given in higher dosage is also used to treat faecal loading/impaction.

If tablet burden is an issue, consider a combined stimulant and softener preparation, for example:

- co-danthramer: 1–2 capsules twice daily or suspension 2.5–5 mL twice daily
- co-danthramer strong: 1–2 capsules twice daily or suspension 2.5–5 mL twice daily.

Patients who do not respond to oral laxatives or where the oral route is inappropriate should be considered for second-line rectal treatment. There are specific clinical situations that should also be considered in the palliative care patient, for example:

- faecal incontinence: danthron (in co-danthramer) should be avoided due to the risk of local skin burn
- bowel obstruction or colic: stimulant laxatives should be avoided
- opioid-induced constipation unresponsive to oral and rectal measures: consider methylnaltrexone injection.

When treating constipation in the dying patient, bowel function may become less of a priority compared to other symptoms as the patient's functional status and conscious level deteriorate. The oral route may become inappropriate.

Nausea and vomiting
Knowledge of the likely cause(s) of nausea and vomiting and the nerve pathways involved provides a useful starting point when deciding on the most appropriate antiemetic. A single antiemetic may be adequate to control symptoms; however, 25% of patients will require a combination of medications. Reversible causes should be treated, e.g. infection, cough, hypercalcaemia, tense ascites (causing excessive pressure on the stomach and bowel), raised intracranial

pressure, emetogenic medications, the sight and smell of foods and anxiety can all exacerbate symptoms.

Table P7 lists possible causes of nausea and vomiting and the antiemetics that may be considered.

TABLE P7

Antiemetics in palliative care

Nerve pathway involved	Possible causes	Consider treatment with
Chemoreceptor trigger zone (D_2, $5HT_3$, acetylcholine) lies outside of the blood–brain barrier and susceptible to chemical changes in the blood	Medications (e.g. opioids, NSAIDs, antibiotics), metabolic (e.g. hypercalcaemia, renal failure) and toxicity (e.g. chemotherapy, radiotherapy)	Haloperidol Metoclopramide Domperidone Granisetron Ondansetron
Gut mucosa (D_2, $5HT_3$, acetylcholine, NK1)	Delayed gastric emptying, gastrointestinal obstruction, colic, tumour mass, gastric irritation and constipation	Metoclopramide, domperidone (prokinetics are contraindicated if colic present or bowel is obstructed), levomepromazine, granisetron/ondansetron, aprepitant, a gastroprotectant and suitable laxative(s). Octreotide may be considered for bowel obstruction associated with large-volume vomits (under specialist supervision)
Vestibular apparatus (H_1, acetylcholine)	Motion sickness	Cyclizine, hyoscine hydrobromide
Cerebral cortex	Emotions, sights, smells and raised intracranial pressure. Repetitive stimulation can lead to 'anticipatory' nausea and vomiting (a type of conditioned behaviour that can be difficult to treat)	Dexamethasone, benzodiazepines

Further reading

Centre for Pharmacy Postgraduate Education (2012). *Palliative Care – An open learning programme for pharmacists and pharmacy technicians*. www.cppe.ac.uk/learning/Details.asp?TemplateID =PALLIATIVE-P-02&Format=P&ID=115&EventID=42008 (accessed 26 April 2015).

Help the Hospices (2011). *Current Learning in Palliative Care –* online tutorials. http://www.hospiceuk.org/what-we-offer/courses-conferences-and-learning-events/e-learning (accessed 15 May 2015).

NICE (2014) *Clinical Knowledge Summaries*. http://cks.nice.org.uk/ (accessed 26 April 2015).

SIGN (2008). *Control of Pain in Adults with Cancer*. Edinburgh: SIGN.

Twycross R, Wilcock A (eds) (2012). *Palliative Care Formulary* (4th edn). Nottingham: Palliativedrugs.com.

Watson M *et al.* (eds) *Palliative Care Adult Network Guidelines Plus*. http://book.pallcare.info/ (accessed 22 September 2015).

REFERENCES

1 Grond S *et al.* (1994). Prevalence and pattern of symptoms in patients with cancer pain: a prospective evaluation of 1635 cancer patients referred to a pain clinic. *J Pain Symptom Manage* 31: 58–69.

2 Department of Transport (2014). *Guidance for Healthcare Professionals on Drug Driving*. https://www.gov.uk/government/publications/drug-driving-and-medicine-advice-for-healthcare-professionals (accessed 21 September 2014).

Pancreatitis

Pancreatitis is an inflammation of the pancreas. This organ plays a vital digestive role in producing enzymes that help to break down food in the small bowel.[1] When inflammation and scarring of the pancreas occur, such as in pancreatitis, the organ is unable to function optimally, which may result in a patient being unable to digest fat and key elements of food.

Types of pancreatitis

There are two types of pancreatitis:

1 acute: where the inflammation may be sudden, after which the pancreas returns to normal
2 chronic (ongoing): where there is a long-standing functional deficit of the pancreas. Chronic pancreatitis is characterised by disabling pain and progressive endocrine and exocrine insufficiency.

Endocrine pancreatic insufficiency results from damage to the endocrine tissue of the pancreatic gland (islets of Langerhans), with failure to produce insulin causing glucose intolerance and diabetes mellitus.[2] Exocrine pancreatic insufficiency results from damage to the acinar cells (exocrine tissue of the pancreatic gland), with failure to produce digestive enzymes causing maldigestion and malabsorption.

Risk factors

Risk factors include the following:

- alcohol: accounts for 70–90% of all cases of chronic pancreatitis, although the exact mechanism is unknown. Only 5–10% of heavy drinkers develop chronic pancreatitis, suggesting that important cofactors are involved

- gallstones: stones of hardened bile that form in a patient's biliary ducts
- idiopathic: chronic pancreatitis is classified as idiopathic after all other possible causes have been ruled out
- autoimmune disease
- obstructive causes
- radiotherapy
- smoking: raises the risk for pancreatic calcification that results in pancreatic duct obstruction and pancreatic tissue damage
- medications: several can cause pancreatitis, including:
  - sodium valproate
  - azathioprine
  - furosemide
  - corticosteroids
  - angiotensin-converting enzyme inhibitors
  - statins
  - didanosine
  - lamivudine
  - oral contraceptives
  - interferon
  - exenatide.

Signs and symptoms of pancreatitis

Symptoms of acute and chronic pancreatitis include severe pain in the upper abdomen, loss of appetite, nausea and vomiting, fever, and swollen tender abdomen.

Additional symptoms for chronic pancreatitis include:

- steatorrhoea, which presents as pale-coloured, oily faeces. This presentation is as a result of the reduced production and secretion of pancreatic enzymes, thereby causing nutrient malabsorption. Malabsorption of all macronutrients occurs; however, fat malabsorption tends to be the most clinically evident.
- failure to gain weight despite routine eating habits and calorie intake. Other symptoms of malabsorption that are less obvious are bloating, flatulence and nausea. Bloating and wind may be due to the passage of undigested carbohydrate into the colon, where fermentation by the colonic flora occurs.

Diagnosis

For a formal diagnosis of pancreatitis the following tests are undertaken:

- pancreatic elastase-1 (faecal elastase) is an enzyme that is not degraded during intestinal transit, is enriched five- to sixfold in the faeces, and is therefore a good test of pancreatic exocrine function[3]
- serum amylase is a digestive enzyme that can be at least three times the normal level in acute pancreatitis
- serum IgG$_4$ is used for diagnosing autoimmune pancreatitis

- serum lipase, a protein released by the pancreas into the small intestine. It assists in the absorption of fat
- serum trypsinogen is produced in the pancreas and released into the small intestine and converted to trypsin, which then starts the process of breaking proteins down to amino acids
- imaging is useful if the above are indeterminate as inflammation, calcium deposits of the pancreas, or changes to the ducts of the pancreas may be seen on an abdominal CT scan.

Treatment

The treatment goals of pancreatitis are to correct the underlying cause, relieve pain and treat malabsorption and impaired blood glucose control. The treatment plan involves a multidisciplinary approach with surgeons, dieticians, endocrinologists, diabetologists, substance misuse specialists and pharmacists, amongst others.

Pain

Pain, secondary to pancreatitis, classically presents as generalised severe abdominal pain at times associated with intense back pain. It is often persistent and refractory to simple analgesia and so at times necessitates admission to hospital to optimise control. There are no current NICE or SIGN guidelines with associated grading for the pharmacological management of this symptom in pancreatitis. Typically the pharmaceutical analgesic plan involves pain control titrated according to the WHO ladder principle (see *Pain management* entry), but in some situations and commonly in acute presentations a top-down approach may be useful to control pain. Adjuvant analgesics, such as amitriptyline, gabapentin or pregabalin, should be considered at an early stage and combinations of drugs are often used. Pancreatic enzyme therapy such as Creon, somatostatin analogues such as octreotide and various antioxidants (vitamins A, D, E or selenium) may be considered as supplements to conventional analgesics in special situations.[4]

Pancreatic enzyme therapy

This has been the subject of several randomised trials and meta-analyses. The proposed mechanism of action is the ability to degrade cholecystokinin (CCK)-releasing factor in the duodenum and thereby lower levels of CCK.[5] An elevated level of CCK has been reported in pancreatitis patients and may generate pain by increasing the pressure in the pancreatic duct.

Somatostatin analogues

Somatostatin analogues inhibit pancreatic secretion by blocking CCK and secretin release and also by a direct inhibitory effect on acinar cells. Whilst an early pilot series of subcutaneous octreotide at a dose of 100 micrograms three times a day showed an effect on pain control, this effect could not be confirmed in a double-blind cross-over study enrolling pancreatitis patients treated with octreotide or placebo.[6]

P

Antioxidants

The proposed analgesic mechanism of action underlying this therapy is an anti-inflammatory and blocking effect of free radicals.[7] The current evidence base in pancreatitis, however, is not sufficient to recommend antioxidant therapy.

Malabsorption

Exocrine insufficiency develops in up to 40% of people with chronic pancreatitis, and can cause malabsorption of fat-soluble vitamins, such as vitamin D.[8]

The deficiency of fat-soluble vitamins appears to have a variable prevalence, and therefore, biochemical assessment of serum fat-soluble vitamin levels is advised and 'blind' routine supplementation should be avoided.

Aggressive nutrition support, such as enteral nutrition, at times is required if malabsorption is severe. Parenteral nutrition is necessary in <1% of cases. Indications include gastric outlet obstruction and when jejunal access is unachievable, complex pancreatic fistulae, and in the severely malnourished patient pre-surgery, where enteral feeding is not possible.

Pancreatic enzyme insufficiency

Pancreatic enzyme replacement therapy (PERT) is recommended by NICE for people with alcohol-related chronic pancreatitis and who have steatorrhoea or have a poor nutritional status, and this recommendation can be reasonably extrapolated to chronic pancreatitis with other causes.[9]

Patients with pancreatic insufficiency need to receive an appropriate dose of PERT, usually starting with a dose of 40 000–50 000 units lipase per meal and 10 000–25 000 units lipase per snack; this is increased in a stepwise manner depending on the patient's response.

Suppression of stomach acid with, for example, a proton pump inhibitor is often required as pancreatic enzymes are denatured at a low pH. Fortunately the majority of pancreatic enzymes on the market are enteric-coated and so are only released once in the high pH of the small bowel.

Blood glucose control

The development of diabetes occurs late into the onset of pancreatitis and occurs as a result of damage to the pancreatic alpha cells (which produce glucagon) and to the islet cells (which produce insulin).

The diabetes that results secondary to pancreatitis should be referred to as type 3 but is often misclassified as type 1 or 2, although it is distinctly different from both of these.[10] Typically those with type 3 diabetes are older than those with type 1 diabetes and have a lower BMI than in type 2 diabetes.

Many patients with type 3 diabetes have difficulty with glucose control. The combination of glucagon deficiency, malnutrition and alcohol intake increases the risk of spontaneous hypoglycaemia.

Hyperglycaemia is also frequent due to unsuppressed hepatic glucose production.

Oral hypoglycaemic drugs are often used for as long as possible due to the risk of insulin-induced hypoglycaemia.

REFERENCES

1 BUPA (2014). *Health Topics: Pancreatitis*. http://www.bupa.co.uk/health-information/directory/p/pancreatitis (accessed 24 July 2014).

2 Kocher HM (2008). Chronic pancreatitis. *Am Fam Physician* 77: 661–662.

3 NICE (2010). *Clinical Knowledge Summaries. Chronic Pancreatitis*. http://cks.nice.org.uk/pancreatitis-chronic (accessed 17 July 2014).

4 Paisley P, Kinsella J (2014). Pharmacological management of pain in chronic pancreatitis. *Scot Med J* 59: 71–79.

5 Olesen S *et al.* (2013). Pharmacological pain management in chronic pancreatitis. *World J Gastroenterol* 19: 7292–7301.

6 Bai Y *et al.* (2008). Prophylactic octreotide administration does not prevent post-endoscopic retrograde cholangiopancreatography pancreatitis: a meta-analysis of randomized controlled trials. *Pancreas* 37: 241–246.

7 Bhardwaj P *et al.* (2009). A randomized controlled trial of antioxidant supplementation for pain relief in patients with chronic pancreatitis. *Gastroenterology* 136: 149–159.

8 Duggan SN, Conlon KC (2013). A practical guide to the nutritional management of chronic pancreatitis. *Pract Gastroenterol* 24–32.

9 Borman P, Beckingham I (2001). ABC of diseases of liver, pancreas and biliary system. *BMJ* 322: 660–663.

10 Cui Y, Andersen DK (2011). Pancreatogenic diabetes: special considerations for management. *Pancreatology* 11: 279–294.

P

Parenteral nutrition: a practical overview

Parenteral nutrition (PN) is used to provide the nutritional needs of patients where there is a failure of the GI tract to perform its normal function of processing and absorbing food, e.g. short-bowel syndrome. It can also be used where enteral nutrition is insufficient to maintain nutritional status, e.g. malabsorption. NICE guidance states that PN should be considered for people who are malnourished or are at risk of being malnourished and meet either of the following criteria:

- inadequate or unsafe oral and/or enteral nutritional intake
- a non-functional, inaccessible or perforated (leaking) GI tract.[1]

PN is not an emergency intervention in adults and there is rarely an indication to start it out of hours or at the weekend.[2] PN is not without risk, e.g. line sepsis, metabolic disorders, compromised immune function, thrombosis and air embolus. Hospitals should have written guidance for the initiation and management of PN and it is important to be aware of these.[2]

PN mixtures can be administered via a peripheral or a central venous catheter. Peripheral lines are most often used if PN is anticipated to last up to 2 weeks. Peripheral cannulas need resiting every 1–2 days.[1] Central venous catheters are used if PN is to be prolonged or in intensive care settings where central lines are used routinely. Central venous catheters should be inserted under sterile conditions and the position of the catheter tip must be confirmed radiologically prior to commencing therapy.[3] Following insertion it is important that the line is cared for correctly to minimise the risk of infection and a lumen should be dedicated to the PN.[2]

A baseline assessment of a range of biochemical markers (Table P8) is needed prior to treatment. The patient's weight should be recorded and nutritional requirements documented in the medical notes. These markers will then need regular reviews, the frequency of which will depend on the individual marker, whether the patient is considered metabolically stable or not, and for any other reason specific to that patient.[3]

TABLE P8
Monitoring parameters

Parameter	Frequency
Sodium, potassium, urea, creatinine	Baseline Daily until stable, then twice weekly
Weight	Baseline Daily until stable and then weekly
Magnesium, phosphate	Baseline Daily if risk of refeeding syndrome Three times a week until stable, then weekly
LFTs	Baseline Twice weekly until stable, then weekly
Glucose	Baseline Once or twice per day (or more if needed) until stable, then weekly
Calcium, albumin	Baseline Weekly
CRP	Baseline Two or three times per week
Zinc, copper	Baseline Every 2–4 weeks depending on result
Iron, ferritin	Baseline Every 3–6 months
Folate, vitamin B_{12}	Baseline Every 2–4 weeks

Refeeding syndrome

The reason for close monitoring, particularly in the first few days, is the concern of refeeding syndrome. As the name suggests, this syndrome can occur when feeding is recommenced, either enterally or parenterally following a period of starvation. During a period of starvation, various electrolytes are lost and there is compensatory movement of the electrolytes, i.e. magnesium, calcium and phosphate, from the cells into the plasma to maintain near-normal plasma levels. When feeding recommences there is an increase in insulin production that causes these electrolytes to move intracellularly and their serum concentrations consequently fall.

The syndrome is characterised by hypophosphataemia, hypomagnesaemia, hypocalcaemia and fluid retention, and there may be a thiamine deficiency, particularly if the patient has a history of alcohol abuse. This can lead to congestive heart failure and life-threatening arrhythmias.

PN for people at high risk of developing refeeding problems should consider:

- starting nutrition support at a maximum of 10 kcal/kg/day, increasing levels slowly to meet or exceed full needs by 4–7 days
- using only 5 kcal/kg/day in extreme cases (for example, BMI $<14\,kg/m^2$ or negligible intake for more than 15 days)
- providing immediately before and during the first 10 days of feeding: oral thiamine 200–300 mg daily (or full-dose daily intravenous vitamin B preparation, if necessary), and a balanced multivitamin/trace element supplement once daily
- providing oral, enteral or intravenous supplements of potassium, phosphate and magnesium unless prefeeding plasma levels are high. Prefeeding correction of low plasma levels is unnecessary.

Monitoring

Baseline measurements should be taken prior to commencement of PN and should then be measured at the intervals shown in Table P8.[1]

The frequency of monitoring of these parameters may also depend on the individual patient. For instance, glucose readings may need to be performed hourly until glycaemic control is achieved in a patient who is metabolically unstable and has impaired glucose tolerance. The patient may need a sliding-scale insulin regimen prescribed to aid glycaemic control. Electrolyte readings may need to be more frequent if the patient shows evidence of refeeding syndrome or other electrolyte disturbances.[4]

It is important that the overall clinical well-being of the patient is taken into account as this can be an indication of an improvement in the patient's condition, or the first sign of a PN-related complication developing.

Drug interactions

Drugs should not be added to the PN admixture, either directly to the bag or via the same catheter. It is imperative that the lumen is dedicated for the PN infusion administration.

The bag should be protected from direct light, so consideration should be given to making sure the patient is not beside a window, or that the PN bag is covered with a bag made of a light-protecting material.

REFERENCES
1 NICE (2006). *Nutrition Support in Adults: Oral nutrition support, enteral tube feeding and parenteral nutrition*. CG32 http://www.nice.org.uk/guidance/cg32/chapter/guidance (accessed 30 September 2014).
2 NCEPOD (2010). *Parenteral Nutrition: A mixed bag*. http://www.ncepod.org.uk/2010pn.htm (accessed 30 September 2014).
3 British Society of Gastroenterology (1996). *Guidelines on Artificial Nutritional Support*. http://www.bsg.org.uk/pdf_word_docs/art_nutrit.pdf (accessed 30 September 2014).
4 *Medicines Information Leaflet* (2001). Oxford: Oxford Radcliffe Hospitals NHS Trust, Medicines Advisory Committee, vol. 2 no. 5.

Patient consultation

The term 'patient consultation' is used here to describe the interaction between patients and health professionals around medicines-related issues. It replaces the term 'patient counselling' as this term is poorly understood outside the pharmacy profession where the word 'counselling' describes a therapeutic relationship of a psychological nature.

Purpose of a consultation

For many years, consultations were regarded as opportunities to educate patients about medicines and highlight risks identified by the pharmacist as important. More recently it has been acknowledged that effective consultations require patient understanding, memory and satisfaction with a consultation. Patient engagement with the pharmacist is key to a successful clinical encounter and supports creation of a shared agenda between the clinician and patient and the development of an agreed explicit goal. NHS Health Education England and the Centre for Postgraduate Pharmacy Education have recently produced a number of resources for pharmacists to support this as part of the drive to focus on a patient-centred approach to consultations.[1]

The NICE *Medicines Adherence* guidance[2] recognises the need for pharmacists to provide patient support around adherence. Effective consultations are an integral part of medicines optimisation to support improved outcomes for patients. In order to improve medicines adherence, an understanding of patients' perspective on their illness, their health goals and their beliefs and concerns about medicines is required. The pharmacist can use this information to tailor the consultation around medicines-related issues for each patient and support patients in addressing their issues of medicines adherence.

Structure of the consultation

In order to make best use of the time allocated for patient consultation, it is helpful to think of the interaction in terms of both content and structure. There are a number of models used for medical patient consultations. Roger Neighbour's five-step model[3] is a helpful guide to developing consultation structure and includes key features such as development of rapport with the patient and agreeing a way forward and safety netting (advising the patient what to do if things go wrong). Neighbour adds that clinicians need time to look after themselves between consultations in order to serve their patients optimally. The Calgary Cambridge model[4] is used by a large number of medical schools in the UK and is also focused on relationship building, gathering information from the patient and explaining, agreeing and planning next steps with the patient.

In a medicines-related consultation, pharmacists are usually focused on ensuring that they have told the patient key information about the medicines prescribed, including how and when to take them, common side effects and key warnings. The recent developments in consultations structure suggest that the pharmacy structure can be improved to engage patients better in their own care.

The medicines-related consultation framework (MRCF)[5] is a validated method of assessing consultations.

The *four e's* structure for consultations

The *four e's* is a structure for consultations,[1] developed from the GROW model, widely used in coaching generally and specifically in health coaching.[6] This model acknowledges the requirements for pharmacists in a medicines-related consultation while ensuring that patients are engaged and their agenda is fully addressed.

The model looks like this:

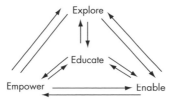

The *four e's* model is built on a foundation of engagement and empathy with patients, and thus the consultation needs to begin with rapport building.

This is most effectively done by introducing yourself by name and asking what medicines-related conversation the patient would like to have with you. This allows patients to refuse a consultation at that time, so you can offer them alternatives for discussion in the future, whether that is rescheduling, giving a medicines helpline number or a website. If the patient agrees to a consultation, you then need to ask the patient what s/he wants to discuss (around medicines) and tell the patient what you would like to cover in the consultation. This conversation will lead to creation of an agreed agenda before the consultation begins.

The first part of the consultation needs to focus on the patient's current knowledge, beliefs and concerns about his or her medicines. If the patient is taking a number of medicines, s/he should be given the opportunity to talk about the medicine that s/he is most interested in first.

Questions that facilitate this part of the consultation are listed below.

Explore

- What do you already know about your medicines?
- What do you want to know?
- What worries/concerns you about your medicine?
- How do you think your medicine helps you?

While pharmacists are adept at providing patient education, this model suggests that education should be tailored to the patient agenda and key safety information given in response to patient lead where possible.

Educate

- Give information in response to patient questions.
- Include safety information as it relates to patient agenda wherever possible.
- Ensure the patient has understood by using a teachback technique, e.g. *I'd like to review what we've discussed to make sure I have explained things clearly. Please let me know what you have understood from our conversation about your medicine.*

In a standard pharmacy consultation, patients are rarely asked whether they are going to take the medicines. There is a tacit assumption that having been prescribed the medication they have already agreed to take it as prescribed. In the UK, up to 50% of medicines are not taken as intended[2] and poor medicines adherence is known to be a global issue. This model acknowledges patient choice in adherence and empowers both the pharmacist and the patient to address the issue within the consultation. In order for this to be effective and to maintain rapport, the pharmacist must respect the patient's decision and support improving health outcomes in a way that is acceptable to the patient, which may include developing or signposting to an alternative strategy.

Empower

The final part of the consultation allows the patient to consider the reality of taking a medicine. Try asking one of the following:

- So, what do you think about taking this medicine now?
- What would you like to do about your medicine now?
- How do you feel about the medicine now?

Regular medicines taking requires development of the 'habit' of medicines taking so that it becomes an automatic part of daily activities, rather than one that has to be thought about every day, which is much more difficult to sustain. Consideration of the reality of how a new medicine fits into an existing medicines regimen or exploring how a new medicines-taking habit can be integrated into the patient's daily activities is important in helping the patient to consider the reality of medicine taking. The following questions are useful in structuring this part of the consultation.

Enable

- How will you fit your medicines into your day? Probe further (to help make the actions real for the patient).
- When will you take them? How will you remember to take them? Where will you keep them?
- How will you know if this system works?
- What will you do to find out if the medicine is working for you?

While the model has been described here in a linear way, the diagram illustrates that the agenda is fluid and education can be included at any time in the consultation.

Closing the consultation

As in Neighbour's model, it is important to ensure that safety information has been received and understood and that the patient knows where to go for additional information or help. It is valuable for both you and the patient to summarise your agreed respective actions following the consultation to reinforce the way forward.

Identifying and supporting patients with adherence issues

Medicines adherence

The WHO identified key factors affecting adherence, including:

- social, economic and cultural, e.g. age, race, medicine cost
- health system and healthcare team
- therapy, e.g. length of treatment, desire for treatment, side effects
- condition treated, e.g. chronic versus acute, disability, severity
- patient, e.g. anxiety, forgetfulness, fear of dependency.

However, while it is known that beliefs about medicines influence adherence, none of the above factors independently predicts poor adherence.

Identifying non-adherence

Patient may express non-adherence openly to the pharmacist or this may be identified through other means, such as irregular ordering or collection of repeat prescription, or widely varying dates of dispensing on medicines brought in on hospital admission. Neither age nor socioeconomic status is a reliable predictor of adherence and, while there is no clear disease-related predictor of adherence, depression, smoking and unhealthy lifestyle choices have been linked to poor adherence in some studies. Effective healthcare systems that support patients appear to improve medication adherence. Patients with knowledge of their disease and medication and high self-efficacy are thought to be more adherent.

There are a number of questionnaires in development that help practitioners and patients to identify issues of non-adherence;

however, these are not widely available. To date, there is no validated simple predictor of medicines adherence that is currently in use in pharmacy consultations. From a pharmacist's perspective, this leaves us with exploration of the patient's beliefs and concerns about medicines, and the practical implications of taking medicines. This can also be considered using the COM-B model[7] of adherence-related behaviour. This includes capability (physical and psychological), opportunity (physical and social) and motivation (automatic/habit and reflective/requiring active thought).

Managing challenges in consultations

Changing consultation style to a more open conversation is inevitably challenging. Common concerns include the difficulty of not giving patients solutions, especially when that is what patients expect of you, managing the rambling patient and managing time to support behaviour change in this type of consultation.

Challenge 1: *I came here for you to tell me what to do!*

While some patients are happy to discuss their options with you, others may consider this question as abrogation of your responsibility as a healthcare practitioner. If patients want you to tell them what to do, it is useful to say that, while you are happy to give your recommendation, your question is asked in recognition that they have choice.

Challenge 2: How to manage the rambling patient

Many pharmacists fear that asking patients open questions will lead to a protracted conversation that may veer off the subject in question. While patients do need uninterrupted time at the beginning of a consultation to tell their story, the *four e's* method helps to prevent rambling as the agenda is agreed *with the patient* at the start of the consultation. This means that, if the patient diverts from the agreed agenda, you can politely remind her of what she said she wanted to speak about to do with medicines, and ask if this is still relevant to her. The patient may tell you that she now has the information she needs, which means you can close the consultation, or it will remind the patient of her question, which she will then reconsider.

Challenge 3: Time

The issue of time is always tricky. Some practitioners find it helpful to introduce this at the beginning of a consultation so that the patient knows how much time you have and you can refer to this during the consultation if you need to and schedule another visit if required.

Further reading

Horne R *et al.* (2005). *Concordance, Adherence and Compliance in Medicines Taking: Report for the National Coordinating Centre for NHS Service Delivery and Organisation R&D*. http://www.nets. nihr.ac.uk/ – data/assets/pdf_file/0007/81394/ES-08-1412-076.pdf (accessed 15 May 2015).

NHS England (2013). *Making Medicines-taking a Better Experience.* http://www.england.nhs.uk/wp-content/uploads/2014/04/mo-ws-report-02-14.pdf (accessed 26 April 2015).

Review: Medication adherence: where are we now? A UK perspective. *Eur J Hosp Pharm* ejhpharm-2013-000373. Published online first: 18 December 2013. http://ejhp.bmj.com/content/early/2013/12/18/ejhpharm-2013-000373.full (accessed 26 April 2015).

World Health Organization (2003). *Adherence to Long-Term Therapies: Evidence for action.* http://www.who.int/chp/knowledge/publications/adherence_full_report.pdf (accessed 26 April 2015).

REFERENCES

1 NHS Health Education England and Centre for Postgraduate Pharmacy Education (2014). *Consultation Skills for Pharmacy Practice: Taking a patient centred approach.* http://www.consultationskillsforpharmacy.com/docs/docb.pdf (accessed 19 January 2015).

2 NICE (2009). *Medicines Adherence. Involving patients in decisions about prescribed medicines and supporting adherence.* NICE guidelines. CG76. http://www.nice.org.uk/guidance/CG76 (accessed 19 January 2015).

3 Neighbour R (2004). *The Inner Consultation* (2nd edn). Milton Keynes: Radcliffe Publishing.

4 Calgary Cambridge (2015). *Teaching and Learning Communication Skills in Medicine.* http://www.gp-training.net/training/communication_skills/calgary/ (accessed 19 January 2015).

5 Abdel-Tawab R *et al.* (2011). Development and validation of the medication-related consultation framework (MRCF). *Patient Educ Counsel* 83: 451–457.

6 Whitmore J (2002). *Coaching for Performance: The new edition of the practical guide (people skills for professionals).* London: Nicholas Brealey.

7 Jackson C *et al.* (2014). Applying COM-B to medication adherence. *Eur Health Psychologist* February: 7–17. http://www.ehps.net/ehp/issues/2014/v16iss1February2014/16_1_EHP_Februay2014%20Jackson%20et%20al.pdf (accessed 19 January 2015).

P

Patient-controlled analgesia

Patient-controlled analgesia (PCA) refers to methods of pain relief that allow a patient to self-administer small doses of an analgesic, usually an opioid, as required. Most often, the term PCA is associated with programmable infusion pumps that deliver opioids intravenously.

Intravenous PCA provides better pain relief than conventional intermittent opioid administration regimens (e.g. intramuscular or subcutaneous administration): although the difference is small, opioid consumption is greater; there are similar opioid-related side effects, but patient satisfaction is higher.[1]

PCA is a safe and effective method of analgesia that is commonly used after major surgery and has the following benefits:[2]

- tailoring of doses to individual requirements
- patient control of delivery of analgesic

- improved patient satisfaction with their pain relief
- less labour-intensive for ward staff
- lower total opioid dose compared with bolus 'rescue' analgesia.

Administration

The patient activates an opioid bolus within preset limits by pressing a hand-held button. The machine is set with a 'lock-out' time during which no further drug can be delivered even if the button is pressed. The standard dosing schedule is a bolus dose, followed by a lock-out period of 5 minutes.

Background infusions may be considered for patients who have previously been taking regular high doses of opioids and occasionally a larger bolus dose may be required for patients with increased analgesic requirements. In such cases, the patient may need to be nursed in a high-dependency environment for greater monitoring.

Some hospitals allow the PCA solutions to remain *in situ* for over 24 hours in accordance with local infection control policies.

Medicines

The most commonly used opioid in PCA is morphine. The usual concentration used is morphine sulfate 1 mg in 1 mL in sodium chloride 0.9%, with the pump delivering a 1-mg bolus dose with a 5-minute lock-out period. Lower doses may be required in renal impairment. Many manufacturers supply prefilled syringes or bags, or vials of morphine sulfate 50 mg in 50 mL.

Alternative regimens

Other medicines used include oxycodone, fentanyl and tramadol:

- oxycodone: 1-mg bolus dose and 5-minute lockout
- fentanyl: 20–40-microgram bolus dose and a 5-minute lockout
- tramadol: 10–20-mg bolus dose and 5-minute lockout.

Monitoring

The pump records the volume of drug administered, the number of times the patient has made requests and the number of doses administered. If the number of successful requests is greatly outweighed by the number of overall requests it may indicate that the patient may not fully understand how to use the pump, or that the patient's pain is not adequately managed.

Patients receiving an opioid by intravenous PCA require regular monitoring and details should be recorded in addition to the standard conventional postoperative recordings, including:

- pain score
- respiratory rate
- nausea or vomiting
- sedation score
- observation of the infusion site.

Additional medicines that should be prescribed

Antiemetics should be prescribed for patients receiving an intravenous PCA.

Simple analgesics, such as paracetamol and NSAIDs, should be prescribed and regularly administered to reduce opioid requirements.

Other opioids may be discontinued during the use of the PCA to minimise side effects.

Naloxone should be available in all areas where PCA is administered to patients.

Some hospitals may have introduced preprinted stickers to place over appropriate sections of the prescription chart, or have order sets of medicines if using e-prescribing, so that these anticipated adjuvant medicines can be quickly and accurately prescribed for the convenience of prescribers and the patient.

Discontinuing the PCA

Intravenous PCA is normally continued until the patient is eating and drinking; most patients require PCA for 2–3 days following surgery. A dose of oral opioid is often administered before PCA is disconnected to ensure adequate pain relief and it is usual to prescribe an oral opioid 'when required' for exacerbations of pain. Other analgesics should continue to be administered regularly, or on a 'when required' basis as appropriate.

REFERENCES

1 Hudcova J et al. (2006). Patient controlled opioid analgesia versus conventional opioid analgesia for postoperative pain. Cochrane Datab Systemat Rev4: CD003348.
2 Macintyre PE et al. (2010). Acute Pain Management: Scientific evidence (3rd edn). Melbourne: ANZCA and FPM. http://www.anzca.edu.au/resources/college-publications/pdfs/Acute%20Pain%20Management/books-and-publications/Acute%20pain%20management%20-%20scientific%20evidence%20-%20third%20edition.pdf (accessed 27 November 2014).

Phaeochromocytoma

Overview	
Definition	Phaeochromocytoma is a tumour of the adrenal gland that causes excess release of catecholamines: adrenaline and noradrenaline
Risk factors	The prevalence of phaeochromocytoma in hypertensive patients attending medical outpatient clinics is 0.1–0.6%[1]
Differential diagnosis	The symptoms vary greatly and are episodic, often non-specific and similar to those of many common conditions such as anxiety. As a result, diagnosis is often delayed[1,2] Differential diagnosis includes: • hyperthyroidism • hypoglycaemia • menopause • heart failure • arrhythmias

	• migraine • stroke • porphyria • panic disorder or anxiety • drug treatment (monoamine oxidase inhibitors, sympathomimetic drugs) • illegal drugs (e.g. cocaine)
Diagnostic tests	The following tests and results may be associated with this syndrome: • an adrenal biopsy that shows phaeochromocytoma • an MIBG scintiscan that shows a tumour • an MRI or abdominal CT scan of abdomen that shows adrenal mass • measurement of catecholamine metabolites either in a 24-hour urine collection or in plasma
Treatment goals	• Removal of tumour • Prevention of hypertensive crisis
Treatment options	• Surgery • Alpha-blocker medication

Pharmaceutical care and counselling

Assess	• Current blood pressure
Essential intervention	The definitive treatment is removal of the tumour by surgery. Secretion of adrenaline and noradrenaline usually returns to normal after surgery. High blood pressure may not be cured in a quarter of patients after surgery, yet control is usually achieved in these people with standard treatments for hypertension. Recurrence of tumour may occur in 10% of cases
Essential intervention	The major aim of medical pretreatment is to prevent catecholamine-induced, serious and potentially life-threatening complications during surgery. These include hypertensive crises, cardiac arrhythmias, pulmonary oedema and cardiac ischaemia. Traditional regimens include the blockade of alpha-adrenoceptors with phenoxybenzamine, prazosin or doxazosin. Phenoxybenzamine is often preferred because it blocks alpha-adrenoceptors non-competitively. This type of blockade offers an advantage, as it avoids drug displacement from alpha-adrenoceptors by excessive increases in catecholamines during surgery
Secondary intervention	Treatment usually lasts for 10–14 days. The initial dose of phenoxybenzamine is 10 mg twice a day, increased every 2–3 days by 10–20 mg to a total daily dose of 1 mg/kg. Doxazosin is given in increasing doses from 1 to 16 mg once a day. A beta-adrenoceptor blocker (e.g. propranolol 40 mg three times daily or atenolol 25–50 mg once daily) can be included after several days of alpha-adrenergic blockade. This addition is especially useful in patients who also have tachycardia. Blockade of beta-adrenoceptors should never be initiated before blockade of alpha-adrenoceptors, since the loss of beta-adrenoceptor-mediated vasodilatation leaves alpha-adrenoceptor stimulation unopposed, which could result in hypertensive crises
Continued monitoring	• Blood pressure • Monitored annually for symptoms of recurrence

REFERENCES

1 Jones AG *et al.*(2012). Phaeochromocytoma. *BMJ* 344: e1042.
2 Lenders JWM *et al.* (2005). Phaeochromocytoma. *Lancet* 366: 665–675.

Pharmacocultural issues

The term pharmacocultural is used here to describe those aspects of medication choice and use influenced by religious and cultural factors.

The UK population contains peoples with diverse faiths and lifestyle philosophies (vegetarian, vegan) and these should be appreciated and respected by pharmacists in their practice.

- Some patients want and need to understand the nature of their prescribed medication – it is essential for informed consent and central to adherence with drug regimens.
- Informing patients about the origins of their medication demonstrates respect for their beliefs and will assist them in making informed decisions about treatments.
- Pharmacists should appreciate that within faiths there are many schools of thought with different interpretations of religious laws.
- Patients and families may place more emphasis on religious needs in times of illness.

Dietary factors

Judaism and Islam strictly forbid pork and other foods derived from pigs within the diet. Hinduism forbids consumption of cow-based products and Jainism requires a strictly vegetarian diet that may also be vegan and exclude root vegetables. Vegetarianism is considered to be spiritually pure in the Buddhist, Sikh and Hindu faiths.[1]

Medicines for Jewish patients

Jewish law permits the oral consumption of porcine and other non-kosher materials in a 'non-edible' manner in the case of any illness. A key point is the distinction made relating to the 'edible' or 'non-edible' nature of a pharmaceutical product. For example, Saliva Orthana is considered an edible product containing the animal-derived active ingredient glucosamine, which is derived from shellfish but is acid-treated and therefore not 'edible'; chondroitin is shark or bovine cartilage and is considered to be edible.

Non-kosher parenteral products, such as porcine/bovine insulin or porcine heparin, may be used by Jewish patients as this is not classed as consumption.

Porcine products present a clear pharmacocultural dilemma; however, there is no exhaustive list of kosher or halal medicines, nor is there a list of unacceptable medicines. Patients can be supported through medicines information centres for up-to-date, specific advice. Note that there are a number of religious authorities within Judaism and Islam, so it is important to establish with patients which authority they follow. For a further explanation of medicines implications in Judaism and Islam, see http://www.medicinesresources.nhs.uk/ upload/documents/Evidence/Medicines%20Q%20&%20A/QA381_ 1KosherandHalal_FINAL.doc.

Blood products

Some Jehovah's Witnesses refuse to accept blood products (red and white blood cells, platelets and plasma) in any circumstances, even at the cost of their life. They may accept so-called minor fractions of blood, such as albumin and globulin, as a personal choice. Anticipated blood loss may be managed by autologous blood transfusion. Epoetin injections and plasma expanders are also considered acceptable for use.[2]

Gelatin

Gelatin is a component of capsules and may be an excipient in other formulations. It can be of animal (meat or fish) or vegetable origin; some manufacturers obtain gelatin from non-animal sources and this will be stated in the product SPC. Many over-the-counter products are now labelled as vegetarian but this may not be acceptable to vegans. Where no differentiation is made, this is usually because varying sources are used, and this should be borne in mind when advising patients.

Muslim patients and Ramadan

Fasting during Ramadan is prescribed for every healthy, adult Muslim, whereas the weak, the sick, children, travellers and menstruating women are among those exempt. Pregnant women are also exempted from fasting if they believe that fasting will harm them or their baby.

Muslims observing the fast are required to abstain from eating and drinking during daylight hours and also from taking oral medicines and injecting intravenous nutritional fluids. Some Muslims who are ill may insist on fasting in any case and this can cause problems if not supervised by health professionals. Advice from pharmacists about changing prescriptions to equally effective drugs that have reduced dosing, such as sustained-release formulations, may be beneficial to the fasting Muslim, to allow dosing during the period between sunset and dawn.[3]

Advice for patients is available at http://www.nhs.uk/Livewell/ Healthyramadan/Pages/faqs.aspx, which includes health and medicines use during Ramadan as part of the frequently asked questions. Be aware that, during Ramadan, Muslim patients often unilaterally change the time and dosage of drugs without taking medical advice.

Diabetics taking oral hypoglycaemic agents or injecting insulin should exercise extreme caution if they decide to fast, and dose adjustments must be considered.

When does Ramadan begin?

The timing of Ramadan varies from year to year and is associated with the ninth lunar month of the Islamic calendar. When Ramadan falls during the summer months the daily period of fasting is extended because of the increased number of daylight hours.

Cultural issues around medicine taking

Patients have a wide variety of beliefs around medicines that are influenced by culture as well as religion. Common cultural beliefs can include receipt of a medicine being the only acceptable conclusion to a consultation and medicine only being useful if its effect on symptoms is immediately obvious. If a patient comes from a culture where antibiotics were always given for minor ailments, it will be difficult to accept the refusal of such treatment by a clinician. In addition to this, some patients are used to being able to purchase medication without consulting any healthcare professional and may feel that pharmacy involvement is an unnecessary barrier to treatment. Conversely, some patients may believe that medicines are generally harmful and will use them only as a last resort, even if the patient appears to be suffering as a result (e.g. use of pain relief). From a pharmacy perspective, consultation with a patient around medicines taking will be more effective if this is borne in mind.

REFERENCES

1 Mynors G *et al.* (2004). *Drugs Derived from Pigs and Their Clinical Alternatives.* Ask about Medicines/Medicines Partnership/Muslim Council of Britain. Booklet supported by educational grant from Sanofi. http://www.scribd.com/doc/80247519/Drugs-Derived-From-Pigs-and-Their-Clinical-Alternatives#scribd (accessed 15 May 2015).

2 Muramoto O (2001). Bioethical aspects of the recent changes in the policy of refusal of blood by Jehovah's Witnesses. *BMJ* 322: 37–39.

3 Ethnicity Online (2014). http://www.ethnicityonline.net (accessed 27 November 2014).

Phenytoin: management and monitoring

Phenytoin is an anticonvulsant drug used in the treatment of epilepsy. It is licensed for the treatment of tonic-clonic seizures (grand mal epilepsy), partial seizures (focal, including temporal-lobe) or a combination of these, and for the prevention and treatment of seizures occurring during or following neurosurgery and/or severe head injury.[1–3]

Pharmacokinetic overview

Oral phenytoin is slowly but almost completely absorbed from the GI tract. The rate of absorption is variable and affected by the presence of food in the stomach. Once absorbed, phenytoin is highly protein-bound (approximately 90%), but may be displaced from plasma proteins by various drugs, e.g. sodium valproate. Protein binding may also be lower in certain patient groups, e.g. those with renal or hepatic disease, neonates and in the third trimester of pregnancy.[4]

The major route of metabolism of phenytoin is oxidation via the liver to an inactive metabolite. This metabolism is a saturable process resulting in a non-linear relationship between the dose of phenytoin and serum concentration. Therefore, small increases in dosage may result in substantial increases in plasma phenytoin concentration and toxicity.[1-3]

Rationale for monitoring

The main indications for phenytoin therapeutic drug monitoring (Table P9) are:

- on initiation of therapy
- during intravenous therapy in status epilepticus
- when there is a loss of seizure control (including an adherence check)
- to monitor the effects of drug interactions
- where formulation changes are made
- when toxicity is suspected.

TABLE P9
Phenytoin drug monitoring information

Half-life	7–42 hours[4]
Pretreatment measures	FBC, U&Es, LFTs[5]
Therapeutic range	40–80 micromol/L (10–20 mg/L)[6]
Sampling time	Middle of dose interval, but this is not critical once steady state is achieved due to the long half-life. Usual time to steady state is 7–10 days
Other monitoring	Megaloblastic anaemia and blood dyscrasias occasionally occur. FBC should be checked periodically. Phenytoin may affect glucose metabolism and therefore should be used with caution in diabetes. LFTs and folic acid should be checked every 6 months[7]

Dose

The adult dose for oral administration starts at 3–4 mg/kg/day. The daily dose is increased if necessary in 25-mg increments, with a minimum interval between dose changes of 7–10 days, until the therapeutic effect is achieved or toxic effects manifest. Dosage must be individualised because there is wide interpatient variability in phenytoin serum concentration from equivalent doses.[1]

In adults in status epilepticus *who are not normally maintained on oral phenytoin*, a loading dose of phenytoin 15–20 mg/kg (the BNF recommends 20 mg/kg to a maximum of 2 g[5]) should be injected slowly intravenously. The rate should not exceed 1 mg/kg/minute to a maximum rate of 50 mg/minute, although the slower rate of 25 mg/minute reduces the likelihood of hypotension. Cardiac monitoring is advised because of the risk of serious arrhythmias. Rate of administration should be further reduced in the elderly or those with heart disease. Blood levels may be checked 2 hours after giving the loading dose to ensure they are in the correct range. The loading dose should be followed by maintenance doses orally or intravenously every 6–8 hours, and serum concentration monitored.[2]

Administration

Injection

Phenytoin can be administered as an intravenous injection or as an intravenous infusion. The intravenous injection route is preferred. Each injection must be preceded and followed by an injection of 5 mL sodium chloride 0.9% through the same needle (this reduces venous irritation due to the alkalinity of the solution). N.B.: Rapid intravenous administration can cause hypotension; ECG and blood pressure monitoring must be carried out. The patient must also be observed for any signs of respiratory depression. It is not recommended to give phenytoin as an intramuscular injection because it may crystallise in the tissue, resulting in very unpredictable absorption. If the intramuscular route *is* to be used, dose adjustment is essential.

- Intravenous injection: withdraw the required dose through a 5 micron filter needle. Replace the filter needle with a large-gauge needle, or intravenous catheter, and inject slowly into a large vein at a rate not exceeding 50 mg/min for adults (but see *Dose* above for more detail).
- Intravenous infusion: the infusion must be given through an in-line filter (0.22–0.50 microns) as there is a risk of precipitation. If the solution is hazy it must not be used. The injection is diluted with sodium chloride 0.9% so that the final concentration does not exceed 10 mg/mL. The infusion is only stable for 1 hour and should be used immediately. It is infused into a large vein at a rate not exceeding 50 mg/min for adults (but see *Dose* above for more detail), via a large-gauge needle or intravenous catheter.[2]

Switching forms

The capsule and injection forms contain phenytoin sodium and the suspension form contains phenytoin base, so when switching between formulations, doses should be changed accordingly (Table P10).[1–3]

TABLE P10

Bioequivalent doses of phenytoin formulations

Injection	Capsule	Suspension
100 mg	100 mg	92 mg*

*N.B.: this relates to molecular weight equivalence, and does not necessarily represent biological equivalence – care should be taken when switching between formulations.

Enteral feeding – phenytoin interaction

Continuous enteral feeds reduce absorption of phenytoin. To avoid this, the feed should be stopped 2 hours before the phenytoin is administered, and recommenced 2 hours after the administration. The nasogastric (NG) tube should be flushed before and after administration. The suspension is thixotropic and cannot be administered under gravity; it has a viscosity 40 times greater than standard enteral feed. Therefore, for NG administration phenytoin suspension should be mixed with an equal volume of a suitable diluent, e.g. water. Even with appropriate flushing and a feeding break, phenytoin is still not well absorbed via the NG route and high doses or alternative agents may need to be considered.

Overdose

The initial symptoms are nystagmus, ataxia and dysarthria. Other signs are tremor, hyperreflexia, lethargy, nausea and vomiting. The patient may become comatose and hypotensive. If death occurs it is due to respiratory and circulatory depression.

Seek specialist advice from the National Poisons Information Service (http://www.toxbase.org). There is no antidote and general supportive measures should be used.[1-3]

Interactions[1-3]

- Drugs that may increase phenytoin serum levels include: amiodarone, antifungal agents (e.g. amphotericin, fluconazole, ketoconazole, miconazole, itraconazole), chloramphenicol, chlordiazepoxide, diazepam, diltiazem, disulfiram, fluoxetine, H2-antagonists, halothane, isoniazid, methylphenidate, nifedipine, omeprazole, oestrogens, phenothiazines, salicylates, sulphonamides, tolbutamide and trazodone.
- Drugs that may decrease phenytoin serum levels include: folic acid, rifampicin, sucralfate, theophylline, vigabatrin and St John's wort.
- Drugs that may either increase or decrease phenytoin serum levels include: carbamazepine, phenobarbital, valproic acid, sodium valproate, antineoplastic agents and ciprofloxacin.
- The effect of phenytoin on the serum concentration of carbamazepine, phenobarbital, valproic acid and sodium valproate is unpredictable.
- Acute alcohol intake may increase phenytoin serum levels, whereas chronic alcoholism may decrease serum levels.
- Tricyclic antidepressants and phenothiazines may precipitate seizures in susceptible patients and phenytoin dosage may need to be adjusted.
- Drugs whose effect is impaired by phenytoin include: antifungal agents, antineoplastic agents, calcium-channel antagonists, clozapine, corticosteroids, ciclosporin, digitoxin, doxycycline, furosemide, lamotrigine, methadone, neuromuscular blockers, oestrogens, oral contraceptives, paroxetine, quinidine, rifampicin, theophylline and vitamin D.
- The effect of phenytoin on warfarin is variable and the patient's INR should be monitored closely.

REFERENCES
1 SPC (2014). *Phenytoin Sodium Flynn Hard Capsules 25 mg, 50 mg, 100 mg and 300 mg.* www.medicines.org.uk (accessed 19 January 2015).
2 SPC (2012). *Epanutin Ready-mixed Parenteral.* www.medicines.org.uk (accessed 19 January 2015).

3 SPC (2013). *Epanutin 30 mg/5 mL Oral Suspension*. www.medicines.org.uk (accessed 19 January 2015).

4 Dollery C (ed.) (1999). *Therapeutic Drugs* (2nd edn). Edinburgh: Churchill Livingstone.

5 Joint Formulary Committee (2014). British National Formulary (68th edn). London: BMJ Group and Pharmaceutical Press.

6 Crawford P (1999). Monitoring requirements with antiepileptic drugs. *Prescriber* 19: 122–123.

7 Dyfed Powys Primary Care Effectiveness Team (2004). *Drug Monitoring Booklet*. Dyfed Powys: National Public Health Service for Wales.

Phosphate

Overview	
Normal range	0.8–1.5 mmol/L
Local range	
Background	• The total plasma phosphate concentration is approximately 3.9 mmol/L in adults.[1] • Two-thirds is organic phosphate, e.g. phospholipids, and one-third is inorganic (the form usually assayed by clinical chemistry laboratories).[2] • Phosphate is found primarily in bone and soft tissue, with less than 1% of the total body store in the extracellular fluid[3]
Recommended nutrient intake	• The average diet provides 1000–2000 mg phosphorus daily,[4] of which 60–80% will be absorbed from the gut.[5] • Dietary sources of phosphorus include: meat, fish, grains, dairy products, seeds, nuts, eggs, most fruits and vegetables and soft drinks

Hypophosphataemia	
Symptoms	• Usually *asymptomatic* • Levels <0.5 mmol/L can produce clinical symptoms Symptoms are non-specific: • Musculoskeletal symptoms – myalgia, muscle weakness, osteomalacia and rhabdomyolysis • Pulmonary symptoms – respiratory failure • Cardiovascular symptoms – acute heart failure
Causes	**Internal redistribution** • The most common cause of hypophosphataemia, resulting from an acute shift from the extracellular to the intracellular compartment • Associated clinical conditions: acute respiratory alkalosis, increased insulin concentration during glucose administration, recovery from diabetic ketoacidosis and the refeeding syndrome associated with feeding of malnourished patients (see *Parenteral nutrition* entry) • These conditions stimulate glycolysis, leading to the formation of phosphorylated glucose compounds and an intracellular shift of phosphate • Rapid cell turnover as a result of malignancy or hungry-bone syndrome can lead to low serum phosphate levels

Increased renal excretion

- Acquired and inherited disorders of the renal tubules as well as some drugs may lead to an increase in the renal excretion of phosphate
- Patients with primary hyperparathyroidism have decreased renal tubular reabsorption, resulting in low serum phosphate levels
- Inherited disorders of vitamin D metabolism may also cause hypocalcaemia and consequently hypophosphataemia
- Some drugs that may cause an increase in renal excretion of phosphate include diuretics, chemotherapy agents, antivirals, antibiotics and antiepileptics

Decreased intake and reduced intestinal absorption

- Dietary phosphorus restriction will only result in hypophosphataemia if the restriction is severe and prolonged or if intestinal absorption is reduced by the long-term use of phosphate binders
- Chronic diarrhoea may also reduce phosphate absorption
- Alcohol misusers may have a prolonged poor intake of phosphate

Assessment	• Mild: 0.65–0.84 mmol/L • Moderate: 0.32–0.64 mmol/L • Severe: <0.32 mmol/L
Treatment*	**Mild hypophosphataemia** • Asymptomatic: no treatment • Symptomatic: Phosphate-Sandoz tablets 2–4 tablets a day for 7–10 days* **Moderate hypophosphataemia** • Asymptomatic: Phosphate-Sandoz tablets 4–6 tablets a day for 7–10 days* • Symptomatic and oral route does not provide an adequate rate of symptom relief: parenteral replacement **Severe hypophosphataemia** • Parenteral replacement
Adminis-tration	• Tablets should be taken orally. The dose should be divided equally to prevent gastrointestinal side effects • Intravenous phosphate: 9 mmol to be infused over 12 hours, which can be repeated as required • In critically ill patients, the phosphate dose can be increased to 500 micromol/kg (max. 50 mmol) infused over 6–12 hours.[6]
Monitoring	• Serum magnesium and potassium: hypomagnesaemia and hypokalaemia promote excessive phosphate excretion • Serum calcium: hypocalcaemia is a common complication of phosphate therapy

Hyperphosphataemia[5]

Symptoms	• Hypocalcaemia • Tetany
Causes	**Renal failure** • Phosphate is cleared through glomerular filtration • 80–95% of the filtered phosphate is reabsorbed by the proximal tubule • Despite maximal suppression of phosphate reabsorption, when glomerular filtration rate falls below 20–25 mL/min, urinary excretion cannot counterbalance the dietary intake

P

	Increase in renal phosphate reabsorption
	• Can occur in the following conditions: hypoparathyroidism, vitamin D toxicity, familial tumoral calcinosis and acromegaly
	Massive acute phosphate load
	• Endogenous or exogenous
	• Endogenous causes result from tissue breakdown, leading to the release of intracellular phosphate into the extracellular fluid. Includes: severe tissue necrosis due to tumour lysis syndrome and rhabdomyolysis. Other causes include lactic acidosis and diabetic ketoacidosis.
	• Exogenous causes include the ingestion of phosphate-containing laxatives
Treatment	**Acute hyperphosphataemia**
	• Cleared rapidly if renal function normal
	• Increase renal phosphate excretion using a sodium chloride 0.9% infusion to expand the extracellular volume
	Chronic hyperphosphataemia
	• Restrict dietary intake
	• Reduce intestinal absorption using phosphate-binding agents
	• Binding agents are split into two categories: calcium-based (e.g. calcium acetate) and calcium-free (e.g. magnesium carbonate or sevelamer)
	• In patients with renal failure, calcium salts are preferred; otherwise aluminium may accumulate to toxic levels
Adminis- tration	• Phosphate-binding agents should be taken with meals to achieve maximal phosphate-binding effect
	• For dosing of individual preparations, see BNF
Monitoring	• Phosphate levels
	• Calcium levels
	• Renal function

*The use of Phosphate-Sandoz in hypophosphataemia is unlicensed. The licensed indications are hypercalcaemia: up to 6 tablets daily, adjusted according to response, and vitamin D-resistant hypophosphataemic osteomalacia: 4–6 tablets daily. Diarrhoea is a common side effect and should prompt a reduction in dosage.[6,7]

TABLE P11

Phosphate content of various preparations[6]

Product	Phosphate content
Phosphate-Sandoz	16.1 mmol/tablet (also contains Na^+ 20.4 mmol and K^+ 3.1 mmol)
Addiphos	40 mmol/20 mL (also contains K^+ 30 mmol, Na^+ 30 mmol – due to the concentration of potassium in Addiphos, availability should be restricted as for strong potassium solutions: see *Potassium* entry)
Phosphate Polyfusor	50 mmol/500 mL

REFERENCES

1 Patel R *et al.* (2013). Management of hypophosphatemia. *Br J Hosp Med* 74: C66–C70.
2 Crook M (1994). Phosphate: an abnormal anion? *Br J Hosp Med* 52: 200–203.
3 Koda-Kimble MA *et al.* (eds) (2004). *Applied Therapeutics: The clinical use of drugs.* London: Lippincott, Williams and Wilkins.
4 European Food Safety Authority (2006). *Tolerable Upper Intake Levels for Vitamins and Minerals.* http://www.efsa.europa.eu/en/ndatopics/docs/ndatolerableuil.pdf (accessed 4 October 2014).
5 Malberti F (2013). Hyperphosphataemia: treatment options. *Drugs* 73: 673–688.
6 Joint Formulary Committee (2014). *British National Formulary* (68th edn). London: BMJ Group and Pharmaceutical Press.
7 Electronic Medicines Compendium (2014). *Summary of Product Characteristics Phosphate-Sandoz Effervescent Tablets.* https://www.medicines.org.uk/emc/medicine/811 (accessed 4 October 2014).

Postoperative nausea and vomiting

Postoperative nausea and vomiting (PONV) is defined as nausea and/or vomiting occurring within 24 hours of surgery.[1] It affects 20–30% of patients undergoing surgery and the consequences can be severe and include:[2]

- aspiration of vomit with depressed consciousness and laryngeal reflexes
- delayed administration of opioid analgesia
- wound disruption after abdominal surgery
- bleeding
- dehydration and electrolyte imbalance
- interference with nutrition
- delayed discharge from theatre recovery
- impact on day surgery and increased nursing time
- general delay in mobilisation and recovery
- patient discomfort, distress and fear about future surgery/anaesthesia.

The cause of PONV is not always clear but is likely to be multifactorial. The assessment of risk can be categorised into those relating specifically to the patient, the type of surgery and the anaesthetic. When deciding to administer prophylaxis or wait until treatment is required, the decision is based on the balance between efficacy of prevention and the incidence of side effects. No single drug is 100% effective in all cases. The use of prophylactic antiemetics in all cases is therefore not always necessary. The use of a high-risk identification tool can be beneficial. A risk stratification method, such as the Apfel score, can be used to determine the likelihood of PONV for each patient. This is a simplified method that includes four positive factors: female gender, non-smoking, history of PONV or motion sickness and postoperative use of opioids. Each of these factors is supposed to elevate the risk by 20%.[3] Local guidelines should be consulted.

Patient factors

The most important risk factors include:

- gender – females are at higher risk of PONV
- previous PONV
- motion sickness, vertigo or Ménière's disease
- PONV in children is usually twice as common as in adults.

Types of surgery

An increased duration of surgery can lead to an increase in PONV, as more drugs are administered to the patient in that time. Each 30-minute increase in duration of surgery increases the risk of PONV by 60%.[1] The following types of surgery increase the risk of PONV:

- major obstetric and gynaecological surgery
- major GI surgery
- ear, nose and throat surgery.

Anaesthetic factors

Anaesthetic factors that have an effect on the incidence of PONV include:

- method of anaesthesia – general is associated with higher risk than either local or epidural
- use of opioids
- etomidate/ketamine
- volatile gases (nitrous oxide) associated with higher incidence than intravenous anaesthetics
- anticholinesterases
- preoperative drug treatment:
  - opioids
  - cancer chemotherapy
  - prostaglandins.

Non-pharmacological intervention

Ensure that:

- the patient is adequately hydrated (which may necessitate intravenous infusion)
- pain is under control with minimal use of opioids
- preoperative fasting recommendations are complied with.

Other methods include psychological techniques, such as suggestion and hypnosis, acupuncture, eating or sucking ginger or mint, and the use of pressurised wristbands, however, there is little evidence to support their use.

Pharmacological intervention

Cyclizine

Cyclizine is a cheap, commonly used drug. Its use is based on anecdotal evidence and, interestingly, there are no real scientific reasons behind its huge use. It has antimuscarinic and antihistamine properties and the few side effects (sedation and dry mouth) and cautions (in glaucoma and heart failure) are related to this mechanism of action.

Dose

The dose is oral/intravenous/intramuscular 50 mg up to three times daily. Cyclizine does not need to be administered strictly every 8 hours and can be given after 4–6 hours if the patient requires, provided the daily maximum of 150 mg is not exceeded.

5HT3 antagonists

Ondansetron, granisetron, tropisetron and dolasetron are specific $5HT_3$ antagonists that block $5HT_3$ receptors in the GI tract and in the central nervous system. They are licensed for the treatment and prophylaxis of PONV and in practice are usually recommended second line after cyclizine.

The dosing for each drug is guided by whether it is treatment or prophylaxis; higher doses are given for prophylaxis.

$5HT_3$ antagonists have few side effects, including headache, transient raised LFTs and constipation due to reduced lower-bowel motility. Patients with signs of subacute intestinal obstruction should be monitored following administration and caution should be taken if the patient is receiving opioids or has a new stoma formed postoperatively.

Dolasetron and tropisetron are reported to have the potential to increase the QT interval and caution should be taken when administering with other drugs that may cause arrhythmias. Ondansetron and granisetron SPCs do not report this interaction; however, in a patient with unstable arrhythmias, antiemetic therapy may be worth considering as a contributory factor.

Metoclopramide

At a 10-mg dose, metoclopramide has been reported as no better than placebo in the management of PONV[4] and is therefore considered to be ineffective for PONV prophylaxis. A treatment dose of 50 mg intravenously would be required to show any reduction in the rate of PONV, but the side effect profile is unsatisfactory.[1]

Its GI motility stimulation properties mean that it is a useful agent as a prokinetic. It can be used in patients who are at risk of developing a postoperative ileus (reduction or lack of peristalsis within the bowel, resulting in poor GI absorption). Due to such properties, care must be taken not to use metoclopramide in patients with a suspected bowel obstruction.

Recent guidance from the MHRA recommends that metoclopramide should be used for no longer than 5 days due to the risks of extrapyramidal disorders and tardive dyskinesia.[5]

Prochlorperazine

There are few clinical studies advocating its use; however, it remains widely used in the prevention and treatment of PONV. Prochlorperazine is only indicated for treatment, and then only as a single dose; however, in some enhanced recovery programmes the use of the buccal formulation is recommended, with a typical regimen being 3 mg three times a day for 5 days post-op.

Dexamethasone

Corticosteroids have been shown to be effective in the prophylaxis of PONV, although their mechanism of action remains unclear. Combination with 5HT$_3$ antagonists may enhance their efficacy. Doses of dexamethasone range from 150 micrograms/kg/24 hours in children up to 8 mg/24 hours in adults.

If the patient is at high risk of PONV, numerous studies have demonstrated that using more than one antiemetic, with differing modes of action, is usually more effective and results in fewer side effects than simply using and increasing the dose of one agent.[6] Clinical trials have shown that the combination of 5HT$_3$ and dexamethasone is the most effective therapy in the prevention of PONV.[1]

REFERENCES

1 McCracken G *et al.* (2008). *Guidelines for the Management of Post-Operative Nausea and Vomiting.* SOGC Clinical Practice Guideline 209. http://sogc.org/wp-content/uploads/2013/07/gui209CPG0807E.pdf (accessed 15 May 2015).
2 UK Key Advances in Clinical Practice Series (2003). The effective prevention and management of post-operative nausea and vomiting. 2nd edition, 2003. London: Aesculapius Medical Press.
3 Pierre S, Whelan R (2013). Nausea and vomiting after surgery. Continuing education in anaesthesia. *Crit Care Pain* 13: 28–32.
4 Henzi ML *et al.* (1999). Metoclopramide in the prevention of postoperative nausea and vomiting: a quantitative systematic review of randomized placebo-controlled studies. *Br J Anaesth* 85: 761–771.
5 MHRA (2013). *Metoclopramide: Risk of neurological adverse effects – restricted dose and duration of use.* http://www.mhra.gov.uk/Safetyinformation/DrugSafetyUpdate/CON300404 (accessed 13 January 2013).
6 Chandrakantan A, Glass P (2011). Multimodal therapies for post-operative nausea and vomiting and pain. *Br J Anaesth* 107(1): i27–i40.

Potassium

Overview	
Normal range	3.5–5.0 mmol/L[1]
Local range	
Background	Potassium is the major intracellular electrolyte. Where an imbalance occurs with the extracellular (serum) concentration, it is important to look at serum concentration over a period of time rather than at an isolated result (a patient may be apparently well, despite having an anomalous high or low potassium serum concentration).
	Blood samples are sometimes haemolysed (the blood cells have disintegrated and released their intracellular contents), and this will result in a falsely high potassium serum concentration. Laboratories highlight this problem, and the potassium result from this sample should be ignored and a further blood sample should be taken. Where close monitoring of potassium levels is crucial, a new sample should be taken as soon as the problem is recognised.

	Patients receiving treatment for acute hyperkalaemia or hypokalaemia should ideally have their potassium level checked at least daily, to check that treatment remains appropriate
Recommended nutrient intake	The reference nutrient intake is 90 mmol/day; however, 40–50 mmol/day is considered adequate for an adult

Hypokalaemia

Symptoms	• Symptoms include muscle weakness, paralysis, respiratory insufficiency, ECG abnormalities and ileus. Chronic hypokalaemia may lead to renal tubular damage. The risk of digoxin toxicity is increased in hypokalaemia
Causes	• GI losses due to diarrhoea, a fistula, persistent vomiting or laxative abuse • Mineralocorticoid excess, e.g. hyperaldosteronism and Cushing's syndrome (see *Cushing's syndrome* entry) • Glucocorticoid therapy, e.g. prednisolone because of mineralocorticoid side effects • Metabolic alkalosis • Drugs, including: aminoglycosides, amphotericin, bicarbonates, corticosteroids, furosemide, insulin, laxatives, levodopa, high-dose penicillins, salbutamol (intravenous), theophylline and thiazides[1]
Assessment	• Renal function and electrolytes (Ur, Cr, K, Na) • Severe hypokalaemia is <2.5 mmol/L • Mild hypokalaemia is >2.5 mmol/L
Treatment	• Severe hypokalaemia requires intravenous therapy; for mild hypokalaemia, oral supplements will normally be sufficient unless vomiting is a problem or the oral route is not available. • Intravenous potassium treatment may involve giving a limited number of infusions to correct a short-term imbalance (e.g. postsurgical) or may be protracted (e.g. as a component of parenteral nutrition). Modest hypokalaemia may require only a single dose of 20–40 mmol of potassium pending the availability of the oral route, whilst a patient with serious potassium losses (e.g. GI fistula) may require 100–200 mmol per day. • The recommended maximum dose of potassium is 2–3 mmol/kg in 24 hours[2]
Administration	**Intravenous potassium chloride** • *Always use a volumetric infusion pump for infusion of potassium.* • In general clinical areas, when given via a peripheral vein, infusion rates in adults should not usually exceed 10 mmol/hour and no more than 20 mmol/hour in emergencies. Administration rates above 20 mmol/hour require cardiac monitoring.[2] Ready-prepared infusion bags containing 20 or 40 mmol/L are available, but solutions above a concentration of 30 mmol/L are associated with an increased risk of phlebitis. As a general principle, ready-prepared bags should be used in preference to preparing bags from concentrated potassium chloride solutions.

P

- In critical care areas (e.g. intensive care units) faster infusion rates or more concentrated solutions may be employed. Because of the risk of thrombophlebitis, more concentrated infusions are generally given via the largest vein available, and ideally by means of a central line. The infusion site should be checked at least every 4 hours for inflammation.[2]
- Infusion rates above 20 mmol/hour require ECG monitoring, whilst infusion rates above 40 mmol/hour present a risk of asystole.
- Concentrated parenteral potassium chloride solutions in ampoules are potentially lethal. Numerous drug errors have occurred with these products, largely because of their availability in clinical areas. For instance, potassium chloride ampoules have been accidentally used in place of sodium chloride 0.9% injection for reconstitution of antibiotic bolus injections. Rapid administration of potassium chloride may be fatal.
- Where infusions have to be prepared using potassium chloride concentrate solution, it is vital to mix the product with vigorous agitation to ensure that additive has dispersed throughout the diluent. It is advised to squeeze and invert the bag 10 times.[2] Failure to do this may result in inadvertent administration of a potassium chloride bolus to the patient, as undispersed concentrated solution will sink towards the outlet of the bag.
- Additions must never be made to an infusion container that has already been connected to a giving set.
- The National Patient Safety Agency issued a Patient Safety Alert on this topic in July 2002, which contained a number of safety measures for implementation in NHS trusts. The key measures were:[3]
  - Restriction of potassium chloride concentrate solutions to pharmacy departments and critical care areas
  - Introduction of a controlled drug-style system for requisition and storage of the product in critical care areas
  - Utilisation of commercially available diluted solutions wherever possible

  Familiarise yourself with the policies for control of use of parenteral potassium chloride in your hospital and the range of products in use locally. Death or harm resulting from a potassium-containing solution is an MHRA 'never event'.[4]

Oral potassium therapy

- Sando-K is typically given as 2 tablets three or four times a day; if serum potassium levels are in the range 2–3 mmol/L, then up to 16 tablets/day may be given[5]
- Liquid and effervescent preparations are preferred. If Slow-K tablets are used, counsel the patient to swallow whole with a full glass of water and remain upright for a few minutes after taking (as this reduces the likelihood of oesophageal ulceration). 'Ghost tablets' may appear in stools[6]
- The potassium content of the various oral preparations available is listed in Table P12 for comparison

TABLE P12

Potassium content of various oral preparations

Product	Potassium content
Sando-K	12 mmol/tablet
Slow-K	8 mmol/tablet
Kay-Cee-L syrup	1 mmol/mL

Monitoring	Monitor serum potassium concentration at least daily and stop treatment when serum potassium levels return to the normal range

Hyperkalaemia

Symptoms	• Include ECG abnormalities, ventricular arrhythmias, and cardiac arrest. • There may also be neuromuscular dysfunction, e.g. muscle weakness and paralysis
Causes	• Excessive intake, e.g. overuse of Lo-Salt (a salt alternative containing 66.6% potassium chloride and 33.4% sodium chloride), inappropriate use of parenteral solutions • Decreased elimination, e.g. in renal failure • Metabolic acidosis • Drugs, e.g. those acting on the renin–angiotensin–aldosterone system: aliskiren, angiotensin-converting enzyme inhibitors, angiotensin II receptor antagonists, aldosterone antagonists, potassium-sparing diuretics, potassium salts, indometacin, trimethoprim, heparins, ciclosporin, tacrolimus[1]
Assessment	• Renal function and electrolytes (Ur, Cr, K, Na), Mg, Ca • A serum potassium concentration of >6.5 mmol/L will usually require urgent treatment, as will those with ECG changes
Treatment	• Give 10 mL calcium gluconate 10% intravenously over 2–3 minutes to stabilise cardiac muscle. N.B.: this does not change serum potassium levels. Repeat as necessary within 5–10 minutes if no effect, dependent on ECG. Duration of action is usually 30–60 minutes so further doses may be necessary if serum potassium remains raised.[7] • Rapidly lower the potassium serum level by giving soluble insulin, e.g. Actrapid insulin 10 units in glucose 50%.[8] The insulin causes uptake of potassium from the extracellular fluid into cells, lowering the level, while the glucose limits the hypoglycaemic effect of the insulin. Higher doses of insulin carry an increased risk of hypoglycaemia. • Nebulised salbutamol (10–20 mg) can also be used in conjunction with the above measures, but should not be used as monotherapy for severe hyperkalaemia.[7] This also moves potassium into the cells. • Dialysis may be an option if these measures are ineffective. • After emergency treatment, or if initial potassium is in the range 5.1–6.4 mmol/L, if possible treat the cause of the hyperkalaemia. This includes stopping any implicated drugs and treating underlying medical conditions. • Calcium Resonium or Resonium A resin may be given but should be stopped when serum potassium concentration falls to 5 mmol/L
Adminis-tration	**Administration of insulin and glucose** • Draw up 50 mL of glucose 50% into a 50 mL syringe from a vial or a 500 mL infusion bag. Infusion bags are preferred to Minijets as they are easier to handle, maintain aseptic technique and are cheaper. • Draw up the prescribed amount of insulin using an insulin syringe (usually 10 units) and add to the 50 mL syringe. Cap the syringe and mix well to disperse the insulin thoroughly. Failure to do this may result in unexpected hypoglycaemia. • Place the syringe in a syringe driver and give intravenously over 5–15 minutes (slower administration reduces thrombophlebitis). Effects are observed within 15–30 minutes and last for 4–6 hours.

Oral/rectal therapy for hyperkalaemia

Continuing treatment with either Calcium Resonium or Resonium A may be appropriate.

- Calcium Resonium should be avoided in patients who have conditions associated with hypercalcaemia.[9]
- Resonium A should be avoided in patients at risk from an increase in sodium load. Neither product should be given if the patient has obstructive bowel disease.[10]
- Both resins can affect the body's balance of magnesium and calcium, and patients should be monitored for disturbances in these electrolytes.
- Antacids and laxatives containing cations, such as magnesium and aluminium, should be avoided during treatment.
- Absorption of lithium and levothyroxine may be reduced.[9,10]
- In the initial stages of treatment of hyperkalaemia, administration by the rectal route as well as orally may help to achieve a rapid lowering of the serum potassium level. If both routes are used initially, it is probably unnecessary to continue rectal administration once the oral resin has reached the rectum.

Oral therapy

- The dose of both Calcium Resonium and Resonium A resins is 15 g three or four times daily.
- Mix the powder with a little water, or mix to a paste with a sweetening vehicle, e.g. jam or honey (do not use fruit squash because of high potassium content).
- Treatment may need to be continued for several days or long-term.[7]

Rectal administration

- Both forms can be given daily as an enema (30 g resin in 150 mL water or 10% dextrose, and retained for at least 9 hours (this may be tricky), and the colon irrigated to remove the resin).
- Some local manufacturing units supply ready-made kits.
- Faecal impaction can sometimes occur with the enema, and lactulose may be used to resolve this. If clinically significant constipation occurs, treatment should be stopped until normal bowel movement returns

Monitoring	Very frequent monitoring of serum potassium level is crucial (every few hours), particularly during the early stages of treatment of severe hyperkalaemia

REFERENCES

1 *Martindale: The Complete Drug Reference* (2015). www.medicinescomplete.com (accessed 15 January 2015).

2 UK Medicines Information (2012). *How Should Intravenous Potassium Chloride be Administered in Adults?* NHS: UKMi Medicines Q&A. www.evidence.nhs.uk (accessed 17 January 2015).

3 NPSA (2002). *Potassium Chloride Concentrate Solutions – Patient safety alert.* http://www.nrls.npsa.nhs.uk/resources/?entryid45=59882 (accessed 17 January 2015).

4 NHS England (2014). *The Never Events List: 2013/14 update.* NHS England: Patient safety domain team. http://www.england.nhs.uk/wp-content/uploads/2013/12/nev-ev-list-1314-clar.pdf (accessed 14 July 2014).

5 SPC (2014). *Sando-K.* www.medicines.org.uk (accessed 17 January 2015).

6   SPC (2014). *Slow-K*. www.medicines.org.uk (accessed 17 January 2015).

7   Renal Association (2012). *Treatment of Acute Hyperkalemia in Adults*. www.renal.org (accessed 14 July 2014).

8   Longmore M *et al.* (eds) (2004). *Oxford Handbook of Clinical Medicine* (6th edn). Oxford: Oxford University Press.

9   SPC (2014). *Calcium Resonium*. www.medicines.org.uk (accessed 17 January 2015).

10 SPC (2014). *Resonium A*. www.medicines.org.uk (accessed 17 January 2015).

Prescription charge exemptions and prepayment certificates

Prescription charge exemptions on medical grounds

People are eligible for free NHS prescriptions if they suffer from specific medical conditions and they hold a valid medical exemption certificate. In NHS England, the specified medical conditions are currently:[1]

- a permanent fistula (for example, caecostomy, colostomy, laryngostomy or ileostomy) that needs continuous surgical dressing or an appliance
- a form of hypoadrenalism (for example, Addison's disease) for which specific substitution therapy is essential
- diabetes insipidus and other forms of hypopituitarism
- diabetes mellitus, except where treatment is by diet alone
- hypoparathyroidism
- myasthenia gravis
- myxoedema (that is, hypothyroidism that needs thyroid hormone replacement)
- epilepsy that needs continuous antiepileptic therapy
- a continuing physical disability, which means you cannot go out without the help of another person
- cancer: undergoing treatment; the effects of cancer; or the effects of cancer treatment.

Such individuals are exempt from all prescription charges, not just for items prescribed for the condition specified. There is variation across other parts of the UK where, for instance, in Wales all prescriptions are free.

Medical exemption certificates are valid for 5 years. Application forms are available at general practitioner surgeries and must be completed and signed by the patient and doctor. The general practitioner sends the completed form directly to:

NHS Help With Health Costs
Medical Exemption
Bridge House
152 Pilgrim Street
Newcastle Upon Tyne
NE1 6SN
UK.

Prepayment certificates

These can be bought for 4- or 12-month periods, and their current price is listed in the *Drug Tariff*.[2] Application forms can be obtained from pharmacies and surgeries, or completed online using the following link: https://apps.nhsbsa.nhs.uk/ppcwebsales/patient.do. Some community pharmacies may sell certificates directly.

REFERENCES

1 NHS England (2014). *Help with Health Costs.* http://www.nhsbsa.nhs.uk /HealthCosts/Documents/HealthCosts/HC11_April_2014.pdf (accessed 23 February 2015).

2 *Drug Tariff Online* (updated monthly). http://www.ppa.org.uk/ppa/edt_intro.htm (accessed 23 February 2015).

Protamine

Protamine sulfate is used to reverse or neutralise the anticoagulant effect of unfractionated and, to a lesser extent, low-molecular-weight heparin (LMWH). It is derived from fish sperm, and acts by binding with heparin to form a salt. 1 mg protamine neutralises 100 units of heparin.[1]

Neutralisation of heparin given by intravenous infusion

Stop the heparin infusion. To calculate the amount of protamine needed, consider the amount of heparin given in the last 2 hours. This is due to the short (60–90 minutes) half-life of heparin. For example, if a patient is receiving 1500 units/hour of heparin and requires reversal, give 30 mg protamine intravenously. This should be given no faster than 5 mg/min, as the risk of severe hypotension and anaphylaxis is increased at faster administration rates. No more than 50 mg protamine should be given in one dose. Protamine has a shorter half-life than heparin (7 minutes), so repeated doses may be required.

Neutralisation of heparin given by subcutaneous injection

As the absorption from subcutaneous injection is slower, the total dose of protamine required is calculated from the total dose of subcutaneous heparin given. Protamine 25–50 mg is given as a slow intravenous bolus, then the remainder is infused over 8–16 hours.[2,3]

Neutralisation of LMWH

For LMWH, the usual recommendation is 1 mg protamine to 100 units LMWH. The anti-Xa activity may not be completely reversed. If the LMWH has been given up to 8 hours prior to the requirement for reversal, protamine in the dose described above can be used. If more than 8 hours has elapsed, lower doses of protamine may be tried. Doses may need to be repeated due to the longer half-life of LMWH.

Risk of allergy

Some patients have an increased risk of allergy to protamine and must be monitored carefully or given antihistamines or corticosteroids pretreatment. These include: previous protamine exposure, patients with diabetes treated with protamine insulin, patients with a fish allergy, men with a vasectomy or infertile who may have protamine antibodies.

The reason for the caution with fish sensitivity and vasectomised males is as follows. When undergoing elective vasectomy, antibodies develop against natural nucleoprotamines (a normal component of human sperm cells) in 22–33% of patients. These antibodies have been shown to cross-react with medicinal protamines, which are extracted commercially from the testes of salmon and certain other fish. There is an increased risk of an allergic reaction developing if these individuals are later exposed to protamine as a medication as cross-reactivity can occur.[4]

REFERENCES

1 SPC (2010). *Protamine Sulphate 10mg/ml Solution for Injection.* http://www.medicines.org.uk/emc/medicine/13567 (accessed 19 November 2014).

2 American College of Chest Physicians (2012). *Antithrombotic Guidelines* (9th edn). http://www.chestnet.org/Guidelines-and-Resources/Guidelines-and-Consensus-Statements/Antithrombotic-Guidelines-9th-Ed (accessed 19 November 2014).

3 British Committee for Standards in Haematology (2012). *Guidelines: Managing bleeding with anti-thrombotic agents.* http://onlinelibrary.wiley.com/store/10.1111/bjh.12107/asset/bjh12107.pdf;jsessionid=2023AF04077F18258798B59461144C9A.f03t01?v=1&t=i2p54js1&s=ba9775e3ebf44b5e80d9e066460d19d1a2f67f4e (accessed 19 November 2014).

4 Watson RA *et al.* (1983). Allergic reaction to protamine: a late complication of elective vasectomy? *Urology* 22: 493–495.

Prothrombin complex concentrates

The two main 4-factor prothrombin complex concentrates (PCC) in use in the UK are Beriplex and Octaplex.[1] They are used for the reversal of bleeding caused by vitamin K antagonists, and for patients bleeding or due for surgery who have a congenital deficiency in the vitamin K-dependent coagulation factors II and X when the specific factors are not available. They contain the vitamin K-dependent clotting factors II, VIII, IX and X, protein C and protein S. The two products differ slightly in the amounts of the factors they contain. As most of the amounts can vary within a range, it is only the factor X that is significantly higher in Beriplex. Both contain small amounts of heparin as an excipient.

They are both blood products (derived from human plasma), so local guidelines on the use of blood products should be followed, with records made of batch number and expiry. They should be used when rapid correction of clotting is required, such as for bleeding or emergency surgery – not for elective surgery or in response to a high INR with no bleeding. The dose of PCC required is based on units of factor IX and is dependent on the INR and the patient's weight.

- Octaplex: a single dose should not exceed 3000 units (120 mL) intravenously at a starting rate of not more than 1 mL/min, increasing to 2–3 mL/min. Higher rates, up to 10 mL/min, have been used, according to the Medusa drug administration guide, but this is not licensed.[2]

- Beriplex: a single dose should not exceed 5000 units given intravenously at a rate of not more than 3 units/kg/min up to a maximum of 210 units/min (approximately 8 mL/min).

It is essential that no blood flows into the syringe containing the product during administration as there is a risk of formation of fibrin clots.

The effect of PCC on coagulation can take up to 30 minutes, but the INR can quickly start to increase again due to the short half-life of the factors. Vitamin K (phytomenadione) 5 mg is therefore given at the same time and this takes effect within 4–6 hours when given intravenously.[3]

The INR should be monitored regularly throughout treatment. Many patients on warfarin will have an underlying hypercoagulable state; PCC can exacerbate this and a thrombus can develop. Disseminated intravascular coagulation (DIC) can also develop as a side effect.[3] PCCs can cause allergy and anaphylaxis and, as they contain heparin, should not be used in patients with a history of HIT, and can actually cause HIT. Other side effects include headache and pyrexia.

Both PCCs can be tried in cases of life-threatening bleeding with the novel oral anticoagulants: dabigatran (a direct thrombin inhibitor), rivaroxaban and apixaban (direct factor Xa inhibitors). There are no extensive trials in patients but there are data from animal and healthy human studies and case reports suggesting they may be of some effect.

The use of the products for patients with a congenital deficiency of any of the vitamin K-dependent coagulation factors is detailed in the SPC.

REFERENCES

1 eMC (2014). www.medicines.org.uk (accessed 1 November 2014).
2 Injectable Medicines Guide (2014). http://www.injguide.nhs.uk/?ID= cb046ef7dab14de7ec7a81755f2f71f01305 (accessed 9 November 2014).
3 Keeling D et al.(2011). Guidelines on oral anticoagulation with warfarin – 4th edition. Br J Haematol 154: 311–324.

Pulmonary function tests

PFTs are non-invasive tests that provide measurable feedback about the function of the lungs. PFTs have both diagnostic and therapeutic roles.

Peak expiratory flow rate

The peak expiratory flow rate (PEFR) is measured using a portable, hand-held peak flow meter, and is the rate at which the air is expelled forcefully from the lungs. PEFR is a useful measure of airway calibre in the management of asthma and is ideally expressed as a percentage

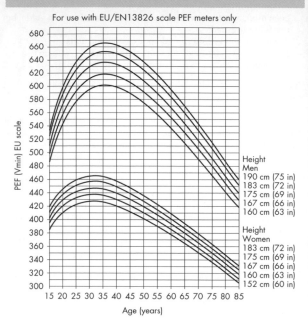

For use with EU/EN13826 scale PEF meters only

Height
Men
190 cm (75 in)
183 cm (72 in)
175 cm (69 in)
167 cm (66 in)
160 cm (63 in)

Height
Women
183 cm (72 in)
175 cm (69 in)
167 cm (66 in)
160 cm (63 in)
152 cm (60 in)

Adapted by Clement Clarke for use with EN13826 / EU scale peak flow meters from Nunn AJ Gregg I, Br Med J 1989:298;1068-70

FIGURE P1   Peak expiratory flow rate – normal values

of the patient's previous best value. In the absence of a previous best result, the PEFR as a percentage of the predicted value is an approximate guide (Figure P1).

When taking a reading, the patient performs three maximum forced expirations, and the best of these three results is recorded on a peak flow chart. Trends in PEFR are used to determine the progression of the disease or the success of treatment.

In acute asthma, PEFR is one of the measures used to determine the severity of the attack (Table P13).

TABLE P13
Severity of asthma as determined by peak expiratory flow rate (PEFR)

PEFR	Severity
50–75% of best or predicted	Moderate
33–50% of best or predicted	Acute severe
<33% of best or predicted	Life-threatening

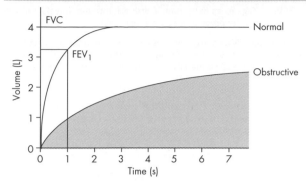

FIGURE P2   An example of a spirometer recording (a spirogram)

PEFR measurement is used by some patients as part of a
self-management plan, e.g. if PEFR drops below a certain percentage
of normal (e.g. <50%), they may have been given instructions to take
a course of oral steroids.

Spirometry

Spirometry is an assessment of lung function by measurement of rate
and volume of air forced out from the lungs immediately after a
maximum inspiration. It is used to differentiate between obstructive
airways disorders (e.g. asthma, COPD) and restrictive disorders (e.g.
interstitial lung diseases).

Relative contraindications for spirometry include haemoptysis of
unknown origin, pneumothorax, unstable angina pectoris, recent
myocardial infarction, thoracic, cerebral or abdominal aneurysms,
recent eye surgery (within 2 weeks due to increased intraocular
pressure during forced expiration), recent abdominal or thoracic
surgical procedures, and patients with a history of syncope associated
with forced exhalation.

Spirometers are the devices used to measure these parameters.
They either produce a spirogram, which is a graph of flow–volume
against time, or they will show the values on a digital display. An
example of a spirogram is shown in Figure P2. Interpretation of
spirometry results should begin with an assessment of test quality.
Failure to meet performance standards can result in unreliable test
results and possible incorrect diagnosis. Reproducibility of the forced
vital capacity (FVC) and the forced expiratory volume (FEV_1) helps
ensure that the results truly represent the patient's lung function.[1]

The main measures obtained by spirometry are as follows:

- FEV_1 is the volume of air that the patient can exhale in the first
  second of forced expiration.
- FVC is the total volume of air that the patient can forcibly exhale in
  one breath.

- FEV_1/FVC gives an indication of airflow limitation. It is the ratio of FEV_1 to FVC, expressed as a percentage.

The FEV_1 and FVC are expressed as a percentage of the predicted normal rate for a person of the same sex, ethnicity, age and height. Tables P14 and P15 contain the reference values for FEV_1 and FVC.

TABLE P14
Predicted values of forced vital capacity (FVC) and forced expiratory volume in 1 second (FEV_1) in men

Male			Height						
			5′ 3″ 160 cm	5′ 5″ 165 cm	5′ 7″ 170 cm	5′ 9″ 175 cm	5′ 11″ 180 cm	6′ 1″ 185 cm	6′ 3″ 190 cm
Age	38–41	FVC	3.81	4.10	4.39	4.67	4.96	5.25	5.54
	years	FEV_1	3.20	3.42	3.63	3.85	4.06	4.28	4.49
	42–45	FVC	3.71	3.99	4.28	4.57	4.86	5.15	5.43
	years	FEV_1	3.09	3.30	3.52	3.73	3.95	4.16	4.38
	46–49	FVC	3.60	3.89	4.18	4.47	4.75	5.04	5.33
	years	FEV_1	2.97	3.18	3.40	6.61	2083	4.04	4.26
	50–53	FVC	3.50	3.79	4.07	4.36	4.65	4.94	5.23
	years	FEV_1	2.85	3.07	3.28	3.50	3.71	3.93	4.14
	54–57	FVC	3.39	3.68	3.97	4.26	4.55	4.83	5.12
	years	FEV_1	2.74	2.95	3.17	3.38	3.60	3.81	4.03
	58–61	FVC	3.29	3.58	3.87	4.15	4.44	4.73	5.02
	years	FEV_1	2.62	2.84	3.05	3.27	3.48	3.70	3.91
	62–65	FVC	3.19	3.47	3.76	4.05	4.34	4.63	4.91
	years	FEV_1	2.51	2.72	2.94	3.15	3.37	3.58	3.80
	66–69	FVC	3.08	3.37	3.66	3.95	4.23	4.52	4.81
	years	FEV_1	2.39	2.60	2.82	3.03	3.25	3.46	3.68

These values apply to Caucasians and should be reduced by 7% for Asians and by 13% for Afro-Caribbeans.

COPD is diagnosed if the postbronchodilator FEV_1/FVC is <70% and the patient has symptoms and risk factors for developing COPD. The severity of the airflow obstruction is determined by the variation of FEV_1 from the predicted, and is classified as mild, moderate, severe or very severe depending on the degree of the reduction of FEV_1 from the predicted value. In a restrictive disorder, the spirometry would show FEV_1 <80% and FVC <80%, but the FEV_1/FVC ratio would be normal (>70%).

Figure P3 gives an example of how spirometry can work in practice.

Reversibility measurements
When airway obstruction is identified on spirometry, reversibility testing is useful in cases of diagnostic doubt, especially to help identify people with COPD or asthma. Response is assessed

TABLE P15
Predicted values of forced vital capacity (FVC) and forced expiratory volume in 1 second (FEV₁) in women

Female			Height						
			4′ 11″	5′ 1″	5′ 3″	5′ 5″	5′ 7″	5′ 9″	5′ 11″
			150 cm	155 cm	160 cm	165 cm	170 cm	175 cm	180 cm
Age	38–41	FVC	2.69	2.91	3.13	3.35	3.58	3.80	4.02
	years	FEV₁	2.30	2.50	2.70	2.89	3.09	3.29	3.49
	42–45	FVC	2.59	2.81	3.03	3.25	3.47	3.69	3.91
	years	FEV₁	2.20	2.40	2.60	2.79	2.99	3.19	3.39
	46–49	FVC	2.48	2.70	2.92	3.15	3.37	3.59	3.81
	years	FEV₁	2.10	2.30	2.50	2.69	2.89	3.09	3.29
	50–53	FVC	2.38	2.60	2.82	3.04	3.26	3.48	3.71
	years	FEV₁	2.00	2.20	2.40	2.59	2.79	2.99	3.19
	54–57	FVC	2.27	2.49	2.72	2.94	3.16	3.38	3.60
	years	FEV₁	1.90	2.10	2.30	2.49	2.69	2.89	3.09
	58–61	FVC	2.17	2.39	2.61	2.83	3.06	3.28	3.50
	years	FEV₁	1.80	2.00	2.20	2.39	2.59	2.79	2.99
	62–65	FVC	2.07	2.29	2.51	2.73	2.95	3.17	3.39
	years	FEV₁	1.70	1.90	2.10	2.29	2.49	2.6	2.89
	66–69	FVC	1.96	2.18	2.40	2.63	2.85	3.07	3.29
	years	FEV₁	1.60	1.80	2.00	2.19	2.39	2.70	2.79

These values apply to Caucasians and should be reduced by 7% for Asians and by 13% for Afro-Caribbeans.

A 47-year-old woman, 5′5″ (165 cm), has an FEV₁ of 1.48 litres and an FVC of 2.6 litres.

$$FEV_1 = \frac{\text{reading (1.48)}}{\text{predicted (2.69)}} \times 100 = 55\% \text{ of predicted normal}$$

$$FVC = \frac{\text{reading (2.6)}}{\text{predicted (3.15)}} \times 100 = 82.5\% \text{ of predicted normal}$$

$$\frac{FEV_1}{FVC} = \frac{\text{reading (1.48)}}{\text{reading (2.6)}} \times 100 = 56.9\%$$

This patient has moderate airflow obstruction (FEV₁ between 50% and 80% of predicted and FEV₁/FVC is <70%). The patient could have either COPD or asthma, and the diagnosis will be dependent on clinical features, history and, if required, bronchodilator reversibility.

FIGURE P3 An example of spirometry interpretation

10–15 minutes after inhalation of a therapeutic dose of salbutamol (four inhalations each of 100 micrograms) administered through a valved spacer device. Asthma can usually be identified if the following are found:

- FEV_1 and FEV_1/FVC ratio returns to normal with drug therapy
- a very large (>400 mL) FEV_1 response to bronchodilators, or to 30 mg oral prednisolone daily for 2 weeks
- serial peak flow measurements showing significant (20% or greater) diurnal or day-to-day variability.

REFERENCE

1 Bellamy D (2005). *Spirometry in Practice: A practical guide to using spirometry in primary care* (2nd edn). London: BTS COPD Consortium.

Pulmonary hypertension and pulmonary arterial hypertension

Our understanding of pulmonary hypertension (PH) has been transformed in recent years. The 'face' of the PH patient has been transformed from a young female (the classic pulmonary arterial hypertension (PAH) patient) having few treatment options and a dismal survival, to an older demographic with numerous comorbidities,[1] and elevated pulmonary pressures, which can complicate a variety of cardiac and respiratory disorders. Understanding of the common pathological processes in certain classes of the disease has led to the development of targeted treatments. It is crucial that pharmacists understand the roles and limitations of specialised drugs and how use of these agents fits into general supportive care. Numerous interactions and adverse effects complicate the use of these specialised treatments.

Diagnostic classification

The diagnostic classification of PH[2] can be seen in Table P16.[3]

TABLE P16

Clinical classification of pulmonary hypertension[4]

Classification group	Sample causes	Comment
Group 1 Pulmonary arterial hypertension (PAH)	• Idiopathic PAH • Heritable PAH – some genotypes have been identified • Drug- and toxin-induced, e.g. anorexigens • Associated with: connective tissue disease, HIV infection, portal hypertension, congenital heart diseases, schistosomiasis, lymphangioleiomyomatosis	Causes in group 1 and group 1′ (PAH) share a common pathophysiology and have proven benefit from therapy acting on the endothelin, nitric oxide and prostacyclin pathways
Group 1′	• Pulmonary veno-occlusive disease	

(Continued)

TABLE P16
(Continued)

Classification group	Sample causes	Comment
Group 2 Pulmonary hypertension (PH) due to left heart disease	• Left ventricular dysfunction • Valvular disease • Congenital/acquired left heart inflow/outflow tract obstruction and congenital cardiomyopathies	In group 2, pulmonary vasodilators may worsen pulmonary oedema and in group 3, ventilation/perfusion mismatching may be worsened by these agents. Targeted therapy should generally not be used. Treatment should be directed at managing underlying cause. Congenital heart disease may have consequent PAH or PH, depending on the exact nature of the disease and any repair. Some of these patients (PAH) may be suitable for targeted therapies
Group 3 PH due to lung disease and/or hypoxaemia	• Chronic obstructive pulmonary disease • Interstitial lung disease • Sleep-disordered breathing	
Group 4 Chronic thromboembolic PH (CTEPH)	• Approximately 4% of patients with pulmonary embolism can develop CTEPH. Ventilation perfusion scan is an important part of the work-up for PH	For CTEPH: a pulmonary endarterectomy can be curative. A recent trial of riociguat in inoperable CTEPH showed benefit[5]
Group 5 PH with unclear multifactorial mechanism	• Haematological disorders • Systemic disorders: sarcoidosis, pulmonary histiocytosis, lymphangioleiomyomatosis	

PAH is defined as a mean pulmonary artery pressure ≥ 25 mmHg and pulmonary capillary wedge pressure ≤ 15 mmHg on right heart catheterisation with exclusion of other causes.[6] If these values are found, further tests are performed to find the underlying cause. During the right heart catheterisation, vasodilator testing with either nitric oxide or epoprostenol will be carried out. The (rare) 'responders' to this test are treated with high-dose nifedipine or diltiazem (depending on heart rate).[4] Non-responders will be treated with specialised treatments with choice based on functional class, ability to comply with complex regimens and methods of administration, interactions and comorbidities (see below).

Disease severity

Disease severity is classified using the New York Heart Association (NYHA) (heart failure) classification.[4] Registry data have shown that treatments leading to improvement or maintenance in functional class translate into improved survival, whilst progression on treatment is associated with worse outcome.[7] The aim of treatment is that the patient improves to class II symptoms; for patients with group 1 PAH the initial choice of targeted therapy will be made depending on the NYHA class (Table P17).

TABLE P17
Functional class and evidence-based targeted therapy

Functional class	Proportion of patients at presentation (UK and Irish registry)	Symptoms	Recommendations for targeted therapy[1]
Class I	15%	Does not limit physical activity	Nil
Class II	15%	Comfortable at rest but slight limitation of physical activity	Ambrisentan, bosentan, sildenafil, tadalafil, riociguat
Class III	67%	Comfortable at rest but marked limitation of physical activity	Ambrisentan, bosentan, sildenafil, intravenous epoprostenol, inhaled iloprost, tadalafil, treprostinil, riociguat
Class IV	18%	Unable to carry out any physical activities without symptoms and may be symptomatic at rest	Intravenous epoprostenol, ambrisentan, bosentan, sildenafil, inhaled or intravenous iloprost, subcutaneous, intravenous or inhaled treprostinil Initial combination therapy

Supportive care

For all types of PH, the importance of supportive treatment cannot be overstated:

1 optimal management of any underlying cause or aggravating factor, e.g. hypothyroidism, infection (particularly pneumonia), anaemia, pulmonary embolism, arrhythmia, non-adherence
2 heart failure management with fluid restriction, salt restriction, diuretics etc.
3 oxygen therapy may be appropriate
4 warfarin is widely used in PAH, with a target INR of approximately 1.5–2 (unless higher is indicated, e.g. in atrial fibrillation). Most of the evidence predates the advent of specialised treatments
5 vaccination (influenza and pneumococcal)
6 physiotherapy
7 psychosocial support/support group network

8 agents to avoid (particularly in class III and IV PAH):
- pregnancy (50% postpartum mortality)
- oestrogen-containing contraceptives are unsuitable (N.B.: bosentan increases clearance of the contraceptive pill)
- cyclizine: anecdotal risk of hypotension and falls
- beta-blockers: may be used if compelling indication in PH
- platelet transfusions
- precipitating medications – anorexigens.

Specialised treatments

Once diagnosis of PAH is confirmed, any reversible factors have been addressed and fluid balance has been optimised, targeted therapy can be instigated. There is a common pathology underlying PAH, involving endothelin, nitric oxide and prostacyclin pathways. Pharmacological agents have been developed to target each of these pathways. Clinical trials have shown the benefit of various combinations; however, the cost means that combinations of more than two agents are not routine practice in the UK.

Phosphodiesterase type-5 (PDE-5) inhibitors

These work on the nitric oxide pathway. Headache and flushing usually subside and hypotension can be avoided by careful titration.[8] Sildenafil has more interaction potential than tadalafil. CYP3A4 inducers and inhibitors have an important effect on sildenafil and slightly less effect on tadalafil kinetics. Bosentan reduces the sildenafil area under the curve by >60%; however, this combination is widely used in practice. Doses used in practice and clinical trials have been ≥80 mg three times a day, although the licensed dose is substantially lower than this.[8] The combination of tadalafil and bosentan has not been as extensively studied. The recently licensed riociguat acts on the same pathway and concomitant use with PDE-5 inhibitors is contraindicated.[8] Nitrates are contraindicated with all of these agents.

Endothelin receptor antagonists

Bosentan, ambrisentan and macitentan block the endothelin receptors A and B in differing ratios.[8] The significance of this difference is not currently fully understood. The main toxicities of these agents are hepatotoxicity and anaemia. The hepatotoxicity of bosentan and ambrisentan is thought to be due to their effects on the bile efflux pump; this is not affected by macitentan.[8] Monthly LFTs (and pregnancy test, where appropriate) are required while on these agents[8] (sitaxentan was withdrawn due to hepatotoxicity). These agents are teratogenic, and effective contraception methods must be used. Bosentan lowers the effectiveness of the oral contraceptive pill.[8]

Prostacyclin analogues

These are complex and demanding therapies, requiring involved administration schedules using sophisticated delivery devices.[8] Iloprost is nebulised up to six times daily using a breath-activated nebuliser. Epoprostenol, iloprost and treprostinil (unlicensed) may be given by continuous intravenous infusion. It is also possible to give treprostinil by continuous subcutaneous infusion; this route has the disadvantage of severe site pain, which is not related to dose. The demands of complying with these treatments (including line care) mean that comparatively few patients can benefit from these treatments.

REFERENCES

1 Peacock A (2013). Clinical year in review – pulmonary hypertension. *Eur Resp Rev* 22: 20–25.

2 Simonneau G *et al.* (2013). Updated clinical classification of pulmonary hypertension.. *J Am Coll Cardiol* 62(Suppl): D34–D41.

3 Ghofrani HA *et al.* (2013). Riociguat for the treatment of chronic thromboembolic pulmonary hypertension.. *N Engl J Med* 369: 319–329.

4 Barst RJ *et al.* (2011). Impact of functional class change on survival in patients with pulmonary arterial hypertension in the reveal registry. *Am J Respir Crit Care Med* 183: A5941.

5 Simonneau G *et al.* (2013). Riociguat for the treatment of Chronic Thromboembolic Pulmonary Hypertension (CTEPH): 1-year results from the CHEST-2 long-term extension study. *Chest* 144(4 Meeting Abstracts): 1023A.

6 Galie N *et al.* (2009). Guidelines for the diagnosis and treatment of pulmonary hypertension. *Eur Respir J* 34: 1219–1263.

7 Ling Y *et al.* (2012). Changing demographics, epidemiology and survival of incident pulmonary arterial hypertension: Results from the Pulmonary Hypertension Registry of the United Kingdom and Ireland. *Am J Respir Crit Care Med* 186: 790–796.

8 eMC (2014). https://www.medicines.org.uk/emc/ (accessed 30 August 2014).

Quinine for muscle cramps

Cramp is a transient, involuntary episode of pain due to muscle spasm, continuing for up to 10 minutes. One-third of people over 60 years suffer from leg cramps: 40% have three or more attacks per week.[1]

Evidence for use of quinine

Mechanism of action is unknown but muscle excitability appears reduced. Quinine has modest efficacy: 25% reduction in frequency,[2,3] although patient response varies. There is no evidence for long-term use.

Choice of treatment

Rule out secondary causes:

- pregnancy
- exercise
- medication – diuretics, salbutamol, raloxifene, nifedipine, phenothiazines, penicillamine, nicotinic acid and statins may aggravate cramps. Review and discontinue or reduce dose if possible
- identify and treat disease, e.g. Baker's cyst, deep-vein thrombosis, dystonia, myoclonus, parkinsonism, metabolic problems.[1]

Reassure patient: idiopathic cramps are common, have no real cause, tend to resolve on their own and won't lead to any serious complications.

Provide advice on self-care measures, such as stretching exercises and massaging the affected area.[1] Simple analgesia can alleviate post-cramp pain.

Consider quinine only if cramps are very painful, frequent enough to affect quality of life or self-care measures have failed.[4] Prescribe only after weighing up the risks of serious adverse effects versus the benefits to the patient.

If appropriate, prescribe 200–300 mg quinine sulfate at bedtime for 4–6 weeks.

Monitor effect by using a sleep or cramp diary. Stop if benefit is not seen. If the patient experiences benefit, continue treatment for another 3 months and review.

If long-term treatment is required, interrupt every 3–6 months to assess for continued effectiveness and ongoing need.[1,2,4,5]

Key prescribing points

- State salt when prescribing: quinine sulfate 200 mg ≅ quinine bisulfate 300 mg.
- For low-dose therapy, no dosage adjustment is required for renal impairment.[6]
- Patients should not have quinine-containing drinks, such as tonic water or bitter lemon.
- Adverse effects are unlikely at these doses but stop treatment if tinnitus, impaired hearing, headache, gastrointestinal symptoms or disturbed vision are experienced. Thrombocytopenia is rare but advise patients to report unexplained bleeding or unusual bruising.
- In overdose, quinine can cause irreversible blindness and death.

Quinine drug interactions

- Quinine may increase risk of ventricular arrhythmias with antipsychotics, antiarrhythmics and moxifloxacin.
- Quinine may increase digoxin levels.
- Antivirals may increase quinine levels.

REFERENCES

1 NICE (2014). *Clinical Knowledge Summaries. Leg cramps.* http://cks.nice.org.uk/leg-cramps (accessed 20 August 2014).
2 Joint Formulary Committee (2014). *British National Formulary* (67th edn). London: BMJ Group and Pharmaceutical Press.
3 El-Tawil S *et al.* (2010). Quinine for muscle cramps. *Cochrane Database of Systemat Rev Issue* 12: (accessed 20 August 2014).
4 MHRA (2010). *Quinine: Not to be used routinely for nocturnal leg cramps.* Drug Safety Update. http://www.mhra.gov.uk/Safetyinformation/DrugSafetyUpdate/CON085085 (accessed 20 August 2014).
5 SPC (2014). *Quinine Sulphate Tablets BP 200mg.* Actavis UK Limited (accessed 20 August 2014).
6 Ashley C, Currie A (eds) (2009). *The Renal Drug Handbook* (3rd edn). Oxford: Radcliffe Medical Press.

R

Rapid tranquillisation

Rapid tranquillisation is a pharmacological strategy that is used over brief intervals of time to help manage acute behavioural disturbance in patients who are unable otherwise to maintain the safety of themselves, others or their environment.[1,2]

Treatment goals

The primary aim is "to anticipate and reduce the risk of violence and aggression". It may be used to avoid or allow cessation of other management strategies, such as seclusion or physical intervention.[3]

Other aims are to reduce the suffering of the service user and to intervene without causing harm (by prescribing safely and monitoring appropriately).[2]

Considerations

The available evidence base is poor. Guidance is based on a mix of evidence and clinical experience and therefore varies across settings and organisations.[2] Person-centred care, including effective risk assessment and risk management strategies should be used to predict and prevent disturbed behaviour where possible.[3]

Risk factors for disturbed behaviour can relate to the service user (e.g. history of disturbed behaviour/trauma, presence of trigger factors/stressors), clinical factors (e.g. effect of alcohol/substances/medication, active mental illness) and the situation itself (e.g. freedom being restricted).[3]

Rapid tranquillisation should only be considered once other management strategies, such as verbal de-escalation, have been ineffective. De-escalation techniques should continue to be used throughout.[3] Clinical need, safety of service users and staff, and advance directives should be considered when deciding which management strategy is indicated, and it must be a proportionate response to the risk posed by the service user.[3]

Identification and treatment of any underlying illness/condition (e.g. psychosis, delirium) should occur alongside rapid tranquillisation, and total daily doses and the possibility of additive adverse effects should be borne in mind.[2]

The medication chosen for rapid tranquillisation is not dictated by any underlying illness; someone with active psychosis may receive an agent other than an antipsychotic for rapid tranquillisation.[2] Arrangements for review of the effect of the medication used and the presentation of the service user should be made in advance.[3]

Staff should be trained to the appropriate resuscitation level, and resuscitation equipment (including oxygen) and medical support must be quickly available if required.[3] Consent and capacity issues must be covered in line with relevant legislation; the Mental Health Act Code of Practice should be followed and any departures from this clearly documented along with rationale.[3]

A physical examination and history (including ECG), and medication and substance history should be carried out prior to undertaking rapid tranquillisation, whenever possible.[1] Privacy and dignity must be maintained for the service user as much as possible. The service user should be debriefed regarding the reasons for the intervention as soon as possible after the event and encouraged to document his or her account of what occurred in the clinical record if s/he wishes.[3]

Medication

The main agents used are benzodiazepines, antipsychotics and antihistamines. Doses need to be individualised to the service user, and will generally be lower in older adults or those with medical comorbidities than those quoted below.[3]

The oral route is preferable; the intramuscular route may be indicated when oral medication is ineffective or has been refused, or where previous experience would suggest it is preferred. Only in exceptional circumstances should the intravenous route be used; senior clinician expertise should be sought prior to doing so.[3]

If the intramuscular route is to be used, lorazepam is the agent of choice if the person is antipsychotic naïve or there is evidence of cardiovascular disease, a prolonged QT interval, or no recent ECG available. Otherwise, a combination of haloperidol and promethazine is recommended;[3] it allows lower doses of both agents to be used, but risks adverse effects from both agents.[2,3]

Prescription considerations:[3]

- Prescribe oral and intramuscular doses separately.
- Do not use two medications from the same class.
- Do not mix medication in the same syringe.

Bioequivalence needs to be borne in mind (e.g. 10 mg of oral haloperidol is approximately equivalent to 6 mg of intramuscular haloperidol). N.B.: BNF and SPC doses may not always match.[1]

Specific SPC cautions, contraindications and requirements (e.g. the need for a baseline ECG prior to use of parenteral haloperidol) should be borne in mind. If medicines are being used off-license, the prescriber should take full responsibility, informed consent should be obtained and documented, and relevant professional guidance should be followed.[3]

Sufficient time should be allowed between doses to elucidate effect (generally 45–60 minutes for oral and 30–60 minutes for intramuscular; but see Table R1), prior to repeating the dose or

TABLE R1

Medication used in rapid tranquillisation[2–4]

Medication	Adult dose	Comments
Oral medication		
Lorazepam	1–2 mg	Recommended to be used in combination with an antipsychotic if psychosis is the underlying cause. Does not accumulate with repeated doses or in hepatic impairment[1]
Olanzapine	10 mg	Not licensed. Slow onset of effect
Risperidone	1–2 mg	Not licensed
Haloperidol	5 mg	SPC recommends a pretreatment ECG and to avoid using concomitantly with other antipsychotics
Promethazine	25 mg	Not licensed. Not recommended by NICE due to lack of UK evidence
Short-acting intramuscular injections		
Lorazepam	2 mg, repeated after 6 hours	May need to be diluted before use depending upon the brand used. Caution in the young/older adults/those with brain damage as disinhibition is more likely
Olanzapine	5–10 mg (usually 10 mg), repeated after 2 hours. Maximum of three injections/day and 20 mg/day (including all formulations)	NICE does not recommend currently due to a lack of UK marketing authorisation. Intramuscular lorazepam should not be used within 1 hour of intramuscular olanzapine, and vice versa
Aripiprazole	9.75 mg (range 5.25–15 mg) repeated after 2 hours. Maximum of three injections/day and 30 mg/day (including all formulations)	Less hypotension than olanzapine but may be less effective
Haloperidol	5 mg (range 2–10 mg), repeated after 4 hours. Maximum of 18 mg/day	NICE recommend as the first-line antipsychotic combination with promethazine
Promethazine	50 mg (may be repeated once after 1–2 hours)	Not licensed. NICE recommend as the first-line agent in combination with haloperdol. May be especially useful if service user is tolerant to benzodiazepines
Intermediate-acting intramuscular injections		
Zuclopenthixol acetate	See SPC	See comments above regarding indications

R

considering moving from oral to intramuscular (only if two doses fail or the person or others are at significant risk), or intramuscular to intravenous administration.[2,3]

The availability of 'rescue' medication needs to be considered. If using an antipsychotic, oral and parenteral forms of an antimuscarinic (e.g. procyclidine) should be quickly available. If using a benzodiazepine, flumazenil should be quickly available.[3]

On occasion, prescribers may elect to use doses exceeding the licensed maximum. In this scenario, specific rationale and risk assessment should be documented; consultation with expert peers may be useful. Monitoring should be more frequent and extensive.[3]

The newer antipsychotics are less likely to cause extrapyramidal adverse effects compared to haloperidol.[2]

Zuclopenthixol acetate is *not* recommended for rapid tranquillisation due to the delay to onset of effect and the long duration of action, nor in those who are antipsychotic-naïve or who are accepting oral medication, but it can be considered for use in the following circumstances:[3]

- There is a previous history of repeated parenteral administration without resolution.
- The service user has responded to zuclopenthixol acetate previously.
- An advance directive is in place indicating this is a preferred management strategy.

Risks

Risks include extrapyramidal adverse effects (especially acute dystonia), oversedation (leading to loss of consciousness/alertness), loss of airway, cardiovascular/respiratory collapse, seizures, neuroleptic malignant syndrome, sudden death, interaction with other medication/substances, issues with comorbidities, injury to the service user/staff and a negative effect on the therapeutic relationship.[1,3]

Cautions

Cautions include pre-existing comorbidities (e.g. QTc prolongation, respiratory issues), hypo-/hyperthermia, stress/extreme emotions, dehydration or extreme physical exertion.[3]

Monitoring

Monitoring should include pulse, blood pressure, temperature, respiratory rate, hydration and consciousness levels.[3]

Parameters should be monitored every 10 minutes initially and then half-hourly until the service user is ambulatory. Any issues detected should prompt increased monitoring, withholding of additional medication and early medical referral.[2]

If consciousness is lost, monitor as if general anaesthesia has been used, including continuous pulse oximetry.[2,3]

If service users refuse to accept monitoring, or remain too behaviourally disturbed for monitoring to be safely undertaken, this should be documented in the clinical record along with any available proxy measures (e.g. being ambulatory, vocalising, looking flushed, becoming unbalanced when standing) used instead.

REFERENCES

1 Bazire S (2014). *Psychotropic Drug Directory: The professionals' pocket handbook and aide memoire*. Dorsington: Lloyd-Reinhold.

2 Taylor D *et al.* (2015). *The Maudsley Prescribing Guidelines in Psychiatry* (12th edn). Chichester: Wiley-Blackwell.

3 NICE (2015). Violence and aggression: short-term management in mental health, health and community settings (NG10) http://www.nice.org.uk/guidance/ng10 (accessed 17 August 2015).

4 eMC (2014). https://www.medicines.org.uk/emc/ (accessed 25 August 2014).

Renal disease: assessment of renal function

Renal function is measured either in terms of creatinine clearance (CrCl) or estimated glomerular filtration rate (eGFR). Serum creatinine alone is not an accurate measure of renal function, as it is affected by factors independent of renal function, including age, gender, race and body size.

Measuring the clearance of an exogenously administered renally cleared marker (e.g. radiolabelled EDTA) is the gold standard in renal function estimation; however, this is expensive and impractical for everyday situations. For this reason, prediction equations using serum creatinine are commonly used to estimate renal function in practice.

Creatinine clearance

The most commonly used method for determining CrCl is the Cockcroft and Gault equation:[1]

$$CrCl \; (mL/min) = \frac{F \times (140 - age) \times weight \; (kg)^*}{serum \; creatinine \; (micromol/L)}$$

where $F = 1.23$ for men, 1.04 for women.

*The use of Cockcroft and Gault in any patient where the patient's actual body weight is not reflective of a normal muscle mass always needs to be interpreted with caution. If the patient is obese ($>20\%$ of ideal body weight (IBW)), IBW must be used because fatty tissue does not produce creatinine:

- for men : IBW (kg) = 50 kg + 2.3 kg for each inch over 5 feet
- for women : IBW (kg) = 49 kg + 1.7 kg for each inch over 5 feet.

In patients with oedema or ascites, IBW should be used, whereas for patients who weigh significantly less than their IBW, actual body weight should be used. In all of these situations there is some degree of inaccuracy.

Renal function gradually declines with age; however, this may not result in an elevated serum creatinine due to a concurrent reduction in muscle mass.

The following examples illustrate why CrCl is a more precise indicator of renal function than serum creatinine alone:

1   70-year-old female, IBW = 45 kg, serum creatinine = 149 micromol/L
2   30-year-old male, IBW = 75 kg, serum creatinine = 149 micromol/L.

Both have the same serum creatinine, but the 70-year-old female has a CrCl of 22 mL/min, whereas the 30-year-old male has a CrCl of 68 mL/min.

eGFR

The Modification of Diet in Renal Disease (MDRD)[2] formula uses serum creatinine in combination with age, sex and race to give an eGFR that is normalised for a body surface area of $1.73 \, m^2$. As eGFR does not require knowledge of the patient's weight, it can easily be reported by laboratories along with serum creatinine, and forms the basis of the classification system for chronic kidney disease.

More recently, NICE[3] has recommended the use of the Chronic Kidney Disease Epidemiology Collaboration (CKD-EPI) equation[4] for determining eGFR. The CKD-EPI equation is based on the same four variables as the MDRD equation, but is proposed to be more accurate at higher eGFR values.

Which method to use for drug dosing?

Most recommendations for dose adjustment in patients with renal impairment are based on CrCl calculated using Cockcroft and Gault. However, eGFR is increasingly being used for the purposes of drug dosing,[5] and it is important to recognise the limitations of this approach: eGFR has not yet been validated for drug dose calculations.

Although CrCl and eGFR are not interchangeable, in practice, for most drugs and for most adults of average build and height, eGFR can be used to determine dosage adjustments in place of CrCl. Exceptions to this include:

- toxic drugs with a narrow therapeutic index, where Cockcroft and Gault should be used in addition to therapeutic drug and clinical response monitoring
- patients at extremes of weight, where either Cockcroft and Gault or the absolute GFR may be used for drug dosing (N.B.: both methods still have limitations in this setting).

An individual's absolute GFR can be calculated from the eGFR as follows:

$$\text{GFR absolute} = \text{eGFR} \times \frac{\text{Individual's body surface area (m}^2)}{1.73}$$

It is extremely important that caution should be used when calculating drug doses in renal impairment, particularly where estimations of renal function using MDRD rather than Cockcroft and Gault would alter a dose recommendation. The risks of drug toxicity or therapeutic failure in an individual patient must always be considered and neither method is validated in acutely unwell patients.

Limitations

Limitations of prediction equations, such as Cockcroft and Gault and MDRD that are based on serum creatinine, include use in:

- extremes of age (not validated)
- extremes of body size
- severe malnutrition or obesity
- oedematous states
- amputation
- disease of skeletal muscle, muscle wasting
- paraplegia or quadriplegia
- pregnancy (not validated)
- rapidly changing serum creatinine, e.g. acute kidney injury (AKI).

Measuring CrCl from a serum creatinine concentration and a timed urine collection may be used to estimate renal function in situations where prediction equations may be inaccurate. A single serum creatinine measurement is taken and urine collected over a fixed period of time, usually 24 hours. The following equation is then applied:

$$\text{CrCl (mL/min)} = \frac{U_{Cr} \times V}{P_{Cr} \times t}$$

U_{Cr} = urine creatinine concentration (micromol/L); V = volume of urine (mL); P_{Cr} = plasma creatinine concentration (micromol/L); t = time (minutes).

N.B.: pay close attention to units and remember that there are 1440 minutes in 24 hours.

The accuracy of a timed urine collection depends on the accurate collection of urine over the time period, which many patients find difficult and inconvenient. Incomplete collection will result in underestimation of renal function.

REFERENCES
1 Cockcroft DW, Gault MH (1976). Prediction of creatinine clearance from serum creatinine. *Nephron* 16: 31–41.

2 Levey AS *et al.* (2006). Using standardized serum creatinine values in the Modification of Diet in Renal Disease Study equation for estimating glomerular filtration rate. *Ann Intern Med* 145: 247–254.

3 NICE (2014). *Chronic Kidney Disease: Early identification and management of chronic kidney disease in adults in primary and secondary care*. NICE guidelines CG182. www.nice.org.uk/guidance/CG182 (accessed 7 September 2014).

4 Levey AS *et al.* (2009). A new equation to estimate glomerular filtration rate. *Ann Intern Med* 150: 604–612.

5 Joint Formulary Committee (2014). *British National Formulary* (68th edn). London: BMJ Group and Pharmaceutical Press.

Renal disease: dosing in renal impairment and renal replacement therapy

The kidney is an important site of excretion for many drugs and/or their metabolites. Reduction in renal function can significantly increase serum concentrations of renally excreted drugs and/or metabolites and cause accumulation and toxicity. A number of other pharmacokinetic and pharmacodynamic changes also occur in renal impairment that may alter efficacy and increase the likelihood of adverse effects.

Pharmacokinetic changes in renal impairment

Absorption (generally less significant)

- Gastrointestinal (GI) oedema may reduce absorption, e.g. oral furosemide; consider converting to intravenous.
- Prolonged gastric emptying.
- Alterations in GI pH due to uraemia or medication, e.g. reduced absorption of iron with proton pump inhibitors.
- Vomiting due to uraemia.
- Phosphate binders/ion exchange resins – may chelate drugs and reduce absorption, e.g. quinolone antibiotics – separate administration times.

Distribution

- Fluid status, e.g. oedema, use of diuretics. Only significant for water-soluble drugs with volume of distribution (V_d) <1 L/kg, e.g. aminoglycosides.
- Reduced protein binding secondary to uraemia and/or low albumin. Results in increased free (active) drug. Clinically important for highly protein-bound drugs (>80%) such as phenytoin and warfarin. Care when interpreting drug levels for highly protein-bound drugs – need to consider increased free levels, e.g. phenytoin.
- Reduced tissue binding secondary to uraemia. Results in increased free (active) drug, e.g. digoxin.

Metabolism

- Hepatic metabolic pathways are generally unaffected, although impact of renal impairment on accumulation of renally cleared active/toxic metabolites needs to be considered.
- Kidneys responsible for activation of vitamin D and metabolism of insulin.
  - In chronic kidney disease (CKD) stages 4/5 use alfacalcidol (1α-hydroxycolecalciferol) as it only requires activation by the liver and not kidneys.
  - Reduced doses of exogenous insulin are required in diabetics as renal function declines.

Excretion

The main pharmacokinetic change is seen in CKD. Many water-soluble drugs and/or metabolites are excreted by the kidney and renal impairment may lead to reduced excretion, accumulation and toxicity unless dose and/or frequency are adjusted. Drugs that are most affected are those with significant renal excretion or active/toxic renally excreted metabolites. Table R2 illustrates how to manage some issues of excretion of drugs; dose reduction depends on:

- degree of renal impairment
- proportion of the drug and/or metabolites cleared by renal excretion
- toxicity
- therapeutic index.

R

Pharmacodynamic changes

Uraemia and renal impairment can increase the risk of side effects of some medications, including:

- increased cerebral sensitivity to sedating medications (even if excretion unaffected) due to increased permeability of blood–brain barrier. Start with low doses and titrate carefully
- increased risk of GI bleeding with non-steroidal anti-inflammatory drugs (NSAIDs) and anticoagulants
- increased risk of hyperkalaemia with potassium-sparing diuretics.

Loading doses

Alterations in V_d and/or tissue binding may require alterations in loading doses, e.g. digoxin may require a lower loading dose in end-stage renal disease due to reduced V_d.

For drugs requiring rapid therapeutic levels that have a prolonged half-life in renal failure (e.g. vancomycin), a loading dose may be needed to achieve steady state in a timely manner, and can be calculated as follows:

$$D = \frac{C_p \times V_d}{FS}$$

D = dose; C_p = desired concentration; V_d = volume of distribution; F = bioavailability; S = salt fraction.

TABLE R2

Drug excretion management issues in renal impairment

Drug characteristics	Management in renal impairment
High renal clearance, wide therapeutic index, e.g. penicillins	• Likely to accumulate; may require either dose reduction or increasing dosing interval
High renal clearance, narrow therapeutic index, e.g. aminoglycosides, lithium, digoxin, glycopeptide antibiotics	• Significant potential for accumulation and toxicity; use alternative where possible • Adjust dose and perform therapeutic drug monitoring (TDM) • Drugs with renally excreted active metabolites (e.g. morphine) should also be used with great care or preferably avoided
Low renal clearance, wide therapeutic index, e.g. lansoprazole	• Generally safe
Low renal clearance, narrow therapeutic index, e.g. theophylline, phenytoin	• Unlikely to be affected, but consider impact of other changes in pharmacokinetics and/or pharmacodynamics • Perform TDM
Drugs titrated against a response, e.g. atenolol, angiotensin-converting enzyme inhibitors	• Use with caution; start with low doses and titrate against response
Stat doses	• Accumulation unlikely • See loading doses section below
Renal clearance needed for efficacy	• Large doses of furosemide required in severe renal impairment as reduced tubular secretion means lower concentrations at site of action • Nitrofurantoin ineffective in CrCl <60 mL/min, as requires urinary excretion to get to site of action

Drug removal by renal replacement therapy

No renal replacement therapy (RRT) method is as effective as a normal kidney; drug doses in RRT should never be larger than in normal renal function.

Factors affecting the removal of a drug by RRT are shown in Table R3.

Key considerations for drug dosing in CKD and on RRT

- use drugs only when there is a definite indication
- avoid nephrotoxins
- degree of renal impairment
- contribution of residual urine output if on RRT
- proportion of drug normally renally excreted
- presence of renally excreted active metabolites

TABLE R3

Factors affecting the removal of a drug by renal replacement therapy

Drug/active metabolite characteristic	Haemodialysis (HD)	Peritoneal dialysis	Continuous venous-venous haemofiltration
Molecular weight[1]	• Clearance by diffusion • <500 Da = likely to be cleared • 500–20 000 Da: clearance depends on dialysis membrane • Low flux = unlikely to be cleared • High flux = more likely to be cleared	• Clearance by diffusion and convection • Poor clearance - small molecular weight more likely to be cleared	• Clearance by convection • Membranes have larger pores than HD • Increased clearance up to 30 kDa
Protein binding	• Low protein binding = more drug available for clearance • High protein binding = not generally removed • (N.B.: consider effect of uraemia on binding)		
Volume of distribution	• <1 L/kg = mostly contained in plasma, more likely to be cleared • >2 L/kg = less contained in plasma, less likely to be cleared		
Water/lipid solubility	• Higher water solubility = higher clearance • Higher lipid solubility = lower clearance		
Amount usually cleared by kidneys	• Higher renal clearance = more likely to be cleared		

R

- proportion of drug and/or metabolites cleared by non-renal routes (e.g. hepatic metabolism)
- toxicity – wide or narrow therapeutic index
- drug removal by RRT
- use TDM where possible
- monitor for effectiveness and toxicity
- available references sources for drug dosing:
  - BNF: limited; little information on RRT
  - SPC (www.medicines.org.uk): more detailed information, but only includes licensed uses. Limited RRT information
  - *Renal Drug Handbook*:[2] detailed, specialist information, including RRT. Includes common practice/off-licence uses. Caution required, as not frequently updated.

REFERENCES

1 UK Medicines Information (UKMi) Q&A 168.5 (2013). *What Factors Need to be Considered When Dosing Patients on Renal Replacement Therapies?* https://www.evidence.nhs.uk/Search?q=What+factors+need+to+be+considered+when+dosing+patients+on+renal+replacement+therapies%22 (accessed 15 May 2015).

2 Ashley C, Currie A (2009). *The Renal Drug Handbook* (3rd edn). Oxford: Radcliffe Publishing.

Renal disease: chronic kidney disease

Overview	
Definition	Diagnosed when there is either impaired kidney function (estimated eGFR <60 mL/min/1.73 m^2), evidence of kidney damage or structural abnormality of the kidney, present for >90 days.[1]
	Markers of kidney damage include leakage of protein (proteinuria) and/or blood (haematuria) into the urine.
	Structural abnormalities include renal stones or prostatic hypertrophy.
	Renal impairment in CKD can range from mild, with minimal or no symptoms, to end-stage renal disease (ESRD) requiring renal replacement therapy (RRT)
Differential diagnosis	Acute kidney injury (AKI) due to potentially reversible causes, e.g. sepsis, urinary tract obstruction, nephrotoxic drugs.
	Acute chronic renal failure – may have features of CKD, but also features of an acute cause for deterioration of renal function, e.g. urinary tract infection
Causes/risk factors[1]	• Diabetes • Hypertension • AKI • Cardiovascular disease (CVD), e.g. ischaemic heart disease, chronic heart failure, peripheral vascular disease • Structural renal tract disease, recurrent renal stones or prostatic hypertrophy • Multisystem diseases with kidney involvement, e.g. systemic lupus erythematosus • Family history of ESRD or hereditary kidney disease (e.g. polycystic kidney disease)

R

Classification[1] Classified according to:

- **Renal function**: using serum creatinine and a prediction equation for eGFR
- **Proteinuria**: using measurement of urinary albumin:creatinine ratio (ACR)

			Urinary albumin: creatinine ratio (ACR) (mg/mmol)		
			<3 Normal to mildly increased	**3–30** Moderately increased	**>30** Severely increased
			A1	A2	A3
eGFR (mL/min/1.73m²)	**> 90** Normal/high	G1	No CKD unless other markers of kidney damage		
	60–89 Mild reduction in young adult	G2			
	45–59 Mild–moderate reduction	G3a			
	30–44 Moderate–severe reduction	G3b			
	15–29 Severe reduction	G4			
	<15 End-stage renal disease	G5			

Increasing risk of adverse outcome

The darker the shading, the greater the risk of an adverse outcome, e.g CKD progression, AKI, all-cause mortality and cardiovascular events

'G' is used to denote the GFR category and 'A' for the ACR category, e.g.:

- A person with an eGFR of 25 mL/min/1.73 m² and an ACR of 15 mg/mmol has CKD stage G4A2
- A person with an eGFR of 50 mL/min/1.73 m² and an ACR of 35 mg/mmol has CKD stage G3aA3

R

Clinical features	The kidney regulates fluid and electrolyte balance, stimulates bone marrow red blood cell production through production of erythropoietin, and helps maintain calcium and phosphate balance by activating vitamin D. It is also responsible for excreting waste products of metabolism (e.g. urea, creatinine, uric acid) and medications.

During the early stages of CKD patients are often asymptomatic; however, as renal function declines, changes to all of these functions occur with the following results:

- **Hypertension:** may cause, or be caused by, CKD. Activation of the renin–angiotensin system occurs in CKD in an attempt to increase renal perfusion. This leads to sodium and fluid retention and hypertension.
- **Proteinuria:** leakage of protein into urine may occur when the glomeruli of the kidney are damaged. Proteinuria is a significant risk factor for progression of CKD and cardiovascular morbidity and mortality.
- **Fluid overload:** due to sodium and fluid retention.
- **Cardiovascular disease:** hypertension and chronic fluid overload can lead to left ventricular hypertrophy and cardiac dysfunction.
- **Uraemia:** accumulation of waste products such as urea can cause nausea, fatigue, itching, restless-leg syndrome and anorexia.
- **Hyperkalaemia:** due to reduced potassium excretion. May be exacerbated by medications, e.g. angiotensin-converting enzyme inhibitors (ACEIs) and angiotensin receptor blockers (ARBs).
- **Anaemia** due to:
  - Reduced erythropoietin production
  - Iron deficiency (poor intake, poor absorption, increased losses)
- **Renal bone disease:** vitamin D from diet and sunlight (colecalciferol) requires hydroxylation by the liver and kidneys to become active (1,25-dihydroxycolecalciferol, calcitriol). Low levels of active vitamin D reduce calcium absorption from the gut. The resulting hypocalcaemia stimulates the production of parathyroid hormone (PTH), which increases calcium release from bones. Untreated, high PTH levels lead to increased bone loss (renal bone disease) and an increased risk of fractures.
- **Hyperphosphataemia** due to reduced phosphate excretion. Reduces calcium absorption from the gut and causes itching.
- **Acidosis:** the kidney regulates acid balance through reabsorption of bicarbonate and production of other buffers to remove hydrogen ions. Metabolic acidosis can occur when the kidney is unable to perform these functions.
- **Bleeding complications:** uraemia increases the risk of gastrointestinal (GI) bleeding and can cause platelet dysfunction

Diagnostic tests	- U&Es, FBC, LFTs, albumin, bicarbonate

- Folate, vitamin B_{12}, iron, ferritin and % transferrin saturation
- Serum calcium, phosphate and PTH
- GFR estimation – usually eGFR
- Plasma glucose (detect undiagnosed diabetes or assess diabetic control)
- Urine dipstick for haematuria
- Urinary ACR
- Renal ultrasound (where appropriate)

Treatment goals	• Early diagnosis and treatment of CKD can delay progression to ESRD, hence screening of at-risk patients is crucial • Establish cause of CKD, particularly if it is treatable (e.g. urinary tract obstruction, nephrotoxic drugs) • Minimise risk factors, e.g. tight glycaemic and blood pressure control. CVD is the most common cause of death in CKD, with CVD-associated mortality risk increasing proportionally with decline in GFR • Slow progression • Manage complications • Appropriate planning for RRT • End-of-life care
Treatment options	**Pharmacological treatments**: most common interventions used to relieve symptoms, replace functions of failing kidneys and slow progression. **Lifestyle advice:** exercise, weight loss, smoking cessation. **Dietary intervention:** restrict/limit potassium, phosphate, salt and fluid intake where appropriate. Supplements may be required in poor intake. **RRT** in ESRD

Medicines optimisation

Blood pressure control	• Aim to keep systolic blood pressure <140 mmHg (120–139 mmHg) and diastolic blood pressure <90 mmHg.[1] • In CKD and diabetes, and in people with an ACR of ≥70 mg/mmol, aim to keep systolic blood pressure <130 mmHg (120–129 mmHg) and diastolic blood pressure <80 mmHg.[1]

R

First-line choice of antihypertensive agent in CKD

	A1 ACR <3 mg/mmol	A2 ACR 3-30 mg/mmol	A3 ACR >30 mg/mmol	ACR >70 mg/mmol
Non-diabetic normotensive				Renin–angiotensin system antagonist*[†]
Non-diabetic hypertensive	Follow National Institute of Health and Care Excellence (NICE) clinical guideline 127[2]		Renin–angiotensin system antagonist*[†]	
Diabetic normotensive	Follow NICE diabetes pathway[3]	Renin–angiotensin system antagonist, irrespective of blood pressure*[†]		
Diabetic hypertens		Renin–angiotensin system antagonist*[†]		

*ACEIs, ARBs or direct renin inhibitors (e.g. aliskiren). ARBs should be used if ACEIs are not tolerated.

[†]Caution if serum potassium >5.0 mmol/L.

Use of ACEI/ARBs is beneficial in CKD, as they reduce renin–angiotensin system activation (a consequence of CKD)

Proteinuria	• ACEIs/ARBs provide additional renoprotective effects (above blood pressure control) by reducing protein leak, and may be used in patents with proteinuria irrespective of initial blood pressure
Fluid overload	• Diuretics (may require large doses of loop diuretics in low GFR) • Fluid restriction
Cardio-vascular risk management	• Follow NICE clinical guideline 181[4] for use of statins in CKD – start at a low dose and increase slowly. • Offer antiplatelet medication where appropriate, but be aware of increased risk of bleeding
Uraemia	• **Itching**: control phosphate and calcium levels; hydrate skin with topical moisturisers; sedating antihistamines • **Restless-leg syndrome**: correct iron deficiency; clonazepam; haloperidol; ropinirole • **Nausea**: antiemetics such as metoclopramide or prochlorperazine • **Gout**: allopurinol
Hyper-kalaemia	• Low-potassium diet • Review medications, i.e. ACEIs/ARBs, potassium-sparing diuretics • Insulin/glucose infusion, sodium bicarbonate and/or nebulised salbutamol are all used in acute hyperkalaemia to increase potassium uptake into cells. May also require calcium gluconate to prevent arrhythmias (see *Potassium* entry) • Ion exchange resins, e.g. Calcium Resonium, exchange calcium ions for potassium ions as it passes through the gut. Always give with a laxative as very constipating. • RRT
Anaemia[5]	In CKD, defined as haemoglobin <110 g/L (<11 g/dL) • Optimise iron levels: often involves intravenous iron due to reduced absorption of oral iron (see *Iron* entry) • Correct folate or vitamin B_{12} deficiencies • Use of an erythropoiesis-stimulating agent to maintain stable haemoglobin 10–12 g/dL (higher levels lack additional benefit and increase risk of harm)
Bone metabolism	• Low-phosphate diet • Phosphate binders,[6] taken with food to bind phosphate in the gut and prevent absorption. Commonly used phosphate binders include calcium acetate, calcium carbonate, aluminium hydroxide, sevelamer and lanthanum • Vitamin D supplementation: initially with colecalciferol or ergocalciferol if vitamin D-deficient. If GFR <30 mL/min/1.73 m^2, use alfacalcidol (1-alpha hydroxycolecalciferol), which does not require activation by kidneys (but still requires activation by liver)[1] • Tertiary (uncontrolled) hyperparathyroidism may require use of calcimimetics, such as cinacalcet and paricalcitol. If severe, surgical removal of the parathyroid glands (parathyroidectomy) may be necessary
Metabolic acidosis	• Consider oral sodium bicarbonate if serum bicarbonate <20 mmol/L. Common dose 500 mg–1 g three times a day
Stress ulceration	• Altered gastric pH in uraemia increases risk of GI bleeding • Consider prophylaxis with H_2-antagonist or proton pump inhibitor

Pharmaceutical care and counselling	
Assess	• Type of renal impairment (e.g. acute or chronic) • Severity of renal impairment: eGFR routinely available, calculate creatinine clearance where possible • RRT method (if applicable) • Residual urine output if on RRT • Choice and dose of medications (see below)
Essential intervention	**Choice of drug in CKD** • Avoid nephrotoxic agents in predialysis patients and patients on RRT with residual renal function • Determine pharmacokinetic and pharmacodynamic effects of renal impairment on drug choice (see *Renal impairment and renal replacement therapy – drug dosing* entry) • Consider using medicines that are metabolised to inactive compounds or excreted by non-renal routes • Renally cleared medicines with a narrow therapeutic index (e.g. aminoglycosides and vancomycin) require careful monitoring and dose adjustment – avoid where possible • Consider reduced efficacy, e.g. nitrofurantoin ineffective in CrCl <60 mL/min, as requires urinary excretion to work
Essential intervention	**Drug dosing in CKD** • Consider proportion that is normally renally cleared • Presence of renally cleared active metabolites • Proportion of drug and/or metabolites cleared through non-renal routes (e.g. hepatic metabolism) • Toxicity – wide or narrow therapeutic index • Drug removal by RRT (see individual *Renal replacement therapy* entries for more information) • Changes in volume of distribution that may require alterations in loading doses (e.g. digoxin)
Essential intervention	**Therapeutic drug monitoring** • Renally cleared, narrow-therapeutic-index medications (e.g. aminoglycosides and vancomycin) require therapeutic drug monitoring and dose adjustment • Caution interpreting levels for highly protein-bound drugs – reduced protein binding due to uraemia will increase amount of unbound (active) drug, e.g. phenytoin
Essential intervention	**Cardiovascular risk management** • Assess in same way as people without CKD; however, some medications (e.g. statins) may require dose modification • Consider increased risk of bleeding with antiplatelets/anticoagulants • Ensure good glycaemic and blood pressure control • Non-pharmacological interventions, e.g. stop smoking, weight management, healthy eating, exercise

R

Essential intervention	**Commencing an ACEIs/ARBs[1]** • Check baseline potassium, creatinine and eGFR • Repeat 1–2 weeks after starting and after each dose increase • If decrease in eGFR of $\geq$25% or increase in creatinine $\geq$30%, investigate other causes (volume depletion, concurrent medication, e.g. non-steroidal anti-inflammatory drugs (NSAIDs)). If no other cause found, stop ACEIs/ARBs or reduce to previously tolerated dose • Stop if serum potassium $\geq$6.0 mmol/L • Titrate to maximum dose where possible
Secondary intervention	**Timing of medications** • Avoid taking phosphate binders at same time as oral iron or some antibiotics (e.g. quinolones) – binds in gut and prevents absorption • Counsel patient and annotate timings on drug chart
Secondary intervention	**Polypharmacy** • May take >10 medications/day • Potential for interactions is very high • Review unnecessary medications/rationalise • Consider adherence aids (or referral to community or domiciliary pharmacy services for assessment)
Secondary intervention	**Fluid restriction** • Polypharmacy may mean a considerable amount of fluid is needed for medication taking, which has an impact on daily fluid allowance • Some medications require addition of fluid, e.g. Movicol/Laxido • Fluid content of intravenous medications
Secondary intervention	**Analgesia in CKD** • Caution with NSAIDs: ↓GFR and ↑GI bleeding risk. Avoid topical use as some systemic absorption occurs. • Paracetamol is generally safe. • Many opiates are renally cleared, therefore accumulation may occur, which may lead to increased cerebral sensitivity – start with low doses and titrate • Impact of renally cleared metabolites, e.g. codeine/morphine have highly active renally cleared metabolites with prolonged half-lives
Secondary intervention	**Over-the-counter medications** • Avoid NSAIDs • Impact of calcium/magnesium in antacids on bone disease control • Some vitamins accumulate in renal disease; also consider vitamin D content • Electrolyte content, e.g. high sodium content in effervescent tablets, potassium content in potassium citrate • Cough/cold remedies containing sympathomimetics in hypertension
Secondary intervention	**Vaccinations** • Annual influenza and 5-yearly pneumococcal vaccination recommended in all patients • All patients on, or being considered for, RRT should be vaccinated against hepatitis B • Caution with live vaccines if on immunosuppressant medications/renal transplant
Further reading	Jogia P, O'Brien M (2009). How to approach prescriptions for patients with renal impairment. *Clin Pharmacist* 179–183. Morlidge C, Richards T (2001). Renal disease (2): managing chronic renal disease. *Pharm J* 266: 655–657.

REFERENCES

1 NICE (2014). *Chronic Kidney Disease: Early identification and management of chronic kidney disease in adults in primary and secondary care*. CG182. www.nice.org.uk/guidance/CG182 (accessed 7 September 2014).

2 NICE (2011). *Hypertension: Clinical management of primary hypertension in adults*. NICE guidelines CG127. www.nice.org.uk/Guidance/CG1277 (accessed 7 September 2014).

3 NICE (2014). *Diabetes Pathway*. www.pathways.nice.org.uk/pathways/diabetes (accessed 7 September 2014).

4 NICE (2014). *Lipid Modification: Cardiovascular risk assessment and the modification of blood lipids for the primary and secondary prevention of cardiovascular disease*. CG181. www.nice.org.uk/guidance/CG181 (accessed 7 September 2014).

5 NICE (2011). *Anaemia Management in People with Chronic Kidney Disease*. CG114. www.nice.org.uk/guidance/CG114 (accessed 7 September 2014).

6 NICE (2013). *Hyperphosphataemia in Chronic Kidney Disease: Management of hyperphosphataemia in patients with stage 4 or 5 chronic kidney disease*. NICE guideline CG157. www.nice.org.uk/guidance/CG157 (accessed 7 September 2014).

Renal replacement therapy: haemodialysis

Overview

Setting	Haemodialysis (HD) can be used either acutely in acute kidney injury to rest the kidneys, or longer term in the treatment of end-stage renal disease.
	HD can be provided:
	• In the hospital setting, usually for acutely unwell patients
	• In satellite units with reduced medical cover
	• In the patient's home, after careful patient selection and training
Vascular access	Access to the patient's blood stream for HD is achieved by one of the following methods:
	Arteriovenous fistula ('fistula'): the radial or brachial artery is surgically joined to an adjacent vein. The higher-pressure arterial blood causes the vein wall to thicken and the lumen to get bigger, creating a vessel of sufficient size and blood flow for dialysis to occur.
	Two needles are usually inserted into the fistula for dialysis – one for the arterial line (taking blood out of the patient) and one for the venous line (returning blood to the patient).
	A fistula may take 3–6 months to be usable, therefore must be planned in advance of the need for dialysis. Complications include stenosis, thrombosis, infection and aneurysm.
	Central venous catheter (CVC or 'line'): usually placed in the internal jugular vein either temporarily or permanently (tunnelled under the skin). CVCs usually have an arterial lumen and a venous lumen.

R

Disadvantages include:

- Relatively narrow calibre, limiting blood flow and dialysis adequacy.
- High risk of infection and thrombosis. Locking with an anticoagulant $\pm$ antibiotic solution (e.g. heparin/vancomycin) may reduce this risk. If CVCs become blocked, locks/infusions of urokinase or alteplase may be used.

Graft: a plastic tube connects the artery to the vein and is used for dialysis. This may be used almost immediately. Disadvantages include an increased infection and thrombosis risk, and a life span of only a few years.

Ideally patients should dialyse with a fistula because they are more durable and less likely to become infected;[1] however, a CVC will be needed if a fistula is not ready or is impossible to create. Grafts are only used if other options have failed

Technology	HD works through a combination of: - **Diffusion** (movement of solutes from fluid with a high to a low concentration across a semipermeable membrane) - **Ultrafiltration** (movement of fluid under pressure across a semipermeable membrane) Blood is removed from the patient via the arterial line of the fistula or CVC and pumped through the dialysis machine via the dialyser or 'kidney'. The patient is usually anticoagulated with either low-molecular-weight heparin or unfractionated heparin to prevent blood from clotting in the dialysis machine. The dialyser contains thousands of hollow fibres made of a semipermeable membrane. Blood is pumped through the fibres, whilst a crystalloid solution (dialysate) is pumped in the opposite direction outside the fibres. The opposing blood and dialysate flow directions increase the amount of diffusion and ultrafiltration that occurs. Different dialysate compositions are used depending on the patient's requirements. Waste products such as urea and creatinine and solutes such as potassium are removed from the blood by diffusion into the dialysate along a concentration gradient (from high to low). Essential minerals (e.g. calcium and bicarbonate) are replaced in the blood by diffusion from the dialysate along a concentration gradient (high in the dialysate, lower in the blood). Excess fluid is removed from the blood by ultrafiltration, with the dialysate compartment having a higher osmolality and being kept at a lower pressure relative to the blood compartment. The dialysed blood is then returned to the patient via the venous line of the fistula or CVC
Common complications	Hypotension, infection, electrolyte disturbance, blood loss, restless-leg syndrome, cramps, nausea and vomiting, headache, angina, arrhythmias
Other information	Length of HD session is gradually increased to 3–5 hours three times a week. Patients are assigned a 'dry weight', equivalent to their weight without excess fluid or hypotension, and are weighed before and after dialysis, with the post weight being as close to their dry weight as possible

Pharmaceutical care for non-specialist pharmacists

Drug dosing on HD	Equations for assessment of estimated glomerular filtration rate (eGFR)/creatinine clearance (CrCl) cannot be used in HD patients.
	Even though drug clearance during HD may be good, as it is an intermittent process performed for a few hours every 2–3 days, drugs are usually dosed for a CrCl of <10 mL/min unless other information is available.[1,2]
	Drug removal by HD is hard to quantify, but is influenced by:[3]
	• Duration of session (longer session = more clearance) • Flow rate (higher flow rate = more clearance) • Dialysate composition • Dialyser porosity ('high-flux' dialysers provide greater clearance than standard dialysers)
	If a drug is likely to be removed by HD it should be given after the session; otherwise it could be removed before it has time to act fully
HD anticoagulation	Caution in patients prescribed anticoagulants for other indications, i.e. venous thromboembolism prophylaxis, warfarin, new oral anticoagulants, fondaparinux.
	Review in patients with bleeding complications or new contraindications to anticoagulation (i.e. recent stroke) – anticoagulant-free dialysis may be needed.
	Patients may develop heparin-induced thrombocytopenia requiring use of different anticoagulants
Fluid restriction	HD patients usually restrict their fluid intake to 500–1000 mL/day, depending on residual urine output. Consider the impact of oral medications needing to be swallowed with fluid and volumes of intravenous medications

R

REFERENCES

1 eMC (2015). www.emc.medicines.org.uk. (accessed 9 February 2015).
2 Ashley C, Currie A (2009). *The Renal Drug Handbook* (3rd edn). Oxford: Radcliffe Publishing.
3 UK Medicines Information (UKMi) Q&A 168.5: *What Factors Need to be Considered When Dosing Patients on Renal Replacement Therapies?* Date prepared: January 2013. http://www.ukmi.nhs.uk/activities/specialistServices/default.asp?pageRef=5 (accessed 14 May 2015).

Renal replacement therapy: haemofiltration

Overview	
Setting	Haemofiltration (HF) is used in the management of severe acute kidney injury in patients who are haemodynamically unstable, e.g. patients with multiple organ failure or shock or requiring vasopressors. For this reason it is usually provided in the critical care setting. It can be either continuous or intermittent depending on the stability of the patient, although continuous is best for very unstable patients.
	The main advantage of continuous HF over intermittent HD is the ability to remove large volumes of fluid over a longer time period, minimising the risk of hypotension
Vascular access	Most HF methods in use are veno-venous. A temporary double-lumen CVC is placed in the femoral, subclavian or internal jugular vein
Technology	HF works through a combination of:
	• Convection (movement of solutes in fluid across a semipermeable membrane under pressure)
	• Ultrafiltration (movement of fluid under pressure across a semipermeable membrane)
	The most common method used is continuous veno-venous haemofiltration (CVVHF), where blood is removed from the patient via one lumen of a venous line and pumped through the dialysis circuit to a semipermeable membrane (the filter).
	The filters used for HF contain thousands of hollow fibres made of a semi-permeable membrane that are very permeable to fluids and solutes (high flux).
	Unlike in HD, dialysate is not used. Instead, a positive hydrostatic pressure created on the blood side of the filter drives water and solutes across the filter membrane into the filtrate compartment. Molecules that are small enough to pass through the membrane (<30 kDa) are dragged across the membrane with the water by the process of convection. The ultrafiltration rate (fluid removal) is controlled by pump speed.
	The filtrate is discarded and an isotonic replacement fluid (haemofiltration fluid) is added to the blood to replace fluid volume and electrolytes. Different haemofiltration fluid compositions are used depending on the patient's requirements and can either be added before the filter (pre-dilution) or after (postdilution). The postdilution method is most common and allows a more accurate fluid balance, but has problems with clotting if the blood becomes too concentrated at the filter. The blood is then returned to the patient via the second lumen of the venous line.
	Advantages of continuous HF over intermittent HD include:
	• Ability to remove larger volume of fluid (up to 3–6 L/day), as it is carried out over a longer time interval
	• Better control of blood pressure and reduced hypotension
	• Better control of fluid balance and reduced hypovolaemia
	• Slower fluid shifts and a more gradual change in electrolytes
	Disadvantages include:
	• Cost
	• Increased complexity and staff training

R

Anti-coagulation	Methods of anticoagulation on HF include: • a prefilter infusion of unfractionated heparin (easily reversed by protamine if needed). Activated partial thromboplastin time (APTT) monitoring is required • infusion of prostaglandins (e.g. epoprostenol) • prefilter infusion of citrate
Common complications	CVC-related infection and thrombosis, haemodynamic instability, blood loss, electrolyte imbalances, hypothermia, effects of anticoagulation (bleeding or specific side effects of the anticoagulant used, e.g. heparin-induced thrombocytopenia)

Pharmaceutical care for non-specialist pharmacists

Drug dosing on HF	Equations for assessment of eGFR/CrCl cannot be used in HF patients.
	Continuous HF generally gives better drug clearance than intermittent HD. During CVVHF drugs are usually dosed for a CrCl of 10–20 mL/min unless other information is available.[1,2]
	Because HF uses convection rather than diffusion, it has a higher rate of removal of larger molecules (up to 30 kDa) compared to HD,[3] as larger molecules have a slower diffusion rate. Therefore, drugs such as vancomycin (molecular weight 1449 Da) have higher clearance on HF than HD.
	Drug removal by HF is hard to quantify, but is influenced by:[3] • permeability of filter membrane • system pressure (pump speed)
	As HF is a continuous process, timing of medication administration in relation to dialysis is not crucial.
	It is important to know whether HF is currently being performed or has stopped (i.e. due to clotting, or because renal function is improving) and consider the effect this will have on drug clearance
HF anti-coagulation	Use of anticoagulation for HF should be avoided in: • coagulopathy • raised international normalised ratio or APTT • thrombocytopenia • high risk of bleeding • new contraindications to anticoagulation (i.e. recent stroke)
	Caution in patients prescribed anticoagulants for other indications, i.e. warfarin, fondaparinux.
	Patients may develop heparin-induced thrombocytopenia requiring use of different anticoagulants
Fluid restriction	Fluid restriction in CVVHF is less of an issue than in intermittent HD, as fluid removal is continuous and larger volumes can be removed

REFERENCES

1 eMC (2014). www.emc.medicines.org.uk (accessed 26 April 2015).

2 Ashley C, Currie A (2009). *The Renal Drug Handbook* (3rd edn). Oxford: Radcliffe Publishing.

3 UK Medicines Information (UKMi) Q&A 168.5: *What Factors Need to be Considered When Dosing Patients on Renal Replacement Therapies?* Date prepared: January 2013. http://www.ukmi.nhs.uk/activities/specialistServices/default.asp?pageRef=5 (accessed 14 May 2015).

Renal replacement therapy: peritoneal dialysis

Overview	
Setting	Peritoneal dialysis (PD) is not as aggressive as haemodialysis (HD) and is performed at home, allowing patients greater flexibility. It is useful for patients likely to have vascular access problems (e.g. diabetics) and people with unstable cardiovascular disease.
	PD requires greater patient involvement than HD, and motivation and home circumstances are important when deciding on patient suitability
Access	Requires intraperitoneal access via a soft flexible catheter (Tenckhoff catheter), inserted surgically into the peritoneum.
	PD catheters have a cuff that promotes fibrous tissue development to secure the catheter and reduce the risk of infection.
	The catheter cannot be used for 2 weeks after insertion to allow healing and reduce the risk of leakage and infection
Technology	PD uses the patient's peritoneal membrane as a semipermeable membrane, and works through a combination of:

- diffusion
- osmosis (movement of water from a less concentrated solution to a more concentrated solution through a semipermeable membrane)
- convection (movement of solutes in fluid across a semipermeable membrane under pressure).

Most dialysates use glucose as the osmotic agent and come in three strengths, weak, medium and strong, with strong solutions providing more fluid removal.

The dialysate also contains solutes such as sodium, potassium, calcium and magnesium.

Diffusion and convection of solutes occur between capillary blood and the dialysate, and fluid is removed from blood by osmosis.

There are two types of PD:

Continuous ambulatory peritoneal dialysis (CAPD)
- Most commonly used.
- Dialysate is warmed to body temperature and instilled into the peritoneal cavity via the catheter by gravity (~10 minutes).
- Volume of dialysate depends on body size, but is usually 2–3 litres.
- Dialysate remains in peritoneum for ~4 hours ('dwell time'), after which the patient connects the catheter to an empty bag and the dialysate is drained out (~10–20 minutes).
- This 'exchange' process is repeated up to 4–5 times per day.
- A dwell time of 8–12 hours is used overnight.

Automated peritoneal dialysis (APD)
- Follows the same principles as CAPD, except that ~6 exchanges of 1.5–3 litres dialysate are performed overnight by a machine and a 12–15-hour dwell time is used in the daytime
- Patients have more freedom during the day, but the machine inhibits night-time mobility.

R

Maintaining sterile technique is critical to prevent infection.

Ways to enhance PD adequacy include:
- increasing bag volumes for CAPD
- increasing frequency of exchanges for CAPD
- increasing the strength of the bag
- increasing dwell time

Common complications	• Peritonitis and catheter exit-site infection. Symptoms and signs of peritonitis include abdominal pain, cloudy peritoneal fluid, fever, nausea and tenderness to palpation. Intraperitoneal administration of antibiotics is often utilised in the treatment of PD peritonitis. Repeated peritonitis episodes can cause dialysis failure due to fibrosis of the peritoneal membrane and formation of adhesions. • Catheter flow or drainage problems, often due to constipation, also caused by catheter misplacement, migration or kinking or fibrin deposition. • Dialysate leakage, hyperglycaemia (due to glucose in dialysate), hernias

Pharmaceutical care for non-specialist pharmacists

Drug dosing on PD	Equations for assessment of estimated glomerular filtration rate/creatinine clearance (CrCl) cannot be used in PD patients. In general, PD provides minimal drug removal and drugs are usually dosed for a CrCl of <10 mL/min unless other information is available.[1,2] Drugs that are small, unbound, uncharged and with a small volume of distribution may have some clearance on PD. Drug removal by PD is influenced by:[3] • dialysate volume • dialysate to plasma osmotic gradient • dwell time • peritoneal perfusion • membrane porosity. Drug clearance is enhanced in patients receiving APD compared to CAPD, and also in those with residual urine output compared to anuric patients. As PD is a continuous process, timing of medication administration in relation to dialysis is not crucial. With PD peritonitis, when an antibiotic that is strongly protein-bound (e.g. teicoplanin) is given intravenously, the amount reaching the peritoneum is low because only unbound drug can be transported into the dialysate. In this situation, administration by the intraperitoneal route is preferred over the intravenous route
Constipation	Constipation can cause catheter flow or drainage problems, and all PD patients should be prescribed regular laxatives. Consider increasing laxatives if constipating medications are prescribed
Fluid restriction	Tends to be less strict than on HD as PD patients usually still pass some urine and dialysis is continuous. However, it is still important to consider the impact of oral medications needing to be swallowed with fluid and volumes of intravenous medications if the patient has poor residual urine output

REFERENCES

1 Electronic Medicines Compendium (2014). www.emc.medicines.org.uk (accessed 14 October 2014).
2 Ashley C, Currie A (2009). *The Renal Drug Handbook* (3rd edn). Oxford: Radcliffe Publishing.
3 UK Medicines Information (UKMi) Q&A 168.5: *What Factors Need to be Considered When Dosing Patients on Renal Replacement Therapies?* https://www.evidence.nhs.uk/Search?q=What+factors+need+to+be+considered+when+dosing+patients+on+renal+replacement+therapies%22 (accessed 15 May 2015).

Rheumatoid arthritis: drugs suppressing the disease process

Traditionally these drugs have been used following NSAID and steroid treatment. Increasingly they are being introduced much earlier in the disease process to prevent irreversible damage despite the potential for adverse effects.

They can be divided into two categories:

1 disease-modifying antirheumatic drugs (DMARDs)
2 cytokine inhibitors, mainly comprising tumour necrosis factor α antagonists (anti-TNFs), which are sometimes called 'biologics'.

All require baseline measurements to be taken prior to commencement, and routine monitoring of various parameters to ensure safe and efficacious use. Disease progression and efficacy of therapy are monitored, typically monthly, by measurement of C-reactive protein and erythrocyte sedimentation rate, amongst others. Any beneficial effect of DMARDs is not usually seen for several months after initiation, whereas anti-TNFs can produce beneficial effects after just a few doses.

It should be noted that many patients suffering from rheumatoid arthritis may have reduced manual dexterity. Assessment of their needs regarding packaging and labelling should be carried out. It may be necessary for them to use larger containers or have easy-to-open lids that aid compliance and discourage the patient from decanting doses into inappropriate containers at home.

The following summarises key information for the common drugs, including dose, common side effects, monitoring requirements and pharmaceutical care issues to facilitate counselling.

Disease-modifying antirheumatic drugs (Tables R4–R11)
Azathioprine pharmaceutical care considerations

- Warn patient to tell doctor immediately if persistent fever, sore throat, bruising, bleeding or other signs of myelosuppression occur.
- Live vaccines should be avoided in patients taking azathioprine. Pneumococcal vaccine and an annual influenza vaccine should be given. Varicella-zoster immunoglobulin should be considered for passive immunisation in non-immune patients if exposed to chickenpox or shingles.[1]

TABLE R4
Azathioprine[1,2]

Dose	• 1 mg/kg daily, increasing after 4–6 weeks to 2–3 mg/kg daily. Use lower doses if there is significant renal or hepatic impairment. If allopurinol is coprescribed, the dose of azathioprine must be reduced by 75%
Examples of possible side effects	• Nausea, flu-like symptoms, hepatitis, cholestatic jaundice, bone marrow suppression, leucopenia, increased susceptibility to infections
Baseline monitoring	• FBC (including platelets), LFTs, U&Es (including serum creatinine)
Routine monitoring	• FBC (including platelets) and LFTs once a week for 6 weeks, then every fortnight until the dose stabilises for 6 weeks, then once a month thereafter. • After each dose, change FBC: LFTs should be repeated after 2 weeks. • U&Es (including serum creatinine) should be monitored every 6 months
Pharmaceutical care considerations	• Warn patient to tell doctor immediately if persistent fever, sore throat, bruising, bleeding or other signs of myelosuppression occur. • Live vaccines should be avoided in patients taking azathioprine. Pneumococcal vaccine and an annual influenza vaccine should be given. Varicella-zoster immunoglobulin should be considered for passive immunisation in non-immune patients if exposed to chickenpox or shingles.[1] • Patients should be warned to avoid excessive exposure to the sun and ultraviolet rays due to possible increased risk of skin cancer. Patients should have their skin examined at regular intervals.[2] • To help avoid problems with GI disturbances patients can be advised to take azathioprine in divided doses or with meals[2]

TABLE R5
Ciclosporin[1,2]

Dose	• 2.5 mg/kg daily in two divided doses. The dose is increased after 6 weeks in 25 mg increments (to a maximum of 4 mg/kg/day) every 2–4 weeks if necessary until clinically effective
Examples of possible side effects	• Hirsutism, gingival hyperplasia, hypertension, renal impairment
Baseline monitoring	• FBC, LFTs, lipids, U&Es (including serum creatinine) and blood pressure. These should be measured on two separate occasions prior to commencement

(Continued)

TABLE R5
(Continued)

Routine monitoring	• U&Es (including serum creatinine) should be measured fortnightly until the dose has been stable for 3 months, then monthly thereafter. FBC and LFTs should be measured monthly until the dose has been stable for 3 months, then 3-monthly thereafter. • Serum lipid profile is measured every 6 months. • Blood pressure should be measured every time the patient attends the monitoring clinic
Pharmaceutical care considerations	• The total daily dose should be taken in two divided doses. Grapefruit or grapefruit juice should be avoided (bioavailability may be increased by up to 45%). • To improve the taste of the solution form, it can be mixed with orange juice (or squash), apple juice or water immediately before taking (and the container rinsed with more to ensure the total dose is taken). The medicine measure provided with the solution must be kept away from other liquids (including water). After use, the outside of the measure should be wiped with a dry tissue only.[2] • Ciclosporin is contraindicated in patients with abnormal renal function or uncontrolled hypertension. NSAIDs should be used with caution if concomitantly prescribed, and in particular the dose of diclofenac should be halved if given with ciclosporin.[1] • Live vaccines should be avoided. The annual influenza vaccine should be given.[1,2] • Prescribing of ciclosporin should always be brand-specific due to possible differences in bioavailability

TABLE R6
Gold, intramuscular (sodium aurothiomalate)[1–3]

Dose	• Before commencing therapy a 10-mg test dose must be given, and the patient observed for 30 minutes for signs of allergy. If no adverse effects are observed a dose of 50 mg weekly is given until a significant response is seen. • Thereafter the dose can be reduced to 50 mg fortnightly until full remission occurs, when the dosing interval can be slowly increased to 6-weekly. • If, after a total dose of 1 g has been administered, no response has occurred, then treatment should be stopped[3]
Examples of possible side effects	• Rashes, pruritus, anaphylaxis, bone marrow suppression, proteinuria

(Continued)

TABLE R6
(Continued)

Baseline monitoring	• FBC, urinalysis, U&Es (including serum creatinine), LFTs
Routine monitoring	• FBC and urinalysis (for proteinuria) at each injection. The result of the previous FBC should be reviewed before giving the next injection. The patient's skin should be inspected for rashes before each injection
Pharmaceutical care considerations	• Warn patients to tell their doctor immediately if any of the following develops: sore throat, fever, infection, unexplained bleeding and bruising, mouth ulcers, metallic taste, rashes, menorrhagia, diarrhoea, breathlessness or cough.[2,3] • Live vaccines should be avoided[1]

TABLE R7
Hydroxychloroquine[2,3]

Dose	• Initially 200 mg twice a day, then maintenance of 200–400 mg daily (maximum dose is 6.5 mg/kg ideal body weight daily, and not more than 400 mg daily)
Examples of possible side effects	• GI disturbances, headache, rashes, pruritus, visual disturbances, hypoglycaemia
Baseline monitoring	• Assessment of eye sight (see BNF: antimalarials 10.1.3 for full guidance)[3] • LFTs, U&Es, FBC
Routine monitoring	• FBC periodically • Assessment of eye sight annually
Pharmaceutical care considerations	• Warn patient to report any visual disturbances. • Avoid antacids for 4 hours before or after a dose.[3] • Patients need to be counselled to recognise the possible symptoms of hypoglycaemia and what action to take if symptoms occur[2]

TABLE R8
Leflunomide[1–3]

Dose	• A loading dose of 100 mg daily for 3 days is given, then 10–20 mg daily. In practice, some rheumatologists do not give a loading dose
Examples of possible side effects	• GI disturbances, alopecia, weight loss, liver abnormalities, hypertension, bone marrow suppression, headache, dizziness, dry skin, tenosynovitis, rash, mouth ulcers, pruritus

(Continued)

TABLE R8
(Continued)

Baseline monitoring	• FBC, LFTs, U&Es, weight and blood pressure
Routine monitoring	• FBC and LFTs fortnightly for the first 6 months, then every 8 weeks. Weight and blood pressure should be assessed every time the patient attends monitoring clinic
Pharmaceutical care considerations	• The recommendation of leflunomide SPC is that it should not be used in conjunction with other DMARDs in routine clinical practice. Leflunomide may inhibit the metabolism of warfarin, phenytoin and tolbutamide. It has an extremely long elimination half-life and interactions with these drugs and with other DMARDs may occur even after leflunomide has been discontinued.[2]
	• For both women and men, effective contraception should be exercised throughout treatment and for women a 2-year period should elapse following cessation of leflunomide before a planned conception (3 months for men). Blood concentrations of its active metabolite should be measured after the discontinuation period before pregnancy occurs. Alternatively the leflunomide washout procedure may be considered (see below), followed by active metabolite monitoring.[1]
	• If alanine transaminase (ALT) level is raised between two and three times the upper limit of normal (ULN), the dose should be reduced from 20 mg to 10 mg and LFTs must be monitored weekly. If the ALT level remains raised at more than twice the ULN, or if a level more than three times the ULN occurs, leflunomide must be stopped and washout procedures initiated. The washout procedure should also be initiated if any severe undesirable side effect of leflunomide occurs or if for any other reason rapid removal of its active metabolite is required.[2]
	• Leflunomide increases susceptibility to infections, which should be treated promptly. Live vaccines are contraindicated.[1]
	• Leflunomide is supplied in a plastic bottle with a desiccant in the lid, and should be supplied to the patient in its original container.

Leflunomide washout procedure

Washout is achieved by administering cholestyramine 8 g three times daily for 11 days. Alternatively, 50 g of activated powdered charcoal may be given four times daily for 11 days. Monitoring of liver enzymes must be maintained after discontinuation until liver enzyme levels have normalised.[3]

It should be noted that the washout procedure is likely to affect the absorption of concurrent drug therapy adversely

TABLE R9
Methotrexate[1]

Dose	• The usual starting dose is 5–10 mg as a single weekly dose; this is increased by 2.5–5 mg every 2–6 weeks as tolerated until the disease stabilises (up to a usual maximum of 25 mg). Lower doses should be used in the frail elderly or if there is significant renal impairment. • Regular folic acid supplements are thought to reduce some side effects. The usual dose of folic acid is 5 mg weekly, often taken the day after the methotrexate, although this varies with local practice. Check your local policy . . . . Methotrexate is sometimes given subcutaneously or intramuscularly if the oral route is not available, if a patient develops GI side effects or if poor absorption is suspected. The dose is usually the same as that given orally, although bioavailability is slightly higher
Examples of possible side effects	• See notes below regarding the patient monitoring booklet
Baseline monitoring	• FBC, U&Es, LFTs and a chest X-ray
Routine monitoring	• U&Es, FBC and LFTs fortnightly until 6 weeks after the last dose increase. Providing the measurements are stable, they can be performed monthly thereafter
Pharmaceutical care considerations	If methotrexate is prescribed with NSAIDs or aspirin, the dose may require careful monitoring as excretion may be reduced; local practice may vary as some rheumatologists do not think the interaction is significant. Patients should be advised to avoid self-medicating with over-the-counter aspirin or NSAID therapies.[3] In July 2004, the National Patient Safety Agency issued a safety alert regarding methotrexate.[4] It was prompted by several safety incidents in which patients died or came to serious harm. The alert concerned agreeing local risk reduction strategies: providing a pretreatment leaflet and a patient handheld monitoring and dosage book; ensuring prescribing and dispensing software were updated to include methotrexate alerts and prompts; and a review of purchasing to ensure the 2.5 mg and 10 mg tablets are of a visually distinguishable shape. Some hospitals only use the 2.5 mg strength.[5] The locally produced patient monitoring booklet will vary in presentation and content from hospital to hospital, and it is worth familiarising yourself with your local version, but there will be a core content that remains constant. The key points that can be used to aid patient counselling are listed below. • The importance of taking methotrexate on the same day each week should be emphasised and this day should be recorded in the booklet. If the dose is missed, it can be taken on one of the two following days, but must not be taken if more than 3 days have elapsed. In either case, the next dose should be taken on the patient's usual day.

R

(Continued)

TABLE R9
(Continued)

	• Patients should speak to their doctor if they have:
	  • any infections, including fever, chills or a sore throat
	  • an unexplained skin rash, ulcerations or soreness of skin
	  • yellowing of the skin/eyes or generalised itching
	  • bleeding gums, black tarry stools or unexplained bleeding or bruising
	  • chest pain, difficulty breathing or a dry, persistent cough
	  • sore mouth or mouth ulcers
	  • severe and continuous diarrhoea, vomiting or stomach pains.
	  • If they come into contact with someone with chickenpox or shingles and they have not had the illness themselves they may need special treatment.
	• Excess alcohol should be avoided, although an occasional drink may not be expected to cause significant side effects, e.g. well within the national daily limits.
	• Read food labels carefully, as foods made from unpasteurised milk, e.g. soft cheese, and uncooked meats, e.g. pâté, may be a source of bacteria, which could increase the risk of infection.
	• Methotrexate can reduce fertility in men and women. It is teratogenic and must be avoided in pregnancy and breastfeeding. For both women and men effective contraception should be exercised throughout treatment and at least a 3-month period should elapse following cessation of methotrexate before a planned conception.
	• Live vaccines should be avoided but the annual influenza vaccination and the pneumococcal vaccine should be given.
	• Co-trimoxazole and trimethoprim should *not* be given concomitantly as serious side effects and fatalities have occurred.
	
	Calcium folinate is a specific antidote for methotrexate and following accidental overdose (see *Methotrexate: calcium folinate rescue regimen* entry).

TABLE R10
Penicillamine[1,2,3]

Dose	• 125–250 mg daily, increasing by 125 mg every 4 weeks to 500 mg daily in divided doses. If no response has occurred after a further 3 months, a dose increase to 750 mg daily could be considered (although a dose of 1.5 g daily is licensed). For patients with renal impairment, therapy should be initiated at a low dose, with intervals between each dose increase of at least 12 weeks
Examples of possible side effects	• Rashes, urticaria, fever, taste disturbance, nausea, proteinuria, bone marrow suppression

(Continued)

TABLE R10
(Continued)

Baseline monitoring	• FBC, U&Es (including serum creatinine) and urinalysis (for proteinuria and haematuria)
Routine monitoring	• FBC and urinalysis fortnightly until the dose has been stable for 3 months, then monthly for both thereafter. Patients should be asked about the presence of rash or oral ulceration every time they attend the monitoring clinic
Pharmaceutical care considerations	• Penicillamine should be taken on an empty stomach at least half an hour before meals or at bedtime.[2] • Warn patients to tell their doctor immediately if a sore throat, fever, unexplained bleeding or bruising, purpura, mouth ulcers, metallic taste or rashes develop.[3] • Penicillamine should be used with caution in patients who have had adverse reactions to gold. Concomitant treatment with gold should be avoided.[2] • If oral iron, digoxin or antacid therapy is coprescribed, a 2-hour administration gap should be left.[2] • NSAIDs and other nephrotoxic drugs may increase the risk of renal damage.[2] • Although cross-reactivity is rare, a patient who is allergic to penicillin may also react to penicillamine[2]

TABLE R11
Sulfasalazine[1–3]

Dose	• Initially 500 mg daily, increasing by 500 mg at weekly intervals to 2–3 g daily in three to four divided doses
Examples of possible side effects	• Nausea, headache, rash, loss of appetite, insomnia, stomatitis, hepatitis, bone marrow suppression
Baseline monitoring	• FBC, U&Es and LFTs
Routine monitoring	• FBC and LFTs every 4 weeks for the first 12 weeks, then 12-weekly thereafter. If, during the first year of treatment, blood results have been stable, 6-monthly tests will suffice for the second year and thereafter monitoring of blood for toxicity could be discontinued. After a dose change, FBC and LFTs should be repeated after 4 weeks. • Patients should be asked about the presence of rash or oral ulceration at each clinic appointment. • U&Es, including urinalysis, should be monitored 4-weekly for 12 weeks
Pharmaceutical care considerations	• Warn patients to tell their doctor immediately if persistent fever, sore throat, unexplained bruising or bleeding occurs. • Urine and tears may be discoloured orange and contact lenses may be stained.[3] • Macrocytosis or pancytopenia due to folic acid deficiency can be reversed by administration of a folic acid supplement[2]

R

Cytokine inhibitors

The NICE guidelines set out eligibility criteria for treatment with anti-TNFs; to comply, the patient must:[5]

1   have active rheumatoid arthritis determined by a disease activity score (DAS28) measured at two points 1 month apart, recording a score >5.1 to confirm ongoing active disease.

2   have trialled at least two standard DMARD therapies (one of which must be methotrexate, unless contraindicated). Trials should have lasted at least 6 months, with 2 months at the recommended maintenance dose, unless toxicity or intolerance required the treatment to be withdrawn or the dose to be limited.

NICE may recommend that additional requirements are met dependant on the drug of choice.

There may be circumstances when other DMARDs are relatively contraindicated, so anti-TNF therapy may be considered very early in the course of the disease and in patients in whom methotrexate has not been used.

Safety of the anti-TNF therapies is unknown or has not been established in pregnancy or lactation and it is recommended that:

- pregnancy should be avoided whilst on cytokine inhibitors and effective contraception is strongly recommended to prevent pregnancy in women of childbearing potential (both sexes should have a washout period before a planned conception)
- the decision to breastfeed should take into consideration the individual circumstances and drug
- consideration should be given to stopping anti-TNF therapy if a patient becomes pregnant whilst on treatment.[6]

All patients should be screened for tuberculosis prior to initiating treatment and monitored for mycobacterial infection during treatment and for 6 months after stopping.[6]

Live vaccines should not be given. It is recommended that juvenile chronic arthritis patients are brought up to date with all immunisations if possible, in agreement with current immunisation guidelines, *before* starting therapy.

As this is an ever-developing area of treatment, please refer to the latest NICE guidance for current recommendations. Tables R12–R14 refer to three of the first-line anti-TNFs.

TABLE R12
Adalimumab[2,3]

Dose	• 40 mg every other week by subcutaneous injection in combination with methotrexate (in monotherapy, the frequency may be increased to weekly depending on response)
Examples of possible side effects	• Injection site pain, respiratory, urinary tract and other infections, headache, dizziness, GI disturbances, rash, pruritus, hyperlipidaemia, worsening heart failure
Baseline monitoring	• Assess for infections or risk factors for infections, especially tuberculosis • Hepatitis B virus should be tested for in patients with risk factors • FBC
Routine monitoring	• Observe for injection site reactions. FBC monitoring
Pharmaceutical care considerations	• Patients should tell their doctor immediately if the following occur: persistent fever, sore throat, weight loss, bruising or bleeding, as these symptoms can be suggestive of blood disorders.[3] • Patients should also be aware to monitor for symptoms of tuberculosis, such as persistent cough, fever or weight loss, and to report these immediately to their doctor.[3] • Patients should carry the relevant alert card provided on initiation of treatment[2]

R

TABLE R13
Etanercept[2,3]

Dose	• 25 mg twice weekly, or 50 mg weekly by subcutaneous injection; it may be given in combination with methotrexate or as monotherapy if methotrexate is contraindicated or not tolerated
Examples of possible side effects	• Injection site reactions, respiratory and other infections, fever, pruritus, worsening heart failure
Baseline monitoring	• Assess for infections or risk factors for infections • Patients should be screened for hepatitis B virus • FBC
Routine monitoring	• Observe for injection site reactions. FBC monitoring
Pharmaceutical care considerations	• Patients should tell their doctor immediately if the following occur: persistent fever, sore throat, weight loss, bruising or bleeding, as these symptoms can be suggestive of blood disorders.[3] • Patients should also be aware to monitor for symptoms of tuberculosis, such as persistent cough, fever or weight loss, and to report these immediately to their doctor.[3] • Patients should be provided with the appropriate patient alert card

TABLE R14
Infliximab[2,3]

Dose	• 3 mg/kg as an intravenous infusion at weeks 0, 2, and 6 and then every 8 weeks thereafter. If the response is inadequate after 12 weeks, refer to product literature for advice on how the dose may be increased.
	• Infliximab must be given in combination with methotrexate when used for rheumatoid arthritis
Examples of possible side effects	• Injection site reactions, respiratory and other infections, fever, pruritus, rash, headache, vertigo, flushing, GI disturbances, fatigue, tachycardia and worsening heart failure
Baseline monitoring	• Assess for infections or risk factors for infections, especially tuberculosis • Patients should be screened for hepatitis B virus • FBC
Routine monitoring	• Observe for injection site reactions, including anaphylaxis (observe patient for 2 hours after infusion). FBC monitoring
Pharmaceutical care considerations	• Patients should tell their doctor immediately if the following occur: persistent fever, sore throat, weight loss, bruising or bleeding, as these symptoms can be suggestive of blood disorders.[3] • Patients should also be aware to monitor for symptoms of tuberculosis, such as persistent cough, fever or weight loss, and to report these immediately to their doctor.[3] • The dose is given as an infusion, which must be prepared in an aseptic suite. An infusion set should be used with an in-line, sterile, non-pyrogenic, low protein-binding filter (pore size 1.2 microns or less).[2] • Patients should be provided with the patient information leaflet and alert card

REFERENCES
1 BSR/BHPR (2008). BSR/BHPR guideline for disease modifying anti-rheumatic drug (DMARD) therapy in consultation with the British association of Dermatologists. http://www.rhuematology.org.uk (accessed 23 August 2014).
2 *Electronic Medicines Compendium* (2014). http://www.medicines.org.uk/emc/ (accessed 23 August 2014).
3 Joint Formulary Committee (2013). *British National Formulary* (66th edn). London: BMJ Group and Pharmaceutical Press.
4 NPSA (2006). *Improving Compliance with Oral Methotrexate Guidelines*. http://www.nrls.npsa.nhs.uk/ (accessed 23 August 2014).
5 NICE (2009). *Rheumatoid Arthritis – The Management of rheumatoid arthritis in adults*. CG79. https://www.nice.org.uk/guidance/cg79 (accessed 5 January 2015).
6 BSR/BHPR (2010). *BSR and BHPR Rheumatoid Arthritis Guidelines on Safety of Anti-TNF Therapies*. http:// www.rheumatology.org.uk (accessed 23 August 2014).

Rockall score for gastrointestinal bleed

Overview

Background
- Designed to predict death based on clinical and endoscopic findings[1]
- Also used to predict rebleeding risk

SCORING SYSTEM[1]

Clinical feature	Score
Age <60 years	0
Age 60–79 years	1
Age ≥80 years	2
Shock: 'no shock', systolic blood pressure (SBP) ≥100 mmHg, pulse <100 beats/min	0
Shock: 'tachycardia', SBP ≥100 mmHg, pulse ≥100 beats/min	1
Shock: 'hypotension', SBP <100 mmHg	2
Comorbidity: no major comorbidity	0
Comorbidity: cardiac failure, ischaemic heart disease, any major comorbidity	2
Comorbidity: renal failure, liver failure, disseminated malignancy	3
Diagnosis: Mallory–Weiss tear, no lesion identified and no stigmata of recent haemorrhage	0
Diagnosis: all other diagnoses	1
Diagnosis: malignancy of upper GI tract	2
Major stigmata of recent haemorrhage: none, or dark spot only	0
Major stigmata of recent haemorrhage: blood in upper GI tract, adherent clot, visible or spurting vessel	2

R

Interpretation[1,2]

Initial pre-endoscopic score (derived from age, score, comorbidity):
- 0: a score of 0 identifies 15% of patients with an acute upper GI bleed at presentation who have an extremely low risk of death (0.2%) and rebleeding (0.2%), and who may be suitable for early discharge or non-admission
- If the initial (pre-endoscopic) score is above 0, there is a significant mortality and endoscopy is recommended for full assessment of bleeding risk:
- 1: predicted mortality 2.4%
- 2: predicted mortality 5.6%

The full Rockall score comprises the initial score plus additional points for endoscopic diagnosis:
  <3: low risk of rebleeding or death and should be considered for early discharge and outpatient follow-up.
  >8: high risk of mortality

REFERENCES

1 SIGN (2008). *Management of Acute Upper and Lower Gastrointestinal Bleeding*. NHS Scotland: SIGN. http://www.sign.ac.uk/pdf/sign105.pdf (accessed 31 July 2014).
2 NICE (2012). *Acute Upper Gastrointestinal Bleeding*. National Clinical Guideline centre: NICE. http://www.nice.org.uk/guidance/cg141/resources/cg141-acute-upper-gi-bleeding-full-guideline2 (accessed 31 July 2014).

S

Sarcoidosis

Overview	
Definition	Sarcoidosis is a condition caused by granulomatous inflammation and can affect virtually any organ.[1] The most commonly affected organs are the lungs (≈80% of patients), the lymph nodes, the eyes and the skin. Granulomas are seen in a number of other conditions and are a collection of immune cells usually formed in response to the presence of an antigen. Sarcoidosis may resolve spontaneously, probably representing clearance of the antigen. In some patients, treatment may be required to bring about resolution or to reduce the damage caused by local inflammation, which may otherwise progress to fibrosis.
	It is likely that a range of antigens may result in sarcoidosis and it is not thought to result from either an infectious or autoimmune process. The pattern of disease and its natural history are thought to represent interplay between: the precipitating antigen, human leukocyte antigen (HLA) class II molecules and T-cell receptors
Risk factors	Sarcoidosis predominantly affects people between the ages of 25 and 40 years. There is a slightly higher incidence in women (male to female ratio of 1:1.2).
	Sarcoidosis is more common in Afro-Caribbeans and in this population more likely to follow a chronic course (the incidence is ≈3-fold higher and prevalence ≈10-fold higher).
	Sarcoidosis has been known to develop during treatment with antitumour necrosis factor (anti-TNF) agents or following chemotherapy
Differential diagnosis	Given the range of organs affected there is considerable scope for initial misdiagnosis.
	Non-specific constitutional symptoms, such as fever, fatigue (which may be very severe), malaise and weight loss, may also be present.
	Granulomas are seen in a number of conditions, including tuberculosis, berylliosis, cat-scratch disease (caused by *Bartonella henselae*), vasculitis and hypersensitivity pneumonitis.
	Pulmonary sarcoidosis may present with bilateral hilar lymphadenopathy (where lymphoma is an important differential), patch infiltrates or pulmonary fibrosis (where interstitial lung disease is an important differential)

Diagnostic tests	
	• The presence of granulomas in a biopsy sample of affected tissue, with the exclusion of other causes of granulomatous inflammation, is desired for diagnosis. Biopsy may not be required if the presentation is peculiar to sarcoidosis, where obtaining the sample would represent an undue risk or where there is sufficient radiological and clinical evidence to support a diagnosis of sarcoidosis confidently.
	• Serum angiotensin-converting enzyme (sACE) may be elevated in ≈60% of patients. An elevated level is supportive of a diagnosis but is neither sensitive nor specific. sACE levels do not reflect disease activity and are of limited value in monitoring progression.
	• Serum immunoglobulin G (IgG) may be elevated in ≈50% of patients. Decreased IgG concentration is uncommon and suggests an alternative diagnosis.
	• Lymphopenia due to relocation of circulating lymphocytes to the site of active disease may occur.
	• Granulomas can produce 1-α hydroxylase, catalysing the conversion of ergocalcitriol to calcitriol and precipitating hypercalcaemia and/or hypercalciuria. Increased urinary calcium concentrations may result in renal stones and renal dysfunction. Ergocalciferol (vitamin D_2) concentration may be low despite elevated calcitriol (vitamin D_3) levels. Assays routinely only measure ergocalciferol levels and should be interpreted cautiously.
	• Pulmonary involvement most commonly presents with a restrictive pattern of spirometry but obstructive patterns may also be seen. Interstitial inflammation or fibrosis will impair gas transfer, with a reduced diffusing capacity of the lung for carbon monoxide (DLCO) or transfer factor for carbon monoxide (TLCO, which provides an estimate of the lung's ability to diffuse gases).
	• Staging based on the appearance of the chest X-ray has been proposed (Scadding stage)
Treatment goals	
	• Sarcoidosis may resolve spontaneously in some patients and watchful waiting may be appropriate. If the likelihood of spontaneous resolution is low or the risk of organ damage high (for example, sarcoidosis involving the central nervous system, eyes or heart) then immunosuppressive treatment may hasten resolution. In some patients, sarcoidosis will not resolve despite treatment and in these patients ongoing immunosuppression is required to reduce the rate of progression.
	• Chronic anterior uveitis may develop without significant symptoms and may be sight-threatening. Routine eye examination is commonly advised in patients suffering with sarcoidosis (recommendations typically 6–12-monthly).
	• Cardiac sarcoidosis is an uncommon complication but can be life-threatening. Some specialists therefore recommend periodic ECGs to identify the development of cardiac abnormalities during follow-up
Treatment options[2]	
	• There are no licensed therapies in sarcoidosis.
	• Corticosteroids are the initial treatment in the majority, typically starting at 20–40 mg prednisolone daily and tapering 1–3 months after initiation to a maintenance dose of 10–20 mg daily. If resolving, treatment will be continued for a period of 6–12 months and then tapered to a stop. Intravenous methylprednisolone (500–1000 mg) is sometimes used for short-course (3–5 days) induction.

S

- Topical corticosteroids (usually potent ones) may be appropriate for some presentations.
- Higher doses of corticosteroids, i.e. 1 mg/kg prednisolone, or initial dosing with 3–5 days' intravenous methylprednisolone (500–1000 mg) has been used in acutely unwell patients.
- In patients in whom a maintenance dose <10 mg prednisolone cannot be achieved then azathioprine or methotrexate are commonly used as steroid-sparing agents.
- Hydroxychloroquine may be useful in some patients but use is generally limited to mild presentations.
- There is limited experience with other immunosuppressive agents, such as leflunomide and mycophenolate mofetil.
- Some evidence supports the use of adalimumab or infliximab in patients with chronic sarcoidosis (>2 years) and treatment-refractory sarcoidosis[3]

Medicines optimisation

Assess	- Is sarcoidosis an adverse reaction to current treatments (particularly anti-TNF-α agents)? - Which organs are affected and how will this affect monitoring of response to, or adverse effects from, treatment?
Corticosteroids	- Relatively long courses with relatively high doses of corticosteroids may be required. Patients should be advised not to stop therapy abruptly and of potential side effects. - Where osteoporosis prophylaxis is indicated, the potential to precipitate or worsen hypercalcaemia or hypercalciuria should be considered and calcium/vitamin D supplementation avoided in some patients or used cautiously in others
Methotrexate[4]	- Methotrexate is the most commonly used steroid-sparing agent in sarcoidosis, typically at doses of 5–20 mg weekly with folic acid 5 mg the following day or 1–5 mg every day apart from the day of treatment to reduce the severity of side effects. It may take up to 6 months for treatment to demonstrate effectiveness and this should be considered when assessing efficacy. - Monitoring of FBC, LFTs and U&Es is consistent with its use in other indications but potential sarcoidosis-related complications should be considered when reviewing blood results, i.e. baseline lymphocytosis reflecting disease activity and potential hepatic dysfunction in hepatic sarcoidosis
Azathioprine	- Azathioprine is possibly as efficacious as methotrexate in sarcoidosis and typically used in the range 50–200 mg daily. - Myalgia, flu-like symptoms and pancreatitis may complicate treatment. - Azathioprine is metabolised by thiopurine S-methyltransferase and high or low levels of activity may predispose to treatment failure or toxicities, respectively. Pretreatment measurement of enzyme activity may be useful. - As with methotrexate, monitoring is consistent with its use in other indications

S

Hydroxychloro-quine	• Gastrointestinal side effects are relatively common and may resolve on dose reduction.
	• Hydroxychloroquine may cause haemolytic anaemia in patients deficient in glucose-6-phosphate-dehydrogenase (G6PD). G6PD deficiency primarily affects those of African or Mediterranean descent and pretreatment measurement of enzyme activity may be useful.
	• Ocular toxicity can occur and may be irreversible. The risk is higher in patients with compromised renal or hepatic function and appears to be related to cumulative dose, with a higher risk in those receiving >6.5 mg/kg/day (hydroxychloroquine has a low volume of distribution and lean body weight should be used if less than actual) or treatment >5 years. Patients should be advised of the need for a baseline eye examination and to seek advice if they experience visual disturbances, especially changes in colour vision, blurred vision, sensitivity to light or the presence of haloes around lights.
	• Hypoglycaemia may occur during treatment and patients should be aware that feeling faint or fainting may be a symptom of this. In diabetic patients antidiabetic therapies may need to be adjusted in light of this

REFERENCES
1 Joint Statement of the ATS/ERS/WASOG (1999). Statement on sarcoidosis *Am J Respir Crit Care Med* 160: 736–755.
2 Baughman RP *et al.* (2012). Therapy for sarcoidosis: evidence-based recommendations. *Exp Rev Clin Immunol* 8: 95–103.
3 Drent M *et al.* (2014). Practical eminence and experience-based recommendations for use of TNF-α inhibitors in sarcoidosis. *Sarcoidosis Vasc Diffuse Lung Dis* 31: 91–107.
4 Cremers JP *et al.* (2013). Multinational evidence-based World Association of Sarcoidosis and Other Granulomatous Disorders recommendations for the use of methotrexate in sarcoidosis: integrating systematic literature research and expert opinion of sarcoidologists worldwide. *Curr Opin Pulm Med* 19: 545–561.

Sclerosants for the management of malignant pleural effusions

Pleurodesis is a treatment to eliminate the space between the tissues in the chest cavity and the pleural membranes to prevent the build-up of fluid. Chemical pleurodesis with a sclerosing agent (i.e. an agent that promotes fibre formation between the pleural membranes) may be used in the management of malignant pleural effusions.

Sterile talc is the chemical sclerosant of choice for pleurodesis. Historically, other agents – bleomycin, doxycycline, tetracycline and minocycline – have been used in the UK for intrapleural administration. Sterile talc is available as an unlicensed product. It has a success rate of approximately 90%.[1]

An intercostal tube is inserted and the pleural effusion is drained. A chest radiograph is then performed to ensure complete lung expansion and to confirm the position of the tube.

Intrapleural administration of sclerosing agents may be painful. A premedication, for example, an anxiolytic, should be administered prior to commencing chemical pleurodesis. After the premedication has been administered, lidocaine solution (3 mg/kg up to a maximum of 250 mg) is instilled via the intercostal tube into the pleural space, followed by the sterile talc. To prepare the talc slurry, 2–5 g of sterile talc is mixed with 40 mL of sterile water in a bladder syringe and instilled. Sterile talc is also available as Steritalc PF Puffer (see instructions below). The tube should then be clamped for 1 hour. The patient will need to change position several times during the procedure to allow dispersion of the talc. After 1 hour, the clamp is released and the fluid is drained off. Common side effects include chest pain and fever. Rare side effects (<1%) include acute respiratory failure.

In practice, some clinicians advise that non-steroidal anti-inflammatory drugs, cyclooxygenase-2 inhibitors and corticosteroids should not be administered to patients for 48 hours before and for up to 5 days after the procedure because of a possible reduction in the inflammatory reaction of the pleura to the sclerosant.

If using Steritalc PF Puffer, which is a medical device containing 4 g sterile talc, it can be administered directly into the pleural cavity as follows:

1 Fix the silicone connector (included) on the internal nozzle of the puffer.
2 Screw the male Luer lock connector to its maximum on the cannula while holding it firmly.
3 Hold the cannula and the puffer together and press smoothly several times on the puffer to spray Steritalc homogeneously into the pleural space.

REFERENCE
1 Roberts ME *et al.* (2010). Management of a malignant pleural effusion. British Thoracic Society Pleural. Guidelines 2010. *Thorax* 65(Suppl. 2): ii32–ii40.

Serotonin syndrome

Serotonin syndrome is a rare, but potentially life-threatening, condition caused by excess serotonergic agonism. It can develop when serotonergic drugs are given in combination, when switching between serotonergic drugs, upon overdose and also with therapeutic doses. Serotonin syndrome usually occurs within hours of initiation or dose change. Very rarely mild symptoms may recur over a period of weeks prior to the development of more severe symptoms.

Diagnosis

Serotonin syndrome is diagnosed if precipitating drugs are identified, no other cause is likely, and at least three of the following symptoms are present:[1]

- mental state changes
- fever

- shivering
- sweating
- agitation/restlessness
- diarrhoea
- myoclonus
- hyperreflexia (more commonly of the lower limbs)
- tachycardia
- ataxia
- tremor.

The Hunter criteria may also be used for diagnosis.[2]

Management

- Discontinue serotonergic agents.
- Seek specialist advice from the National Poisons Information Service.[3]
- Carry out supportive care to normalise vital signs.
- Consider:
  - benzodiazepines, e.g. 1–2 mg lorazepam by slow intravenous injection every 30 minutes
  - serotonin antagonists, e.g. cyproheptadine orally 4–8 mg every 2–4 hours (max. 0.5 mg/kg/day).

Symptoms often resolve within 24–36 hours with adequate supportive care but may persist following agents with long half-lives or those with active metabolites.

Managing risk

The risk of serotonin syndrome developing is reduced by avoiding the use of serotonergic drugs in combination (Table S1). Care must be taken when switching, especially between selective serotonin reuptake inhibitors (SSRIs) and monoamine oxidase inhibitors (MAOIs).

Tramadol may cause serotonin syndrome, particularly when it is used at high doses (patients with low weight should use 0.7 mg/kg body weight[4]) or in combination with other drugs increasing serotonin concentrations.

TABLE S1

Drug combinations to be avoided or used with caution due to increased risk of serotonin syndrome developing[5]

Drug	Interacting combination	Comment
Almotriptan	Lithium or other 5-HT$_{1B/1D}$ agonists	Some combinations contraindicated by manufacturers
MAOIs	Bupropion, pethidine, rizatriptan, sumatriptan, SSRIs, tramadol	
MAOIs	Tricyclic antidepressants, venlafaxine	Avoid due to severe cases of serotonin syndrome reported
St John's wort	Psychotropic drugs (e.g. SSRIs), triptans	
Lithium	MAOIs, SSRIs, sumatriptan, tricyclic antidepressants, tramadol, venlafaxine	Use with caution and monitor closely for symptoms of serotonin syndrome
SSRIs	Tramadol, triptans	
Venlafaxine	Fluoxetine, paroxetine	

REFERENCES

1 Sternbach H (1991). The serotonin syndrome. *Am J Psychiatry* 148: 705–713.
2 Dunkley EJ *et al.* (2003). The Hunter serotonin toxicity criteria: simple and accurate diagnostic decision rules for serotonin toxicity. *QJM* 96: 635–642.
3 National Poisons Information Service. http://www.toxbase.org (accessed 16 September 2015).
4 SPC (2015). *Tramadol.* http://www.medicines.org.uk (accessed 2 January 2015).
5 Neil K (2003). Drug interactions and serotonin syndrome: tramadol with MAOIs. *Prescriber* 19: 18–24.

Systemic inflammatory response syndrome due to sepsis scoring system

Background

Systemic inflammatory response syndrome (SIRS) is the term given to the inflammatory process seen in response to an insult, which can be either infectious or non-infectious in origin. Causes of SIRS can include infection, trauma and ischaemia. The term SIRS does not necessarily mean an infection is present

SCORING SYSTEM – SIRS (TWO OR MORE OF THE FOLLOWING)	
Clinical feature	**Score**
Temperature <36°C or >38°C	1
Heart rate >90 beats/min	1
Respiratory rate >20 breaths/min or $PaCO_2$ <4.2 kPa	1
White cell count <4 or >12 $\times$ 10^9/L	1

Definition of SIRS plus sepsis[1]

Infection (suspected or diagnosed) plus any of the following:

- Temperature <36°C or >38°C
- Heart rate >90 beats/min
- Respiratory rate >20 breaths/min or $PaCO_2$ <4.2 kPa
- White cell count <4 or >12 $\times$ 10^9/L
- Blood pressure <90 mmHg or mean <65 mmHg
- O_2 saturations <90% on air or oxygen
- Creatinine >175 micromol/L or urine output <0.5 mL/kg/hour for 2 hours despite adequate fluid resuscitation
- Abnormal LFTs
- Platelets <100 $\times$ 10^9/L or coagulopathy (INR >1.5)
- Lactate >1 mmol/L
- Decreased capillary refill
- Ileus
- Acutely altered mental state

Interpretation[2]

Guidelines for the management of sepsis, severe sepsis and septic shock have been developed by the Surviving Sepsis Campaign, and include the following in the first 6 hours:

1. Initial resuscitation:
   i. central venous pressure 8–12 mmHg
   ii. mean arterial pressure $\geq$65 mmHg
   iii. urine output $\geq$0.5 mL/kg/hour.
2. Diagnosis:
   i. obtain appropriate cultures in order to identify causative organism *before* antibiotics are administered (e.g. respiratory secretions, cerebrospinal fluid, wound swabs, urine)
   ii. at least two blood cultures (sample peripherally and centrally if vascular access device is in place)
   iii. imaging where appropriate.
3. Antibiotic therapy:
   i. initial intravenous antibiotics *within 1 hour of recognition of severe sepsis*
   ii. consider spectrum of activity, penetrations and local formulary when starting empiric antibiotics
   iii. review antibiotics every 24 hours against received culture and sensitivity results and consider de-escalation to a narrow-spectrum agent
   iv. stop antibiotics if SIRS subsequently deemed to be due to a non-infectious cause.
4. Source control:
   i. consider source of infection and possible control measures, e.g. abscess drainage, removal of vascular access device.
5. Fluid therapy:
   i. use crystalloid for initial fluid resuscitation
   ii. do *not* use hydroxyethyl starches for fluid resuscitation
   iii. consider albumin in patients requiring large volumes of crystalloid.
6. Vasopressors:
   i. use noradrenaline first-line
   ii. add vasopressin to noradrenaline to raise mean arterial pressure or in an attempt to reduce noradrenaline doses.
7. Inotropes:
   i. dobutamine may be added to vasopressors when myocardial dysfunction is present.
8. Corticosteroids·
   i. do not use steroids if fluid resuscitation and vasopressors have achieved haemodynamic stability
   ii. if hydrocortisone is appropriate, give 200 mg/day via continuous infusion.
9. Venous thromboembolism (VTE) prophylaxis:
   i. ensure VTE risk assessed and prophylactic doses of low-molecular-weight heparin prescribed as appropriate
   ii. if pharmacological methods are contraindicated, consider mechanical prophylaxis.
10. Stress ulcer prophylaxis:
   i. give either a proton pump inhibitor (preferably) or H_2 antagonist.

REFERENCES

1 Dellinger RP *et al.* (2013). Surviving sepsis campaign: international guidelines for management of severe sepsis and septic shock. *Crit Care Med* 41: 580.
2 Townsend S *et al.* (eds) (2005). *Implementing the Surviving Sepsis Campaign*. Mount Prospect: Society of Critical Care Medicine.

Sodium

Overview	
Normal range	135–146 mmol/L
Local range	
Background	Sodium is the major extracellular electrolyte and its role and metabolism are closely related to the body's water balance
Reference nutrient intake[1]	70 mmol/day (1.6 g sodium, or about 4 g sodium chloride)

Hypernatraemia	
Symptoms	Thirst, reduced salivation and lacrimation, fever, tachycardia, hypertension, headache, dizziness, restlessness, irritability and weakness. Hypernatraemia can lead to central nervous system dehydration, manifesting as somnolence, confusion, convulsions, coma, respiratory failure and death
Causes	• Fluid loss with inadequate water intake, e.g. diarrhoea, vomiting, burns, coma • Incorrect fluid replacement in patients dependent on intravenous therapy • Osmotic diuresis, e.g. diabetic ketoacidosis • Excessive fluid loss due to diabetes insipidus • Primary aldosteronism • Drugs that can cause hypernatraemia include: demeclocycline, clonidine, corticosteroids, lactulose, methyldopa, oestrogens, oral contraceptives and sodium bicarbonate
Treatment	If due to dehydration or there is only mild sodium excess, rehydrating the patient should correct this and sodium intake may be restricted. Water given orally is the preferred route
	If hypernatraemia is severe, intravenous fluids may be needed. There is some debate as to whether to use glucose 5% or sodium chloride 0.9% (sodium chloride 0.9% can cause less marked fluid shifts and is relatively hypotonic to a hypernatraemic individual).
	If the hypernatraemia is drug-induced, discontinuing or changing the drug therapy may alleviate the condition

Hyponatraemia	
Classification	The severity of hyponatraemia can be classified by the serum sodium concentration:[2] • Mild hyponatraemia: serum sodium concentration is 125–134 mmol/L. • Moderate hyponatraemia: serum sodium concentration is 115–124 mmol/L. • Severe hyponatraemia: serum sodium concentration is <115 mmol/L
Symptoms	• Dilutional hyponatraemia can be asymptomatic but headache, confusion, nausea, vomiting, somnolence and weakness can manifest. If there is plasma volume contraction as well as sodium depletion, postural hypotension and circulatory insufficiency may occur

S

Causes	• Reduced water excretion, e.g. in renal impairment • SIADH, which may be drug-induced (see *Syndrome of inappropriate secretion of antidiuretic hormone* entry) • Excessive oral fluid intake • Inappropriate intravenous administration of hypotonic fluids • Certain disease states, e.g. nephrotic syndrome, heart failure, liver cirrhosis, renal failure, adrenocortical insufficiency and acquired immunodeficiency syndrome • Drugs that can cause hyponatraemia include: amphotericin, angiotensin-converting enzyme inhibitors, carbamazepine, cyclophosphamide, desmopressin, diuretics, heparin, lithium, non-steroidal anti-inflammatory drugs (NSAIDs), selective serotonin reuptake inhibitors (SSRIs), opioids, tolbutamide and vasopressin[3]
Treatment	Fluid restriction is often all that is necessary. If due to SIADH, the hyponatraemia may be drug-nduced. Sodium chloride supplementation is sometimes used. If sodium depletion is mild or moderate, e.g. in salt-losing bowel or renal disease, Slow Sodium is used at doses of 4–8 tablets daily (40–80 mmol or 2.4–4.8 g). In severe cases up to 20 tablets daily (200 mmol or 12 g) have been used. For control of muscle cramps during routine maintenance haemodialysis, 10–16 tablets per dialysis is usual. Patients should swallow each tablet whole with at least 70 mL water/tablet, and be counselled about 'ghost' tablets appearing in their stools.[4] Acute symptomatic hyponatraemia (water intoxication), where serum sodium concentration falls below 120 mmol/L, is treated aggressively with intravenous hypertonic or isotonic sodium chloride solution. Furosemide is often given, especially if fluid overload is likely to be a problem. The aim is for the patient to be asymptomatic, and to achieve a sodium serum concentration of 120–130 mmol/L. Care should be taken to increase sodium levels gradually, as central nervous system toxicity can occur if correction is too rapid. It is important to avoid the development of hypernatraemia

TABLE S2

Sodium content of various preparations

Product	Sodium content[3]
Slow Sodium MR tablets	600 mg (approx. 10 mmol)
Sodium chloride 0.9% intravenous infusion	9 g/L (150 mmol)
Sodium chloride 0.18% and glucose 4%	30 mmol/L
Sodium chloride 0.45% and glucose 2.5%	75 mmol/L
Sodium chloride 0.45% and glucose 5%	75 mmol/L
Ringer's solution	147 mmol/L
Sodium lactate intravenous infusion, compound (Hartmann's solution for injection, Ringer's lactate solution for injection)	131 mmol/L
Sodium bicarbonate capsules	500 mg (6 mmol)

REFERENCES

1 *Martindale: The Complete Drug Reference* (2014). www.medicinescomplete.com (accessed 1 November 2014).
2 NICE (2011). Hyponatraemia – CKS. http://cks.nice.org.uk/hyponatraemia (accessed 1 November 2014).
3 Joint Formulary Committee (2014). *British National Formulary* (68th edn). London: BMJ Group and Pharmaceutical Press.
4 Summary of Product Characteristics (2014). *Slow Sodium*. http://www.medicines .org.uk (accessed 1 November 2014).

Sterile larvae

Larval therapy (also known as 'maggot therapy' or 'biosurgery') is a method of wound debridement that, after having been used for centuries, has been reintroduced relatively recently into modern medicine by doctors and wound care specialists.[1] It can be used as a bridge between debridement procedures, or for debridement of chronic wounds when surgical debridement is not available or cannot be performed.[2] Larval therapy can be used for debridement of acute or chronic necrotic, infected or sloughy wounds and has been used in the treatment of pressure ulcers, chronic venous ulceration and diabetic ulcers.[2] It can also be used to maintain a clean wound after debridement if the wound is considered prone to resloughing.[1]

In the UK, the maggots used in larval therapy are the live sterile larvae of *Lucilia sericata*, also known as the common greenbottle fly. Outside of the UK, *Lucilia cuprina*, also known as the Australian sheep blow fly, are used as well.[2]

Mode of action

The sterile larvae work by releasing a mixture of natural proteolytic enzymes and components that break down the necrotic tissue (healthy tissue is left unharmed) into a liquid form that they can then easily remove and digest.[3] During this process the larvae also take up bacteria, particularly Gram-positive bacteria, which are then destroyed within their gut.[1] Larval therapy has been shown to be successful at eliminating MRSA from wounds[1] and the movement of the larvae is also thought to accelerate wound healing by promoting the formation of granulation tissue.[4]

Disadvantages of larval therapy

Some patients experience an increased amount of wound pain and this may be particularly so for those patients with poor circulation.[1] Pain associated with the therapy may limit its use in about 20% of patients.[2] It has also been suggested that maggots should not be applied to wounds that have a tendency to bleed easily or that communicate with a body cavity or any internal organ.[3]

Availability

In the UK, larval therapy is prescribable on the NHS; however, it should be noted that randomised trials have not found consistent reductions in the time to wound healing compared with standard wound therapy.[2]

In the UK, larval therapy is produced by a company called Biomonde. Larvae are available as either a Biobag dressing or loose within a retention system.

The advantage of the Biobag dressing is that the larvae remain sealed within the dressing throughout the treatment, making the application and removal of larvae significantly easier for clinicians and also allowing for inspection of the wound during treatment.[1]

The loose larvae are particularly useful when the exact extent of the wound is unknown (e.g. the depth).

It has been demonstrated that loose and Biobag larvae are equally effective in terms of debriding the wound.[1] The quantity of larvae required to treat a wound effectively is dependent on the area of the wound and the amount of slough, which is expressed as a percentage of the wound area covered. Once these two factors have been assessed a 'larvae calculator'[5] is used to calculate the quantity of sterile larvae necessary.[4]

Practical points

There are some important practical points to remember regarding larval therapy.

- Metronidazole is known to kill larvae and so it is important to ensure that, for at least 2 days prior to larval therapy being initiated, it is not administered to the patient.[4]
- Larval therapy has a 3- or 4-day treatment cycle (depending on the preparation of larvae used) and so care must be taken to ensure that subsequent supplies are ordered the day before needed so that they can be reared and delivered in time for optimum application. This is ideally on the day of delivery; however, they may be stored at 6–25°C for 24 hours.
- Any dressings used to secure the sterile larvae in place must not be occlusive, as the larvae need a constant oxygen supply to survive.
- When the larvae are removed from a wound they should be bagged as clinical waste and incinerated according to local policy.[1,4]
- Full guidance and instructions on all aspects of treatment with larvae therapy can be found at the Biomonde website.[1]

REFERENCES

1 Biomonde (2015). http://biomonde.com/en/ (accessed 30 January 2015).
2 Up To Date (2014). *Principles of Wound Debridement*. http://www.uptodate.com/contents/basic-principles-of-wound-management?source=machineLearning&search=principles+of+wound+debridement&selectedTitle=1%7E150&sectionRank=2&anchor=H55268712#H55268712 (accessed 30 January 2015).
3 *Martindale: The Complete Drug Reference* (2014). www.medicinescomplete.com (accessed 30 January 2015).
4 Thomas S, McCubbin P (2002). Use of maggots in the care of wounds. *Hosp Pharm* 9: 267–271.
5 Biomonde Sizing Ordering Guide (2015). http://biomonde.com/attachments/article/7/BM48_EN_08_0914_IP.PDF (accessed 21 February 2015).

Stroke and transient ischaemic attack

Overview	
Definition: stroke	Stroke is defined by the WHO as a clinical syndrome consisting of 'rapidly developing clinical signs of focal (at times global) disturbance of cerebral function, lasting more than 24 hours or leading to death with no apparent cause other than that of vascular origin'.[1] The 'stroke of God's hande' was the phrase physicians used in the late 16th century to describe what is now simply called a stroke or a cerebrovascular accident (CVA)
Definition: TIA	A transient ischaemic attack (TIA) is defined as stroke symptoms and signs that resolve within 24 hours.[2] However, in the majority of TIAs the symptoms usually resolve within minutes, or a few hours at the most, and anyone with continuing neurological signs when first assessed should be presumed to have had a stroke
Classification	Broadly, a stroke can be classified as either ischaemic or haemorrhagic. **Ischaemic stroke**: about 70% of strokes are ischaemic and are caused by a blood clot formed as a result of either cardioembolic or atherosclerotic vascular disease. **Haemorrhagic stroke**: results from the rupture of blood vessels in the brain with the leakage of blood, causing damage. The most common cause is primary intracerebral haemorrhage (PIH), which accounts for about 10% of all patients presenting with acute stroke. Subarachnoid haemorrhage (SAH) accounts for approximately 5%, with an overall survival rate of about 50%[3]
Assessment	All people with suspected stroke should be admitted directly to a specialist acute stroke unit following initial assessment, either from the community or from the Accident and Emergency department. The unit is staffed by a coordinated multidisciplinary team (MDT) with a special interest in stroke care.[4] Pharmacists are part of this MDT and should contribute to regular MDT meetings that occur for goal setting
Diagnostic tests	• Face Arm Speech Test (FAST) is a common validated tool used to screen for a diagnosis of stroke or TIA outside the hospital setting. A stroke should be suspected if a person exhibits any of these symptoms. • Recognition Of Stroke In Emergency Room (ROSIER).[4] A stroke is likely if a person scores >0 in the absence of hypoglycaemia. • Non-contrast CT scanning is quick and can easily identify haemorrhagic stroke, which is of use when identifying patients who may be suitable for thrombolysis. A CT scan, however, is not sensitive for early ischaemic stroke (less than 6 hours from onset) or small areas of ischaemia. • MRI is more sensitive than CT to early stroke and small strokes but is expensive and takes longer to perform and process the results. • Carotid imaging (Doppler ultrasound) – about 80% of TIAs require scanning of the arteries around the throat, which provide blood supply to the brain.[5,6] This is due to carotid artery stenosis (CAS), which may be a cause of ischaemic stroke. 'Carotid imaging' is the

S

- most common way of assessing the blood flow in the carotid arteries and diagnosing CAS. If blood flow is sufficiently impaired, patients will be referred to the vascular team and offered surgery (carotid endarterectomy) to improve carotid blood flow.
- ECG monitoring – used for identification of atrial fibrillation (AF), which is a risk factor for stroke and to establish if the stroke is cardioembolic in origin (see *Atrial fibrillation* entry)

Treatment goals	Time is the most important factor in the treatment of stroke. There is evidence that rapid treatment improves outcomes after stroke. Thrombolysis with alteplase in acute ischaemic stroke has been shown to reduce the risk of permanent disability from a stroke significantly[7]

Treatment of acute ischaemic stroke

Thrombolysis	<ul><li>Intravenous thrombolysis uses the recombinant human tissue plasminogen activator alteplase.</li><li>Licensed indication: treatment of acute ischaemic stroke in adults if treatment is started as early as possible within 4 1/2 hours of onset of stroke symptoms *and* intracranial haemorrhage (ICH) has been excluded by appropriate imaging techniques (e.g. CT).[7]</li><li>Dose: 0.9 mg alteplase/kg body weight (maximum of 90 mg) intravenously over 60 minutes with 10% of the total infused dose administered as an initial intravenous bolus. The treatment effect is time-dependent; therefore, earlier treatment increases the probability of a favourable outcome. Beyond 4 1/2 hours after onset of stroke symptoms there is a negative benefit–risk ratio associated with alteplase administration (increased risk of ICH) and so it should not be administered.[8]</li><li>If patients wake from sleep with stroke symptoms, then they will generally be excluded as it is nearly impossible to say at which point during their sleep they had a stroke.</li><li>Contraindications: <18 and >80 years of age. Other exclusion criteria are mainly related to patients who have an increased risk of haemorrhage. These include the prior use of all anticoagulants, including the novel oral anticoagulants (NOAC) drugs</li></ul>
Aspirin and anticoagulant treatment	<ul><li>Once a diagnosis of PIH has been excluded by CT scan, all patients with an acute stroke should be given aspirin 300 mg orally or, if dysphagic, this can be given rectally or via an enteral feeding tube. This should be continued until 2 weeks after the onset of stroke symptoms, at which time long-term secondary prevention should be initiated.</li><li>Anyone who is allergic to, or genuinely intolerant of, aspirin, should be given an alternative antiplatelet agent (e.g. clopidogrel 300 mg as a single loading dose and then continued at 75 mg daily). If there is a history of dyspepsia associated with aspirin, a proton pump inhibitor (PPI) should be given in addition to the aspirin.[3,4]</li><li>Anticoagulation treatment should not be used routinely for the treatment of acute stroke</li></ul>
Anticoagulation for comorbidities	<ul><li>For patients in AF, anticoagulation should be deferred for 2 weeks after onset of symptoms of stroke and replaced with 300 mg aspirin daily during this period.</li></ul>

	• In people with prosthetic heart valves, and who are at significant risk of haemorrhagic transformation, anticoagulation treatment should be stopped for 1 week after onset of stroke and substituted with aspirin 300 mg daily.
	• Patients with stroke and symptomatic proximal deep-vein thrombosis (DVT) or pulmonary embolism (PE) should receive anticoagulation treatment in preference to treatment with aspirin unless there are other contraindications to anticoagulation[4]
Statin therapy	• Immediate initiation of a statin is not recommended in people with acute stroke and the consensus is that it is safe to start one after 48 hours. People already taking a statin may continue with their treatment[4]
Blood pressure (BP) control	• Antihypertensive treatment is only recommended in acute stroke if there is a hypertensive emergency (BP >220/120 mmHg) or for people suitable for thrombolysis but who need a reduction in their BP to ≤185/110 mmHg.[1,4] If treatment is indicated, intravenous antihypertensive drugs with a short half-life should be used, e.g. glyceryl trinitrate or labetalol. BP should be reduced cautiously and abrupt lowering is to be avoided
Thrombo-prophylaxis	• Heparins are not routinely used in the treatment of acute stroke, due to the increased risk of ICH[3]

Treatment of haemorrhagic stroke

Cessation of antiplatelets/ anticoagulants	• Following brain imaging confirmation of PIH, all antiplatelets or anticoagulants should be discontinued. A baseline full blood count and clotting screen should be done and clotting levels in those receiving anticoagulation treatment (and who have an elevated INR) should be returned to normal as soon as possible. Reversal is usually achieved using a combination of prothrombin complex concentrate and intravenous vitamin K.[4]
	• At present, there is no antidote for the NOACs, so patients admitted with PIH taking these drugs need to be managed with supportive care.[3]
	• Patients with haemorrhagic stroke and symptomatic DVT or PE should be treated with either anticoagulants or a caval filter[4]
Statin therapy	• Is not recommended routinely as there may be an increased risk of ICH in patients being treated with statins.[9] Current practice is only to use statins where the risk of further ischaemic vascular events outweighs the risk of further haemorrhage, but even then, only once the haemorrhage has resolved[1]
SAH	• Patients diagnosed as having an SAH should be referred to a tertiary neuroscience centre. For prevention of ischaemic neurological deficits, patients may be started on oral nimodipine 60 mg every 4 hours (within 4 days of onset of SAH) and continued for 21 days unless there are specific contraindications[3,10]

Treatment of TIA

Assessment
- People experiencing a TIA should be assessed rapidly in order to minimise the chances of a full stroke occurring. It is crucial that these people are referred for further investigation within a specialist TIA clinic since the risk of subsequent stroke is greatest in the first few days.[3,5]
- The risk of subsequent stroke is made using a validated scoring system, such as ABCD[2] (see *ABCD[2] scoring system* entry)

Secondary prevention of stroke and TIA

Pharmacists have an opportunity to improve patients' adherence in taking their secondary prevention medication and should counsel patients on the importance of adherence with drug treatment and how to take their medicines. Changes in lifestyle are also important and people should be given both written and verbal information on smoking cessation, alcohol consumption, diet and exercise

Antiplatelet therapy
Antiplatelet medicines used in secondary prevention are usually started 2 weeks after the acute event and should be continued lifelong. Occasionally, they may be started earlier if the patient is discharged from hospital within this time period.

- Aspirin, modified-release (m/r) dipyridamole and clopidogrel are the three current treatment options used in secondary prevention following TIA or ischaemic stroke.
- After the 2-week course of aspirin 300 mg daily, patients who have experienced an ischaemic stroke should receive clopidogrel 75 mg daily, to be continued indefinitely. For people in whom clopidogrel is either contraindicated or not tolerated, the combination of aspirin 75 mg daily and dipyridamole m/r 200 mg twice daily should be used.[11]
- Clopidogrel is not licensed for the management of TIA but many stroke units will also use clopidogrel in TIA patients for the secondary prevention of stroke.[5,12] Others will follow NICE guidance, which recommends the combination of aspirin 75 mg daily and dipyridamole m/r 200 mg twice daily for this indication.[11] For people who have a contraindication or intolerance to aspirin, dipyridamole MR alone is recommended as a treatment option

PPIs
- There is pharmacological evidence that omeprazole and esomeprazole may reduce the efficacy of clopidogrel, so the combination should be avoided and an alternative PPI, e.g. lansoprazole, used if needed.[12]

Anticoagulation
- Patients who have had a cardioembolic stroke (e.g. patients with AF) should be anticoagulated after imaging to exclude ICH, unless contraindicated. This is usually not until 14 days after the onset of stroke symptoms, as there is a concern that anticoagulation may increase the risk of haemorrhagic transformation of the initial infarct. Treatment can be started earlier, especially in minor or non-disabling strokes, at the discretion of the stroke physician. Anticoagulation may be with an NOAC (e.g. apixaban, dabigatran, rivaroxaban) or a vitamin K antagonist (e.g. warfarin).

S

	• In patients with AF, aspirin 300 mg daily should be continued until warfarin has been started and the INR is in therapeutic range (usually 2–3); then the aspirin can be stopped. The NOACs have the advantage of fast onset of action and aspirin can be stopped on their initiation.
	• The decision of starting treatment with an oral anticoagulant should be made after an informed discussion between the clinician and the patient, and a comparison should be made regarding the risks and benefits of the different NOACs available and warfarin.[13–15]
	• Risk stratification is important to determine which patients have a stroke risk that is significant enough to justify the bleeding risk associated with oral anticoagulants. The CHA_2DS_2-VASc is a validated tool, used to score people in non-valvular AF and assess their risk of stroke[16]

See CHA_2DS_2-VASc and HAS-BLED scoring, below

Hypertension	• Hypertension is the single most important modifiable risk factor for stroke. A target BP of <130/80 mmHg should be aimed for in all patients with stroke or TIA. Poststroke hypertension is common and in most cases a patient's BP will return to baseline in the first 4–10 days after stroke. Ideally, BP-lowering treatment should be initiated after stroke or TIA prior to hospital discharge or at 2 weeks, whichever is the soonest.[3]
	• In the PROGRESS trial, BP lowering using the combination of perindopril and indapamide in patients with a history of stroke or TIA was shown to reduce the incidence of both recurrent stroke and major vascular events.[17]
	• Hypertensive patients <55 years old and not of African or Caribbean origin should be started on an ACE inhibitor, e.g. perindopril, or an angiotensin-II receptor blocker if an ACE inhibitor is not tolerated.
	• For patients >55 years old and African or Caribbean patients of any age, first-line treatment should be with a calcium-channel blocker, such as amlodipine, or a thiazide-like diuretic, such as indapamide[17]

Lipid-lowering therapy	• All patients who have had an ischaemic stroke or TIA should be prescribed a statin, irrespective of cholesterol level.[18] Evidence suggests that the vasoprotective effects of statins extend further than just cholesterol reduction. In the Heart Protection Study, the addition of simvastatin 40 mg daily, irrespective of initial cholesterol levels, was shown to reduce the risk of ischaemic stroke by 25%.[19] Note that the dose of simvastatin may need halving if coprescribed with some drugs, e.g. certain calcium-channel antagonists. In the SPARCL study, atorvastatin 80 mg daily was also shown to reduce the risk of stroke.[9]
	• The first-line treatment often used is therefore simvastatin 40 mg daily, but high-intensity statins, e.g. atorvastatin 80 mg daily, can be used if target cholesterol levels are not achieved, i.e. total cholesterol <4.0 mmol/L and low-density lipoprotein cholesterol <2.0 mmol/L.[3]
	• The SPARCL study also showed that the risk of haemorrhagic stroke was increased for those on a statin; therefore, statins are not routinely used for secondary prevention in patients with a history of PIH[3]

Rehabilitation and long-term management

In addition to knowing what secondary prevention measures are required for patients who have had a stroke, pharmacists should also be aware and be able to advise on how medications will be administered. Patients may now need help in taking their medicines, so it is important to review this prior to discharge, e.g. if there are dexterity problems a patient may need a compliance aid, such as easy-open tops or a monitored-dosage system. Patients may also now be unable to take their medicines in the same form as before their stroke due to difficulties in swallowing

Dysphagia	• The majority of patients who develop swallowing difficulties (dysphagia) following a stroke will recover; however, a proportion will have persistent abnormal swallowing problems that may become chronic.[3] Patients may require enteral feeding tubes to ensure that they receive adequate fluid and nutrition.
	• Aspiration pneumonia is a major risk in patients with dysphagia, and so to administer medicines safely to patients with dysphagia it is important to find out what the patient's swallowing status is. Speech and language therapists assess patients to check for safe swallowing. They may ask for patients to be kept nil-by-mouth (NBM) if patients have an unsafe swallow or advise for patients to be tried on thickened fluids/modified diets. If NBM, medicines would need to be given by other routes, e.g. topically, rectally or parenterally.
	• Most of the secondary prevention medicines used in stroke, however, are in tablet/capsule form and very few are available as either liquids or dispersible preparations. There is therefore little choice and many tablets will need to be crushed and dispersed in water for administration via a nasogastric tube or mixed with food/thickened fluids. Any change to a drug's licensed formulation will deem the medicine off-licence, as there is a risk of increased side effects and potential differences in bioavailability. There is also a possibility for interactions between enteral feeds and medication (e.g. with perindopril, a gap of 2 hours should be left before and after feeds), so pharmacists should liaise with the dietician to organise times for feeding and medicine administration to cause the least disruption.
	• Pharmacists should help to rationalise and tailor drug therapy to the patient's swallowing requirements by endorsing prescription charts/discharge letters with information for nurses/carers on the safest method of administering a patient's medications. Pharmacists should be familiar with the resources available to check whether a drug can be safely crushed or if a suitable alternative can be recommended
Sialorrhoea and xerostomia	• Sialorrhoea (drooling or excessive saliva secretion) can increase a patient's risk of aspiration. The drug options for treating sialorrhoea are limited and most are unlicensed for this use. Antimuscarinics, such as hyoscine and glycopyrronium, are generally prescribed and preparations are available for topical, oral and parenteral use.
	• A large proportion of stroke patients will develop xerostomia (dry mouth) and this can lead to oral infections and contribute to dysphagia. Administration of an artificial saliva spray may help to reduce any discomfort

Spasticity and spasms	• Patients with poststroke general spasticity can be managed with skeletal muscle relaxants, such as baclofen, tizanidine or gabapentin, but they all have the disadvantage of causing drowsiness so should be started at a low dose and titrated up according to response.
	• Patients with focal spasticity affecting one or more joints should be treated where appropriate with intramuscular botulinum toxin in conjunction with weeks of rehabilitation therapy from a specialist MDT service[3]
Depression and anxiety	• Mood disturbance is common after stroke and may present as depression or anxiety. All patients entering stroke rehabilitation should be screened for depression using a validated tool and observed regularly for mood changes.[3] It is important to manage and treat poststroke depression, especially during rehabilitation, as if left untreated this may impact on a patient's recovery.
	• At present there is no evidence to determine the choice of drug treatment but in practice most experience poststroke is with the use of SSRIs. Patients started on an SSRI should be prescribed a low dose initially and monitored regularly for improvement in mood and any adverse effects
Pain	• Pain symptoms poststroke may be due to different causes, e.g. neuropathic, musculoskeletal, spasticity and depression. A patient's pain should initially be assessed using a validated tool and regularly monitored thereafter.[3]
	• Neuropathic pain should be treated in accordance with the recommendations from the NICE guidance on neuropathic pain. A choice of amitriptyline, gabapentin or pregabalin should be offered as initial treatment, starting with low doses and titrating to the maximum tolerated dose that controls the patient's pain. If satisfactory pain reduction is not achieved with first-line treatment, another drug should be used instead of, or in combination with, the original drug.[20]
	• Shoulder pain is common and is the most important specific musculoskeletal pain problem after stroke. It is often associated with subluxation of the joint and, in the later stages, spasticity. Treatment with simple analgesic drugs taken regularly should be tried first-line if needed

CHA_2DS_2-VASc score (risk of stroke in valvular atrial fibrillation)

Background	• $CHADS_2$ was replaced in practice in 2011 with CHA_2DS_2-VASc (pronounced 'chads-two-vasc') as a scoring system used to determine the long-term risk of stroke in valvular AF, the name coming from an acronym for the risk factors shown in the table (see below).[21] The subscript '2' is used for criteria that score 2.
	• The scoring system was increased, with three additional risk factors, as the revised system was found to be more sensitive. Patients with a CHA_2DS_2-VASc score of 0 were found to be less likely to have a thromboembolic event than those with a $CHADS_2$ score of 0, and those with a CHA_2DS_2-VASc score of 1 were also less likely to have a thromboembolic event than those with a $CHADS_2$ score of 1

S

TABLE S3
CHA$_2$DS$_2$-VASc scoring

Clinical feature	Score
Congestive heart failure or left ventricular dysfunction	1
Hypertension	1
Age $\geq$ 75 years	2
Diabetes mellitus	1
Stroke or TIA or thromboembolism	2
Vascular disease (prior myocardial infarction, peripheral artery disease or aortic plaque)	1
Age 65–74 years	1
Sex category (i.e. female gender)	1
Maximum score	**9**

Interpretation

CHA$_2$DS$_2$-VASc score	Recommended antithrombotic therapy
0	Either aspirin 75–325 mg daily or no antithrombotic therapy.
	Preferred: no antithrombotic therapy rather than aspirin
1	Either oral anticoagulant or aspirin 75–325 mg daily.
	Preferred: oral anticoagulant rather than aspirin
$\geq$2	Oral anticoagulant

A vitamin K antagonist, e.g. warfarin, is first-line oral anticoagulant with INR range 2.0–3.0 (target 2.5). NOAC drugs may be considered if warfarin is not suitable; the risk of bleeding needs to be considered when considering the choice and dose of a NOAC (see HAS-BLED score, below).

HAS-BLED score

Atrial fibrillation increases the risk of stroke by fivefold, and anticoagulant therapy reduces the risk of stroke and all-cause mortality, although there is a bleeding risk associated with anticoagulant therapy.[21] The HAS-BLED tool can be used to assess and score an individual's bleeding risk in patients with AF who are starting, or have started, anticoagulation.[22] It can be used to support a clinical decision to commence antithrombotic therapy, in conjunction with the CHA$_2$DS$_2$-VAS$_c$ score to estimate risk of stroke in AF versus the risk of a bleed[23] (see CHA$_2$DS$_2$-VAS$_c$ above).

HAS-BLED is an acronym, with a score of 1 given to each measure in Table S4. Scores range from 0 to 9; scores of $\geq$3 indicate a high risk of bleeding, for which caution and regular review of the patient are recommended.[24]

TABLE S4
HAS-BLED scoring

	Scores
Hypertension (uncontrolled systolic blood pressure >160 mmHg)	1
Abnormal liver and/or renal function:	1
Liver: cirrhosis, bilirubin >2 $\times$ upper limit of normal (ULN) with aspartate transaminase/alanine transaminase/alkaline phosphatase >3 $\times$ ULN	
Renal: chronic dialysis, renal transplant, serum creatinine $\geq$2.3 mg/dL (200 micromol/L)	1

(Continued)

TABLE S4

HAS-BLED scoring (*Continued*)

Stroke – previous history	1
Bleeding history or predisposition	1
Labile INRs (therapeutic time in range <60%)	1
Elderly (age >65 years)	1
Drugs and/or alcohol usage:	1
Drugs: other antiplatelet agents or NSAIDs	1
Alcohol: >8 units/week	
Maximum score	9

REFERENCES

1   SIGN (2008). A National Clinical Guideline: Management of patients with stroke or TIA: assessment, investigation, immediate management and secondary prevention. 108. www.sign.ac.uk (accessed 13 May 2015).

2   Aho K *et al.* (1980). Cerebrovascular disease in the community: results of a WHO collaborative study. *Bull WH O* 58: 113–130.

3   Intercollegiate Stroke Working Party, Royal College of Physicians (2012). *National Clinical Guideline for Stroke* (4th edn). www.sign.ac.uk (accessed 13 May 2015).

4   NICE (2008). *Stroke: Diagnosis and initial management of acute stroke and transient ischaemic attack (TIA)*. Clinical guideline 68. https://www.nice.org.uk/guidance/cg68 (accessed 13 December 2014).

5   NICE (2013). *ESUOM23: Transient ischaemic attack: clopidogrel.* http://www.nice.org.uk/advice/esuom23/resources/non-guidance-transient-ischaemic-attack-clopidogrel-pdf (accessed 13 December 2014).

6   Department of Health (2007). *National Stroke Strategy.* http://clahrc-gm.nihr.ac.uk/cms/wp-content/uploads/DoH-National-Stroke-Strategy-2007.pdf (accessed 13 December 2014).

7   NICE (2012). Technology appraisals (TA264*). Alteplase for treating acute ischaemic stroke* (review of technology appraisal guidance 122). https://www.nice.org.uk/guidance/ta264 (accessed 13 December 2014).

8   SPC (2014). *Actilyse.* https://www.medicines.org.uk/emc/medicine/308 (accessed 10 October 2014).

9   The Stroke Prevention by Aggressive Reduction in Cholesterol Levels (SPARCL) (2006). Investigators high-dose atorvastatin after stroke or transient ischaemic attack. *N Engl J Med* 355: 549–559.

10 SPC (2014). *Nimotop.* https://www.medicines.org.uk/emc/medicine/8086 (accessed 10 October 2014).

11 NICE (2010). Technology appraisal (TA210). *Clopidogrel and Modified-release Dipyridamole for the Prevention of Occlusive Vascular Events.* http://www.nice.org.uk/guidance/ta210 (accessed 13 December 2014).

12 SPC (2014). *Plavix.* https://www.medicines.org.uk/emc/medicine/24207 (accessed 10 October 2014).

13 NICE (2013). Technology appraisal (TA275). *Apixaban for the Prevention of Stroke and Systemic Embolism in People with Non-Valvular Atrial Fibrillation.* http://www.nice.org.uk/guidance/ta275 (accessed 13th December 2014).

14 NICE (2012). Technology appraisal (TA249). *Dabigatran Etexilate for the Prevention of Stroke and Systemic Embolism in Atrial Fibrillation.* http://www.nice.org.uk/guidance/ta249 (accessed 13 December 2014).

15 NICE (2012). Technology appraisal (TA256). *Rivaroxaban for the Prevention of Stroke and Systemic Embolism in People with Atrial Fibrillation.* http://www.nice.org.uk/guidance/ta256 (accessed 13 December 2014).

16 NICE (2014). Clinical guideline (CG180). *Atrial Fibrillation: The management of atrial fibrillation.* http://www.nice.org.uk/guidance/cg180 (accessed 13 December 2014).

17 Progress Collaborative Group (2001). Randomised trial of a perindopril based blood pressure lowering regimen among individuals with previous stroke or TIA. *Lancet* 358: 1033–1041.

18 NICE (2011). Clinical guideline (CG127) *Hypertension: Clinical management of primary hypertension in adults.* http://www.nice.org.uk/guidance/cg127 (accessed 13 December 2014).

19 Heart Protection Study Collaborative Group (2002). MRC/BHF heart protection study of cholesterol lowering with simvastatin in high-risk individuals: a randomised placebo-controlled trial. *Lancet* 360: 7–22.

20 NICE (2013). Clinical guideline CG173 *Neuropathic Pain – Pharmacological management: the pharmacological management of neuropathic pain in adults in non-specialist settings.* https://www.nice.org.uk/guidance/cg173 (accessed 13 December 2014).

21 Camm AJ *et al.* (2010). Guidelines for the management of atrial fibrillation. The Task Force for the Management of Atrial Fibrillation of the European Society of Cardiology (ESC). *Eur Heart* 31: 2369–2429.

22 You JJ *et al.* (2012). Antithrombotic therapy for atrial fibrillation: antithrombotic therapy and prevention of thrombosis, 9th edn: American College of Chest Physicians evidence-based clinical practice guidelines. *Chest* 141: e531S–e575S.

23 NICE (2014). *Atrial Fibrillation: The management of atrial fibrillation.* Clinical Guideline 180. Available at: www.nice.org.uk/guidance/CG180 (accessed 6 May 2015).

24 Pisters R *et al.* (2010). A novel user-friendly score (HAS-BLED) to assess one-year risk of major bleeding in atrial fibrillation patients: the Euro Heart Survey. *Chest* 138: 1093–1100.

S

Suppositories

If the rectal route is selected for administration of medication, it is useful to be aware of current thought on which way round a suppository should be inserted.

Traditionally the pointed or round end is inserted first, and most patient information leaflets provided by manufacturers use this method in their explanation to patients. If one is self-administering, this may be the easiest way to insert. The rationale is that the round end enters the anal sphincters more easily than the blunt end, and the flat end is easier to push against.

In hospital most suppositories are inserted by nurses. Many nursing textbooks advocate insertion of suppositories blunt-end first, on the basis of a single study that suggested retention was better, with less need to introduce a finger into the anal canal.[1] However, the change in practice has been more recently criticised in that it was based on the results of a single small study, with no statistical analysis.[2]

It may not make a great deal of difference which way round the suppository enters the rectum, as long as it is retained there long enough to dissolve. It is probably easier to self-administer round end first, and it is equally easy for a nurse to administer either way round.

Caution must be exercised when administering suppositories post colorectal surgery, as there is a risk of perforating anastomoses. Some consultants will not consider the rectal route even after minor colorectal surgery.

REFERENCES
1 Abd-el-Maeboud KH *et al.* (1991). Rectal suppository: commonsense and mode of insertion. *Lancet* 338: 798.
2 Kyle G (2012). Practice questions: Should a suppository be inserted with the blunt end or the pointed end first, or does it not matter? *Nurs Times* 105: 16.

Surgical pharmacy

The role of the pharmacist in surgery should not be underestimated. The multidisciplinary care of patients who come into hospital for surgical procedures should always include pharmaceutical input.

The key areas for the pharmacist to be involved in are:

- management of long-term medication in the perioperative period
- postoperative nausea and vomiting
- pain control
- thromboprophylaxis
- antibiotic prophylaxis.

The pharmacist should become integrated as part of the multidisciplinary team and be prepared to accept responsibility for writing protocols, procedures and guidelines for use by the nursing and medical staff. These protocols should then be reinforced on the wards and audited in practice.

When beginning work on the surgical wards, it is important to become familiar with the different surgical procedures and understand the principles of the terminology. Examples of commonly used suffixes and meanings are:

−oscopy = to view using scope (colonoscopy)

−ectomy = the surgical removal of (nephrectomy)

−otomy = the surgical incision of (laparotomy)

−ostomy = to create a hole, also referred to as stoma, surgically.

e.g. *laparoscopic cholecystectomy* is the removal of the gallbladder (cholecyst) using a surgical scope method.

It is important to understand the surgical procedure that the patient is undergoing to identify any implications for changes in medication, e.g. stopping alpha-blocker therapy post transurethral resection of the prostate.

The importance of an accurate medicines reconciliation

The pharmacy team is responsible for patients' medication throughout the admission, which starts with ensuring an accurate drug history before surgery. The optimum place to take the drug history is the preadmission clinic and now more pharmacists have a key role in this area. This allows time before the patient goes to theatre to advise on stopping, withholding or changing long-term medication. Ideally, the documentation should be available for the anaesthetist and surgeon prior to the procedure.

The important details to find out are: name of medicine, form, strength, dose, frequency and, if known, the indication for its use. This should be established for all routinely taken medication, including over-the-counter, herbal and homeopathic medicines. Use of illegal drugs should also be documented if possible. Find out if any medicines have been recently stopped or changed; e.g. prior to surgery it is important to know if a long course of steroids has only recently stopped as replacement with intravenous hydrocortisone may still be required.

If the medication history has been recorded in the preadmission clinic, it is important to check that nothing has changed in the time between the clinic and admission.

Once all this information is established the management of the medicines throughout the perioperative period can be planned and tailored to meet the patient's ongoing needs and to prepare for a safe and effective discharge (see *'Nil-by-mouth' – management of long-term medicines during surgery* entry).

Many surgical specialties have now adopted the enhanced recovery after surgery (ERAS) approach.[1] This encompasses perioperative pathways as part of a multidisciplinary approach to improve patient outcomes of surgery.[2] Pharmacists can play an important role in this, particularly in terms of medicines optimisation, pain management and fluid management.

Thromboprophylaxis

Patients undergoing surgical procedures are at an increased risk of a VTE. There is a vast amount of literature to support the routine use of prophylaxis, which reduces the risk of DVT and PE. Equally, there are data to reassure that the use of anticoagulants at the time of surgery causes little or no increase in the rate of clinically important bleeding.[3,4] It should be noted that the combination of NSAIDs and prophylactic heparin is a common necessity in surgical patients; however, consideration should always be given to the patient's risk of bleeding and renal dysfunction.

Surgical units should have thromboprophylaxis protocols which are easy to apply in practice and which take into consideration:

- acute and chronic clinical risks
- previous thromboembolic episodes
- risk associated with type of surgery
- assessment of the risk of VTE versus bleeding.[3]

The risk of VTE should be viewed as two separate categories: patient risk and surgical risk.

Patient risks
- age over 60 years
- active cancer or cancer treatment
- dehydration
- immobility (pre-existing/postoperative)

- hypercoagulable state – this includes all the thrombophilic diseases, such as low coagulation inhibitors (antithrombin, protein C or S); activated protein C resistance (factor V Leiden); high coagulation factors (I, II, VIII, IX, XI); antiphospholipid syndrome or high homocysteine. Any patients undergoing surgery with these conditions are usually discussed with the haematologist to ensure appropriate prophylaxis
- obesity – if the body mass index is greater than $30 \, \text{kg/m}^2$, the risk of VTE is three times greater
- pregnancy – the risk of VTE postpartum within 6 weeks or through pregnancy is increased by 10 times
- oestrogen therapy – the use of the combined oral contraceptive pill (COCP), hormone replacement therapy, raloxifene or tamoxifen confers an additional VTE risk. Stopping the COCP can be considered and discussed with the patient; however, the risk of becoming pregnant and using less effective contraception must be taken into account. The perioperative use of these drugs should be in accordance with local policy, combined with appropriate thromboprophylaxis. There is no evidence that low-dose progestogens increase the risk and therefore they do not need to be stopped prior to surgery
- coexisting illness (heart failure, myocardial infarction, sepsis) – medical patients have an increased risk of DVT even without undergoing a surgical procedure, so it is important to increase the level of the thromboprophylaxis in these patients.

Surgical risk

- Surgical procedure lasting longer than 90 minutes.
- Acute surgical admission.
- Pelvic or lower-limb surgery – the risk can be increased by up to 30%.
- Major abdominal surgery, including gynaecological and colorectal.

Extended thromboprophylaxis may be indicated in patients for up to 35 days postprocedure following hip or knee replacements and abdominal surgery for cancer treatment.[5]

Thromboprophylaxis should be considered in terms of both pharmacological and mechanical methods. Only after assessing each individual patient's risks should the appropriate therapy be prescribed.

Mechanical prophylaxis

The choice should be based on individual factors. It is important to be aware of the contraindications of use. Mechanical prophylaxis is recommended as first-line, with pharmacological methods used as an adjuvant in higher-risk patients.

- antiembolic stockings/graduated compression stockings. If correctly sized and fitted, VTE risk can be reduced by up to 50%.

- intermittent pneumatic compression devices and foot pumps increase the venous outflow in the lower limbs and hence reduce venous stasis.

Pharmacological prophylaxis

The choice should be based on local policy, licensed indication and individual factors.

Heparins and fondaparinux

Low-molecular-weight heparins (LMWH) are the agents most commonly used, as they require once-a-day administration, as opposed to unfractionated heparin, which is administered three times daily. The timing of administration needs to be considered, particularly if patients are to have surgery under a spinal or epidural anaesthetic because there is a risk of spinal haematoma. To avoid this risk, the LMWH is administered in the evening. Removal of an epidural catheter should be delayed for 10–12 hours postadministration of the LMWH, and the administration of LMWH should not be within 6 hours of the insertion or removal of an epidural catheter.

The duration of treatment is variable. It is an unfortunate paradox that most patients are continued on LMWH until discharge, when in reality they may go home to a state of immobility, or they may be back to a fully mobile state well before discharge (see *Low-molecular-weight heparin* entry). Fondaparinux sodium is a synthetic pentasaccharide that inhibits activated factor X. It is licensed for prophylaxis in patients undergoing major orthopaedic surgery of the legs. It has more recently been superseded by the NOACs. However, it still has a useful role in patients where heparins are contraindicated.

NOACs

NOACs include direct thrombin inhibitors (dabigatran) and factor Xa inhibitors (rivaroxaban and apixaban). Currently all agents are only licensed for use as prevention of VTE in patients undergoing hip or knee replacements.[6] Dose and duration of course are dependent on patient factors and type of surgery. Timing and initiation of therapy must be considered due to the associated bleeding risk. NOACs can be used after LMWHs to complete the recommended course if a patient is nil-by-mouth following surgery.

Antibiotic prophylaxis

Refer to your local guidelines that should be in place to ensure appropriate prescribing of antibiotics for surgical procedures, which take into account local antibiotic resistance patterns. Antibiotic prophylaxis presurgery is important in the prevention of surgical site infections (SSIs), which are a type of healthcare-associated infection. At least 5% of patients undergoing a surgical procedure develop SSIs.[7] Other factors may predispose the patient to an increased risk of postoperative infections, most commonly, urinary tract infections and chest infections.

The risk factors for postoperative infection include:

- the patient's overall state of health (respiratory comorbidities increase the risk of chest infections and so patients should be highlighted for postoperative physiotherapy)
- age
- decreased blood supply to the operation site (e.g. in diabetic patients postamputation)
- foreign material in the wound
- concomitant medication (long-term antibiotics and corticosteroids)
- operative and environmental factors (these include the surgeon's skill and theatre cleanliness).

Antibiotics should not routinely be used to prevent such infections but precautions should be in place to reduce this risk, i.e.:

- early mobilisation
- adequate hydration
- chest physiotherapy
- medicines optimisation (e.g. review of opioid use to allow adequate mobilisation).

Operations are classified into 'clean' (elective, no trauma, no break in technique), 'clean contaminated', 'contaminated' or 'dirty – infected' (the latter may include spillage from the GI tract and traumatic emergency). Usually antibiotic prophylaxis is given to patients in the clean contaminated category and further doses that constitute treatment may be given for contaminated or dirty surgery.[8]

The choice of antibiotic is related to the bacteria that would most likely be found at the site of surgery. Generally a broad-spectrum antibiotic that covers both anaerobic and aerobic bacteria is recommended.

The timing of administration of antibiotics is important to ensure optimum blood levels at the time of incision. The route of choice is usually intravenous to ensure adequate serum antibiotic concentration is achieved. However, it is common practice to give a dose of oral ciprofloxacin 1 or 2 hours before an endoscopic retrograde cholangiopancreatography. 'Stat' doses of antibiotics should have minimal adverse effects on the patient, and should be clearly documented in the anaesthetic records. Care must be taken to review the appropriateness of the antibiotic agent used and the duration of therapy should be kept to a minimum (a single dose is usually sufficient).[6]

Pain management

When managing pain postoperatively, use the World Federation of Societies of Anaesthesiologists analgesic ladder (see *Pain management* entry). Begin with a strong opioid and step down as the patient's pain improves, adding in adjuvant therapies as necessary.

Regular analgesia initially is better than when required as acute pain is much more difficult to manage if it becomes out of control.[9]
An extensive review of postoperative pain and pain relief after major surgery indicates that about 1 in 5 patients experienced severe pain and only poor or fair pain relief after surgery.[10]

Many procedures will use an epidural or patient-controlled opioid analgesia immediately postoperatively. These two methods have good evidence to support their use, both in patient compliance and in reducing length of hospital stay and improving outcomes (see *Patient-controlled analgesia* and *Epidural analgesia in the postoperative period* entries).

The efficacy of analgesics in acute pain is documented in greater detail in the Oxford league table of analgesic efficacy, where the analgesics are graded according to their number needed to treat (NNT: i.e. number of patients who need to receive the active drug for one to achieve at least 50% relief of pain compared with placebo over a 4–6-hour treatment period). More information can be found on the Bandolier website: http://www.medicine.ox.ac.uk/bandolier.
The most effective drugs have a low NNT of just over 2. A combination of a simple analgesic with weak opioids improves the NNT and this theory should be put into practice by administering coanalgesics such as paracetamol and NSAIDs.

Oral administration of medication may not be practical perioperatively; therefore, use of intravenous paracetamol or suppositories may be appropriate. Suppositories should be used with caution when patients have had colorectal surgery as the anastomosis (surgical join between two sections of bowel) may be low in the GI tract, or the anatomy of the bowel may have changed. Check that rectal administration is an accepted local policy in these cases. The intravenous COX-2 inhibitor parecoxib is also licensed for short-term treatment of postoperative pain; however, caution needs to be taken in patients with impaired renal function and cardiovascular/cerebrovascular risk factors.

As soon as the patient is able to tolerate oral medicines, the epidural or patient-controlled analgesia can be changed to oral strong opioids or stepped down to a weak opioid, with the continued use of the NSAID and paracetamol as appropriate.

REFERENCES

1 ERAS Society (2014) http://www.erassociety.org (accessed 27 November 2014).
2 Niranjan N *et al.* (2014). *Enhanced Recovery After Surgery – Current trends in peri-operative Care. Update in anaesthesia.* www.anaesthesiology.org (accessed 7 October 2014).
3 SIGN (2014). *Prophylaxis of Venous Thromboembolism.* www.sign.ac.uk (accessed 7 October 2014).
4 Geerts WH *et al.* (2004). Prevention of venous thromboembolism. The seventh 4. ACCP conference on antithrombotic and thrombolytic therapy. *Chest* 126: 338S–400S.
5 NICE (2010). *Venous Thromboembolism: Reducing the risk.* www.nice.org.uk/guidance/cg92 (accessed 7 October 2014).

6   Electronic Medicines Companion (2014). www.medicines.org.uk/emc/ (accessed 7 October 2014).

7   NICE (2008). *Surgical Site Infection: Prevention and treatment of surgical site infection*. www.nice.org.uk/guidance/cg74 (accessed 7 October 2014).

8   Rahman MH, Anson J (2004). Perioperative antibacterial prophylaxis. *Pharm J* 272: 743–745.

9   Millen S, Sheikh C (2003). Anaesthesia and surgical pain relief. *Hosp Pharmacist* 10: 442–450.

10 Dolin S *et al.* (2002). Effectiveness of acute postoperative pain management: I. Evidence from published data. *BMJ Anaesth* 89: 409–423.

Synacthen (tetracosactide) tests

Synacthen contains tetracosactide acetate, which consists of the first 24 amino acids in natural adrenocorticotrophic hormone (ACTH), and displays the same physiological properties as ACTH.

Synacthen can provoke hypersensitivity or an anaphylactic reaction, and is contraindicated in patients with allergic disorders, e.g. asthmatics. If a reaction occurs, it is most likely within 30 minutes of the injection, so the patient should be closely monitored during this time and staff prepared to respond as appropriate to the situation.

The short Synacthen test

The short Synacthen test or 30-minute Synacthen diagnostic test is used:

- to check the ability of the adrenal cortex to respond to an acute maximal ACTH stimulus
- in the investigation of Addisonian disorders (see *Addison's disease* entry)
- to check for hypopituitarism.

Dose

Table S5 shows the dose for adults and children.

TABLE S5
Dose of tetracosactide for the short Synacthen test

Age	Dose
Adults	250 micrograms
Children	Standard test: 145 microgram/m^2 (max. 250 microgram)[1,2] Low-dose test: 300 ng/m^2

Procedure

A blood sample is taken to measure the baseline plasma cortisol concentration and then the tetracosactide injection is given by intravenous or intramuscular injection.[1] Another blood sample is taken exactly 30 minutes after the injection. In tests for hypopituitarism, a further blood sample is taken at 60 minutes postinjection.

Adrenocortical function can be regarded as normal if the postinjection plasma cortisol concentration rises by 200 nmol/L (70 micrograms/L) or more, but check local policy.

Long Synacthen tests

Long Synacthen tests may be used in the investigation of adrenocortical insufficiency:

- following inconclusive results of the 'short' 30-minute test
- to check whether adrenal failure is primary or secondary
- following unilateral adrenalectomy for Cushing's syndrome
- following long-term steroid therapy.

In practice, long Synacthen tests may offer little additional information that cannot be obtained from a short Synacthen test. Synacthen depot is not licensed for children under 3 years of age due to the presence of benzyl alcohol in the formulation.

Procedure

A blood sample is taken to measure the baseline plasma cortisol concentration and then 1 mg tetracosactide depot intramuscular injection is given.[3] Further blood samples are taken at 30 minutes, 1, 2, 3, 4 and 5 hours after the injection.

If adrenocortical function is normal, baseline plasma cortisol (normally >200 nmol/L) doubles in the first hour and then continues to rise slowly, as shown in Table S6.

TABLE S6
Anticipated cortisol serum concentrations following a long Synacthen test

Time	nmol/L
1st hour	600–1250
2nd hour	750–1500
3rd hour	800–1550
4th hour	950–1650
5th hour	1000–1800

If plasma cortisol rises more slowly than indicated above, this may be the result of Addison's disease, secondary adrenocortical insufficiency due to a disorder of hypothalamopituitary function or overdose of corticosteroids.

A 3-day test is sometimes performed with 1 mg tetracosactide depot intramuscular injection given each day. If the plasma cortisol level is >500 nmol/L at the end of the test, then adrenal insufficiency is likely to be secondary rather than primary.

REFERENCES
1 SPC (2011). *Synacthen Ampoules 250 mcg*. www.medicines.org.uk (accessed 13 May 2015).
2 *BNFC* (2014). London: British Medical Association and Royal Pharmaceutical Society of Great Britain.
3 SPC (2011). *Synacthen Depot*. www.medicines.org.uk (accessed 13 May 2015).

Syndrome of inappropriate secretion of antidiuretic hormone

Overview

Definition	Hyponatraemia is defined as an excess of water in relation to sodium in the extracellular fluid. It is the most common electrolyte imbalance in hospital inpatients, with 15–20% showing sodium serum concentrations of <135 mmol/L. Syndrome of inappropriate secretion of antidiuretic hormone (SIADH) is the most frequent cause of euvolaemic hyponatraemia
Risk factors	The risk of SIADH rises with increasing age. There are also a myriad of causes that can be categorised as related to malignant diseases, pulmonary diseases and disorders of the central nervous system. In addition, a variety of drugs can stimulate the release of arginine vasopressin or potentiate its action. These include: • SSRIs and tricyclic antidepressants • carbamazepine • NSAIDs • antipsychotics
Differential diagnosis	The differential diagnoses of SIADH include other hyponatraemic conditions, which can be divided into those that cause impairment in urinary water excretion and those in which renal handling of water is normal. All patients with hyponatraemia should have a plasma osmolality measured to confirm hypo-osmolality. Other possibilities include: • acute renal failure • chronic renal failure • addison's disease and adrenal crisis • diabetic ketoacidosis • hypothyroidism and myxoedema coma
Diagnostic tests	• Low plasma Na^+ (<135 mmol/L) • Low plasma osmolality (<275 mOsmol/L) • Submaximally dilute urine osmolality (>100 mOsmol/kg)
Treatment goals	• Return to normal plasma sodium range (135–145 mmol/L)
Treatment options	• Fluid restriction • Demeclocycline • Tolvaptan

Pharmaceutical care and counselling

Assess	The treatment of SIADH and the rapidity of correction of hyponatremia depend on the degree of hyponatraemia, on whether the patient is symptomatic and on whether it is acute (<48 hours) or chronic[1]
Essential intervention	Emergency (symptomatic, severe and acute <48 hours): The goal is to correct hyponatraemia at a rate that does not cause neurological complications. The objective is to raise serum Na^+ levels by 0.5–1 mEq/hour, and not more than 10–12 mEq in the first 24 hours. Administration of hypertonic sodium chloride 3% is used (2.7% is more widely available in the UK), but its use should be restricted to emergency circumstances, and both neurological symptoms and serum Na^+ should be monitored frequently to achieve the desired target and to prevent overcorrection[2]

	Water restriction. The degree of restriction depends on the prior water intake, the expected ongoing fluid losses, and the degree of hyponatraemia. Water restriction to about 500–1500 mL/day is usually prescribed. The main drawback of fluid restriction is poor compliance due to an intact thirst mechanism.[2]
Secondary intervention	Demeclocycline is a tetracycline derivative that causes a partial nephrogenic diabetes insipidus. Its limitations include a slow onset of action (2–5 days) and an unpredictable treatment effect. It is used off-licence; however, it is cheap and easy to administer and therefore is the first-line choice for medical therapy. The dose is initially 0.9–1.2 g, given daily in divided doses, reduced to 600–900 mg daily for maintenance[3]
Secondary intervention	Tolvaptan is a selective vasopressin V_2-receptor antagonist (there are usually excessive levels of vasopressin in the pathophysiology of most types of SIADH). Tolvaptan aims to prevent the excess water absorption that causes hyponatraemia by blocking these effects. When taken orally there is an increase in urine excretion, resulting in decreased urine osmolality and increased serum sodium concentrations.[4] The dose is 15 mg once daily, increased as required to max. 60 mg daily.[3]
	Due to the expense of 'vaptans', the need to start in the hospital and a lack of clear long-term benefit, they are only recommended when traditional measures, such as fluid restriction, have been unsuccessful.
Continued monitoring	• Plasma Na^+ • Volume status

REFERENCES
1 Ellison DH, Berl T (2007). The syndrome of inappropriate diuresis. N Engl J Med 356: 2064–2072.
2 Thomas CP (2014). Syndrome of Inappropriate Antidiuretic Hormone Secretion. Medscape. http://emedicine.medscape.com/article/246650-overview (accessed 19 November 2014).
3 Joint Formulary Committee (2014). British National Formulary (68th edn). London: BMJ Group and Pharmaceutical Press.
4 Verbalis J et al. (2011). Efficacy and safety of oral tolvaptan therapy in patients with the syndrome of inappropriate antidiuretic hormone secretion. Eur J Endocrinol 163: 725–732.

Syringe pumps

Syringe pumps are portable, battery-operated devices for delivering medicines by continuous subcutaneous infusion. The most common clinical use for syringe pumps is in the palliative care setting where the administration by this route can be helpful in the management of symptoms when the oral route cannot be used (Tables S7 and S8). Typically patients may present with one or more of the following:

- intestinal obstruction
- difficulty swallowing
- persistent nausea with or without vomiting
- mouth, throat and oesophageal lesions
- unconsciousness or fluctuating consciousness
- malabsorption

TABLE S7

Potential advantages and disadvantages of using a syringe pump in palliative care

Advantages	Disadvantages
Ability to control more than one symptom through a single infusion	Reliance on trained health professionals
Reduces need for *when required* bolus injections	Site discomfort
Stability of medication doses over 24 hours	Risk of psychological dependence
Reduces oral medication burden	Portable – but adds practical burden
Portable device	Stigma of being associated with dying

TABLE S8

Preferred sites to insert a subcutaneous needle for a syringe pump

Preferred sites		Sites to avoid
Chest wall		Active radiotherapy sites
Outer thighs		Broken, inflamed or infected skin
Upper arms		Lymphoedematous limbs/ascites
Abdomen		Near bony prominence/joints
Scapula (consider if the patient is agitated and may pull the infusion out)		

- an unsatisfactory response to oral medications, for example, intractable pain despite upwards titration of analgesia, and where the rectal, sublingual or transdermal routes of administration are inappropriate.

In 2010, the National Patient Safety Agency issued guidance on the technical standards that syringe pumps had to comply with in order to improve their safety in clinical practice.[1] The commonly used Graseby syringe drivers (MS16a and MS26) were not compliant with these standards and have now been replaced by other models. One of the most popular is the CME Medical T34 (formerly known as the McKinley T34).

Ask your palliative care team for a copy of their syringe pump clinical guidelines for more information.

Clinically screening the prescription

Medicines used together in a syringe pump should be checked for compatibility. Combinations may be compatible only at certain concentrations; therefore, the concentration of each medication in the syringe should be compared with compatibility data, not the dose. Standard reference sources include *The Syringe Driver*[2] and the *Palliative Care Formulary*[3] and online at: http://www.pallcare.info/.

The BNF carries some limited information about compatibilities in the section 'Prescribing in palliative care'.[4] Consider the following when there is a lack of compatibility data:

- Medicines with a similar pH are more likely to be compatible.
- Medicines commonly used in a syringe pump are acidic in solution; therefore more alkaline medications such as dexamethasone, diclofenac, furosemide, ketorolac and phenobarbital can cause compatibility problems if added. A second syringe pump should be considered to administer such medicines.
- Exposure of the syringe mixture to extremes of temperature and light can affect stability and should be avoided where possible.
- In general, medications tend to be more stable in lower concentrations in solution. Therefore, use a larger syringe with more diluent where possible.
- Medications with long durations of action can be given equally well as a bolus subcutaneous or intravenous injection once or twice daily, for example dexamethasone and levomepromazine. This avoids the need to add to a continuous subcutaneous infusion that may affect stability.
- Skin irritation around the needle site, poor symptom control or an unexpected loss of symptom control may result from medications becoming unstable when mixed together. Frequent checks of the syringe pump contents for precipitation or discoloration, as well as the patient's condition, are essential.

Medicines are commonly prescribed for pain, nausea and/or vomiting, agitation and distress, and respiratory tract secretions. If a range of doses is prescribed, the lowest possible dose of medication should be used to control the symptom. Bolus subcutaneous doses of medicines should be prescribed for 'when required' use to treat breakthrough of any of the patient's symptoms. It is also good practice to anticipate symptoms and prescribe medications in case of future need. Patients with evidence of abnormal renal or liver function, as well as frail, elderly patients may require dose adjustments. The prescription should be reviewed daily in light of any 'when required' bolus doses given and the dose of the medicines in the syringe pump adjusted accordingly. Patients must be referred to the palliative care team where symptoms remain uncontrolled.

Medicines doses and their frequencies may vary between organisations; ask your palliative care team for a copy of their syringe pump clinical guidelines for more information, and make contact with your local palliative care pharmacist for support.

Preparing and monitoring the syringe pump

The preparation of a syringe pump is a complex process that is undertaken by healthcare professionals who are trained to do so, for example nurses and doctors.

Pharmacy staff can offer help in some basic aspects of monitoring of the syringe pump while it is in use, including:

- the needle is firmly in place and there are no signs of skin inflammation

- the solutions in the syringe and line are clear
- the battery light is flashing green
- the pump is silent; there is no alarm sounding.

The palliative care team must be contacted urgently if there is a concern that the pump may be malfunctioning.

Offering general advice to the patient and relative/carer

Pharmacy staff can offer the following advice:

- Avoid spilling liquids on the syringe pump, or dropping it, and report if the battery light stops flashing green or the alarm sounds.
- Support the syringe pump when mobile, for example carry it in a pocket or holster.
- Do not lose the syringe pump; most palliative care teams have arrangements for returning pumps that are no longer required.
- Check the patient and relative/carer have been offered an information leaflet by their palliative care team.

Medicines reconciliation of syringe pumps

There is a substantial body of evidence that shows when patients move between care providers that risk of miscommunication and unintended changes to medicines remain a significant problem.[5] This is particularly challenging for patients receiving medicines via a syringe pump. Routine sources of information used to reconcile medicines, e.g. discharge letters and discharge medication labels, may not be helpful as they will often state doses as a range, and they may not distinguish medicines currently being administered from those prescribed in case of future anticipatory needs. This can lead to medication errors, a failure in symptom control and the possibility of readmission.

Pharmacists should check with their palliative care team what arrangements are in place to facilitate medicines reconciliation and identify how they may be able to help; for example, encouraging the patient and relative/carer to carry important information about their medications if they have to move.

REFERENCES

1 National Patient Safety Agency (2010). *Rapid Response Report*. NPSA/2010/RRR019 2010 www.nrls.npsa.nhs.uk (accessed 13 May 2015).

2 Dickman A, Schneider J (eds) (2011). *The Syringe Driver: Continuous subcutaneous infusions in palliative care* (3rd edn). Oxford: Oxford University Press.

3 Twycross R *et al.* (eds) (2011). *Palliative Care Formulary* (4th edn). Palliative-drugs.com. Oxon: Radcliffe Press.

4 Joint Formulary Committee (2014). *British National Formulary* (68th edn). London: BMJ Group and Pharmaceutical Press.

5 Royal Pharmaceutical Society (2012). *Keeping Patients Safe When they Transfer Between Care Providers – Getting the medicines right*. http://www.rpharms.com/previous-projects/getting-the-medicines-right.asp (accessed 11 December 2014).

T

Theophylline

Theophylline is a xanthine derivative, which exerts its therapeutic effect by relaxing bronchial smooth muscle and is used to manage reversible airways obstruction. Theophylline also stimulates the central nervous system and cardiac muscle, and acts on the kidneys to produce diuresis.[1]

Pharmacokinetic overview

Different brands of modified-release theophylline have differing release characteristics and bioavailabilities, therefore patients should not swap brands without supervision.[2]

The difference in bioavailability of modified-release formulations can be up to 20%. Twice-daily dose regimens of theophylline achieve peak plasma levels between 4 and 8 hours. Theophylline is 40–60% bound to plasma proteins.[1,3]

Theophylline is metabolised in the liver and many diseases, drugs and even dietary preferences can affect the rate of elimination. These factors are important because theophylline has a narrow therapeutic range.[1,3]

Rationale for monitoring

Pharmacokinetic variations between individuals, such as age, disease, smoking status, diet and drug interactions, all affect serum concentration levels of theophylline. Doses should be adjusted for patients individually and serum concentration monitored to avoid toxicity and ensure effectiveness (see Table T1).[1]

Theophylline may have a bronchodilator effect at 'subtherapeutic' serum concentrations; ensure the patient is being treated rather than serum levels meeting the therapeutic range.[2]

Serious toxicity is related to high serum theophylline concentrations; the patient may not present with any minor symptoms first.[1]

Dose

The adult dose of oral theophylline is initiated with a modified-release preparation. Doses range from 175 mg to 500 mg twice daily, adjusted according to clinical response and serum concentration levels.[2]

Table T2 provides guidance for any action from a given plasma concentration, but local policy should always be followed.

TABLE T1

Drug monitoring information

Half-life[1]	Adult (healthy): 7–9 hours (elderly: 10 hours, smokers: 4–5 hours)
	Children: 3–5 hours
Pretreatment measures[2]	Liver function tests (LFTs), smoking status, weight (and height for obese patients to calculate ideal body weight)
	Also consider age and assess for cor pulmonale and heart failure
Therapeutic range	10–20 mg/L (55–110 micromol/L)[2]
Sampling time of plasma theophylline concentrations[2]	Initiation of oral treatment: after 5 days
	Dose adjustments to oral treatment: after at least 3 days
	(Oral theophylline levels should be taken 4–6 hours postdose).
	Intravenous (aminophylline):
	1 Prior to infusion (if the patient has been taking theophylline or aminophylline orally); if possible, wait for results.
	2 After infusion initiation: 4–6 hours, then every 24 hours

TABLE T2

Action to be taken based on plasma theophylline concentration[3]

Plasma level (mg/L)	Result	Action
<5	Too low	Increase dose by 25%
5–20	Correct	Maintain dose providing patient is clinically responding
20–25	Too high	Decrease dose by 10%
25–30	Too high	Miss next dose and decrease subsequent doses by 25%
>30	Too high	Miss next two doses and decrease subsequent doses by 50%

Administration of intravenous aminophylline

Aminophylline (a mixture of theophylline and ethylenediamine) is given intravenously to relieve bronchospasm in asthma and chronic obstructive pulmonary disease.[3]

A loading dose of 250–500 mg (5 mg/kg) aminophylline may be given if the patient has not been treated previously with oral theophylline. This is given by slow intravenous injection over a minimum of 20 minutes. This can be followed by a maintenance infusion.[2]

No loading dose is required for patients who have been receiving oral theophylline; after checking levels, commence a maintenance infusion.

The maintenance aminophylline infusion should be given at a rate of 500–700 micrograms/kg/hour (300 micrograms/kg/hour in the elderly, in cor pulmonale, heart failure or liver disease). The rate can be adjusted according to plasma theophylline concentration.[2]

To prevent overdosing in obese patients the ideal body weight based on the patient height should be used to calculate the dose.[2]

It is useful to recommend the use of a standard-strength solution, e.g. 500 mg aminophylline in 500 mL of glucose 5% or sodium chloride 0.9%.[2] The rate of infusion can be adjusted according to response and concentration levels.

Toxicity

Side effects are common, e.g. nausea, vomiting, diarrhoea and palpitations, and can occur even when the serum concentration is within the normal range.[1]

At higher serum concentrations, more serious side effects are observed, such as tremor, cardiac arrhythmias and seizures. Hypokalaemia may also occur and can be exacerbated by other hypokalaemic drugs.[1,2]

Treatment

Seek specialist advice from the National Poisons Information Service (http://www.toxbase.org). The stomach should be emptied. It may be necessary to give repeated doses of activated charcoal. Monitor the ECG and maintain fluid balance. Check serum theophylline concentration every 4 hours after ingestion and at 4–12-hourly intervals thereafter if symptoms are severe.[1,3]

Interactions

Examples of drugs that increase serum concentration of theophylline include:

- allopurinol, cimetidine, ciprofloxacin, diltiazem, erythromycin, fluconazole, interferon-alfa, oral contraceptives, nifedipine, norfloxacin, verapamil.[2]

Examples of drugs that decrease serum concentration of theophylline include:

- barbiturates, carbamazepine, phenytoin, rifampicin, ritonavir, sulfinpyrazone, St John's wort, tobacco smoking.[2,4]

When ciprofloxacin or erythromycin is added to the prescription of a patient receiving theophylline it is a recommended precaution to reduce the dose of theophylline by 25–50% for the duration of the antibiotic course.[4]

A pragmatic approach with a modified-release preparation is to omit either the morning or the nighttime dose if each individual dose cannot be halved. Remember to reinstate the original theophylline dose when the interacting drug is withdrawn.

Avoid concomitant use of theophylline and fluvoxamine. If this is not possible, the dose of theophylline should be halved.[2]

Smoking tobacco and cannabis can cause a reduction in theophylline levels. Patients who stop smoking should have plasma theophylline levels monitored carefully.[4]

REFERENCES

1 Brayfield A (ed.) (2014). *Martindale: The complete drug reference*. www.medicines complete.com (accessed 25 November 2014).

2 Joint Formulary Committee (2014). *British National Formulary* (68th edn). London: BMJ Group and Pharmaceutical Press.

3 eMC (2014). www.medicines.org.uk/emc (accessed 25 November 2014).

4 Baxter K, Preston CL (eds) (2014). *Stockley's Drug Interactions*. www.medicines complete.com (accessed 25 November 2014).

Thunderclap headache

Thunderclap headaches are very severe and have a sudden onset; typically they peak within 60 seconds. The pain may fade after 60 minutes but some headaches can last for several days.

Thunderclap headaches may be primary or secondary. There are many causes[1] and treatment will depend on the cause of the headache. Patients presenting with a thunderclap headache should be referred urgently to an emergency department for consideration of a secondary cause, as it may be caused by a subarachnoid haemorrhage.[2]

Some of the common causes of a thunderclap headache are:[3]

- subarachnoid headache
- reversible cerebral vasoconstriction syndrome: there is no evidence-based treatment, patients should rest, and all vasoactive substances should be stopped and avoided. Nimodipine has been used in an unlicensed capacity to treat this, although evidence is scarce. A suggested dose is 30–60 mg orally every 4 hours or 0.5–2 mg/hour intravenously if the oral regimen fails or images showed cerebral vasospasm.[4]

Less common causes include: intracerebral haemorrhage, cerebral venous sinus thrombosis, arterial dissection, pituitary apoplexy, infection.

REFERENCES

1 Devenney E *et al.* (2014). A systematic review of causes of sudden and severe headache (thunderclap headache): should lists be evidence based? *J Headache Pain* 15: 49.

2 SIGN Guideline 107 (2008) *Diagnosis and Management of Headache in Adults*. http://www.sign.ac.uk/guidelines/fulltext/107/ (accessed 18 November 2014).

3 Ducros A *et al.* (2013). Clinical review: thunderclap headache. *BMJ* 346: e8557.

4 Lu SR *et al.* (2004). Nimodipine for treatment of primary thunderclap headache. *Neurology* 62: 1414–1416.

Thyroid function

The thyroid gland produces hormones that are essential for the function and maintenance of all body systems. Since disorders of thyroid function are common (especially in women) it is important for pharmacists to be aware of the monitoring requirements.

Thyroid function tests

Table T3 shows the ranges of the markers used to measure thyroid function, although there may be some local variations depending on the assay used by the laboratory.

TABLE T3
Normal ranges of thyroid hormones[1]

Hormone	Range
Thyroid-stimulating hormone (TSH)	0.3–4.2 munits/L
Free triiodothyronine (T_3) (FT_3)	3–9 picomol/L
Free levothyroxine (T_4) (FT_4)	10–26 picomol/L
Total serum T_3 (TT_3)	1.3–3.1 nanomol/L
Total serum T_4 (TT_4)	66–174 nanomol/L

Hypothyroidism

There are three types of hypothyroidism:

1 primary hypothyroidism: failure of the thyroid gland to produce thyroid hormone, due to disease (usually autoimmune)
2 secondary hypothyroidism: failure of the anterior pituitary gland to produce TSH
3 tertiary hypothyroidism: failure of the hypothalamus to produce thyroid-releasing hormone (TRH).

Monitoring therapy

Table T4 indicates the monitoring requirements for patients treated for hyperthyroidism. In hypothyroidism expect to see the following biochemical results:[2,3]

- TSH: raised
- FT_4: lowered.

TABLE T4
Monitoring in hypothyroidism[3]

Half-life	7 days[4]
Pretreatment measures	Prior to commencing therapy with levothyroxine, an ECG is useful because changes induced by hypothyroidism may be confused with evidence of ischaemia
Sampling time	Monitoring should be 6–8 weeks after a dose change, and once stable, should be checked annually. The blood sample may be collected at any time of the day
Other monitoring	Monitor for side effects, and correction of signs and symptoms of hypothyroidism. Toxicity symptoms include diarrhoea, tachycardia, insomnia and tremors

Treatment of hypothyroidism

Oral levothyroxine (T_4) is the treatment of choice for primary and secondary hypothyroidism. The normal starting dose is

50–100 micrograms (or 25 micrograms in the elderly and patients with ischaemic heart disease). The dose can be increased by 25–50 microgram increments every 6–8 weeks according to response.

The tablets should be taken 30 minutes before breakfast as a single daily dose because the presence of food can affect the absorption of levothyroxine. Similarly, if patients are also taking calcium supplements they should allow a 4-hour gap between the T_4 dose and the calcium preparation.

Liothyronine sodium injection is used to treat severe hypothyroidism and hypothyroidism myxoedema coma. It has also been used to maintain organ viability (unlicensed) in brain-dead organ donors (a dose of 0.6 micrograms/kg has been given approximately 2 hours before harvesting from heart donors).[5,6]

Oral liothyronine is rarely used, but can be useful when a rapid response is needed. It has a similar action to levothyroxine, but is more rapidly metabolised. It can precipitate arrhythmias and so must be used with caution in the elderly.

20 micrograms liothyronine $\equiv$ 100 micrograms levothyroxine[7]

Hyperthyroidism

In hyperthyroidism expect to see the following biochemical results:[3]

- TSH: significantly lowered
- TT_4: raised
- TT_3: raised
- FT_4: raised
- FT_3: raised.

The most common cause of hyperthyroidism is Graves' disease (caused by antibodies developing to TSH receptors). Other causes include:

- toxic nodular goitre
- thyroiditis
- iodine-induced hyperthyroidism
- amiodarone-induced hyperthyroidism
- TSH-secreting pituitary adenoma (rare).

Treatment of hyperthyroidism

Treatment involves giving an antithyroid agent that blocks the production of thyroid hormones. The treatment of choice is carbimazole, which is given as a single daily oral dose at a dose titrated to reduce FT_4 levels.

Some endocrinologists use a block-replacement regimen. In this case a carbimazole dose of 40–60 mg daily is given to block production of endogenous T_4, and supplemental levothyroxine is given to prevent hypothyroidism. This strategy cannot be used in pregnancy because T_4 does not cross the placenta, whereas carbimazole does, therefore fetal hypothyroidism can develop.[8]

Monitoring

Table T5 indicates the monitoring requirements for patients treated for hyperthyroidism.

If oral carbimazole is not tolerated (usually if the patient develops a rash or pruritus), propylthiouracil is given orally in divided doses. The usual starting dose is 150–400 mg daily and the maintenance dose is 50–100 mg daily.

Carbimazole and propylthiouracil may be used in pregnancy, although they both cross the placenta and should be used in the lowest possible dose after assessing the mother's needs against the risk to the foetus.[9]

Carbimazole and propylthiouracil may cause agranulocytosis and patients should be warned to report any signs of infection, especially a sore throat. The estimated incidence of agranulocytosis is 0.3 cases per 1000 patient-years of treatment in European populations.[10]

TABLE T5

Monitoring in hyperthyroidism[3]

Pretreatment	Consider a baseline white blood cell count for patients at risk of agranulocytosis, e.g. the elderly, patients taking other drugs that may cause agranulocytosis
During treatment	• Thyroid function test: periodically. • Creatine kinase (CK) if myalgia occurs. • LFTs: if hepatic side effects occur. • White blood cells: if signs of neutropenia or agranulocytosis occur, e.g. sore throat, mouth ulcers, bruising, fever or exercise tiredness

Radioactive iodine (^{131}I)

If this treatment is being used then carbimazole and propylthiouracil should be stopped at least 4 days before the dose of ^{131}I (as sodium iodide solution) is given and restarted at least 3 days after treatment.[5]

Thyrotoxicosis

Long-acting beta-blockers, such as atenolol, propranolol or nadolol may be used to relieve many of the symptoms of thyrotoxicosis, especially palpitations, tremor and anxiety.

Beta-blocker treatment is short-term, usually for 2–6 weeks, until the antithyroid agent is effective and the symptoms have resolved.[5]

REFERENCES

1 British Thyroid Association (2008). *Diagnosis and Management of Primary Hypothyroidism*. http://www.british-thyroid-association.org/news/Docs/ hypothyroidism_statement.pdf (accessed 25 April 2015).

2 NHS Lanarkshire Acute Division (2005). *Thyroid Function Tests*. http:// www.show.scot.nhs.uk/monklands/index.htm?/monklands/ClinicalServices/ labServices/Biochem/notes/TFTS.html (accessed 18 August 2005).

3 Dyfed Powys Primary Care Effectiveness Team (2004). *Drug Monitoring Booklet*. Dyfed Powys: National Public Health Service for Wales.

4 Dollery C (ed.) (1999). *Therapeutic Drugs* (2nd edn). Edinburgh: Churchill Livingstone.

5 MacFarlane I (2000). Endocrinology – thyroid disease. *Pharm J* 265: 240–244.

6 Jeevanandam V *et al.* (1994). Reversal of donor myocardial dysfunction by triiodothyronine replacement therapy. *J Heart Lung Transplant* 13: 681–687.

7   Joint Formulary Committee (2014). *British National Formulary* (68th edn).
    London: BMJ Group and Pharmaceutical Press.
8   SPC (2014.) *NeoMercazole Tablets*. http:// emc.medicines.org.uk/ (accessed
    13 August 2014).
9   SPC (2014). *Propylthiouracil Tablets, Cell-tech*. http://emc.medicines.org.uk/
    (accessed 13 August 2014).
10 CSM/MHRA (1999). Reminder: agranulocytosis with anti-thyroid drugs. *Curr
    Probl Pharmacovig* 25: 3.

Tinzaparin dosing in pulmonary embolism and deep-vein thrombosis

Dose

Tinzaparin is a low-molecular-weight heparin (LMWH) licensed for
the treatment of DVT and PE. It is administered by subcutaneous
injection at a dose of 175 units/kg body weight once a day. Peak
activity is seen around 4 hours postdose and its effects last for 24
hours. If a patient presents acutely unwell, requiring urgent
anticoagulation, and an accurate weight and renal function cannot be
obtained, the first dose of tinzaparin can be prescribed and
administered without knowing an exact weight or renal function. For
subsequent doses it is important to know an accurate weight and
renal function using creatinine clearance (CrCl) to ensure the correct
dose is used.

Patients with a CrCl as low as 20 mL/min can use the standard
dose of tinzaparin and, although antifactor Xa monitoring is
recommended for patients with CrCl between 20 and 30 mL/min, it
frequently does not happen in practice. There are no data on the use
of tinzaparin at CrCl below 20 mL/min and its use below this level is
therefore unlicensed.

Preparations

Preparations containing tinzaparin 20 000 units/mL are used to
deliver treatment doses (the lower-strength 10 000 units/mL
preparations are used for prophylactic doses). Graduated syringes are
available as 10 000 units in 0.5 mL, 14 000 units in 0.7 mL and 18 000
units in 0.9 mL. There is also a 2 mL multidose vial of 20 000
units/mL, but this does contain benzyl alcohol so should not be used
for premature babies or neonates and use should be avoided in
children under 3 years and pregnant and breastfeeding women.[1]

Administration

Doses should be rounded to the nearest 1000 units for ease of
measurement, especially if patients are self-administering. There is an
air bubble in the syringe and this should be left in if administering the
whole syringe, but will need to be expelled if only a portion of the
syringe is required – this can be the cause of much discussion amongst
nurses but the bubble is insignificant and should not cause concern.

Larger patients may need to administer the contents of more than
one syringe to get the required dose. When checking prescriptions for

these patients it is important to check what syringes they have been using and what volume from each they have been administering to avoid dosing errors.

Duration of treatment

Some patients will remain on tinzaparin for the duration of their treatment course, usually 3–6 months for a first DVT or provoked PE, as detailed in NICE CG144.[2] These would include active intravenous drug users, where warfarin is not considered safe; pregnant patients, where warfarin may cause damage to the fetus; and patients with cancer, where LMWH has been shown to be superior to warfarin.

Warfarin initiation

Warfarin can be initiated at the same time as tinzaparin using an appropriate loading regimen (see *Warfarin treatment and monitoring* entry). Tinzaparin should be continued for at least 6 days and until the INR is >2 on two subsequent occasions. This is due to the hypercoagulable state that warfarin, in high doses, induces in its first few days. Stopping the tinzaparin too early can lead to an extension of the existing thrombus.

REFERENCES

1 SPC (2014). *Innohep 20,000 IU/mL and Innohep Syringe 20,000 IU/mL*. http://www.medicines.org.uk/emc/medicine/5176 (accessed 18 September 2015).
2 NICE (2012). *Venous Thromboembolic Diseases: The management of venous thromboembolic diseases and the role of thrombophilia testing*. http://www.nice.org.uk/guidance/cg144 (accessed 19 November 2014).

Tobramycin: monitoring and management

Tobramycin is an aminoglycoside antibiotic produced by *Streptomyces tenebrarius*. It is used clinically as the sulfate salt.[1] It has a similar spectrum of activity to gentamicin and is particularly active against Gram-negative organisms, and inhibits bacterial growth through inhibition of protein synthesis. Like other aminoglycosides, it is not active against anaerobic bacteria; it has no activity against mycobacteria, including *Mycobacterium tuberculosis*. It has the advantage of having a greater intrinsic activity against *Pseudomonas aeruginosa* and can therefore be used to treat some gentamicin-resistant *Pseudomonas* strains.[1]

Pharmacokinetic overview

Tobramycin has a very poor oral bioavailability and is therefore given intravenously or by intramuscular injection. It is distributed throughout bodily fluids and tissues in a similar manner to gentamicin and is excreted via the kidneys, with high concentrations in the urine.

Tobramycin crosses the placenta. It is not known to be harmful in pregnancy, but it is recommended only where the benefits clearly outweigh the risks. It is excreted into breast milk and is therefore not recommended in breastfeeding mothers.[2]

Dose

Initial dosing is based on a patient's weight and renal function. CrCl, calculated using the Cockcroft and Gault equation, should be used to estimate renal function. As with other aminoglycosides, actual body weight is used in calculations, except for those patients who are obese (see *Gentamicin* entry). Like gentamicin, dosing is either as a multiple-daily-dosing regimen or a once-daily (unlicensed) dosing regimen. It is important to follow your local policy.

Multiple daily dosing

For adult patients with normal renal function, the dose is 3–5 mg/kg in three divided doses; it is recommended that the higher dose is used in life-threatening infections.[3] Table T6 shows the initial doses in renal impairment.

TABLE T6
Recommended doses in renal impairment

CrCl (mL/min)	Recommended dose[4]
20–50	1–2 mg/kg, then according to serum levels
10–20	1 mg/kg, then dose according to serum levels
<10	1 mg/kg, then dose according to serum levels

Subsequent doses can be adjusted by either reducing the dose administered every 8 hours (Table T7) or by increasing the dosage interval (Table T8).

TABLE T7
Tobramycin dose adjustment in renal impairment[2]

CrCl (mL/min)	Adjusted dose at 8-hourly intervals	
	50–60 kg	60–80 kg
>70	60 mg	80 mg
40–69	30–60 mg	50–80 mg
20–39	20–25 mg	30–45 mg
10–19	10–18 mg	15–24 mg
5–9	5–9 mg	7–12 mg
<4	2.5–4.5 mg	3.5–6 mg

Predose (trough) and peak serum concentrations should be checked around the third or fourth dose and dose adjustments made accordingly.

Once-daily dosing

Many hospitals use once-daily dosing regimens. In patients with cystic fibrosis, 10 mg/kg once a day up to a maximum dose of 660 mg is recommended.[5] Levels should be checked before the second dose, and then doses adjusted accordingly (Table T9).

TABLE T8
Dose frequency adjustment of tobramycin in renal impairment

CrCl (mL/min)	Normal dose at prolonged interval
	50–60 kg: dose is 60 mg
	60–80 kg: dose is 80 mg
>70	Every 8 hours
40–69	Every 12 hours
20–39	Every 18 hours
10–19	Every 24 hours
5–9	Every 36 hours
<4	Every 48 hours (when dialysis is not performed)

Therapeutic drug monitoring

TABLE T9
Drug monitoring information

Therapeutic range	Multiple daily dosing: peak: <10 mg/L[3]
	Pre-dose (trough): <2 mg/L[3]
	Once-daily dosing: pre-dose <1 mg/L
Sampling time	Peak: 60 minutes post-dose (required for multiple daily dosing only)
	Trough: pre-dose
Other monitoring	U&Es at least 2–3 times a week, urine output, consideration of auditory monitoring in those receiving repeated courses

Administration

Tobramycin may be given by intravenous infusion, intravenous bolus over 3–5 minutes or by intramuscular injection. If given as an infusion (recommended for once-daily dosing), tobramycin should be diluted in 50–100 mL sodium chloride 0.9% or glucose 5% and given over 20–60 minutes.[2,6]

Overdose

Specialist advice should be sought.[7] Most common features are nephrotoxicity, ototoxicity and neuromuscular blockade as well as electrolyte imbalance (e.g. hypocalcaemia, hypokalaemia). Nephrotoxicity may be reversible. Ototoxicity may be irreversible and may present as hearing loss or deafness or as vestibular toxicity (dizziness, vertigo). U&Es, aminoglycoside concentrations and assessment of auditory and vestibular function should be undertaken. Haemodialysis should be considered in those with acute renal failure. As onset of nephrotoxicity and ototoxicity may be delayed, patients should be reviewed at 48 hours and 1 week.[7]

Drug interactions[2,3]

The risk of ototoxicity is increased by use with loop diuretics and vancomycin. Tobramycin is known to potentiate the actions of warfarin and enhance the effects of non-depolarising muscle relaxants. Use of tobramycin with general anaesthetics (e.g. succinylcholine, tubocurarine) may potentiate neuromuscular blockade and cause respiratory paralysis. Tobramycin antagonises the effects of pyridostigmine and neostigmine.

REFERENCES

1 Grayson M et al. (eds) (2010). Kucers' The Use of Antibiotics (6th edn). London: Hodder Arnold.

2 eMC (2014). SPC Tobramycin 40 mg/mL Injection. http://www.medicines.org.uk/emc (accessed 24 August 2014).

3 Joint Formulary Committee (2014). British National Formulary (68th edn). London: BMJ Group and Pharmaceutical Press.

4 Ashley C, Dunleavy A (2014). Renal Drug Database. https://www.renaldrugdatabase.com (accessed 23 August 2014).

5 Cystic Fibrosis Trust (2009). Antibiotic Treatment for Cystic Fibrosis (3rd edn). https://www.cysticfibrosis.org.uk/media/82010/CD_Antibiotic_treatment_for_CF_May_09.pdf (accessed 7 January 2015).

6 Gray A, Wright J, Goodey V, Bruce L. (eds) (2011). Injectable Drugs Guide. London: Pharmaceutical Press.

7 National Poisons Information Service (2014). Toxbase. http://www.toxbase.org (accessed 17 August 2014).

Travel recommendations

An increase in easier, cheaper and more readily available international travel has led to ever more patients seeking advice on travel health. The following list identifies validated sources of travel health information; the list is not comprehensive, and links may be subject to change.

For patients

- Comprehensive disease-specific prevention (including vaccination) and general travel health advice from NHS Scotland: http://www.fitfortravel.nhs.uk/home.aspx.
- Country-specific clinical information and health risks: http://www.nathnac.org/ds/map_world.aspx.
- General travel information from NHS Choices: http://www.nhs.uk/livewell/travelhealth.
- Healthy holidays section of NHS Choices (with a focus on UK holidays): http://www.nhs.uk/LiveWell/Healthyholidays/Pages/Healthyholidayshome.aspx7.
- General advice on travelling in pregnancy: http://www.nhs.uk/Conditions/pregnancy-and-baby/Pages/travel-pregnant.aspx.

For healthcare professionals

- Comprehensive resource, including general and disease-specific information, regular clinical updates, country-specific advice and outbreak surveillance: http://nathnac.org/pro/ (non-24-hour telephone advice also available on 020 3447 5943).
- Travel vaccination and malaria prophylaxis: http://www.mims.co.uk/TravelTables (free registration required).
- Full travel health information: http://www.travax.nhs.uk/ (requires registration, for which a fee may be payable).
- Country and patient subgroup-specific information (e.g. disaster relief workers) on travel diseases and prevention, including patient counselling points and a 'healthy travel packing list': http://wwwnc.cdc.gov/travel/.

Other useful resources

- Public Health England: Immunisation against Infectious Disease (The Green Book): https://www.gov.uk/government/collections/immunisation-against-infectious-disease-the-green-book.
- Information on the European Health Insurance Card (EHIC) and link to the online application: http://www.nhs.uk/nhsengland/Healthcareabroad/pages/Healthcareabroad.aspx.
- Home Office advice on travelling abroad with controlled drugs: https://www.gov.uk/travelling-controlled-drugs.

Tuberculosis

Tuberculosis (TB) is an infectious disease, usually caused by the bacillus *Mycobacterium tuberculosis*, which most commonly affects the lungs but may affect almost any part of the body. The disease is spread in the air by people with active pulmonary TB infection. In general, a relatively small proportion of people infected with *M. tuberculosis* will develop TB disease; however, the probability of developing TB is much higher among people infected with HIV. Untreated disease has a high mortality rate and remains a major global health problem.[1] In the UK, the incidence of notified cases is 12.3/100 000 and is concentrated in deprived areas and people born abroad.[2] People suffering from any form of active TB must be notified to the 'proper officer' under Public Health Law (usually the Consultant in Communicable Disease in England and Wales, or the equivalent in Scotland and Northern Ireland) within 3 working days.[3]

The management of TB should be undertaken by expert clinicians and specialist nurses. Pharmacists need to be aware of the issues surrounding the treatment of TB and must be able to give advice on the monitoring requirements of the medication used to treat this disease. Patient adherence to the medicine regimen is vital for successful treatment outcomes and pharmacists can play an important role.

Diagnosing active tuberculosis

Diagnosing pulmonary TB is usually made on a clinical and microbiological basis. Typical signs and symptoms include:[4]

- cough – with or without mucus
- haemoptysis
- breathlessness – gradual increase
- weight loss – gradual
- anorexia
- fever – often with night sweats
- malaise
- cachexia.

Chest X-ray

Often this is the first indication of the presence of TB because the symptoms may be non-specific. Chest X-ray appearance suggestive of TB should lead to further diagnostic investigation.[5]

Microbiological investigations[6]

Culturing *M. tuberculosis* is the gold standard for diagnosing TB and multiple sputum samples should be sent to the microbiology laboratory.

1 Initially a smear test is performed, which will provide results within 24 hours, and identify patients who are 'smear-positive' (mycobacteria present in sputum), and who are thought to be the most infectious.
2 Sputum is incubated to culture and identify the specific mycobacteria present – it may take several weeks for a positive result.
3 Susceptibility testing on positive cultures is performed to identify strains resistance to antitubercular drugs – this may require multiple weeks for a result.
4 Nucleic acid amplification (molecular) tests may be used to provide considerably more rapid detection and susceptibility testing from specimen or culture but are comparatively expensive and not offered routinely for all patients – a decision is made on clinical and epidemiological grounds.

Treatment of active tuberculosis

The aim of treatment is to eradicate the infection in the individual and to control the spread of the disease. The recommended drug regimens in the UK are listed in the BNF section 5.1.9.[7] The standard unsupervised 6-month regimen for adults is summarised in

Tables T10 and T11. Combination preparations are commonly used to improve adherence, unless one of the components cannot be given because of resistance or tolerance. Drugs may also be given as individual components if liquid formulations are required.

TABLE T10

Standard adult unsupervised 6-month tuberculosis treatment regimen using combination preparations

Initial phase, 2-month period only	
Drug	Adult dose
Rifater (rifampicin, isoniazid and pyrazinamide)	Body weight <40 kg: 3 tablets daily
	Body weight 40–49 kg: 4 tablets daily
	Body weight 50–64 kg: 5 tablets daily
	Body weight ≥65 kg: 6 tablets daily
Ethambutol (may be omitted if the risk of isoniazid resistance is low)	15 mg/kg daily
4-month continuation phase	
Drug	Adult dose
Rifinah (rifampicin and isoniazid) following initial treatment with Rifater	Body weight <50 kg: 3 tablets daily of Rifinah 150
	Body weight ≥50 kg: 2 tablets daily of Rifinah 300

Longer treatment courses are required for meningeal TB and infection with resistant organisms.

Monitoring therapy

Before treatment commences the following should be established:

- body weight of the patient – this is vital to ensure the correct dose is prescribed
- hepatic function (LFTs) – a pretreatment baseline is required
- renal function (U&Es): the dose of ethambutol and pyrazinamide should be adjusted in renal impairment
- visual acuity: ethambutol can cause optic neuropathy. This is more common in the elderly and renally impaired. Advise the patient to report changes in colour vision and visual field.

During treatment LFTs should continue to be monitored frequently in high-risk patients, e.g. weekly for 4 weeks, then monthly thereafter.

- Rifampicin commonly causes a transient rise in hepatic enzymes, usually within the first 8 weeks of therapy; however, less than 1% lead to hepatotoxicity.
- Pyrazinamide can cause hepatotoxicity; this tends to be dose-related.
- Isoniazid commonly causes an asymptomatic rise in hepatic enzymes, usually within the first 8 weeks, but less than 5% develop hepatitis, the risk increasing with patient age.[9]

TABLE T11

Standard adult unsupervised 6-month tuberculosis treatment regimen if combination preparations are not appropriate

Initial phase, 2-month period only			
Drug	Paediatric dose	Adult dose	Common side effects[8]
Isoniazid	10 mg/kg daily (max. dose 300 mg)	300 mg daily	Transient rise in LFTs, peripheral neuropathy
Rifampicin	<50 kg: 15 mg/kg daily (max. dose 450 mg)	Body weight <50 kg: 450 mg daily Body weight ≥50 kg: 600 mg daily	GI upset, transient rise in LFTs, reddish discoloration of bodily fluids, 'influenza-like' syndrome
Pyrazinamide	<50 kg: 35 mg/kg daily (max. dose 1.5 g)	Body weight <50 kg: 1.5 g daily Body weight ≥50 kg: 2 g daily	Nausea, vomiting, arthralgia. Transient rise in LFTs (leading to hepatotoxicity), rash
Ethambutol (may be omitted if the risk of isoniazid resistance is low)	20 mg/kg daily	15 mg/kg daily	Optic neuritis, red/green colour blindness
4-month continuation phase			
Drug	Paediatric dose	Adult dose	
Isoniazid	10 mg/kg daily (max. dose 300 mg)	300 mg daily	
Rifampicin	<50 kg: 15 mg/kg daily (max. dose 450 mg)	Body weight <50 kg: 450 mg daily Body weight ≥50 kg: 600 mg daily	

If the AST/ALT level exceeds five times the ULN or if the bilirubin level rises, treatment with rifampicin, isoniazid and pyrazinamide should be stopped. If the patient is not unwell, wait until the patient's liver function returns to normal, then rechallenge with the drugs one at a time. The following regimen may be used:[10]

1 Isoniazid 50 mg/day, increasing daily to 300 mg/day after 2–3 days. If there is no reaction after a further 2–3 days, rifampicin should be added.

2 Rifampicin 75 mg/day, increasing to 300 mg/day after 2–3 days, and then to 450 mg/day (for patients <50 kg) or 600 mg/day (for patients ≥50 kg). If there is no reaction after a further 2–3 days, pyrazinamide should be added.

3 Pyrazinamide 250 mg/day, increasing to 1 g/day after 2–3 days and then to 1.5 g/day (for patients <50 kg) or 2 g/day (for patients ≥50 kg).

If there is a reaction, the offending drug should be withdrawn and consideration should be given to an alternative regimen. If the patient is unwell or infectious and the AST/ALT exceeds five times the ULN then, provided they are not clinically contraindicated, streptomycin and ethambutol may be given whilst the process of rechallenge is undertaken as before.

Drug interactions

Potential clinically significant drug interactions to consider include:[7]

- rifampicin: antiarrhythmics, various antiretroviral agents, azole antifungals, antacids, oral anticoagulants, phenytoin, lamotrigine, calcium-channel blockers, immunosuppressants, oral contraceptive pill, corticosteroids
- isoniazid: carbamazepine.

Adherence

Patient adherence to their drug regimen is necessary to ensure successful treatment. The following should be considered:

- patient counselling about medication, including potential side effects, duration of therapy, taking rifampicin on an empty stomach and the importance of adherence
- use of combination products, e.g. Rifinah and Rifater
- intermittent dosing at higher doses three times a week. Doses are listed in BNF section 5.1.9
- supervised treatment (directly observed therapy or DOT) for non-compliant patients. Patients are dosed three times weekly as above, but the administration is supervised.

Multidrug-resistant tuberculosis

Multidrug-resistant tuberculosis (MDR-TB) is defined as resistance to at least isoniazid and rifampicin.[11] The proportion of TB cases with MDR-TB in the UK has remained stable over the last few years at 1.6%, with the large majority of patients born outside the UK.[2] Patients with MDR-TB will require a different combination of drugs and a longer period of treatment. Five different drug types are generally used to treat MDR-TB and usually include:

- a first-line oral agent to which the isolated organism is sensitive
- an injectable second-line (or reserve) drug, typically an aminoglycoside
- a quinolone
- two other second-line drugs, unless it is possible to substitute one of these for pyrazinamide or ethambutol, depending on sensitivity results.

Table T12 gives details of drugs used in MDR-TB.

TABLE T12
Drugs used in multidrug-resistant tuberculosis[12]

Drug	Paediatric dose	Adult dose	TDM	Common side effects
Amikacin	15 mg/kg intravenously daily	15 mg/kg intravenously daily (maximum dose 1 g daily)	Yes	Ototoxicity and nephrotoxicity (increased risk with prolonged exposure), neuromuscular blockade, electrolyte abnormalities
Bedaquiline	Not currently recommended	400 mg orally daily for 2 weeks, then 200 mg three times a day for 22 weeks	No	Arthralgia, chest pain, nausea, headache, haemoptysis, QTc interval prolongation in patients at risk
Capreomycin	15 mg/kg intramuscularly daily	15 mg/kg intramuscularly daily (maximum dose 1 g daily)	No	Ototoxicity and nephrotoxicity (increased risk with prolonged exposure), eosinophilia
Clarithromycin	See BNFC dose for respiratory infections[13]	500 mg twice daily (orally or intravenously)	No	Nausea, diarrhoea, vomiting, abdominal pain, headache, taste perversion, QTc interval prolongation in patients at risk
Clofazimine	1 mg/kg orally daily[13]	100–200 mg orally daily (up to 300 mg daily)	No	Red skin discolouration, GI upset, ichthyosis and dry skin, pruritus, rash, photosensitivity reactions
Co-amoxiclav	See BNFC dose for respiratory infections	1.2 g intravenously or 625 mg orally 8-hourly	No	Rash, urticaria, GI upset, candidiasis
Cycloserine	10–20 mg/kg/day orally in two divided doses (maximum daily dose 1 g)	250–500 mg orally twice daily	Yes	Confusion, dizziness, somnolence
Delamanid	Not currently recommended	18–64 years: 100 mg orally twice daily for 24 weeks >65 years: no data available	No	Dermatitis, urticaria, GI upset, dizziness, insomnia, paraesthesias, tremor, haemoptysis, QTc interval prolongation in patients at risk

TABLE T12
(Continued)

Drug	Paediatric dose	Adult dose	TDM	Common side effects
Imipenem/cilastatin	20–40 mg/kg (maximum dose 2 g) intravenously 8-hourly	>50 kg: 1 g intravenously 12-hourly <50 kg: 15 mg/kg intravenously 12-hourly	No	Rash, urticaria, GI upset, thrombophlebitis, eosinophilia, transient rise in LFTs, transient rise in serum urea/creatinine
Levofloxacin	>5 years: 10 mg/kg once daily <5 years: 7.5–10 mg/kg once daily Both intravenously or orally	500–1000 mg intravenously or orally once daily	Yes	Nausea, vomiting, diarrhoea, dizziness, headache, transient rise in LFTs, QTc interval prolongation in patients at risk
Linezolid	10 mg/kg three times daily in children up to 11 years of age and 10 mg/kg (maximum dose 600 mg) twice daily in older children[13] Both intravenously or orally	600 mg intravenously or orally once daily	Yes	GI upset, headache, transient rise in LFTs, candidiasis, myelosuppression and neuropathy with prolonged use
Meropenem	1 month to 12 years: 10–20 mg/kg intravenously 8-hourly. If >50 kg use adult dose	1 g intravenously 8-hourly (with co-amoxiclav)	No	Rash, pruritus, GI upset, thrombocytopenia, headache, transient rise in LFTs
Moxifloxacin	7.5–10 mg/kg orally once daily	400 mg intravenously or orally once daily	Yes	Nausea, vomiting, headache, dizziness, taste perversion, transient rise in LFTs, QTc interval prolongation in patients at risk
Ofloxacin	15–20 mg/kg orally once daily (maximum dose 400 mg)	400 mg intravenously or orally twice daily	Yes	Nausea, vomiting, headache, dizziness, taste perversion, transient rise in LFTs, QTc interval prolongation in patients at risk

T

(continued)

TABLE T12
(Continued)

Drug	Paediatric dose	Adult dose	TDM	Common side effects
Para-aminosali-cylate sodium	50 mg/kg/day orally (maximum dose 12 g) in two to four divided doses. Higher doses have been used	150 mg/kg/day orally, usually 8–12 g/day in two to four divided doses	No	GI upset, hypersensitivity reactions, including fever and rash
Protionamide	15–20 mg/kg orally once daily (maximum dose 1 g)	15–20 mg/kg orally once daily (max. dose 1 g)	No	GI upset, including nausea, vomiting, diarrhoea, anorexia, excessive salivation, metallic taste, stomatitis, abdominal pain and transient rise in LFTs
Rifabutin	5 mg/kg orally once a day	300–450 mg orally once daily	Yes	GI upset, neutropenia, uveitis, transient rise in LFTs, rash, reddish discolouration of bodily fluids
Streptomycin	15 mg/kg intramuscularly once daily (maximum dose 1 g daily) initially then reduce to thrice weekly	15 mg/kg intramuscularly once daily (maximum dose 1 g daily) initially, then reduce to thrice weekly. If >59 years: 10 mg/kg once daily (maximum dose 750 mg daily) initially, then reduce to 15 mg/kg thrice weekly	Yes	Nephrotoxicity, ototoxicity, rashes and urticaria, eosinophilia
Thiacetazone	No information	150 mg daily	No	GI upset, dizziness, rash. Contraindicated if HIV-positive

Diagnosis of latent tuberculosis[14]

Latent TB may reactivate in later life, often associated with a weakened immune system due to disease, drugs or older life. The Mantoux (tuberculin skin) test and interferon-gamma release assay (IGRA) are used to identify individuals with latent TB.

The Mantoux test involves injecting tuberculin purified protein derivative (PPD) intradermally and measuring the individual's skin reaction 48–72 hours after injection. The greater the reaction, the more likely an individual is infected with TB. In the UK, the standard strength of tuberculin PPD used is 2 TU/0.1 mL, with 0.1 mL injected per test. Reading the test involves measuring the diameter of the area of induration (not erythema) in millimetres with a ruler. Interpretation of the result is described in Table T13. It is possible to obtain a false-negative result due to immunosuppression, viral illness or live viral vaccines. The Mantoux does not provide the ability to distinguish between previous bacillus Calmette-Guérin (BCG) vaccination and latent TB, and requires an experienced operator to perform the test and the individual to return for a second visit.

TABLE T13
Interpretation of the Mantoux test

Diameter of induration	Positivity	Interpretation
Less than 6 mm	Negative	No previous TB infection or BCG vaccination
>6 mm, but <15 mm	Positive	Previous TB infection or BCG vaccine or exposure to non-tuberculous bacteria
≥15 mm	Strongly positive	Suggests TB infection or disease

There are currently two IGRA tests commercially available and both involve stimulating an individual's blood with a synthetic antigen and measuring the amount of interferon-gamma produced by T cells or the number of active T cells. IGRAs can be used to diagnose latent TB alone or in a two-step strategy after a Mantoux test.[15] IGRAs are more expensive than the Mantoux and are not readily available in all areas; however, they do not require an individual to return for a second visit for interpretation. IGRAs provide the ability to distinguish between previous BCG vaccination and latent (or active) TB infection and can reduce the number of individuals offered chemoprophylaxis when there is no vaccination record or scar.

Treatment of latent tuberculosis

Chemoprophylaxis should be offered, consisting of isoniazid for 6 months or a combination of isoniazid and rifampicin for 3 months. Doses are as for the treatment regimen described in Table T11. If there is a high risk of exposure to MDR-TB, seek specialist advice.

Miscellaneous points

Pregnancy and breastfeeding

Standard treatment is compatible with pregnancy and breastfeeding. Streptomycin and other aminoglycosides should be avoided as they may be ototoxic in the foetus. For second-line drugs consult specialist literature.

Unconscious patients[16]

- Rifampicin and isoniazid may be given intravenously or via a nasogastric tube.
- Pyrazinamide tablets may be crushed and dispersed in water (unlicensed) and given via a nasoenteric tube.
- Ethambutol tablets may be crushed and dispersed in water (unlicensed) and given via a nasogastric tube.
- Streptomycin may be given intramuscularly.

Isoniazid

Isoniazid may cause peripheral neuropathy and pyridoxine 10 mg daily should be prescribed for patients at high risk, e.g. those who are alcoholics, diabetics, HIV-positive, in chronic renal failure or the malnourished.

REFERENCES

1 WHO (2013). *Global Tuberculosis Report 2013*. http://apps.who.int/iris/bitstream/ 10665/91355/1/9789241564656_eng.pdf (accessed 13 September 2014).

2 Public Health England (2014). *TB in the UK 2014 Report*. https://www.gov.uk/ government/publications/tuberculosis-tb-in-the-uk (accessed 13 September 2014).

3 Public Health England (2014). *Tuberculosis and Other Mycobacterial Diseases: Diagnosis, screening, management and data*. https://www.gov.uk/government/ collections/tuberculosis-and-other-mycobacterial-diseases-diagnosis-screening-management-and-data (accessed 13 September 2014).

4 Campbell IA, Bah-Sow O (2006). Pulmonary tuberculosis: diagnosis and management. *BMJ* 332: 1194–1197.

5 NICE (2011). Clinical guideline 117. *Tuberculosis: Clinical diagnosis and management of tuberculosis, and measures for its prevention and control*. http://www.nice.org.uk/guidance/cg117 (accessed 13 September 2014).

6 Health Protection Agency (2013). *Molecular Diagnosis of Tuberculosis (TB): Information for health care professionals*. https://www.gov.uk/government/ publications/tuberculosis-tb-molecular-diagnosis (accessed 13 September 2014).

7 Joint Formulary Committee (2014). *British National Formulary* (68th edn). London: BMJ Group and Pharmaceutical Press.

8 eMC (2014). http://www.medicines.org.uk/emc/ (accessed 1 November 2014).

9 Larson ASM, Graziani AL (2014). *Isoniazid Hepatotoxicity. Up to date 2014*. http://www.uptodate.com/contents/isoniazid-hepatotoxicity?source=see_link (accessed 21 October 2014).

10 Pozniak AL *et al.* (2011). British HIV Association guidelines for the treatment of TB/HIV coinfection 2011. *HIV Med* 12: 517–524.

11 Lange C *et al.* (2014). Management of patients with multi-drug resistant/extensively drug-resistant tuberculosis in Europe: a TBNET consensus statement. *Eur Respir J* 44: 23–63.

12 Potter JL, Capstick T (2014). TB drug monographs. A UK based resource to support the monitoring and safe use of anti-tuberculosis drugs and second line treatment of multidrug-resistant tuberculosis. http://www.tbdrugmonographs.co.uk/ (accessed 1 November 2014).

13 Paediatric Formulary Committee (2014). *British National Formulary* 2014–15. London: BMJ Group and Pharmaceutical Press.bWHO (2014). *Companion Handbook to the WHO Guidelines for the Programmatic Management of Drug-resistant Tuberculosis*. Available at: http://apps.who.int/iris/bitstream/10665/130918/1/ 9789241548809_eng.pdf?ua=1 (accessed 11 May 2015).

14 Public Health England (2011). *The Green Book: Tuberculosis*; Chapter 32. https:// www.gov.uk/government/publications/tuberculosis-the-green-book-chapter-32 (accessed 13 September 2014).

15 Public Health England (2011). *Health Protection Agency Position Statement on the Use of Interferon gamma Release Assay Tests for Tuberculosis: Draft interim guidance.* https://www.gov.uk/government/publications/tuberculosis-tb-interferon-gamma-release-assay-tests (accessed 13 September 2014).

16 Pharmaceutical Press (2014). *Handbook of Drug Administration via Enteral Feeding Tubes.* https://www.medicinescomplete.com/mc/tubes/current/index.htm (accessed 7 November 2011).

T

V

Vancomycin

Vancomycin is a glycopeptide antibiotic with bactericidal activity against aerobic and anaerobic Gram-positive bacteria. It is usually reserved to treat resistant staphylococcal infections (in particular, methicillin-resistant *Staphylococcus aureus* (MRSA)) in patients who have not responded or are allergic to penicillins/cephalosporins.[1] Check your local antibiotic policy to see when vancomycin is used in your hospital.

Vancomycin is absorbed poorly from the gastrointestinal (GI) tract and therefore is given as an intravenous infusion. The exception is for the treatment of *Clostridium difficile* and enterocolitis, where vancomycin is given orally, acting locally in the GI tract.[2]

Pharmacokinetic properties

Vancomycin readily diffuses into most tissues. However, it does not penetrate into the cerebrospinal fluid in a healthy patient. In meningitis, where the meninges are inflamed, therapeutic concentrations may be achieved. Vancomycin is excreted renally.[1]

Rationale for monitoring

Early impure formulations of vancomycin resulted in high levels of ototoxicity and nephrotoxicity. Therapeutic drug monitoring was recommended on the basis that toxicity could be avoided if serum concentrations were below 40 mg/L.[3] Due to the increased prevalence of MRSA and other resistant bacteria, monitoring is now aimed at ensuring drug levels are therapeutic to prevent treatment failure.[4]

Dosing

Practice varies with regard to dosing of intravenous vancomycin; consult your local guideline. Dosing recommendations made here are based on a newer method of dosing devised to reach therapeutic concentrations rapidly.[4]

Loading dose

To reach therapeutic concentrations rapidly, a loading dose of vancomycin should be given irrespective of renal function. This is dose-banded with regard to the body weight of the patient (Table V1).

TABLE V1

Vancomycin loading dose guidance[4]

Patient's actual body weight (kg)	<60	60–90	>90
Loading dose	1000 mg	1500 mg	2000 mg

Maintenance dose

After the loading dose, a maintenance dose is needed based on the patient's renal function, with the patient's creatinine clearance calculated using the Cockcroft and Gault equation (see *Renal function – assessment* entry). In patients who are at the extremes of weight, anuric or in acute renal failure, creatinine clearance is less accurate and clinical judgement is needed. If a patient's creatinine is less than 60 mmol/L use 60 mmol/L in the equation to avoid overestimating renal function.

In obese patients calculate creatinine clearance using a maximum body weight, which is the ideal body weight (IBW) × 1.2.

- For men: IBW (kg) = 50 kg + 2.3 kg for each inch over 5 feet
- For women: IBW (kg) = 49 kg + 1.7 kg for each inch over 5 feet

Table V2 shows suggested maintenance doses.

Monitoring and dose adjustment

Fluid balance should be monitored along with at least twice-weekly urea and electrolytes. It is now common practice to monitor only trough levels (pre-dose) of vancomycin and the timing of this first level is shown in Table V2.

The *BNF* recommends a trough serum concentration of 10–15 mg/L vancomycin for most infections and 15–20 mg/L in more resistant or deep-seated infections or less sensitive MRSA strains.[5]

If the vancomycin assay is in the desired range, continue with the current dose and repeat another pre-dose level after 3–4 days provided renal function remains stable. If the assay is not in the desired range, refer to Table V3 for further information.

Side effects of vancomycin

Vancomycin has an infusion rate-related side effect known as 'red-man syndrome', which exhibits as flushing of the skin and a potentially dangerous drop in blood pressure. This usually can be avoided by administering vancomycin no faster than 10 mg/min.

Ototoxicity and nephrotoxicity are recognised side effects of vancomycin associated with higher doses of vancomycin.

TABLE V2

Vancomycin maintenance dose guidance[4]

Calculated creatinine clearance	Maintenance dose	Time after loading dose to start maintenance dose	Recommended infusion fluid volume for each dose (either sodium chloride 0.9%* or glucose 5%)	Advised duration of infusion for dose	Time of first vancomycin pre-dose level
>110 mL/min	1.5 g every 12 hours†	12 hours	500 mL	150 minutes	Before fourth dose
90–110 mL/min	1.25 g every 12 hours	12 hours	250 mL	150 minutes	Before fourth dose
75–89 mL/min	1 g every 12 hours	12 hours	250 mL	120 minutes	Before fourth dose
55–74 mL/min	750 mg every 12 hours	12 hours	250 mL	90 minutes	Before fourth dose
40–54 mL/min	500 mg every 12 hours	12 hours	100 mL	60 minutes	Before fourth dose
30–39 mL/min	750 mg every 24 hours	24 hours	250 mL	90 minutes	Before fourth dose
20–29 mL/min	500 mg every 24 hours	24 hours	100 mL	60 minutes	Before fourth dose
10–19 mL/min	500 mg every 48 hours	48 hours	100 mL	60 minutes	Before second dose
<10 mL/min oliguric or anuric	Check levels 48 hours after loading dose. Redose with 1 g when levels <15 mg/L	Only redose when levels <15 mg/L	250 mL	120 minutes	48 hours after dose

*Be mindful of patient's sodium requirements (each 100 mL of sodium chloride 0.9% contains 15 mmol of sodium).
† Patients under 45 kg should be given a maximum starting dose of 1.25 g every 12 hours.

V

TABLE V3
Vancomycin dose adjustment guidance

Pre-dose (trough) serum concentration	Adjustment needed to maintenance dose	When to take subsequent level
Less than 5 mg/L	Increase the dose by two dosing levels from current dosing schedule in Table V2	Before fourth dose
5–10 mg/L	Increase by one dosing level in Table V2	Before fourth dose
10–15 mg/L	If aiming for 10–15 mg/L: continue at current dose	After 3–4 days
	If aiming for 15–20 mg/L: increase by one dosing level in Table V2	Before fourth dose
15–20 mg/L	If aiming for 10–15 mg/L: decrease by one dosing level in Table V2	Before fourth dose
	If aiming for 15–20 mg/L: continue at current dose	After 3–4 days
20–25 mg/L	Decrease by one dosing level in Table V2	Before fourth dose
25–30 mg/L	Omit next dose and decrease by two dosing levels in Table V2	Before fourth dose
>30 mg/L	Omit any further doses and seek specialist advice	

Interactions

Careful monitoring is required if vancomycin is given with other nephrotoxic drugs, e.g. amphotericin, streptomycin, neomycin, gentamicin, kanamycin, amikacin, tobramycin, bacitracin, polymyxin B, colistin and cisplatin. Loop diuretics may increase the risk of ototoxicity.

Anaesthetic drugs given with intravenous vancomycin can cause hypersensitivity reactions.[5]

Counselling

Warn the patient of its offensive taste when given orally.

REFERENCES

1 Summary of Product Characteristics (2014). *Vancomycin Hydrochloride 500 mg and 1 g Powder for Concentrate for Infusion*. Hospira UK. http://www.medicines.org.uk (accessed 23 August 2014).
2 Summary of Product Characteristics (2014). *Vancocin Matrigel Capsules 125 mg*. Flynn Pharma. http://www.medicines.org.uk (accessed 23 August 2014).
3 Tobin CM *et al.* (2002). Vancomycin therapeutic drug monitoring: is there a consensus view? The results of a UK National External Quality Assessment Scheme (UK NEQAS) for antibiotic assays questionnaire. *Antimicrob Chemother* 50: 713–718.
4 Thomson A *et al.* (2009). Development and evaluation of vancomycin dosage guidelines designed to achieve new target concentrations. *Antimicrob Chemother* 63: 1050–1057.
5 Joint Formulary Committee (2014). *British National Formulary* (online). London: BMJ Group and Pharmaceutical Press. http://www.medicinescomplete.com (accessed on 23 August 2014).

V

Venofer

Overview[1] (see also *Iron: guidance on parenteral dosing and administration* entry)			
Form	Iron (III) (as iron (III)–hydroxide sucrose complex)		
Dose	• Total dose required (mg iron) $$= [\text{body weight (kg)} \times (\text{target haemoglobin (Hb)} - \text{actual Hb (g/L)}) \times 0.24] + X$$ $X = 500$ mg and is the milligrams of iron required to replace the body's iron stores (or depot iron) and is only applicable for patients 35 kg and above. The target Hb for these patients is 150 g/L. For patients with a body weight below 35 kg, a 15 mg/kg dose should be used for X and the target Hb is 130 g/L. The dose should be rounded down to the nearest 5 mg. • Total single dose should not exceed 200 mg of iron • Should not be administered more than three times a week • If total dose exceeds maximum allowed single dose, the administration should be split		
Adminis-tration routes	**Intravenous drip infusion**	**Intravenous instalments**	**Intramuscular**
	Yes	Yes	No
Administration	• Dilute in sodium chloride 0.9% • Each 50 mg of iron should be diluted in a maximum of 50 mL of sodium chloride 0.9% • Administer at a rate of 100 mg of iron in at least 15 minutes	• Administer by slow intravenous injection at not more than 20 mg (1 mL) per minute	
Monitoring	• Patients should be monitored for signs and symptoms of hypersensitivity reactions during and following each administration[2] • Observe patient for adverse effects for at least 30 minutes following each injection • If hypersensitivity reactions or signs of intolerance occur during administration, the treatment must be stopped immediately		

REFERENCE
1 eMC (2014). *Summary of Product Characteristics Venofer (Iron Sucrose)*. https://www.medicines.org.uk/emc/medicine/24168 (accessed 27 August 2014).
2 MHRA Drug Safety Update (2013). *Intravenous iron and serious hypersensitivity reactions: strengthened recommendations*. https://www.gov.uk/drug-safety-update/intravenous-iron-and-serious-hypersensitivity-reactions-strengthened-recommendations (accessed 29 August 2015).

Vitamins and minerals

Many patients are interested in dietary supplements. When dealing with queries, it is useful to be aware of the current recommended daily amounts (RDA) of these substances and also what is considered the maximum safe dose if patients are taking non-prescribed vitamins and minerals (Table V4).

TABLE V4

Role, sources and recommended daily amounts of vitamins and minerals[1] (reproduced by kind permission of the Food Standards Agency)

Supplement	Role	Natural sources	Adult RDA	FSA, maximum recommended safe daily amount
Beta-carotene (precursor of vitamin A)	See vitamin A. Beta-carotene's importance to an individual depends upon the level of preformed vitamin A in the diet	Kidney, liver, eggs, some fruit and vegetables, especially dried mixed fruit	N/A	No more than 7 mg
Boron	Boron's function is unknown but it may be involved in the utilisation of various elements (including calcium, copper, magnesium), glucose, triglycerides, reactive oxygen and oestrogen	Green vegetables, fruit and nuts	1–13 mg	No more than 6 mg
Calcium	Calcium provides rigidity in the form of calcium phosphate in bones, is a component in the maintenance of cell structure, is a cofactor for many enzymes (e.g. lipase) and it has a role in the blood-clotting mechanism. Changes in the concentration of intracellular calcium, in response to a physiological stimulus, e.g. a neurotransmitter, can act as an intracellular signal causing events such as cell aggregation, muscle contraction and cell movement, secretion, transformation and cell division	Milk, cheese and other dairy foods, green leafy vegetables (e.g. broccoli, cabbage and okra, but not spinach), soya bean products, nuts, bread and anything made with fortified flour, fish where the bones are eaten, e.g. sardines and pilchards	700 mg	No more than 1500 mg
Chromium	It has been shown to potentiate insulin action and thereby affect metabolism of carbohydrate, lipids and protein	Trace element found in the air, water and soil, plants and animals	25 microgram	No more than 10 mg

(continued)

V

TABLE V4
(Continued)

Supplement	Role	Natural sources	Adult RDA	FSA, maximum recommended safe daily amount
Cobalt	It is an essential trace element, being an integral part of vitamin B$_{12}$	Fish, nuts, green leafy vegetables, e.g. broccoli, spinach and cereals, e.g. oats	Daily amount obtained from vitamin B$_{12}$	No more than 1.4 mg
Copper	It is involved in the function of several enzymes, e.g. monoamine oxidase. It is thought to be required for infant growth, host defence mechanisms, bone strength, red and white blood cell maturation, iron transport, cholesterol and glucose metabolism, myocardial contractility and brain development	Nuts, shellfish and offal, e.g. liver	1.2 mg	No more than 3 mg
Fluoride	It contributes to the formation of strong teeth and increases resistance to tooth decay	As a trace element, it is present in all animals, plants and water. Fish and tea are particularly good sources. In some parts of the UK fluoride is added to drinking water to improve dental health	It is not clear how much fluoride is needed for good health	Supplementation is not recommended if fluoride concentration of drinking water >0.7 ppm (700 microgram/L)
Folic acid	Folate coenzymes are involved in phases of amino acid metabolism, purine and pyrimidine synthesis and the formation of S-adenosylmethionine	Green leafy vegetables, peas, chickpeas, yeast extract, brown rice and some fruit, e.g. oranges and bananas	200 microgram (400 microgram if pregnant)	No more than 1 mg
Germanium	It has no known biological function. There is a suggestion that it may have an involvement in carbohydrate metabolism	Beans, tomato juice, oysters, tuna and garlic	N/A	N/A

V

	Function	Food sources		
Iodine	Iodine forms part of the thyroid hormones, levothyroxine (T_4) and triiodothyronine (T_3). Therefore, it has an involvement in the maintenance of metabolic rate, cellular metabolism and integrity of connective tissue	Sea fish and shellfish	0.14 mg	No more than 0.5 mg
Iron	The majority of functional iron is present in haem proteins, e.g. haemoglobin, myoglobin and cytochromes, which are involved in oxygen transport or mitochondrial electron transfer	Liver, meat, beans, nuts, dried fruit, e.g. dried apricots, wholegrains, e.g. brown rice, fortified breakfast cereals, soya bean flour and most dark green leafy vegetables, e.g. watercress, curly kale and spinach	Male: 8.7 mg Female: 14.8 mg	No more than 17 mg
Magnesium	It is a cofactor for many enzyme systems. It is needed for protein synthesis, for both anaerobic and aerobic energy generation and for glycolysis. It has a role in cell division. It may be necessary for the maintenance of an adequate supply of nucleotides. It is involved in the movement of potassium in myocardial cells. It is involved in the metabolism of vitamin D, and is essential for the synthesis and secretion of parathyroid hormone	Green leafy vegetables, e.g. spinach, nuts, bread, fish, meat and dairy foods	Male: 300 mg Female: 270 mg	No more than 400 mg
Manganese	It is a component of a number of enzymes, e.g. glycosyltransferases	Bread, nuts, cereals and green vegetables, e.g. peas and runner beans, and tea	1–10 mg	No more than 10 mg
Molybdenum	It is required in metalloenzymes, which exploit the variable valency states of molybdenum, e.g. xanthine oxidase and sulfite oxidase	Peas, leafy vegetables, e.g. broccoli and spinach, and cauliflower	0.1–0.3 mg	N/A

(continued)

V

TABLE V4
(Continued)

Supplement	Role	Natural sources	Adult RDA	FSA, maximum recommended safe daily amount
Nickel	Nickel influences iron absorption and metabolism and may be an essential component of the haemopoietic process	Lentils, oats and nuts	N/A	N/A
Phosphorus	It is required for phospholipids that are major constituents of most biological membranes, and for nucleotides and nucleic acids. Phosphorus is involved in carbohydrate, fat and protein metabolism and is essential for bone health. Most metabolic processes derive their energy from the phosphate bonds of adenosine triphosphate and other high-energy phosphate compounds. Phosphorus intake influences the parathyroid–vitamin D axis, which maintains the body's calcium balance	Red meat, dairy foods, fish, poultry, bread, rice and oats	550 mg	No more than 2400 mg
Potassium	Together with sodium, it is needed to maintain normal osmotic pressure within cells. Extracellular potassium concentration is a critical determinant of neuromuscular excitability. Potassium is also a cofactor for numerous enzymes, and is required for secretion of insulin	Fruit, e.g. bananas, vegetables, pulses, nuts and seeds, milk, fish, shellfish, beef, chicken, turkey, liver and bread	3.5 g	No more than 3.7 g

V

Selenium	The biologically active form of selenium is selenocysteine that is incorporated into selenoproteins. These help protect against oxidative damage and are involved in the production of T_3. They are involved in antioxidant and transport functions, and in the maintenance of the intracellular redox state	Brazil nuts, bread, fish, meat and eggs	Male: 75 microgram Female: 60 microgram	No more than 350 microgram
Silicon	Silicon is involved in the formation of bone and connective tissues	Grains, e.g. oats, barley and rice	N/A	No more than 700 mg
Sodium chloride	Together with potassium, it is an essential mineral for regulating body fluid balance. Sodium is the major determinant of extracellular volume. Chloride is also involved in maintaining fluid balance as it is a component of gastric and intestinal secretions	Rock salt	1.6 g	No more than 2.3 g
Tin	There is no known biological function for tin. There is a suggestion that it may contribute to the structure and function of metalloenzymes	Fresh and tinned foods. The amount varies dependent on the amount of tin in the soil where the food is grown	N/A	No more than 13 mg
Vanadium	No specific function has been identified. It may function as an oxidation-reduction catalyst	Seafood, meat, dairy foods, cooking oils, fresh fruit and vegetables	N/A	N/A
Vitamin A (retinol)	It is essential to the processes of vision, reproduction, embryonic development, morphogenesis, growth and cellular differentiation. Vitamin A metabolites are involved in the control of gene expression	Liver, cheese, eggs, oily fish (such as mackerel), milk, fortified margarine and yoghurt	Male: 0.7 mg Female: 0.6 mg	No more than 1.5 mg. Caution in pregnancy

(continued)

V

V

TABLE V4
(Continued)

Supplement	Role	Natural sources	Adult RDA	FSA, maximum recommended safe daily amount
Vitamin B₁ (thiamine)	It is a coenzyme in several enzymatic reactions. It may also be involved in the stimulation of neuronal cells and other excitable tissues, e.g. skeletal muscle	Pork, vegetables, milk, cheese, peas, fresh and dried fruit, eggs, wholegrain breads and some fortified breakfast cereals	Male: 1 mg Female: 0.8 mg	No more than 100 mg
Vitamin B₂ (riboflavin)	It promotes normal growth and assists in the synthesis of steroids, red blood cells and glycogen. It helps to maintain the integrity of mucous membranes, skin, eyes and the nervous system. It is involved in the production of adrenaline and is thought to aid the absorption of iron	Milk, eggs, fortified breakfast cereals, rice and mushrooms	Male: 1.3 mg Female: 1.1 mg	No more than 40 mg
Vitamin B₃ (niacin)	It is the functional factor of two important coenzymes, NAD and NADP, which activate over 200 dehydrogenases essential to electron transport and other cellular respiratory reactions. It is involved in the oxidation of fats and carbohydrates, and also the synthesis of steroids	Beef, pork, chicken, wheat flour, maize flour, eggs and milk	Male: 17 mg Female: 13 mg	No more than 500 mg
Vitamin B₅ (pantothenic acid)	It fulfils several roles in cellular metabolism, including the synthesis of many essential molecules	Chicken, beef, potatoes, porridge, tomatoes, liver, kidney, yeast, eggs, broccoli and wholegrains, e.g. brown rice and wholemeal bread	N/A	No more than 200 mg

Vitamin B$_6$ (pyridoxine)	It is a cofactor in the metabolism transformation of amino acids. It can modify the action of steroid hormones. It is essential for the manufacture of prostaglandins and the formation of red blood cells. It is involved in cellular replication and antibody production. It is necessary for the function of the nervous system and is involved in the biosynthesis of several neurotransmitters, including serotonin, gamma-aminobutyric acid (GABA), dopamine and noradrenaline and has a role in the regulation of mental processes and mood. It is also involved in sodium–potassium balance, histamine metabolism, the conversion of tryptophan to niacin, absorption of vitamin B$_{12}$ and the production of hydrochloric acid in the GI tract	Liver, pork, chicken, turkey, cod, bread, whole cereals, e.g. oatmeal, wheatgerm (found in cereals and cereal products) and rice, eggs, vegetables, soya beans, peanuts, milk, potatoes and some fortified breakfast cereals	Female: 1.2 mg Male: 1.4 mg	Between 10 mg and 200 mg for short-term use only is considered safe
Vitamin B$_{12}$ (cobalamin)	It serves as a cofactor for several enzymes required for the cellular import and metabolism of folate and even-chained fatty acid synthesis	Meat products and certain algae, e.g. seaweed	1.5 microgram	No more than 2 mg

(continued)

V

TABLE V4
(Continued)

Supplement	Role	Natural sources	Adult RDA	FSA, maximum recommended safe daily amount
Vitamin C (ascorbic acid)	It is a reducing agent and an antioxidant, involved in prevention of damage from free radicals. It is involved in the synthesis of collagen, neurotransmitters and carnitine. It is an enzyme cofactor, and increases the GI absorption of non-haem iron	Strawberries, peppers, broccoli, Brussels sprouts, sweet potatoes, oranges and kiwi fruit	40 mg	No more than 100 mg
Vitamin D: vitamin D$_2$ (ergocalciferol) and vitamin D$_3$ (colecalciferol)	It regulates calcium and phosphate metabolism and is involved in the regulation of parathyroid hormone synthesis	Oily fish, liver and eggs, fortified foods, e.g. margarine, breakfast cereals, bread and powdered milk	10 microgram	No more than 25 microgram
Vitamin E (D-α-tocopherol)	Current information suggests that the effects of vitamin E are consistent with an antioxidant role. It is thought to have a role in the maintenance of membrane integrity in virtually all cells of the body	Soya, corn and olive oil, nuts and seeds, and wheatgerm	Male: 4 mg Female: 3 mg	No more than 540 mg (800 units)
Vitamin H (biotin/ coenzyme R)	It is an essential cofactor for enzymes involved in the synthesis of fatty acids, the catabolism of branched-chain amino acids and the gluconeogenic pathway. It may also have a role in the regulation of gene expression	Kidney and liver, eggs, some fruit and vegetables, especially dried mixed fruit	0.01–0.2 mg	No more than 0.9 mg

Vitamin K: vitamin K_1 (phylloquinone) Vitamin K_2 (menaquinone) Vitamin K_3 (menadione) Vitamin K_4 (menadiol)	It catalyses the carboxylation of a number of protein factors involved in blood clotting, including prothrombin. It is thought to be involved in the limitation of bone growth, and the mobilisation and deposition of bone calcium. It may be involved in reabsorption of calcium by the kidney tubules. Vitamin K-dependent proteins are also thought to have roles in cell signalling and brain lipid metabolism	Green leafy vegetables, e.g. broccoli and spinach, and in vegetable oils and cereals. Small amounts can also be found in meat (such as pork), and dairy foods, e.g. cheese	1 microgram	No more than 1 mg
Zinc	It is required for the synthesis and stabilisation of genetic material and is necessary for cell division and the synthesis and degradation of carbohydrates, lipids and proteins	Meat, shellfish, milk and dairy foods, e.g. cheese, bread and cereal products, e.g. wheatgerm	Male: 5.5–9.5 mg Female: 4–7 mg	No more than 25 mg

V

Prescribed doses (e.g. in deficiency states, alcoholic liver disease) will vary considerably from what is considered necessary for a healthy lifestyle, i.e. the Food Standards Agency (FSA) maximum recommended safe daily amount.

For detailed information on this topic, visit the FSA websites at http://www.food.gov.uk and www.nhs.uk/livewell/healthy-eating.

REFERENCE
1 Food Standards Agency (2003). *Safe Upper Levels for Vitamins and Minerals: Report of the expert group on vitamins and minerals*. http://cot.food.gov.uk/sites/default/files/cot/vitmin2003.pdf (accessed 13 December 2014).

von Willebrand disease

Overview	
Definition	von Willebrand disease is a bleeding disorder caused by reduced functioning of von Willebrand factor. von Willebrand factor is a plasma glycoprotein responsible for normal haemostasis
Diagnosis	The disease tends to be diagnosed when patients present bleeding, usually mucocutaneously, or bleeding more after a surgical procedure or postdelivery
Treatment goals	• Stopping or preventing bleeding episodes
Treatment options	• Desmopressin • Tranexamic acid • von Willebrand factor

Pharmaceutical care and counselling

Desmopressin[1]

Desmopressin works by increasing factor VIII levels and von Willebrand factor levels by causing a release from stores. This usually results in levels 2–5 times the patient's pretreatment level

Dose	• Intravenous dose is 0.3–0.4 micrograms/kg body weight diluted in 50 mL sodium chloride 0.9% and infused over 20 minutes depending on the product used • One product is licensed for subcutaneous use • This can be repeated every 12 hours if cover is still required
Side effects	• Include flushing and hypotension, which tend to be harmless. Fluid retention should be managed by fluid restriction for 24 hours postdose, usually to around 1 litre
Contra-indications	• Unstable angina • Decompensated cardiac insufficiency
Pharmacist interventions	• Pharmacists can ensure the dose of desmopressin is correct based on a patient's weight and is given an appropriate time prior to a procedure, ideally immediately before. The pharmacist should ensure the patient is aware of potential side effects and knows to restrict fluid intake. For patients undergoing surgery, ensuring tranexamic acid is also prescribed is important

Tranexamic acid	
Tranexamic acid[2]	Tranexamic acid is an antifibrinolytic drug
Dose	The local fibrinolytic dose of 1–1.5 grams (2–3 tablets) 2–3 times a day is recommended for patients with von Willebrand disease undergoing surgery, usually starting before surgery. If using the intravenous form, 0.5–1 grams 2–3 times a day is recommended.
Pharmacist interventions	• Pharmacists can ensure that patients know how to take the medication and what side effects to expect, and ensure a reduced dose is used in patients with renal dysfunction

von Willebrand disease	
von Willebrand factor[3]	• If von Willebrand factor is required, there are specific brands that contain the factor alone or brands containing factor VIII and von Willebrand factor. The combined product with factor VIII is more common and should be used for acute bleeding episodes or emergency surgery according to British Committee for Standards in Haematology guidance.[3] • This should be given on the guidance of a haematologist

REFERENCES

1 SPC (2014). *DDAVP/Desmopressin Injection*. www.medicines.org.uk (accessed 31 October 2014).
2 SPC (2014). *Cyklokapron Tablets and Injection*. www.medicines.org.uk (accessed 31 October 2014).
3 Laffan MA *et al.* (2014). The diagnosis and management of von Willebrand disease: a United Kingdom Haemophilia Centre Doctors Organization guideline approved by the British Committee for Standards in Haematology. *Br J Haematol* 167: 453–465.

V

Warfarin treatment and monitoring

The oral anticoagulant warfarin is the most widely used agent for long-term anticoagulation in the UK. The other coumarin drugs, acenocoumarol and phenindione, are used occasionally in people who cannot tolerate warfarin and the information in this entry (apart from dosing details) can also be applied to the use of these drugs.

The action of warfarin

Warfarin is a vitamin K antagonist that reduces the hepatic production of vitamin K-dependent active coagulation factors II, VII, IX and X, along with the regulatory anticoagulant proteins C and S, in a dose-related way. This action results in prolongation of the prothrombin time ('bleeding time') and a decreased tendency to form blood clots. Warfarin therefore acts to prevent enlargement of existing blood clots and formation of new clots. All patients treated with warfarin require dose titration to achieve a target intensity of anticoagulation, with dosage determined individually for each patient.

Monitoring of warfarin is a *pharmacodynamic* rather than *pharmacokinetic* measure.

Bleeding and the international normalised ratio

The overwhelming treatment risk with warfarin is uncontrolled bleeding. The desired targets or ranges for intensity of anticoagulation have been defined for which a highly protective antithrombotic effect is combined with an acceptable risk of bleeding – the so-called 'Goldilocks range' (Table W1). Intensity of anticoagulation is expressed as the international normalised ratio (INR), which is the prothrombin time expressed as a ratio (clotting time for patient plasma divided by the clotting time for control plasma) corrected by a standardising factor: the higher the INR value, the greater the level of anticoagulation and the greater the risk of bleeding.

Length of treatment

The recommended initial treatment duration after a first episode of confirmed VTE is 3 months. Treatment beyond 3 months may be indicated in patients with unprovoked VTE depending on risk of VTE recurrence and bleeding.[2]

TABLE W1

Indications for warfarin and international normalised ratio (INR) targets[1]

Indication	Target (desired range) INR
Prophylaxis of venous thromboembolism in high-risk patients	2.5 (2.0–3.0)
Treatment of VTE (including thromboembolism associated with antiphospholipid syndrome, although warfarin is contraindicated in pregnancy)	2.5 (2.0–3.0)
Recurrent VTE whilst receiving warfarin within therapeutic range	3.5 (3.0–4.0)
Prophylaxis of cardiac thromboembolism	
Atrial fibrillation (AF)	2.5 (2.0–3.0)
Heart valve disease (mitral stenosis or regurgitation with a history of systemic embolism, left atrial thrombus or left atrial enlargement), cardiomyopathy	2.5 (2.0–3.0)
Mechanical heart valves – range dependent on prosthesis thrombogenicity and patient risk factors for thrombosis[1]	2.5–3.5 (2.0–4.0)
Bioprosthetic heart valves (some patients)	2.5 (2.0–3.0)
Cardioversion (for 3 weeks before and 4 weeks after)	2.5 (2.0–3.0) To reduce cardioversion cancellations due to low INR on the day of the procedure, a target of 3.0 (2.5–3.5) can be used prior to the procedure

Prophylaxis of thrombosis in patients with mechanical heart valves and patients with recurrent thromboembolism will be lifelong.

Prophylaxis in patients with AF at risk of stroke (as determined by the CHA_2DS_2VASc score: see *Atrial fibrillation* entry) is lifelong, irrespective of the duration of AF or if sinus rhythm is achieved.[3]

W

Warfarin and antiplatelet therapy

The routine combination of warfarin and an antiplatelet agent is not recommended due to the increased risk of bleeding. However, in patients with a high cardiovascular thrombotic risk, warfarin plus aspirin or clopidogrel may be indicated.[4] Unless there is a high bleeding risk, warfarin plus aspirin for at least 12 months is indicated in patients who have had a myocardial infarction (MI) who otherwise need anticoagulation and who:

- have had the condition managed medically
- have undergone balloon angioplasty
- have undergone coronary artery bypass grafting (CABG).

For patients who need warfarin and have had an MI and undergone percutaneous intervention (PCI) with a bare metal stent or drug-eluting stent, warfarin should be combined with clopidogrel for at least 12 months.

Patients with mechanical heart valves who have had an embolic event despite good INR control should also be considered for warfarin plus antiplatelet therapy.[1]

Anticoagulation services

The anticoagulation of patients is usually the responsibility of a consultant haematologist or sometimes a general practitioner. Some services are hospital-based, whilst others are delivered directly within primary care under the auspices of the primary care organisation. Pharmacists are often involved in the management and delivery of these services. It is important to familiarise yourself with the model of service delivery in your locality.

Patient education

Patients must understand the implications, risks and benefits of oral anticoagulation when commencing treatment with warfarin.
A well-informed patient will find it easier to accept the regimen of clinic appointments, blood tests and the precautions to be observed.

In the UK, all NHS patients are supplied with the yellow Anticoagulant Therapy Record booklet (the 'yellow book'). The booklet contains a diary for recording INR results, dosing instructions for the patient, clinic appointment dates and information about the safe use of warfarin.

The following points should be included in discussion with patients:

- the reason for treatment, i.e. their diagnosis
- how warfarin works (delays clotting time), the benefits of treatment and likely length of treatment
- warfarin tablets – strengths are colour-coded:
  - 0.5 mg is white
  - 1 mg is brown
  - 3 mg is blue
  - 5 mg is pink
- explain the need to keep a selection of the available strengths in order to manage dose changes and make sure patients know they can use any combination of tablets that provide the required dose
- take the dose at the same time each day, usually around 6 p.m., to allow dose adjustments to be made on the day of clinic visits
- explain why everybody needs different doses and the likely pattern of blood tests required (i.e. blood tests daily or on alternate days initially, decreasing over weeks eventually to every 8 or 12 weeks if stable)
- the increased risk of bleeding and bruising and the need to see a doctor urgently if serious bleeding occurs, e.g. uncontrolled nose bleeds, blood in urine, conjunctival haemorrhage, vaginal bleeding

- patients should make sure that healthcare professionals are aware of the anticoagulation prior to any invasive procedures or dental work
- interactions with medicines – patients should always make prescribers and pharmacists aware they are taking warfarin and should seek advice before using any non-prescribed medicinal substances. The major interaction problems are covered in the booklet (see Table W4, below)
- the need to maintain a consistent diet should be stressed. Most dietary sources of vitamin K (e.g. spinach, broccoli, avocado) do not significantly affect the INR if eaten in moderate quantities. Cranberry juice should be avoided due to the risk of elevated INR. Products containing gingko biloba may also increase the risk of bleeding. St John's wort, ginseng and garlic may reduce blood levels of warfarin
- alcohol should be consumed only in moderation according to the usual recommended safe limits (the Department of Health advises a maximum of 3–4 units per day for men and 2–3 units per day for women)
- the need for adequate contraceptive measures in women of childbearing potential.

Initiation of therapy (induction of anticoagulation)

Anticoagulation with warfarin takes 72–96 hours to develop fully. An extremely rapid blockade of clotting factors (and rapid increase in INR) can result in a hypercoagulable state due to rapid reduction in protein C and S levels.

Patients requiring rapid anticoagulation (active VTE, heart valve insertion, acute-onset AF) should be treated with a parenteral anticoagulant until therapeutic anticoagulation is achieved with warfarin.

Historical 10 mg loading regimens have not been shown to be superior to 5 mg loading regimens in achieving a stable level of anticoagulation.[1] And in the elderly or in patients without active thrombosis or in those taking amiodarone, 10 mg loading regimens do increase the risk of high out-of-range INRs during the initiation phase.[1]

A suitable 5 mg loading regimen for elderly patients or those starting warfarin for stroke prevention in AF is given below.[5]

- Ensure the baseline INR is <1.4.
- Give 5 mg daily for 4 days.
- Check INR on day 5 and adjust according to Table W2.
- Check INR on day 8 and adjust according to Table W2.
- Check INR on day 15 (or day 12) and make fine dose adjustments as appropriate.

In patients receiving concomitant amiodarone (particularly in the elderly), initiation with a 5 mg loading regimen may result in

W

TABLE W2
Dose adjustments of warfarin following 5 mg induction[5]

Day 5 INR	Dose (day 5–7)	Day 8 INR	Dose (from day 8)
≤1.7	5 mg	≤1.7	6 mg
		1.8–2.4	5 mg
		2.5–3.0	4 mg
		>3.0	3 mg for 4 days
1.8–2.2	4 mg	≤1.7	5 mg
		1.8–2.4	4 mg
		2.5–3.0	3.5 mg
		3.1–3.5	3 mg for 4 days
		>3.5	2.5 mg for 4 days
2.3–2.7	3 mg	≤1.7	4 mg
		1.8–2.4	3.5 mg
		2.5–3.0	3 mg
		3.1–3.5	2.5 mg for 4 days
		>3.5	2 mg for 4 days
2.8–3.2	2 mg	≤1.7	3 mg
		1.8–2.4	2.5 mg
		2.5–3.0	2 mg
		3.1–3.5	1.5 mg for 4 days
		>3.5	1 mg for 4 days
3.3–3.7	1 mg	≤1.7	2 mg
		1.8–2.4	1.5 mg
		2.5–3.0	1 mg
		3.1–3.5	0.5 mg for 4 days
		>3.5	Omit for 4 days
>3.7	Omit days 5, 6 and 7	<2.0	1.5 mg for 4 days
		2.0–2.9	1 mg for 4 days
		3.0–3.5	0.5 mg for 4 days

excessive INRs; close monitoring and dose reduction are advised in these patients.

For younger patients with active thromboembolism (acute VTE) who are not taking amiodarone, a 10 mg loading regimen may be required. An example of such a regimen is given in Table W3.

Some outpatient anticoagulant clinics may initiate with 3 mg daily for 1 week, followed by dose increases of 1 mg daily at weekly intervals until a therapeutic INR is achieved. However, this regimen can delay therapeutic anticoagulation for some weeks and the impact of this on the patient's thrombotic risk should be evaluated before it is employed.

Maintenance doses

The daily dose of warfarin required to achieve an INR within usual ranges can be anything from 1 mg to 15 mg, although doses above or below this are sometimes required. Warfarin sensitivity varies widely

TABLE W3

Example of a warfarin induction dosing regimen in patients with active thrombosis[6]

Day	INR	Warfarin dose (mg)
1	<1.4	10
2	<1.8	10
	1.8	1
	>1.8	0.5
3	<2.0	10
	2.0–2.1	5
	2.2–2.3	4.5
	2.4–2.5	4
	2.6–2.7	3.5
	2.8–2.9	3
	3.0–3.1	2.5
	3.2–3.3	2
	3.4	1.5
	3.5	1
	3.6–4.0	0.5
	>4.0	0
	Predicted maintenance dose	
4	<1.4	>8
	1.4	8
	1.5	7.5
	1.6–1.7	7
	1.8	6.5
	1.9	6
	2.0–2.1	5.5
	2.2–2.3	5
	2.4–2.6	4.5
	2.7–3.0	4
	3.1–3.5	3.5
	3.6–4.0	3
	4.1–4.5	Omit the next day's dose, then give 2 mg
	>4.5	Omit the next 2 days' doses, then give 1 mg

W

between individuals, and within the same person, due to variables such as age, diet, diseases and drugs. Intercurrent illness such as influenza can cause dramatic changes in INR requiring significant dose adjustment.

Computer software is now widely used for dose prediction. These programs base predictions on previous response to therapy, although sound clinical judgement and experience are also required to use software safely.

Reversal of anticoagulation[1]

In patients with an elevated INR, the cause should be investigated. In the case of over anticoagulation (INR >5.0) without bleeding, warfarin should be withheld for 1–2 days. In the presence of a very high INR (>8.0), 1–5 mg of oral vitamin K should be given. Vitamin K (1–5 mg orally) may also be considered in patients with an INR between 5.0 and 8.0 if they are at increased risk of bleeding. Correction of INR should be achieved within 24 hours. The INR should be checked the day after administration of vitamin K in case a further dose is required. Higher doses of vitamin K should be avoided when correcting an elevated INR, as they can lead to overcorrection and resistance to re-anticoagulation.

Patients with major bleeding (limb- or life-threatening bleeding) should be managed with a four-factor prothrombin complex concentrate plus 5 mg intravenous vitamin K (see *Prothrombin complex concentrates* entry).

Patients with non-major bleeding can be managed with 1–3 mg intravenous vitamin K and temporary warfarin omission/dose reduction. Intravenous vitamin K produces a more rapid correction of the INR (within 6–8 hours) compared with oral administration. It should *not* be given intramuscularly due to the risk of haematoma formation or subcutaneously due to inconsistent correction.

Intravenous vitamin K can be given as a slow bolus injection over 3–5 minutes or as an infusion over 20–30 minutes, diluted in 50 mL glucose 5%.[7,8]

Drug interactions

Prescription monitoring for interacting medications is essential for treatment with warfarin. Serious bleeding may result from poorly managed drug therapy. Table W4 lists commonly interacting drugs, although this is not exhaustive: if in doubt, consult the BNF[9] or *Stockley's Textbook of Drug Interactions*.[10]

'When required' therapy

Regular dosing with interacting drugs may be acceptable if managed knowingly by the anticoagulant clinic. However, patients should be strongly warned about the risks of 'when required' dosing (e.g. analgesics), which might cause an increased risk of bleeding.

Pregnancy and lactation

Warfarin must *not* be taken during pregnancy because the drug is teratogenic. Subcutaneous low-molecular-weight heparin is used where treatment or prevention of deep-vein thrombosis/pulmonary embolism is required. Warfarin is safe when breast-feeding because the drug does not pass into breast milk. Acenocoumarol and phenindione should be avoided.

TABLE W4
Drug interactions with warfarin and suggested action

Drugs to avoid wherever possible	
Aspirin	• See section above on warfarin and antiplatelet therapy
Analgesics	• Non-steroidal anti-inflammatory drugs (NSAIDs), ketorolac (postoperative)
Antifungals and antibacterials	• Miconazole
Others	• Enteral feeds containing vitamin K
Consider dose adjustment	
Ulcer healing	• Cimetidine, omeprazole, esomeprazole
Antiarrhythmics	• Amiodarone, propafenone
Lipid lowering	• Fibrates, fluvastatin
Antiepileptics	• Carbamazepine, phenobarbital, primidone, phenytoin
Dependency	• Disulfiram
Antibiotics and antifungals	• Aztreonam, chloramphenicol, ciprofloxacin, clarithromycin, co-trimoxazole, erythromycin, griseofulvin, levofloxacin, metronidazole, neomycin, ofloxacin, rifampicin, sulphonamides
Thyroid	• Levothyroxine
Gout	• Allopurinol
Others	• Aminoglutethimide, barbiturates, ciclosporin, mercaptopurine, oral contraceptive steroids
Monitor INR	
Antiarrhythmics	• Quinidine
Lipid-lowering agents	• Colestyramine, simvastatin, rosuvastatin
Antidepressants	• Selective serotonin reuptake inhibitor
Antibiotics and antifungals	• Consult BNF if not listed above
NSAIDs	• All drugs in this class
Others	• Anabolic steroids, corticosteroids, hormone antagonists, ifosfamide, influenza vaccine, sucralfate

W

Discontinuation of therapy

It has been demonstrated that, when warfarin is no longer indicated and the drug is discontinued, dosing may be stopped abruptly without fear of rebound hypercoagulability.[11] Thromboembolism occurring after cessation of therapy is likely to be due to ongoing clotting disorder and not cessation of warfarin *per se*.

REFERENCES
1 Keeling D *et al.* (2011). Guidelines on oral anticoagulation with warfarin – fourth edition. *Br J Haematol* 154: 311–324.
2 NICE (2012). CG 144. *Venous Thromboembolic Diseases: The management of venous thromboembolic diseases and the role of thrombophilia testing*. http://www.nice.org.uk/Guidance/CG144 (accessed 3 September 2014).

3 NICE (2014). CG 180. *Atrial Fibrillation: The management of atrial fibrillation*. http://www.nice.org.uk/Guidance/CG180 (accessed 3 September 2014).

4 NICE (2013). CG 172. *MI – Secondary Prevention: Secondary prevention in secondary and primary care for patients following a myocardial infarction*. http://www.nice.org.uk/guidance/CG172 (accessed 3 September 2014).

5 Tait RC *et al.* (1998). A warfarin induction regimen for out-patient anticoagulation in patients with atrial fibrillation. *Br J Haematol* 101: 450–454.

6 Fennerty A *et al.* (1984). Flexible induction dose regimen for warfarin and prediction of maintenance dose. *Br Med J* 288: 1268–1270.

7 Summary of Product Characteristics (2012). *Konakion MM*. http://www.medicines.org.uk/emc/medicine/1698 last updated 17.08.12 (accessed 3 September 2014).

8 Gray A, Wright J, Goodey V, Bruce L (eds) (2011). *Injectable Drugs Guide*. London: Pharmaceutical Press.

9 Joint Formulary Committee (2014). *British National Formulary* (68th edn). London: BMJ Group and Pharmaceutical Press.

10 Baxter K and Preston CL (2013). *Stockley's Drug Interactions* (10th edn). London: Pharmaceutical Press.

11 Baglin TP *et al.* (2005). Guidelines on oral anticoagulation (warfarin): third edition – 2005 update. *Br J Haematol* 132: 277–285.

Wells score for deep-vein thrombosis

Background

The Wells score is a clinical prediction rule for estimating the probability of deep-vein thrombosis (DVT) and pulmonary embolism (PE) that looks at various risk factors and clinical signs associated with thromboembolic disease.

When a patient presents with signs or symptoms of DVT, the patient's general medical history should be assessed and a physical examination carried out to exclude other causes.

If a DVT is suspected, NICE recommends the use of the adapted two-level DVT Wells score to estimate the clinical probability of DVT[1,2]

SCORING SYSTEM

Clinical feature	Score
Active cancer (treatment ongoing, within previous 6 months or palliative)	1
Paralysis, paresis or recent plaster immobilisation of the lower extremities	1
Recently bedridden for 3 days or more or major surgery within 12 weeks requiring general or regional anaesthesia	1
Localised tenderness along the distribution of the deep venous system	1
Entire leg swollen	1
Calf swelling at least 3 cm larger than the asymptomatic side	1
Pitting oedema confined to the symptomatic leg	1
Collateral superficial veins (non-varicose)	1
Previously documented DVT	1
An alternative diagnosis is at least as likely as DVT	−2

Interpretation

DVT unlikely – 1 point or less
DVT likely – 2 points or more

The following procedure is then appropriate to confirm diagnosis:

- a proximal leg ultrasound scan carried out within 4 hours of being requested and, if the result is negative, a D-dimer test

  or

- a D-dimer test and an interim 24-hour dose of a parenteral anticoagulant (if a proximal leg vein ultrasound scan cannot be carried out within 4 hours) and a proximal leg vein ultrasound scan carried out within 24 hours of being requested.[2]

NICE provides additional detailed guidance on interpretation of test results, possible alternative diagnoses and further action that should be taken

REFERENCES
1 Wells PS *et al.* (2003). Evaluation of D-dimer in the diagnosis of suspected deep-vein thrombosis. *N Engl J Med* 349: 1227–1235.
2 NICE (2012). *Venous Thromboembolic Diseases: The management of venous thromboembolic diseases and the role of thrombophilia testing.* (CG 144.) http://www.nice.org.uk/guidance/cg144 (accessed 28 January 2015).

Wells score for pulmonary embolism

Background

The Wells score is a clinical prediction rule for estimating the probability of DVT and PE that looks at various risk factors and clinical signs associated with thromboembolic disease.

When a patient presents with signs or symptoms of PE, the patient's general medical history should be assessed and a physical examination and chest X-ray carried out to exclude other causes.

If a PE is suspected, NICE recommends the use of the adapted two-level PE Wells score to estimate the clinical probability of PE.[1,2]

W

SCORING SYSTEM

Clinical feature	Score
Clinical signs and symptoms of DVT (minimum of leg swelling and pain with palpation of the deep veins)	3
An alternative diagnosis is less likely than PE	3
Heart rate >100 beats/min	1.5
Immobilisation for more than 3 days or surgery in the previous 4 weeks	1.5
Previous DVT/PE	1.5
Haemoptysis	1
Malignancy (on treatment, treated in the last 6 months, or palliative)	1

Interpretation

PE unlikely – 4 points or less
PE likely – more than 4 points

The following procedure is then appropriate to confirm diagnosis:

- an immediate computed tomography pulmonary angiogram (CTPA)

    or

- immediate interim parenteral anticoagulant therapy followed by a CTPA if a CTPA cannot be carried out immediately.[2]

NICE provides additional detailed guidance on interpretation of test results, possible alternative diagnoses and further action that should be taken.

REFERENCES

1 Wells PS *et al.* (2000). Derivation of a simple clinical model to categorize patients' probability of pulmonary embolism: increasing the models utility with the SimpliRED D-dimer. *Thromb Haemost* 83: 416–420.

2 NICE (2012). *Venous Thromboembolic Diseases: The management of venous thromboembolic diseases and the role of thrombophilia testing.* (CG 144.) http://www.nice.org.uk/guidance/cg144 (accessed 28 January 2015).

W

Yellow Card scheme

In 1964, the UK Committee on Safety of Drugs provided doctors and dentists with pre-paid yellow postcards with which to report adverse reactions to drugs, thus creating the Yellow Card scheme. Remodelled Yellow Cards may now be found in National Health Service prescription pads, the BNF, and the *Monthly Index of Medical Specialities* (MIMS), or may be obtained from the MHRA. Yellow Cards may also be completed online at https://yellowcard.mhra. gov.uk. Access to this site and the drug analysis prints (listing all reactions reported for a particular medicine) can also be found via: http://www.mhra.gov.uk/Safetyinformation/Reportingsafety problems/Reportingsuspectedadversedrugreactions/index.htm.

Action taken by the MHRA

Once a specific problem has been identified for a medicine, the MHRA may take action in a number of ways. It may publish the findings and advice to prescribers in *Drug Safety Update*, a bulletin used to disseminate information about ADRs to healthcare professionals. Analysis of ADR reports received by the MHRA may also result in the withdrawal of drugs from the market or the amendment of product licences. For example, domperidone was amended from a 'pharmacy' medicine to a 'prescription-only medicine' in 2014 because of QT-interval prolongation and arrhythmias.[1] The MHRA may also publish warnings in the BNF to highlight particular aspects of drug safety.[2] Examples include warnings about the use of beta-blockers in asthmatics, the risks of atypical femoral fractures with bisphosphonates, and the need for all intravenous iron preparations to be administered by trained staff with resuscitation facilities immediately available due to risks of serious hypersensitivity reactions.

Underreporting of ADRs

Underreporting of ADRs is a consistent problem. It has been suggested that the incidence of reporting of serious ADRs is at best in the order of 10% and for non-serious ADRs it is estimated at 2–4%.[3] Even though Yellow Card scheme reporting rates are low in the UK,

Y

they compare favourably with schemes in other countries. The data obtained through the Yellow Card scheme are therefore incomplete and indeed, many serious and fatal reactions are never brought to the attention of the regulatory authorities. Factors considered to dissuade potential reporters from completing an ADR report include:[4–6]

- the reaction not being considered severe enough
- the reaction is well known
- familiarity with the suspect drug concerned
- concern over potential legal implications
- the reaction may be predictable or expected
- ignorance of how to report an ADR
- lack of time, lethargy or complacency
- lack of feedback following previous reports
- failure to identify the presence of an ADR
- guilt because of patient suffering and lack of confidence in making a report.

The concept of a fee has been proposed as a method of stimulating reporting and research has shown that a fee-based incentive can increase reporting rates, but upon withdrawal of the fee, reporting rates fall substantially.[7]

The data collected in the Yellow Card scheme are also open to significant bias and caution should be exercised in their interpretation. Reports of reactions appearing in the medical or lay press may result in numerous similar reports being submitted via the Yellow Card scheme. In turn, this may result in a 'false-positive' or 'true-positive' sign that a problem exists. An example of a 'false-positive' is the association of autism with measles, mumps and rubella (MMR) vaccination.

The lessons of the practolol-induced oculomucocutaneous syndrome, from the 1970s, are worth noting. Following publication of a report on this syndrome in the medical press, over 200 reports of a similar nature were subsequently submitted via the Yellow Card scheme. Prior to the publication of the first report only one report had been made to the MHRA in 4 years.[4] This suggests that either practitioners had failed to associate a serious syndrome with a patient's drug therapy, or that they had, but were unwilling to report it either because it was unrecognised or for other reasons.

Intensive monitoring of medicines

The new EU pharmacovigilance legislation has introduced a Europe-wide 'additional monitoring' scheme. Medicines included on the additional monitoring list are being monitored particularly closely by regulatory authorities and must have an inverted black triangle (as previously used in the UK) displayed in their patient information leaflet and SPCs, together with the following sentence:

▼ This medicinal product is subject to additional monitoring

A medicine is included on the additional monitoring list if:

- it contains a new active substance
- it is a biological medicine, such as a vaccine or a medicine derived from plasma (blood)
- it has been given a conditional approval (where the company that markets the medicine must provide more data about it) or approved under exceptional circumstances (where there are specific reasons why the company cannot provide a comprehensive set of data)
- the company that markets the medicine is required to carry out additional studies: for instance, to provide more data on long-term use of the medicine, or on a rare side effect seen during clinical trials.

A medicine is included on the list when it is approved for the first time and could be added at any time during its lifecycle. A medicine usually remains under additional monitoring for 5 years or until the EMA's Pharmacovigilance Risk Assessment Committee (PRAC) is satisfied that it can be removed from the list.

Black-triangle drugs are identified in the BNF, MIMS and SPC documents and all promotional materials aimed at healthcare professionals or patients. A current list of black-triangle drugs is maintained by the EMA and is available via the MHRA website.[8]

The limitations of clinical trials mean that the detection of rare ADRs, be it due to underlying pathology, drug–drug interactions, drug–disease interactions, delayed onset, or to their bizarre or unexpected nature, may not occur until long after the drug has been marketed. Reporting of ADRs to newly marketed drugs, i.e. those marked with a black triangle, is particularly important.

Monitoring of established drugs

Once drugs are no longer under additional monitoring, the black triangle is removed and the emphasis on ADR surveillance alters. Relatively minor or well-documented reactions become less significant and, instead of reporting all reactions, the MHRA requests that only serious or unusual reactions be reported. Any reaction that is fatal, life-threatening, disabling, incapacitating or which results in or prolongs hospitalisation should be reported, even if well recognised.[2] These data are especially of value when comparing drugs in the same class. Examples of 'serious' reports that are of particular interest to the MHRA include anaphylaxis, blood disorders, convulsions, endocrine disturbances, effects on fertility, haemorrhage from any site, jaundice, hepatic abnormalities, renal abnormalities, ophthalmic disorders, severe central nervous system effects and severe skin reactions. Further information on reporting is available on the MHRA website.[9]

The MHRA is extremely interested in gathering information about possible ADRs to herbal medicines and would like all suspected reactions to be reported.

ADRs in children

In September 2014, the MHRA introduced new guidance on reporting suspected adverse drug reactions in children. The advice on which suspected ADRs to report in children is now the same as for adults (i.e. you are no longer requested to report all suspected ADRs for children):

- all suspected ADRs that are serious or result in harm. Serious reactions are those that are fatal, life-threatening, disabling or incapacitating, those that cause a congenital abnormality or result in hospitalisation, and those that are considered medically significant for any other reason
- all suspected ADRs associated with new drugs and vaccines (identified by the black-triangle symbol: ▼).

Problems with MHRA Yellow Card data

Although the data received by the MHRA are of great value to pharmacovigilance, there are limitations to their use.[10] For example, reporting rates for drugs tend to be at their highest following their introduction to the market, particularly as they are marked with black triangles. Furthermore, owing to underreporting and because the number of patients taking a drug is unknown, it is impossible to calculate the incidence of specific ADRs and it is only possible to hypothesise about identified problems. It is not uncommon for unusual or unexpected reactions to be reported at the expense of well-recognised, albeit more serious, reactions.

Other methods of pharmacovigilance

Whilst the Yellow Card scheme is of great importance, many ADRs come to light via other routes. Robust and systematic methods employed in pharmacovigilance include case-control studies, cohort studies and case-registry studies. These methods, rather than relying on spontaneous reports, focus on individual drugs with the aim of identifying ADRs. For example:

- the Prescription Event Monitoring (PEM) scheme is run by the Drug Safety Research Unit in Southampton and is designed to target particular drugs[11]
- Clinical Practice Research Datalink, which enables many types of observational research, including pharmacoepidemiology studies.[12]

REFERENCES

1 MHRA (2014). *Domperidone (Motilium) can no Longer be Bought without a Prescription.* http://www.mhra.gov.uk/NewsCentre/Whatsnew/CON452545 (accessed 27 November 2014).

2 Joint Formulary Committee (2014). *British National Formulary* (68th edn). London: BMJ Group and Pharmaceutical Press.

3 Rawlins MD (1995). Pharmacovigilance: paradise lost, regained or postponed. *J R Coll Phys Lond* 29: 41–49.

4 Inman WHW (ed.) (1980). *Monitoring for Drug Safety*. Lancaster: MTP Press, pp. 26–27.

5 Belton KJ *et al.* (1995). Attitudinal survey of adverse drug reaction reporting by medical practitioners in the United Kingdom. *Br J Clin Pharmacol* 39: 223–226.

6 Bateman DN *et al.* (1992). Attitudes to adverse drug reaction reporting in the northern region. *Br J Clin Pharmacol* 34: 421–426.

7 Feely J *et al.* (1990). Stimulating reporting of adverse drug reactions by using a fee. *BMJ* 300: 22–23.

8 MHRA (2014). *Black Triangle Scheme – New medicines and vaccines subject to EU-wide additional monitoring*. http://www.mhra.gov.uk/Safetyinformation/ Howwemonitorthesafetyofproducts/Medicines/BlackTriangleproducts/index.htm (accessed 27 November 2014).

9 MHRA (2014). *The Yellow Card Scheme*. http://www.mhra.gov.uk/Safety information/Howwemonitorthesafetyofproducts/Medicines/TheYellowCard Scheme/ (accessed 27 November 2014).

10 Edwards JG, Anderson I (1999). Systematic review and guide to selection of selective serotonin uptake inhibitors. *Drugs* 57: 527.

11 Drug Safety Research Unit (2014). http://www.dsru.org (accessed 27 November 2014).

12 Clinical Practice Research Datalink (2014). http://www.cprd.com/home/ (accessed 27 November 2014).

Y

Z

Zinc

Normal range: 10–24 micromol/L

Local lab range . . . .

The reference nutrient intake per day is 9.5 mg (males) and 7 mg (females).[1]

The micronutrient zinc is one of the most important trace elements in our diet and has an essential role in human physiology. Zinc is essential for enzyme activities within the body and also contributes to protein structure and regulates gene expression. It is found in a variety of foods, such as beef, poultry and grains, and is absorbed from the GI tract and distributed throughout the body.[2]

In the body zinc is stored in the prostate and testes (male), muscle, liver and kidney, bones and skin (the highest concentrations occur in hair, eyes, male reproductive organs and bone). Lower levels are present in liver, kidney and muscle. In blood 80% is found in erythrocytes. Plasma zinc levels range from 70 to 110 microgram/dL and about 50% of this is loosely bound to albumin.[3]

Individuals who may be at greater risk of zinc deficiency include: smokers, alcoholics, diabetics, anyone taking large amounts of vitamin B_6 and people on non-nutritious or very-low-calorie diet plans. Zinc levels are also depleted by excessive sweating. Zinc may accumulate in renal failure.

Zinc deficiency

Symptoms[3]

Severe deficiency causes skin lesions, alopecia, diarrhoea, increased susceptibility to infections and failure to thrive in children. Symptoms of less severe deficiency include distorted or absent perceptions of taste and smell and poor wound healing.

Causes

Causes include:

- inadequate diet or malabsorption
- parenteral nutrition.[4]

Excessive loss of zinc can also occur in trauma, burns and protein-losing conditions.[5]

Treatment

Zinc supplements should only be given when there is good evidence of deficiency (hypoproteinaemia spuriously lowers zinc plasma concentration).[5] Plasma levels are unreliable as they may be low, e.g. in infection or trauma without deficiency.

Treatment with oral supplements is usual unless the patient is in the critical care setting. The usual treatment is with Solvazinc, dosed at:[3,5]

- adults and children >30 kg: 1 tablet in water 1–3 times daily
- children 10–30 kg: 1/2 tablet 1–3 times daily
- children <10 kg: 1/2 tablet daily.

It is advisable to take with or after food to reduce the adverse effect on the GI tract. Supplementation continues until clinical improvement occurs, or it may be ongoing in severe malabsorption, metabolic disease or non-resolving zinc-losing states.[5]

Side effects[3,5]

Side effects of treatment include: abdominal pain, dyspepsia, nausea, vomiting, diarrhoea, gastric irritation, gastritis, irritability, headache and lethargy.

Interactions[3,5]

Zinc reduces the absorption of quinolone antibiotics. The absorption of tetracycline antibiotics, oral iron, penicillamine and trientine is reduced by zinc and the absorption of zinc is reduced by these drugs. When both zinc and tetracycline are being given, an interval of at least 3 hours should be allowed between preparations.

Preparations

Total parenteral nutrition (TPN) contains zinc within the trace elements. Baseline zinc requirement in micromoles can be calculated [0.3 × weight (kg)]. A suggested dose for intravenous nutrition is elemental 6.5 mg zinc (100 micromol) daily.[5] Table Z1 shows the zinc content of available preparations.

Other uses of zinc

The use of zinc in patients with leg ulcers has been assessed in a systematic review and found to be no better than placebo; therefore, unless the patient is shown to be deficient, there is no indication for its use.[6]

TABLE Z1

Zinc content of various preparations

Product	Zinc content[5]
Solvazinc	125 mg zinc sulfate monohydrate ≡ 45 mg elemental zinc (0.7 mmol/tablet)
Additrace	10 mL ≡ 100 micromoles of zinc
Zinc sulfate injection	14.6 mg/mL zinc sulfate (1 mL ≡ 50 micromoles elemental zinc)

Zinc is an effective treatment for Wilson's disease.[2] Zinc supplementation has been shown to reduce the duration and severity of diarrhoea and to prevent subsequent episodes in children in developing countries.[7] It has also been used in combination with antioxidants to slow the progression of age-related macular degeneration.[2]

REFERENCES

1 European Food Safety Authority (2006). *Tolerable Upper Intake Levels for Vitamins and Minerals*. http://www.efsa.europa.eu/en/ndatopics/docs/ndatolerableuil.pdf (accessed 4 October 2014).

2 Saper R, Rash R (2009). Zinc: an essential micronutrient. *Am Fam Physician* 79: 768–772.

3 eMC (2014). *Summary of Product Characteristics. Solvazinc Effervescent Tablets*. https://www.medicines.org.uk/emc/medicine/ 25407 (accessed 4 October 2014).

4 Longmore M *et al.* (eds) (2004). *Oxford Handbook of Clinical Medicine* (6th edn). Oxford: Oxford University Press.

5 Joint Formulary Committee (2014). *British National Formulary* (68th edn). London: BMJ Group and Pharmaceutical Press.

6 Wilkinson EAJ, Hawke CI (1998). Does oral zinc aid the healing of chronic leg ulcers? A systematic literature review. *Arch Dermatol* 134: 1556–1560.

7 WHO; UNICEF (2004). *Clinical Management of Acute Diarrhoea*. http://whqlibdoc. who.int/hq/2004/WHO_FCH_CAH_04.7.pdf (accessed 4 October 2014).

Z

Appendix 1
Glossary of terms

ABGs	arterial blood gases
ABPA	allergic bronchopulmonary aspergillosis
ABW	actual body weight
ACBS	Advisory Committee on Borderline Substances
ACE	angiotensin-converting enzyme
ACE 111	Addenbrookes cognitive examination 111
ACEI	angiotensin-converting enzyme inhibitor
ACR	albumin:creatinine ratio
ACTH	adrenocorticotrophic hormone
ADH	antidiuretic hormone
ADR	adverse drug reaction
AF	atrial fibrillation
AIDS	acquired immunodeficiency syndrome
AIN	acute interstitial nephritis
AKI	acute kidney injury
ALP	alkaline phosphatase
ALT	alanine aminotransferase or alanine transaminase
AMD	age-related macular degeneration
APD	automated peritoneal dialysis
APLS	antiphospholipid antibody syndrome
APS	antiphospholipid syndrome
APTT	activated partial thromboplastin time
ARB	angiotensin receptor blocker
AREDS	Age-Related Eye Disease Study
ART	antiretroviral therapy
AST	aspartate transaminase
ATN	acute tubular necrosis
AV	atrioventricular
AVPU	alert, voice, pain, unresponsive
BCG	bacillus Calmette-Guérin
BHIVA	British HIV Association
BMD	bone mineral density
BMI	body mass index

BNF	*British National Formulary*
BP	blood pressure
BSA	body surface area
BTS	British Thoracic Society
BV	blood volume
Ca	calcium
CABG	coronary artery bypass graft
CAPD	continuous ambulatory peritoneal dialysis
CAS	carotid artery stenosis
CBG	capillary blood glucose
CCK	cholecystokinin
CCR	chemokine receptor
CD	Crohn's disease
CF	cystic fibrosis
CFTR	cystic fibrosis transmembrane regular
CHF	congestive heart failure
CINV	chemotherapy-induced nausea and vomiting
CIPOLD	Confidential Inquiry into Premature Deaths of People with Learning Disabilities
CK	creatine kinase
CKD	chronic kidney disease
CKD-EPI	Chronic Kidney Disease Epidemiology Collaboration
COCP	combined oral contraceptive pill
COPD	chronic obstructive pulmonary disease
COSHH	Control of Substances Hazardous to Health
COX-2	cyclooxygenase-2
Cr	creatinine
CrCl	creatinine clearance
CRP	C-reactive protein
CSII	continuous SC insulin infusion
CT	computed tomography
CTD-ILD	connective tissue disease-interstitial lung disease

CTEPH	chronic thromboembolic pulmonary hypertension
CTPA	computed tomography pulmonary angiogram
CVA	cerebrovascular accident
CVC	central venous catheter
CVD	cardiovascular disease
CVVHF	continuous venous-venous haemofiltration
CYP450	cytochrome P450
DAFNE	dose adjustment for normal eating
DCCT	Diabetes Control and Complications Trial
DDW	dose-determining weight
DI	diabetes insipidus
DIG	Digitalis Investigation Group
DigCl	digoxin clearance
DIP	desquamative interstitial pneumonia
DKA	diabetic ketoacidosis
DLCO	diffusing capacity of the lung for carbon monoxide
DM	diabetes mellitus
DMARD	disease-modifying antirheumatic drug
DIC	disseminated intravascular coagulation
DOT	directly observed therapy
DSM-V	*Diagnostic and Statistical Manual of Mental Disorders*
DVLA	Driver and Vehicle Licensing Agency
DVT	deep-vein thrombosis
DXA	dual-energy X-ray absorptiometry
ECF	extracellular fluid
ECG	electrocardiogram
eGFR	estimated glomerular filtration rate
EHIC	European Health Insurance Card
EMA	European Medicines Agency
eMC	electronic Medicines Compendium
ERAS	enhanced recovery after surgery
ESC	European Society of Cardiology
ESR	erythrocyte sedimentation rate
ESRD	end-stage renal disease
EWS	early warning score

FAST	Face Arm Speech Test
FBC	full blood count
FDA	Food and Drug Administration
FEV_1	forced expiratory volume in 1 second
FPG	fasting plasma glucose
FRAX	Fracture Risk Assessment Tool
FSA	Food Standards Agency
FT_3	free triiodothyronine
FT_4	free levothyroxine
FTU	fingertip unit
FVC	forced vital capacity
G6PD	glucose-6-phosphate-dehydrogenase
GABA	gamma-aminobutyric acid
GGT	gamma-glutamyltransferase or gamma-glutamyltranspeptidase
GI	gastrointestinal
GKI	glucose−potassium−insulin
GORD	gastro-oesophageal reflux disease
GP	general practitioner
Hb	haemoglobin
HbA_{1C}	glycosylated haemoglobin
Hct	haematocrit
HD	haemodialysis
HDL	high density lipoprotein
HDU	High Dependency Unit
HF	heart failure
HF	haemofiltration
HHS	hyperosmolar hyperglycaemia state
HIT	heparin-induced thrombocytopenia
HIV	human immunodeficiency virus
HLA	human leukocyte antigen
HONK	hyperosmotic non-ketotic acidosis
HONS	hyperosmotic non-ketotic acidosis
HP	hypersensitivity pneumonitis
HPA	hypothalamic−pituitary−adrenocortical
HRCT	high-resolution computed tomography
HSE	Health and Safety Executive
hypo	hypoglycaemia
IBD	inflammatory bowel disease
IBS	irritable bowel syndrome
IBW	ideal body weight

ICH	intracranial haemorrhage
ICS	inhaled corticosteroid
ICU	intensive care unit
IE	infective endocarditis
IFCC	International Federation of Clinical Chemistry
Ig	immunoglobulin
IGRA	interferon-gamma release assay
IHD	ischaemic heart disease
IIP	idiopathic interstitial pneumonia
ILD	interstitial lung disease
IM	intramuscular
IMCA	Independent mental capacity advocate
INR	international normalised ratio
IPF	idiopathic pulmonary fibrosis
IV	intravenous
JBDS	Joint British Diabetes Societies
LABA	long-acting beta-2 agonist
LAMA	long-acting muscarinic antagonist
LDL	low-density lipoprotein
LMWH	low-molecular-weight heparin
LOLA	L-ornithine and L-aspartate
LTRA	leukotriene antagonist
LVSD	left ventricular systolic dysfunction
MAOI	monoamine oxidase inhibitor
MCV	mean corpuscular volume
MDRD	Modification of Diet in Renal Disease
MDR-TB	multidrug-resistant tuberculosis
MDT	multidisciplinary team
MEWS	medical early warning score
MHRA	Medicines and Healthcare products Regulatory Agency
MI	myocardial infarction
MIMS	*Monthly Index of Medical Specialities*
MMR	measles, mumps and rubella
MODY	maturity-onset diabetes of the young
MRC	Medical Research Council
mMRC	modified Medical Research Council
MR	modified-release
MRI	magnetic resonance imaging
MRSA	methicillin-resistant *Staphylococcus aureus*

MS	multiple sclerosis
NaCl	sodium chloride
NBM	nil/nothing-by-mouth
NEWS	National Early Warning Score
NG	nasogastric
NICE	National Institute for Health and Care Excellence
NK1	neurokinin 1
NMDA	*N*-methyl-D-aspartate
NMS	neuroleptic malignant syndrome
NNRTI	non-nucleoside reverse transcriptase inhibitors
NOAC	new oral anticoagulant
NOS	nitric oxide synthetase
NPSA	National Patient Safety Agency
NRT	nicotine replacement therapy
NRTI	nucleoside reverse transcriptase inhibitor
NSAID	non-steroidal anti-inflammatory drug
NSIP	non-specific interstitial pneumonia
NSTEMI	non-ST-segment-elevation myocardial infarction
NTM	non-tuberculous mycobacteria
NYHA	New York Heart Association
OGTT	oral glucose tolerance test
OTC	over-the-counter
PAH	pulmonary arterial hypertension
PBC	primary biliary cirrhosis
PCA	patient-controlled analgesia
PCC	prothrombin complex concentrate
PCEA	patient-controlled epidural analgesia
PCI	percutaneous intervention
PCV	packed cell volume
PD	peritoneal dialysis
PE	pulmonary embolism
PEFR	peak expiratory flow rate
PEG	percutaneous endoscopic gastrostomy
PEG/J	percutaneous endoscopic gastrostomy-jejunostomy
PEM	Prescription Event Monitoring
PERT	pancreatic enzyme replacement therapy

PFT	pulmonary function test
PI	protease inhibitor
PIH	primary intracerebral haemorrhage
PLCH	pulmonary Langerhans' cell histiocytosis
PN	parenteral nutrition
PONV	postoperative nausea and vomiting
PPD	purified protein derivative
PPI	proton pump inhibitor
PRAC	Pharmacovigilance Risk Assessment Committee
PSA	prostate specific antigen
PSC	primary sclerosing cholangitis
PT	prothrombin time
PTH	parathyroid hormone
PV	plasma volume
RBC	red blood count
RB-ILD	respiratory bronchiolitis-associated interstitial lung disease
RCC	red cell count
RDA	recommended daily amount
ROSIER	Recognition Of Stroke In Emergency Room
RRT	renal replacement therapy
RSV	respiratory syncytial virus
RV	residual volume
SABA	short-acting beta-2 agonist
sACE	serum angiotensin-converting enzyme
SAH	subarachnoid haemorrhage
SAMA	short-acting muscarinic antagonist
SBP	systolic blood pressure
SBP	spontaneous bacterial peritonitis
SC	subcutaneous
SDC	serum digoxin concentration
SHIFT	Systolic Heart failure treatment with the If inhibitor Ivabradine Trial
SIADH	syndrome of inappropriate antidiuretic hormone secretion
SIGN	Scottish Intercollegiate Guidelines Network
SIRS	systemic inflammatory response syndrome

SPAF	stroke prevention in atrial fibrillation
SPARCL	Stroke Prevention with Aggressive Reductions in Cholesterol Levels
SPC	Summary of Product Characteristics
SSRI	selective serotonin reuptake inhibitor
SVCO	superior vena cava obstruction
T_3	triiodothyronine (liothyronine)
T_4	thyroxine (levothyroxine)
TB	tuberculosis
TC	topical corticosteroid
TCA	tricyclic antidepressant
TDM	therapeutic drug monitoring
TENS	transcutaneous electrical nerve stimulation
TIA	transient ischaemic attack
TIBC	total iron-binding capacity
TIPS	transjugular intrahepatic portosystemic shunt
TLC	total lung capacity
TLCO	transfer factor of the lung for carbon monoxide
TOE	transoesophageal echocardiogram
TNF	tumour necrosis factor
TPMT	thiopurine S-methyl transferase
TPN	total parenteral nutrition
TRH	thyroid-releasing hormone
TSH	thyroid-stimulating hormone
TTE	transthoracic echocardiogram
TT_3	total serum triiodothyronine
TT_4	total serum thyroxine
U	urea
U&Es	urea and electrolytes
UC	ulcerative colitis
UIP	usual interstitial pneumonia
ULN	upper limit of normal
UPDRS	Unified Parkinson's Disease Rating Scale
UTI	urinary tract infection
V/Q	ventilation/perfusion
VRIII	variable-rate intravenous insulin infusion
VTE	venous thromboembolism
WHO	World Health Organization

Appendix 2
Laboratory reference ranges

Always use the reference ranges quoted by your local laboratory.

Analyte	Serum/plasma concentration
Bicarbonate	23–31 mmol/L
Albumin	39–50 g/L
Calcium	2.1–2.6 mmol/L
Creatinine	62–133 micromol/L
Phosphate	0.8–1.5 mmol/L
Potassium	3.6–5.0 mmol/L
Sodium	137–145 mmol/L
Total protein	63–82 g/L
Urea	2.5–7.5 mmol/L
Plasma glucose (fasting) 2 hours after a meal/75 q glucose	3.8–5.5 mmol/L Maximum 7.8 mmol/L
Troponin I high sensitivity	<50 ng/L
Troponin T	<0.2 microgram/L

Liver enzymes	Serum/plasma concentration
Alanine transaminase or alanine aminotransferase (ALT)	7–56 units/L
Alkaline phosphatase (ALP)	30 300 units/L (adult) 100–390 units/L (ages 3–15 years) Up to 500 units/L (age 3 years and under, and growth spurts)
Aspartate transaminase (AST or aspartate aminotransferase)	5–40 units/L
Bilirubin	3–17 micromol/L
Gamma-glutamyltransferase or gamma-glutamyltranspeptidase (GGT)	15–73 units/L (male) 12–43 units/L (female)

Enzymes and markers	Serum/plasma concentration
Amylase	30–110 units/L
Creatine kinase (CK)	Maximum 170 units/L
prostate specific antigen (PSA)	<2.5 microgram/L if aged <50 years <3.5 microgram/L if aged 50–59 years <4.5 microgram/L if aged 60–69 years <6.5 microgram/L if aged 70 years or more

Blood gases and acid–base state (arterial blood)	Range
Actual bicarbonate	22–30 mmol/L
Standard bicarbonate	22–26 mmol/L
Base excess	−3 to +3 mmol/L
pCO_2	4.67–6.0 kPa
pO_2	11.3–14.0 kPa
pH	7.35–7.45

Lipids	Serum/plasma concentration
Serum cholesterol	Desirable <5.0 mmol/L
High-density lipoprotein (HDL)	Desirable >0.8 mmol/L
Low-density lipoprotein (LDL)	Desirable <4.3 mmol/L
Triglycerides (fasting)	Desirable <1.8 mmol/L

Trace elements	Serum/plasma concentration
Copper	13–26 micromol/L
Iron	Males: 11–28 micromol/L Females: 7–26 micromol/L
Magnesium	0.6–0.95 mmol/L
Zinc	10–24 micromol/L
Carotene	0.9–5.6 micromol/L

Thyroid function	Range
Thyroxine-binding globulin	7.0–18.0 mg/L
Free T_4 (thyroxine)	11.8–32.5 pmol/L
Free T_3 (triiodothyronine)	2.8–6.6 pmol/L
Thyroid-stimulating hormone (TSH)	0.3–6.0 mu/L

White cells	Adults	Children	Infants
Total count ($\times 10^9$/L)	3.0–11.0	4.5–13.5	10.0–26.0
Differential counts (% and $\times 10^9$/L)			
Neutrophils	40–75% (2.0–7.5)	(2.0–6.0)	
Lymphocytes	20–45% (1.5–4.0)	(5.5–8.5)	
Monocytes	2–10% (0.2–0.8)	(0.7–1.5)	
Eosinophils	1–6% (0.04–0.4)	(0.3–0.8)	
Basophils	<1.0% (<0.01–0.1)	(<0.01–0.1)	

Red cells	Men	Women	Children	Infants
Haemoglobin (Hb) (g/dL)	13.0–18	11.5–16.5	3–6 years: 12.0–14.0	13.0–19.5
			10–12 years: 11.5–14.5	
Red cell count (RCC) $\times 10^{12}$/L	4.5–6.5	3.8–5.8	3–6 years: 4.1–5.5	4.0–6.0
			10–12 years: 4.0–5.4	
Packed cell volume (PCV) or haematocrit (Hct) (%)	0.4–0.54	0.37–0.47	3–6 years: 0.36–0.44	0.44–0.64
			10–12 years: 0.37–0.45	
Mean cell volume (MCV) (femtolitres: fL)	76–100	76–100	3–6 years: 73–89	106 (mean)
			10–12 years: 77–91	
Mean corpuscular Hb (MCH) (pg)	27–32	27–32	24–30	24–30
Mean corpuscular Hb concentration (MCHC) (%)	31–35	31–35	31–35	31–35
Red cell distribution width (RDW)	10.9–15.7	10.9–15.7	10.9–15.7	10.9–15.7

Platelets ($\times 10^9$/L)	150–400
Plateletcrit (PCT) (%)	0.150–0.320
Mean platelet volume (MPV) (fl)	6.3–10.1

Miscellaneous	Range
D-dimer	<50 mg/dL
Serum ferritin	Male: 28–365 microgram/L
	Female: 6–159 microgram/L
	Children: 10–150 microgram/L
Serum vitamin B_{12}	193–982 ng/L
Serum folate	3.0–17 microgram/L
Red cell folate	80–727 microgram/L
Erythrocyte sedimentation rate (ESR)	Male:
	17–50 years: 0–5 mm in first hour
	>50 years: 2–10 mm in first hour
	Female:
	17–50 years: 0–7 mm in first hour
	>50 years: 5–15 mm in first hour
Reticulocytes	0–2%
HbA_{1c}	4.6–6 %

Appendix 3
Imperial–metric height conversion

Imperial	Metric (cm)
4′	122
4′ 2″	127
4′ 4″	132
4′ 6″	137
4′ 8″	142
4′ 10″	147
5′	152
5′ 2″	157
5′ 4″	163
5′ 6″	168
5′ 8″	173
5′ 10″	178
6′	183
6′ 2″	188
6′ 4″	193
6′ 6″	198
6′ 8″	203
6′ 10″	208
7′	213

Appendix 4
Imperial–metric weight conversion

Imperial	Pounds	Metric (kg)	Imperial	Pounds	Metric (kg)
6 st	84	38.2	10 st 4 lb	144	65.5
6 st 2 lb	86	39.1	10 st 6 lb	146	66.4
6 st 4 lb	88	40.0	10 st 8 lb	148	67.3
6 st 6 lb	90	40.9	10 st 10 lb	150	68.2
6 st 8 lb	92	41.8	10 st 12 lb	152	69.1
6 st 10 lb	94	42.7	11 st	154	70.0
6 st 12 lb	96	43.6	11 st 2 lb	156	70.9
7 st	98	44.5	11 st 4 lb	158	71.8
7 st 2 lb	100	45.5	11 st 6 lb	160	72.7
7 st 4 lb	102	46.4	11 st 8 lb	162	73.6
7 st 6 lb	104	47.3	11 st 10 lb	164	74.5
7 st 8 lb	106	48.2	11 st 12 lb	166	75.5
7 st 10 lb	108	49.1	12 st	168	76.4
7 st 12 lb	110	50.0	12 st 2 lb	170	77.3
8 st	112	50.9	12 st 4 lb	172	78.2
8 st 2 lb	114	51.8	12 st 6 lb	174	79.1
8 st 4 lb	116	52.7	12 st 8 lb	176	80.0
8 st 6 lb	118	53.6	12 st 10 lb	178	80.9
8 st 8 lb	120	54.5	12 st 12 lb	180	81.8
8 st 10 lb	122	55.5	13 st	182	82.7
8 st 12 lb	124	56.4	13 st 2 lb	184	83.6
9 st	126	57.3	13 st 4 lb	186	84.5
9 st 2 lb	128	58.2	13 st 6 lb	188	85.5
9 st 4 lb	130	59.1	13 st 8 lb	190	86.4
9 st 6 lb	132	60.0	13 st 10 lb	192	87.3
9 st 8 lb	134	60.9	13 st 12 lb	194	88.2
9 st 10 lb	136	61.8	14 st	196	89.1
9 st 12 lb	138	62.7	14 st 2 lb	198	90.0
10 st	140	63.6	14 st 4 lb	200	90.9
10 st 2 lb	142	64.5	14 st 6 lb	202	91.8

Imperial	Pounds	Metric (kg)	Imperial	Pounds	Metric (kg)
14 st 8 lb	204	92.7	16 st 10 lb	234	106.4
14 st 10 lb	206	93.6	16 st 12 lb	236	107.3
14 st 12 lb	208	94.5	17 st	238	108.2
15 st	210	95.5	17 st 2 lb	240	109.1
15 st 2 lb	212	96.4	17 st 4 lb	242	110.0
15 st 4 lb	214	97.3	17 st 6 lb	244	110.9
15 st 6 lb	216	98.2	17 st 8 lb	246	111.8
15 st 8 lb	218	99.1	17 st 10 lb	248	112.7
15 st 10 lb	220	100.0	17 st 12 lb	250	113.6
15 st 12 lb	222	100.9	18 st	252	114.5
16 st	224	101.8	18 st 2 lb	254	115.5
16 st 2 lb	226	102.7	18 st 4 lb	256	116.4
16 st 4 lb	228	103.6	18 st 6 lb	258	117.3
16 st 6 lb	230	104.5	18 st 8 lb	260	118.2
16 st 8 lb	232	105.5	18 st 10 lb	262	119.1

Index